# NURSING RESEARCH

## Methods and Critical Appraisal for Evidence-Based Practice

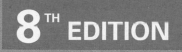

**8**TH EDITION

## Geri LoBiondo-Wood, PhD, RN, FAAN

Professor and Coordinator, PhD in Nursing Program
University of Texas Health Science Center at Houston
School of Nursing
Houston, Texas

## Judith Haber, PhD, APRN, BC, FAAN

The Ursula Springer Leadership Professor in Nursing
Associate Dean for Graduate Programs
New York University
College of Nursing
New York, New York

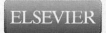

ELSEVIER

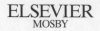
3251 Riverport Lane
St. Louis, Missouri 63043

---

**Notices**

Knowledge and best practices in this field are constantly changing. As new research and experience broaden our understanding, changes in research methods, professional practices, or medical treatment may become necessary.

Practitioners and researchers must always rely on their own experience and knowledge in evaluating and using any information, methods, compounds, or experiments described herein. In using such information or methods they should be mindful of their own safety and the safety of others, including parties for whom they have a professional responsibility.

With respect to any drug or pharmaceutical products identified, readers are advised to check the most current information provided (i) on procedures featured or (ii) by the manufacturer of each product to be administered, to verify the recommended dose or formula, the method and duration of administration, and contraindications. It is the responsibility of practitioners, relying on their own experience and knowledge of their patients, to make diagnoses, to determine dosages and the best treatment for each individual patient, and to take all appropriate safety precautions.

To the fullest extent of the law, neither the Publisher nor the authors, contributors, or editors, assume any liability for any injury and/or damage to persons or property as a matter of products liability, negligence or otherwise, or from any use or operation of any methods, products, instructions, or ideas contained in the material herein.

---

**Library of Congress Cataloging-in-Publication Data**

Nursing research (LoBiondo-Wood)
  Nursing research: methods and critical appraisal for evidence-based practice / [edited by] Geri LoBiondo-Wood, Judith Haber. -- 8th edition.
      p. ; cm.
  Includes bibliographical references and index.
  ISBN 978-0-323-10086-1 (alk. paper)
  I. LoBiondo-Wood, Geri, editor of compilation. II. Haber, Judith, editor of compilation. III. Title.
  [DNLM: 1. Nursing Research--methods. 2. Evidence-Based Nursing--methods. 3. Research Design. WY 20.5]
  RT81.5

  610.73072--dc23
                                                                                2013023802

*Executive Content Strategist:* Lee Henderson
*Senior Content Development Specialist:* Jennifer Ehlers
*Publishing Services Manager:* Jeff Patterson
*Senior Project Manager:* Anne Konopka
*Design Direction:* Amy Buxton

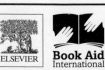
Printed in China
Last digit is the print number:   9   8   7   6   5   4   3

# ABOUT THE AUTHORS

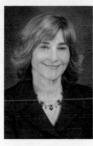

**Geri LoBiondo-Wood**, PhD, RN, FAAN, is Professor and Coordinator of the PhD in Nursing Program at the University of Texas Health Science Center at Houston, School of Nursing (UTHSC-Houston) and former Director of Research and Evidence-Based Practice Planning and Development at the MD Anderson Cancer Center, Houston, Texas. She received her Diploma in Nursing at St. Mary's Hospital School of Nursing in Rochester, New York; Bachelor's and Master's degrees from the University of Rochester; and a PhD in Nursing Theory and Research from New York University. Dr. LoBiondo-Wood teaches research and evidence-based practice principles to undergraduate, graduate, and doctoral students. At MD Anderson Cancer Center, she developed and implemented the Evidence-Based Resource Unit Nurse (EB-RUN) Program, a hospital-wide program that involves all levels of nurses in the application of research evidence to practice. She has extensive national and international experience guiding nurses and other health care professionals in the development and utilization of research. Dr. LoBiondo-Wood is an Editorial Board member of *Progress in Transplantation* and a reviewer for *Nursing Research, Oncology Nursing Forum, Oncology Nursing,* and *Nephrology Nursing Journal.* Her research and publications focus on chronic illness and oncology nursing.

Dr. LoBiondo-Wood has been active locally and nationally in many professional organizations, including the Oncology Nursing Society, Southern Nursing Research Society, the Midwest Nursing Research Society, and the North American Transplant Coordinators Organization. She has received local and national awards for teaching and contributions to nursing. In 1997, she received the Distinguished Alumnus Award from New York University, Division of Nursing Alumni Association. In 2001 she was inducted as a Fellow of the American Academy of Nursing and in 2007 as a Fellow of the University of Texas Academy of Health Science Education. In 2012 she was appointed as a Distinguished Teaching Professor of the University of Texas System.

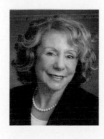

**Judith Haber**, PhD, APRN, BC, FAAN, is the Ursula Springer Leadership Professor in Nursing and Associate Dean for Graduate Programs in the College of Nursing at New York University. She received her undergraduate nursing education at Adelphi University in New York, and she holds a Master's degree in Adult Psychiatric–Mental Health Nursing and a PhD in Nursing Theory and Research from New York University. Dr. Haber is internationally recognized as a clinician and educator in psychiatric–mental health nursing. She has extensive clinical experience in psychiatric nursing, having been an advanced practice psychiatric nurse in private practice for over 30 years, specializing in treatment of families coping with the psychosocial sequelae of acute and chronic catastrophic illness. Her NIH-funded program of research addressed physical and psychosocial adjustment to illness, focusing specifically on women with breast cancer and their partners and, more recently, breast cancer survivorship. Dr. Haber is also committed to an interprofessional program of clinical scholarship related to improving oral-systemic health outcomes and leads the *Oral Health Nursing Education and Practice (OHNEP)* program funded by the DentaQuest Foundation as well as the HRSA-funded *Teaching Oral Systemic Health (TOSH)* program.

Dr. Haber has been active locally and nationally in many professional organizations, including the American Nurses Association, the American Psychiatric Nurses Association, and the American Academy of Nursing. She has received numerous local, state, and national awards for public policy, clinical practice, and research, including the APNA Psychiatric Nurse of the Year Award in 1998 and 2005 and the APNA Outstanding Research Award in 2005. She received the 2007 NYU College of Nursing Distinguished Alumnus Award, the 2011 NYU Distinguished Teaching Award, and the 2013 NYU Alumni Meritorious Service Award. In 1993, she was inducted as a Fellow of the American Academy of Nursing and in 2012 as a Fellow in the New York Academy of Medicine.

# CONTRIBUTORS

**Julie Barroso, PhD, ANP, APRN, BC, FAAN**
Professor and Research Development
  Coordinator
Duke University School of Nursing
Durham, North Carolina

**Ann M. Berger, PhD, APRN, AOCNS, FAAN**
Professor and Dorothy Hodges Olson Endowed
  Chair in Nursing
Director PhD Program
University of Nebraska Medical Center
Omaha, Nebraska

**Nancy Bergstrom, PhD, RN, FAAN**
Theodore J. and Mary E. Trumble Professor
  in Aging Research
Director, Center on Aging
Associate Dean for Research
School of Nursing
University of Texas Health Science
  Center at Houston
School of Nursing
Houston, Texas

**Carol Bova, PhD, RN, ANP**
Associate Professor of Nursing and Medicine
Graduate School of Nursing
University of Massachusetts–Worcester
Worcester, Massachusetts

**Maja Djukic, PhD, RN**
Assistant Professor
New York University College of Nursing
New York, New York

**Stephanie Fulton, MSIS, AHIP**
Executive Director, Research Medical Library
The University of Texas MD Anderson
  Cancer Center
Houston, Texas

**Mattia J. Gilmartin, PhD, RN**
Senior Research Scientist
New York University College of Nursing
New York, New York

**Carl A. Kirton, DNP, ANP-BC, ACRN**
Senior Vice President, Patient Care Services
North General Hospital
Adjunct Clinical Associate Professor
College of Nursing
New York University
New York, New York

**Nancy E. Kline, PhD, RN, CPNP, FAAN**
Director, Clinical Inquiry, Medicine
Patient Services
Boston Children's Hospital
Boston, Massachusetts
Adjunct Clinical Assistant Professor
College of Nursing
New York University
New York, New York

**Barbara Krainovich-Miller, EdD, RN,
PMHCNS-BC, ANEF, FAAN**
Professor and Associate Dean, Academic and
  Clinical Affairs
New York University College of Nursing
New York, New York

**Ann Kurth, PhD, RN, FAAN**
Professor and Executive Director
NYUCN Global Division
New York University College of Nursing
New York, New York

**Marianne T. Marcus, EdD, RN, FAAN**
John P. McGovern Distinguished Professor
  in Addictions Nursing
Assistant Dean, Department Chair
University of Texas Health Science
  Center at Houston
School of Nursing
Houston, Texas

**Melanie McEwen, PhD, RN, CNE**
Associate Professor
University of Texas Health Science Center
    at Houston
School of Nursing
Houston, Texas

**Helen J. Streubert, EdD, RN, ANEF**
President
College of Saint Elizabeth
Morristown, New Jersey

**Susan Sullivan-Bolyai, DNSc, CNS, RN, FAAN**
Associate Professor
Director, Florence S. Downs Doctoral Program
    in Research and Theory Development
College of Nursing
New York University

**Marita Titler, PhD, RN, FAAN**
Professor and Chair, Division of Nursing
    Business and Health Systems
Rhetaugh G. Dumas Endowed Chair
Associate Dean, Office of Clinical Scholarship
    and Practice Development
Division of Nursing Business and Health
    Systems
University of Michigan School of Nursing
Ann Arbor, Michigan

**Mark Toles, PhD, RN**
Postdoctoral Scholar
Claire M. Fagin Fellow, John A. Hartford
    Foundation
Duke University School of Nursing
Durham, North Carolina

# REVIEWERS

**Tom Christenbery, PhD, RN, CNE**
Assistant Professor of Nursing
Vanderbilt University School of Nursing
Nashville, Tennessee

**Betsy Frank, PhD, RN, ANEF**
Professor Emerita
Indiana State University College of Nursing,
    Health, and Human Services
Terre Haute, Indiana

**Mary Tod Gray PhD, RN**
Professor
East Stroudsburg University
East Stroudsburg, Pennsylvania

**Sharon Kitchie, PhD, RN, CNS-BC**
Instructor
Keuka College
Keuka Park, New York

**Madelaine Lawrence, PhD, RN**
Associate Professor
Queens University of Charlotte
Charlotte, North Carolina

**Christina B. McSherry, PhD, RN, CNE**
Assistant Professor of Nursing
William Paterson University
Wayne, New Jersey

**Sue Ellen Odom, RN, DSN, CNE**
Professor
Department Chair, BSN Program
Clayton State University
Morrow, Georgia

**Teresa M. O'Neill, PhD, APRN, RNC**
Professor
Our Lady of Holy Cross College
New Orleans, Louisiana

**Sharon Souter, PhD, RN, CNE**
Dean and Professor
University of Mary Hardin-Baylor
Belton, Texas

**Molly J. Walker, PhD, RN, CNS, CNE**
Professor
Angelo State University
San Angelo, Texas

**Fatma Youssef, DNSc, MPH, RN**
Marymount University
Malek School of Health Professions
Arlington, Virginia

The foundation of the eighth edition of *Nursing Research: Methods and Critical Appraisal for Evidence-Based Practice* continues to be the belief that nursing research is integral to all levels of nursing education and practice. Over the past 28 years since the first edition of this textbook, we have seen the depth and breadth of nursing research grow, with more nurses conducting research and using research evidence to shape clinical practice, education, administration, and health policy.

The Institute of Medicine has challenged all health professionals to provide care based on the best available scientific evidence. This is an exciting challenge to meet. Nurses are using the best available evidence, combined with their clinical judgment and patient preferences, to influence the nature and direction of health care delivery and document outcomes related to the quality and cost-effectiveness of patient care. As nurses continue to develop a unique body of nursing knowledge through research, decisions about clinical nursing practice will be increasingly evidence based.

As editors, we believe that all nurses need not only to understand the research process but also to know how to critically read, evaluate, and apply research findings in practice. We realize that understanding research, as a component of evidence-based practice and quality improvement practices, is a challenge for every student, but we believe that the challenge can be accomplished in a stimulating, lively, and learner-friendly manner.

Consistent with this perspective is a commitment to advancing implementation of evidence-based practice. Understanding and applying nursing research must be an integral dimension of baccalaureate education, evident not only in the undergraduate nursing research course but also threaded throughout the curriculum. The research role of baccalaureate graduates calls for evidence-based practice and quality improvement competencies; central to this are critical appraisal skills—that is, nurses should be competent research consumers.

Preparing students for this role involves developing their critical thinking skills, thereby enhancing their understanding of the research process, their appreciation of the role of the critiquer, and their ability to actually critically appraise research. An undergraduate course in nursing research should develop this basic level of competence, which is an essential requirement if students are to engage in evidence-informed clinical decision making and practice. This is in contrast to a graduate-level research course in which the emphasis is on carrying out research, as well as understanding and appraising it.

The primary audience for this textbook remains undergraduate students who are learning the steps of the research process, as well as how to develop clinical questions, critically appraise published research literature, and use research findings to inform evidence-based clinical practice. This book is also a valuable resource for students at the master's and doctoral levels who want a concise review of the basic steps of the research process, the critical appraisal process, and the principles and tools for evidence-based practice and quality improvement. This text is also a key resource for doctor of nursing practice (DNP) students who are preparing to be experts at leading evidence-based and quality initiatives in clinical settings. Furthermore, it is an important resource for practicing nurses who strive to use research evidence as the basis for clinical decision making and development of evidence-based policies, protocols, and standards, rather than rely on tradition, authority, or trial and error. It is also an important resource for nurses who collaborate with nurse-scientists in the conducting of clinical research and evidence-based practice.

Building on the success of the seventh edition, we maintain our commitment to introducing evidence-based practice, quality improvement processes and research principles to baccalaureate students, thereby providing a cutting-edge, research consumer foundation for their clinical practice. *Nursing Research: Methods and Critical Appraisal for Evidence-Based Practice* prepares nursing students and practicing nurses to become knowledgeable nursing research consumers by doing the following:

- Addressing the evidence-based practice and quality improvement role of the nurse, thereby embedding evidence-based competence in the clinical practice of every baccalaureate graduate.
- Demystifying research, which is sometimes viewed as a complex process.
- Using an evidence-based approach to teaching the fundamentals of the research process.
- Adding a new chapter on the role of theory in research and evidence-based practice.
- Providing a new chapter on systematic reviews and clinical guidelines that presents the processes and critical appraisal of reviews and clinical practice guidelines as they relate to supporting evidence-based practice.
- Offering two chapters on current strategies and tools for developing an evidence-based practice.
- Concluding with a new chapter on quality improvement and its application to practice.
- Teaching the critical appraisal process in a user-friendly, but logical and systematic, progression.
- Promoting a lively spirit of inquiry that develops critical thinking and critical reading skills, facilitating mastery of the critical appraisal process.
- Developing information literacy, searching, and evidence-based practice competencies that prepare students and nurses to effectively locate and evaluate the best available research evidence.
- Elevating the critical appraisal process and research consumership to a position of importance comparable to that of producing research. Before students become research producers, they must become knowledgeable research consumers.
- Emphasizing the role of evidence-based practice and quality initiatives as the basis for informing clinical decision making and nursing interventions that support nursing practice, demonstrating quality and cost-effective outcomes of nursing care delivery.
- Presenting numerous examples of recently published research studies that illustrate and highlight each research concept in a manner that brings abstract ideas to life for students new to the research and critical appraisal process. These examples are a critical link for reinforcement of evidence-based concepts and the related research and critiquing process.
- Presenting five published articles, including a Cochrane Report, in the Appendices; references to these articles are woven throughout the text as exemplars of research and evidence-based practice principles.
- Showcasing, in **Research Vignettes,** the work of renowned nurse researchers whose careers exemplify the links among research, education, and practice.
- Providing numerous pedagogical chapter features, including **Learning Outcomes, Key Terms, Key Points,** new **Critical Thinking Challenges, Helpful Hints, Evidence-Based**

**Practice Tips,** revised **Critical Thinking Decision Paths,** and numerous tables, boxes, and figures. At the end of each chapter that presents a step of the research process we feature a revised section titled **Appraising the Evidence,** which reviews how each step of the research process should be evaluated from a consumer's perspective and is accompanied by an updated **Critiquing Criteria** box.

- Offering an **Evolve site** with interactive review questions that provide chapter-by-chapter review in a format consistent with that of the NCLEX® Examination.
- Offering a **Study Guide** that promotes active learning and assimilation of nursing research content.
- Presenting **Evolve Resources for Instructors** that include a test bank, TEACH lesson plans, PowerPoint slides with integrated audience response system questions, and an image collection. Evolve resources for both students and faculty also include a research article library with appraisal exercises for additional practice in reviewing and critiquing as well as content updates.

The eighth edition of *Nursing Research: Methods and Critical Appraisal for Evidence-Based Practice* is organized into four parts. Each part is preceded by an introductory section and opens with an exciting Research Vignette by a renowned nurse researcher.

**Part I, Overview of Research and Evidence-Based Practice,** contains four chapters: Chapter 1, "Integrating Research, Evidence-Based Practice, and Quality Improvement Processes," provides an excellent overview of research and evidence-based practice processes that shape clinical practice. The chapter speaks directly to students and highlights critical thinking and critical reading concepts and strategies, facilitating student understanding of the research process and its relationship to the critical appraisal process. The chapter introduces a model evidence hierarchy that is used throughout the text. The style and content of this chapter are designed to make subsequent chapters more user friendly. The next two chapters address foundational components of the research process. Chapter 2, "Research Questions, Hypotheses, and Clinical Questions," focuses on how research questions and hypotheses are derived, operationalized, and critically appraised. Numerous clinical examples illustrating different types of research questions and hypotheses maximize student understanding. Students are also taught how to develop clinical questions that are used to guide evidence-based inquiry. Chapter 3, "Gathering and Appraising the Literature," showcases cutting-edge literacy content, providing students and nurses with the tools necessary to effectively search, retrieve, manage, and evaluate research studies and their findings. This chapter also develops research consumer competencies that prepare students and nurses to critically read, understand, and appraise a study's literature review and framework. Chapter 4, "Theoretical Frameworks for Research," is a new user-friendly theory chapter that provides students with an understanding of how theories provide the foundation of research studies as well as evidence-based practice projects using research and clinical exemplars.

**Part II, Processes and Evidence Related to Qualitative Research,** contains three interrelated qualitative research chapters. Chapter 5, "Introduction to Qualitative Research," provides a framework for understanding qualitative research designs and literature as well as the significant contribution of qualitative research to evidence-based practice. Chapter 6, "Qualitative Approaches to Research," presents, illustrates, and showcases major qualitative methods using examples from the literature as exemplars. This chapter highlights the questions most appropriately answered using qualitative methods. Chapter 7, "Appraising Qualitative Research," synthesizes essential components of and criteria for critiquing qualitative research reports.

**Part III, Processes and Evidence Related to Quantitative Research,** contains Chapters 8 to 18. This group of chapters delineates the essential steps of the quantitative research process, with published clinical research studies used to illustrate each step. Links between the steps and their relationship to the total research process are examined. These chapters have been streamlined to make the case for linking an evidence-based approach with essential steps of the research process by teaching students how to critically appraise the strengths and weaknesses of each step of the research process and then weave them together in a synthesized critique of a research study. The steps of the quantitative research process, evidence-based concepts, and critical appraisal criteria are synthesized in Chapter 18. Chapter 11, a new and unique chapter, addresses the use of the various types of systematic reviews that support an evidence-based practice as well as the development and application of clinical guidelines to support clinical practice.

**Part IV, Application of Research: Evidence-Based Practice,** contains three chapters that present a unique showcase of evidence-based practice models and tools to use in effectively solving patient problems. Chapter 19, "Strategies and Tools for Developing an Evidence-Based Practice," is a vibrant, user-friendly, evidence-based toolkit with "real-life" exemplars that capture the totality for implementing high-quality, evidence-informed nursing care. It "walks" students and practicing nurses through clinical scenarios and challenges them to consider the relevant evidence-based practice "tools" they would use to develop and answer the questions that emerge from clinical situations. Chapter 20, "Developing an Evidence-Based Practice," offers a dynamic presentation of important evidence-based practice models that promote evidence-based decision making. These models can be applied, step by step, at the organizational or individual patient level as frameworks for implementing and evaluating the outcomes of evidence-based health care. Chapter 21, "Quality Improvement," is a new and unique, user-friendly chapter that outlines the steps of the quality improvement process with information from current guidelines from organizations that support practice based on evidence. Together, these chapters provide an inspirational conclusion to a text that we hope will motivate students and practicing nurses to advance their evidence-based practice knowledge base and clinical competence, thereby preparing to make an important contribution to improving health care delivery.

Stimulating critical thinking is a core value of this text. Innovative chapter features such as Critical Thinking Decision Paths, Evidence-Based Practice Tips, Helpful Hints, and Critical Thinking Challenges enhance critical thinking and promote the development of evidence-based decision-making skills. Consistent with previous editions, we promote critical thinking by including sections called "Appraising the Evidence," which describe the critical appraisal process related to the focus of the chapter. Additionally, Critiquing Criteria are included in this section to stimulate a systematic and evaluative approach to reading and understanding qualitative and quantitative research literature and evaluating its strengths and weaknesses. Extensive resources are provided on the Evolve site that can be used to develop critical thinking and evidence-based knowledge and skills.

The development and refinement of an evidence-based foundation for clinical nursing practice is an essential priority for the future of professional nursing practice. The eighth edition of *Nursing Research: Methods and Critical Appraisal for Evidence-Based Practice* will help students develop a basic level of competence in understanding the steps of the research process that will enable them to critically analyze research studies, judge their merit, and judiciously apply evidence in clinical practice. To the extent that this goal is accomplished, the next generation of nursing professionals will have a cadre of clinicians who inform their practice using theory and research evidence, combined with their clinical judgment, and specific to the health care needs of patients and their families in health and illness.

**Geri LoBiondo-Wood**
Geri.L.Wood@uth.tmc.edu

**Judith Haber**
jh33@nyu.edu

# TO THE STUDENT

We invite you to join us on an exciting nursing research adventure that begins as you turn the first page of the eighth edition of *Nursing Research: Methods and Critical Appraisal for Evidence-Based Practice*. The adventure is one of discovery! You will discover that the nursing research literature sparkles with pride, dedication, and excitement about the research dimension of professional nursing practice. Whether you are a student or a practicing nurse whose goal is to use research evidence as the foundation of your practice, you will discover that nursing research and a commitment to evidence-based practice positions our profession at the forefront of change. You will discover that evidence-based practice is integral to meeting the challenge of providing quality biopsychosocial health care in partnership with patients and their families/significant others, as well as with the communities in which they live. Finally, you will discover the richness in the "Who," "What," "Where," "When," "Why," and "How" of nursing research and evidence-based practice, developing a foundation of knowledge and skills that will equip you for clinical practice and making a significant contribution to quality patient outcomes!

We think you will enjoy reading this text. Your nursing research course will be short but filled with new and challenging learning experiences that will develop your evidence-based practice skills. The eighth edition of *Nursing Research: Methods and Critical Appraisal for Evidence-Based Practice* reflects cutting-edge trends for developing evidence-based nursing practice. The four-part organization and special features in this text are designed to help you develop your critical thinking, critical reading, information literacy, and evidence-based clinical decision-making skills, while providing a user-friendly approach to learning that expands your competence to deal with these new and challenging experiences. The companion Study Guide, with its chapter-by-chapter activities, serves as a self-paced learning tool to reinforce the content of the text. The accompanying Evolve Web site offers review material to help you tie the chapter material together and apply it to ten research articles. The site also offers review questions to help you reinforce the concepts discussed throughout the book.

Remember that evidence-based practice skills are used in every clinical setting and can be applied to every patient population or clinical practice issue. Whether your clinical practice involves primary care or specialty care and provides inpatient or outpatient treatment in a hospital, clinic, or home, you will be challenged to apply your evidence-based practice skills and use nursing research as the foundation for your evidence-based practice. The eighth edition of *Nursing Research: Methods and Critical Appraisal for Evidence-Based Practice* will guide you through this exciting adventure, where you will discover your ability to play a vital role in contributing to the building of an evidence-based professional nursing practice.

**Geri LoBiondo-Wood**
Geri.L.Wood@uth.tmc.edu

**Judith Haber**
jh33@nyu.edu

# ACKNOWLEDGMENTS

No major undertaking is accomplished alone; there are those who contribute directly and those who contribute indirectly to the success of a project. We acknowledge with deep appreciation and our warmest thanks the help and support of the following people:

- Our students, particularly the nursing students at the University of Texas Health Science Center at Houston School of Nursing and the College of Nursing at New York University, whose interest, lively curiosity, and challenging questions sparked ideas for revisions in the eighth edition.
- Our chapter contributors, whose passion for research, expertise, cooperation, commitment, and punctuality made them a joy to have as colleagues.
- Our vignette contributors, whose willingness to share evidence of their research wisdom made a unique and inspirational contribution to this edition.
- Our colleagues, who have taken time out of their busy professional lives to offer feedback and constructive criticism that helped us prepare this eighth edition.
- Our editors, Lee Henderson, Jennifer Ehlers, and Anne Konopka, for their willingness to listen to yet another creative idea about teaching research in a meaningful way and for their timely help with manuscript preparation and production.
- Our families: Brian Wood, who now is pursuing his own law career and over the years has sat in on classes, provided commentary, and patiently watched and waited as his mother rewrote each edition, as well as provided love, understanding, and support. Lenny, Andrew, Abbe, Brett and Meredith Haber and Laurie, Bob, Mikey, Benjy, and Noah Goldberg for their unending love, faith, understanding, and support throughout what is inevitably a consuming—but exciting—experience.

**Geri LoBiondo-Wood**

**Judith Haber**

# CONTENTS

## PART III    PROCESSES AND EVIDENCE RELATED TO QUANTITATIVE RESEARCH

## PART IV    APPLICATION OF RESEARCH: EVIDENCE-BASED PRACTICE

## APPENDICES

## GLOSSARY, 575

## INDEX, 585

# PART I

# Overview of Research and Evidence-Based Practice

Research Vignette: *Ann M. Berger*

# RESEARCH VIGNETTE

## IMPROVING SUPPORTIVE CARE FOR CANCER PATIENTS AND THEIR FAMILIES

**Ann M. Berger, PhD, APRN, AOCNS, FAAN**
**Professor and Dorothy Hodges Olson Endowed Chair in Nursing**
**University of Nebraska Medical Center**
**Omaha, Nebraska**

My introduction to using the research process to improve nursing care of oncology patients began during my Master of Science in Nursing program. A required assignment quickly ignited a passion in me to promote quality supportive care to patients with cancer. I worked with a Clinical Nurse Specialist colleague to develop and test the Oral Assessment Guide (OAG). The OAG uses a reliable and valid scoring method to quantify changes in the mouth that result from cytotoxic chemotherapy. We collaborated with PhD-prepared nurses throughout the development process and published our findings (Eilers, Berger, & Petersen, 1988). The OAG has been translated into several languages and is now used around the world to guide oral care for oncology patients. This project demonstrated the value of using quantitative methods to assess symptoms that are secondary to cancer treatment. The process serves as an excellent example of translating nursing research into real-world practice to improve patient outcomes.

After I participated in that research study, I realized that clinical researchers perform an essential role in advancing quality care! As a researcher, I knew I would have opportunities to investigate other common and significant clinical problems and advance knowledge in those areas. I began my PhD program and focused on the symptom of cancer-related fatigue (CRF). This symptom has been a challenge for clinical scientists to study because it is a perception, and therefore, difficult to define and measure (Barsevick et al., 2010).

My research trajectory developed in scope from individual efforts to working with teams, collaborating with multidisciplinary colleagues and on guideline panels to advance the science of symptom management in cancer patients and survivors. My initial opportunity to serve as a principal investigator was on my dissertation study. With funding awarded from the Oncology Nursing Foundation (ONF), I embarked on a descriptive study of fatigue and factors influencing fatigue during breast cancer adjuvant chemotherapy (Berger, 1998; Berger & Farr, 1999). I used a reliable and valid quantitative scale to measure subjective CRF and wrist actigraphs to objectively measure 24-hour activity/rest rhythms. Study findings enhanced the knowledge and understanding of relationships between activity/rest rhythms and CRF at various times during and after chemotherapy. Analysis of quantitative data revealed that symptoms, including disturbed sleep, predicted higher CRF over time, and therefore, were targets for interventions to reduce CRF (Berger & Walker, 2001a; Berger & Walker, 2001b). At that time, researchers had not conducted studies targeting sleep to improve sleep and CRF in patients with cancer.

I worked with a clinical psychologist to develop a behavioral therapy (BT) intervention to improve sleep and reduce fatigue. We pilot tested it after obtaining funding from the ONF. Based on positive results, I was awarded NIH funding to test the "Individualized Sleep Promotion Plan" (ISPP) in a larger sample. This randomized controlled trial (RCT) enrolled women with breast cancer a few days before their first chemotherapy treatment. The control group received equal time and attention and information about healthy eating. We were pleased that the ISPP group had significantly better sleep than the control group, but were disappointed that there were no differences between the groups on CRF (Berger et al., 2009; Berger, Kuhn et al., 2009a, 2009b). Implications for research and practice were that CRF did not respond to an intervention designed and demonstrated to improve a different symptom; in this case, sleep.

While conducting the RCT, I worked collaboratively with the Oncology Nursing Society (ONS), and we were awarded NIH-NCI funding to convene a conference on *Sleep-Wake Disturbances in Cancer Patients and their Caregivers*. The conference brought together multi-disciplinary leaders with a record of studying sleep in cancer patients, and each researcher was invited to sponsor the attendance of a PhD student interested in the topic. An ONS State-of-the-Science publication summarized participants' contributions to the conference and became the foundation for directing attention to sleep-wake disturbances in clinical, educational, and research settings (Berger et al., 2005). The conference attendees collaborated to promote the importance of discovering new knowledge about sleep in cancer patients and caregivers in order to build the evidence to establish guidelines for practice. That knowledge is gained by examining quantitative data from individuals experiencing the symptom.

Recognizing that evidence-based practice is the foundation of excellent patient care, I accepted an invitation from the National Comprehensive Cancer Network (NCCN) to serve as the Team Leader of the NCCN CRF guidelines panel (Berger et al., 2010). This organization supports an annual review of the evidence and update of the guidelines (www.nccn.org). When reviewing interventions tested to reduce CRF, critical elements include the definition, measurement, and analyses used to quantify CRF. Every year, newly published intervention studies, such as the one I described above, are reviewed for their scientific merit. Studies with methods judged to be of poor quality do not contribute to the advancement of evidence for the management of CRF.

I also serve as a researcher on the ONS-Putting Evidence into Practice (PEP) Sleep/Wake intervention team that evaluates results of quantitative data from studies to rate the evidence to reduce sleep-wake disturbances in adults with cancer (Page, Berger, & Eaton, 2009). ONS supports 19 ONS-PEP teams and influences the growth and development of symptom management research to improve care provided to patients with cancer (www.ons.org). ONS also conducts a Research Priorities survey every 4 years and the results of the survey are used to update the ONS Research Plan (Berger, Cochrane, & Mitchell, 2009). As a leader involved in these important activities, I collaborated with the teams to identify priorities for oncology research to improve patient care.

My journey as a clinical scientist has been an exciting one. I have personally witnessed advances in the science of cancer symptom management, in particular CRF and sleep-wake disturbances. I am confident that nurses who come after me will continue to test interventions and provide evidence of best practices, which will reduce these distressing symptoms that interfere with quality of life.

# REFERENCES

Barsevick, A. M., Cleeland, C., Manning, D. C., et al. (2010). ASCPRO recommendations for the assessment of fatigue as an outcome in clinical trials. *Journal of Pain and Symptom Management, 39*(6), 1086–1099.

Berger, A. (1998). Patterns of fatigue and activity and rest during adjuvant breast cancer chemotherapy. *Oncology Nursing Forum, 25*(160), 51–62.

Berger, A., Abernathy, A., Atkinson, A., et al. (2010). Cancer-related fatigue: clinical practice guidelines in oncology. *Journal of the National Comprehensive Cancer Network, 8*(8), 904–930.

Berger, A., Cochrane, B., & Mitchell, S. A. (2009). The 2009–2013 research agenda for oncology nursing. *Oncology Nursing Forum, 36*(5), E274–E282. doi:10.1188/09.

Berger, A., & Farr, L. (1999). The influence of daytime inactivity and nighttime restlessness on cancer-related fatigue. *Oncology Nursing Forum, 26*(1053), 1663–1671.

Berger, A., Kuhn, B. R., Farr, L., et al. (2009a). Behavioral therapy intervention trial to improve sleep quality and cancer-related fatigue. *Psycho-Oncology, 18*(6), 634–646.

Berger, A., Kuhn, B. R., Farr, L., et al. (2009b). One-year outcomes of a behavioral therapy intervention trial on sleep quality and cancer-related fatigue. *Journal of Clinical Oncology, 27*(35), 6033–6040.

Berger, A., Parker, K., Young-McCaughan, S., et al. (2005). Sleep wake disturbances in people with cancer and their caregivers: state of the science. *Oncology Nursing Forum, 32*(6), E98–E126.

Berger, A., & Walker, S. N. (2001a). An explanatory model of fatigue in women receiving adjuvant breast cancer chemotherapy. *Nursing Research, 50*(1), 42–52.

Berger, A., & Walker, S. N. (2001b). An explanatory model of fatigue in women receiving adjuvant breast cancer chemotherapy [corrected] [published erratum appears in *Nuring Research, 50*(3), 164]. *Nursing Research,* 50(1166), 42–52.

Eilers, J., Berger, A., & Petersen, M. C. (1988). Development, testing, and application of the oral assessment guide. *Oncology Nursing Forum, 15*(365), 325–330.

Page, M., Berger, A., & Eaton, L. (2009). Sleep-wake disturbances. In L. Eaton & J. M. Tipton (Eds.), *Putting evidence into practice* (pp. 285–297). Pittsburgh, PA: Oncology Nursing Society.

# Integrating Research, Evidence-Based Practice, and Quality Improvement Processes

*Geri LoBiondo-Wood and Judith Haber*

## ⊖volve WEBSITE

*Go to Evolve at http://evolve.elsevier.com/LoBiondo/ for review questions, critiquing exercises, and additional research articles for practice in reviewing and critiquing.*

## LEARNING OUTCOMES

*After reading this chapter, you should be able to do the following:*

- State the significance of research, evidence-based practice, and quality improvement.
- Identify the role of the consumer of nursing research.
- Define evidence-based practice.
- Define quality improvement.
- Discuss evidence-based and quality improvement decision making.
- Explain the difference between quantitative and qualitative research.

- Explain the difference between the types of systematic reviews.
- Identify the importance of critical reading skills for critical appraisal of research.
- Discuss the format and style of research reports/articles.
- Discuss how to use a quantitative evidence hierarchy when critically appraising research studies.

## KEY TERMS

| | | | |
|---|---|---|---|
| abstract | critique | levels of evidence | qualitative research |
| clinical guidelines | evidence-based | meta-analysis | quantitative research |
| consensus guidelines | guidelines | meta-synthesis | research |
| critical appraisal | evidence-based practice | quality improvement | systematic review |
| critical reading | integrative review | | |

We invite you to join us on an exciting nursing research adventure that begins as you read the first page of this chapter. The adventure is one of discovery! You will discover that the nursing research literature sparkles with pride, dedication, and excitement about this dimension of professional nursing practice. As you progress through your educational program, you are taught how to ensure quality and safety in practice through acquiring knowledge of the various sciences and health care principles. Another critical component of clinical knowledge is research knowledge as it applies to practicing from an evidence base.

Whether you are a student or a practicing nurse whose goal is to use **research** as the foundation of your practice, you will discover that nursing research, **evidence-based practice,** and **quality improvement** processes position our profession at the cutting edge of change and improvement in patient outcomes. You will also discover the cutting edge "who," "what," "where," "when," "why," and "how" of nursing research, and develop a foundation of evidence-based practice knowledge and competencies that will equip you for twenty-first–century clinical practice.

Your nursing research adventure will be filled with new and challenging learning experiences that develop your evidence-based practice skills. Your critical thinking, critical reading, and clinical decision-making skills will expand as you develop clinical questions, search the research literature, evaluate the research evidence found in the literature, and make clinical decisions about applying the "best available evidence" to your practice. For example, you will be encouraged to ask important clinical questions such as: "What makes a telephone education intervention more effective with one group of patients with a diagnosis of congestive heart failure but not another?" "What is the effect of computer learning modules on self-management of diabetes in children?" "What research has been conducted in the area of identifying barriers to breast cancer screening in African-American women?" "What is the quality of studies conducted on telehealth?" "What nursing-delivered smoking cessation interventions are most effective?" This book will help you begin your adventure into evidence-based nursing practice by developing an appreciation of research as the foundation for evidence-based practice and quality improvement.

## NURSING RESEARCH, EVIDENCE-BASED PRACTICE, AND QUALITY IMPROVEMENT

Nurses are constantly challenged to stay abreast of new information to provide the highest quality of patient care (IOM, 2011). Nurses are challenged to expand their "comfort zone" by offering creative approaches to old and new health problems, as well as designing new and innovative programs that make a difference in the health status of our citizens. This challenge can best be met by integrating rapidly expanding research and evidence-based knowledge about biological, behavioral, and environmental influences on health into the care of patients and their families.

It is important to differentiate between research, evidence-based practice, and quality improvement. **Research** is the systematic, rigorous, critical investigation that aims to answer questions about nursing phenomena. Researchers follow the steps of the scientific process, which are outlined later in this chapter and discussed in detail in each chapter of this textbook. There are two types of research: quantitative and qualitative. The methods used by nurse researchers are the same methods used by other disciplines; the difference is that nurses study questions relevant to nursing practice. The conduct of research provides knowledge that is reliable and useful for practice. Research studies published in journals, are read and evaluated for use in clinical practice. The findings of studies provide evidence that is evaluated, and its applicability to practice is used to inform clinical decisions.

**Evidence-based practice** is the collection, evaluation, and integration of valid research evidence, combined with clinical expertise and an understanding of patient and family values and preferences, to inform clinical decision making (Sackett et al., 2000). Research studies are gathered from the literature and assessed so that decisions about application to practice can be made, culminating in nursing practice that is evidence based. For example, to help you understand the importance of evidence-based practice, think about one of the latest reports from the Cochrane Collaboration by Murphy and colleagues (2012), which assessed whether follow-up affects the psychological well being of women following miscarriage (see Appendix E). Based on their search and synthesis of the literature, they put forth several conclusions regarding the implications for practice and further research for nurses working in the field of maternal child care.

**Quality improvement** (QI) is the systematic use of data to monitor the outcomes of care processes as well as the use of improvement methods to design and test changes in practice for the purpose of continuously improving the quality and safety of health care systems (Cronenwett et al., 2007). While research supports or generates new knowledge, evidence-based practice and QI uses currently available knowledge to improve health care delivery. When you first read about these three processes you will notice that they all have similarities. Each begins with a question. The difference is that in a research study the question is tested with a design appropriate to the question and specific methodology (i.e., sample, instruments, procedures, and data analysis) used to test the research question and contribute to new, generalizable knowledge. In the evidence-based practice and QI processes, a question is used to search the literature for already completed studies in order to bring about improvements in care.

All nurses share a commitment to the advancement of nursing science by conducting research and using research evidence in practice. Scientific investigation promotes accountability, which is one of the hallmarks of the nursing profession and a fundamental concept of the American Nurses Association (ANA) Code for Nurses (ANA, 2004). There is a consensus that the research role of the baccalaureate and master's graduate calls for the skills of **critical appraisal**. That is, nurses must be knowledgeable consumers of research, who can evaluate the strengths and weaknesses of research evidence and use existing standards to determine the merit and readiness of research for use in clinical practice (AACN, 2008; QSEN, 2012). Therefore to use research for an evidence-based practice and to practice using the highest quality processes, you do not have to conduct research; however, you do need to understand and appraise the steps of the research process in order to read the research literature critically and use it to inform clinical decisions.

As you venture through this text, you will see the steps of the research, evidence-based practice, and QI processes. The steps are systematic and orderly and relate to the development of evidence-based practice. Understanding the step-by-step process that researchers use will help you develop the assessment skills necessary to judge the soundness of research studies.

Throughout the chapters, terminology pertinent to each step is identified and illustrated with examples from the research literature. Five published research studies are found in the appendices and used as examples to illustrate significant points in each chapter. Judging the study's strength and quality, as well as its applicability to practice is key. Before you can judge a study, it is important to understand the differences among studies. There are many different study designs that you will see as you read through this text and the appendices. There are standards not only for critiquing the soundness of each step of a study, but also for judging the strength and quality of evidence provided by a study and determining its applicability to practice.

This chapter provides an overview of research study types and appraisal skills. It introduces the overall format of a research article and provides an overview of the subsequent chapters in the book. It also introduces the QI and evidence-based practice processes, a level of evidence hierarchy model, and other tools for helping you evaluate the strength and quality of evidence provided by a study. These topics are designed to help you read research articles more effectively and with greater understanding, so that you can make evidence-based clinical decisions and contribute to quality and cost-effective patient outcomes. The remainder of this book is devoted to helping you develop your evidence-based practice expertise.

## TYPES OF RESEARCH: QUALITATIVE AND QUANTITATIVE

Research is classified into two major categories: qualitative and quantitative. A researcher chooses between these categories based primarily on the question being asked. That is, a researcher may wish to test a cause-and-effect relationship, or to assess if variables are related, or may wish to discover and understand the meaning of an experience or process. A researcher would choose to conduct a **qualitative research** study if the question to be answered is about understanding the meaning of a human experience such as grief, hope, or loss. The meaning of an experience is based on the view that meaning varies and is subjective. The context of the experience also plays a role in qualitative research. That is, the experience of loss as a result of a miscarriage would be different than the experience from the loss of a parent.

Qualitative research is generally conducted in natural settings and uses data that are words or text rather than numeric to describe the experiences being studied. Qualitative studies are guided by research questions and data are collected from a small number of subjects, allowing an in-depth study of a phenomenon. For example, Seiler and Moss (2012) explored the experiences of nine nurse practitioners involved in providing health care to the homeless (see Appendix C). Although qualitative research is systematic in its method, it uses a subjective approach. Data from qualitative studies help nurses to understand experiences or phenomena that affect patients; these data also assist in generating theories that lead clinicians to develop improved patient care and stimulates further research. Highlights of the general steps of qualitative studies and the journal format for a qualitative article are outlined in Table 1-1. Chapters 5 through 7 provide an in-depth view of qualitative research underpinnings, designs, and methods.

Whereas qualitative research looks for meaning, **quantitative research** encompasses the study of research questions and/or hypotheses that describe phenomena, test relationships, assess differences, seek to explain cause-and-effect relationships between variables, and test for intervention effectiveness. The numeric data in quantitative studies are summarized and analyzed using statistics. Quantitative research techniques are systematic, and the methodology is controlled. Appendices A, B, and D illustrate examples of different quantitative approaches to

| TABLE 1-1 | STEPS OF THE RESEARCH PROCESS AND JOURNAL FORMAT: QUALITATIVE RESEARCH |
|---|---|
| **RESEARCH PROCESS STEPS AND/OR FORMAT ISSUES** | **USUAL LOCATION IN JOURNAL HEADING OR SUBHEADING** |
| Identifying the phenomenon | Abstract and/or in introduction |
| Research question study purpose | Abstract and/or in beginning or end of introduction |
| Literature review | Introduction and/or discussion |
| Design | Abstract and/or in introductory section or under method section entitled "Design" or stated in method section |
| Sample | Method section labeled "Sample" or "Subjects" |
| Legal-ethical issues | Data collection or procedures section or in sample section |
| Data collection procedure | Data collection or procedures section |
| Data analysis | Methods section under subhead "Data Analysis" or "Data Analysis and Interpretation" |
| Results | Stated in separate heading: "Results" or "Findings" |
| Discussion and recommendation | Combined in separate section: "Discussion" or "Discussion and Implications" |
| References | At end of article |

answering research questions. Table 1-2 indicates where each step of the research process can usually be located in a quantitative research article, and where it is discussed in this text. Chapters 2, 3, and 8 through 18 describe processes related to quantitative research.

The primary difference is that a qualitative study seeks to interpret meaning and phenomena, whereas quantitative research seeks to test a hypothesis or answer research questions using statistical methods. Remember as you read research articles that, depending on the nature of the research problem, a researcher may vary the steps slightly; however, all of the steps should be addressed systematically.

## CRITICAL READING SKILLS

To develop an expertise in evidence-based practice, you will need to be able to critically read all types of research articles. As you read a research article, you may be struck by the difference in style or format between a research article and a clinical article. The terms of a research article are new, and the focus of the content is different. You may also be thinking that the research article is hard to read or that it is too technical and boring. You may simultaneously wonder, "How will I possibly learn to appraise all the steps of a research study, the terminology, and the process of evidence-based practice? I'm only on Chapter 1. This is not so easy; research is as hard as everyone says."

Try to reframe these thoughts with the "glass is half-full" approach. That is, tell yourself, "Yes, I can learn how to read and appraise research, and this chapter will provide the strategies for me to learn this skill." Remember that learning occurs with time and help. Reading research articles can be difficult and frustrating at first, but the best way to become a knowledgeable research consumer is to use critical reading skills when reading research articles. As a student, you are not expected to understand a research article or critique it perfectly the first time. Nor are you expected to develop these skills on your own. An essential objective of this book is to help you acquire critical reading skills so that you can use research in your practice.

**TABLE 1-2    STEPS OF THE RESEARCH PROCESS AND JOURNAL FORMAT: QUANTITATIVE RESEARCH**

| RESEARCH PROCESS STEPS AND/OR FORMAT ISSUE | USUAL LOCATION IN JOURNAL HEADING OR SUBHEADING | TEXT CHAPTER |
|---|---|---|
| Research problem | Abstract and/or in article introduction or separately labeled: "Problem" | 2 |
| Purpose | Abstract and/or in introduction, or end of literature review or theoretical framework section, or labeled separately: "Purpose" | 2 |
| Literature review | At end of heading "Introduction" but not labeled as such, or labeled as separate heading: "Literature Review," "Review of the Literature," or "Related Literature"; or not labeled or variables reviewed appear as headings or subheadings | 3 |
| Theoretical framework (TF) and/or conceptual framework (CF) | Combined with "Literature Review" or found in separate section as TF or CF; or each concept used in TF or CF may appear as separate subheading | 3, 4 |
| Hypothesis/research questions | Stated or implied near end of introduction, may be labeled or found in separate heading or subheading: "Hypothesis" or "Research Questions"; or reported for first time in "Results" | 2 |
| Research design | Stated or implied in abstract or introduction or in "Methods" or "Methodology" section | 8, 9, 10 |
| Sample: type and size | "Size" may be stated in abstract, in methods section, or as separate subheading under methods section as "Sample," "Sample/Subjects," or "Participants"; "Type" may be implied or stated in any of previous headings described under size | 12 |
| Legal-ethical issues | Stated or implied in sections: "Methods," "Procedures," "Sample," or "Subjects" | 13 |
| Instruments | Found in sections: "Methods," "Instruments," or "Measures" | 14 |
| Validity and reliability | Specifically stated or implied in sections: "Methods," "Instruments," "Measures," or "Procedures" | 15 |
| Data collection procedure | In methods section under subheading "Procedure" or "Data Collection," or as separate heading: "Procedure" | 14 |
| Data analysis | Under subheading: "Data Analysis" | 16 |
| Results | Stated in separate heading: "Results" | 16, 17 |
| Discussion of findings and new findings | Combined with results or as separate heading: "Discussion" | 17 |
| Implications, limitations, and recommendations | Combined in discussion or as separate major headings | 17 |
| References | At end of article | 4 |
| Communicating research results | Research articles, poster, and paper presentations | 1, 20 |

---

**BOX 1-1    HIGHLIGHTS OF CRITICAL READING STRATEGIES**

**Strategies for Preliminary Understanding**
- Keep a research text and a dictionary by your side.
- Review the text's chapters on the research process steps, critiquing criteria, key terms.
- List key variables.
- Highlight or underline new terms, unfamiliar terms, and significant sentences.
- Look up the definitions of new terms and write them on the photocopy.
- Review old and new terms before subsequent readings.
- Highlight or underline identified steps of the research process.

**Strategies for Comprehensive Understanding**
- Identify the main idea or theme of the article; state it in your own words in one or two sentences.
- Continue to clarify terms that may be unclear on subsequent readings.
- Before critiquing the article, make sure you understand the main points of each step of the research process.

**Strategies for Analysis Understanding**
- Using the critiquing criteria, determine how well the study meets the criteria for each step of the research process.
- Determine which level of evidence fits the study.
- Write cues, relationships of concepts, and questions on the article .
- Ask fellow students to analyze the same study using the same criteria and then compare results.
- Consult faculty members about your evaluation of the study.

**Strategies for Synthesis Understanding**
- Review your notes on the article and determine how each step in the article compares with the critiquing criteria.
- Type a one-page summary in your own words of the reviewed study.
- Briefly summarize each reported research step in your own words using the critiquing criteria.
- Briefly describe strengths and weaknesses in your own words.

---

Remember that becoming a competent critical thinker and reader of research, similar to learning the steps of the research process, takes time and patience.

Critical reading is a process that involves the following levels of understanding and allows you to assess a study's validity. Box 1-1 provides strategies for these levels:
- Preliminary: familiarizing yourself with the content—skim the article
- Comprehensive: understanding the researcher's purpose or intent
- Analysis: understanding the terms and parts of the study
- Synthesis: understanding the whole article and each step of the research process in a study—assess the study's validity

Learning the research process further develops critical skills. You will gradually be able to read an entire research article and reflect on it by identifying assumptions, identifying key concepts and methods, and determining whether the conclusions are based on the study's findings. Once you have obtained this critical appraisal competency, you will be ready to synthesize the findings of multiple research studies to use in developing evidence-based practice. This will be a very exciting and rewarding process for you. To read a research study critically will require several readings. As you analyze and synthesize an article, you will begin the appraisal process that will help determine a study's worth. An illustration of how to use critical reading strategies is provided by the example in Box 1-2, which contains an

## BOX 1-2    EXAMPLE OF CRITICAL APPRAISAL READING STRATEGIES

**Introductory Paragraphs, Study's Purpose and Aims**

Despite important advances in its management, cancer pain remains a significant clinical problem (Apolone et al., 2009; McGuire, 2004; van den Beuken-van Everdingen et al., 2007). In a meta-analysis, cancer pain was found in 64% of patients with metastatic disease, 59% of patients receiving antineoplastic therapy, and 33% of patients who had received curative cancer treatment (van den Beuken-van Everdingen et al., 2007). Cancer pain also has a negative effect on patients' functional status (Ferreira et al., 2008; Holen et al., 2008; Vallerand et al., 2007) and is associated with psychological distress (Cohen et al., 2003; Vallerand et al., 2005). The effect of cancer pain on an individual's quality of life (QOL) can be significant and extend beyond disturbances in mood and physical function (Burckhardt & Jones, 2005; Dahl, 2004; Fortner et al., 2003).

The purposes of this randomized clinical trial were to test the effectiveness of two interventions compared to usual care in decreasing attitudinal barriers to cancer pain management, decreasing pain intensity, and improving pain relief, functional status, and QOL. The aims of this study are consistent with the study purpose: Given the limitations of previous intervention studies, additional research is warranted using approaches that can be implemented in the outpatient setting.

**Literature Review—Concepts**
Cancer pain and quality of life
Cancer pain interventions

The effect of cancer pain on an individual's quality of life (QOL) can be significant and extend beyond disturbances in mood and physical function (Burckhardt & Jones, 2005; Dahl, 2004; Fortner, et al., 2003).

In a meta-analysis of the benefits of patient-based psychoeducational interventions for cancer pain management, Bennett, Bagnall, and Closs (2009) concluded that, compared to usual care, educational interventions improved knowledge and attitudes, and reduced average and worst pain intensity scores. However, those interventions had no effect on medication adherence or in reducing pain's level of interference with daily activities.

**Conceptual Framework**

Change theory, specifically the Transtheoretical Model (Prochaska & DiClemente, 1984), is a useful conceptual framework for coaching. In this model, behavioral change is a function of a person's state of readiness or motivation to modify a particular behavior. Motivational interviewing is a nonauthoritarian counseling technique that can assist patients in recognizing and resolving ambivalence about making constructive behavioral changes. It matches the patients' readiness to change and can motivate the patient to move through the stages of the Transtheoretical Model: precontemplation (unaware of need for change), contemplation (thinking about change), preparation (actively considering change), action (engaging in changing behavior), and maintenance (maintaining a changed behavior) (Fahey et al., 2008; Prochaska & DiClemente, 1984).

**Methods**
**Design**

The study used a randomized clinical trial.

**Specific Aims and Hypotheses**

The authors hypothesized that the motivational-interviewing–based coaching group would demonstrate greater benefit (i.e., decreasing attitudinal barriers; decreasing pain intensity; and improving pain relief, functional status, and QOL) than either the conventional education or usual care groups.

**Subject Recruitment and Accrual**

A convenience sample was obtained by recruiting patients from six outpatient oncology clinics. Patients were eligible to participate if they were able to read and understand English, had access to a telephone, had a life expectancy longer than 6 months, and had an average pain intensity score of 2 or higher as measured on a 0-10 scale, with higher scores indicating more pain. Patients were excluded if they had a concurrent cognitive or psychiatric condition or substance abuse problem that would prevent adherence to the protocol, had severe pain unrelated to cancer, or resided in a setting where the patient could not self-administer pain medication (e.g., nursing home, board and care facility).

| BOX 1-2 | **EXAMPLE OF CRITICAL APPRAISAL READING STRATEGIES—cont'd** |
|---------|--------|
| **Procedure** | The study was approved by the institutional review board and research committee at each of the sites. Patients were identified by clinic staff and screened for eligibility by the research associate, who then approached eligible patients, explained the study, and obtained written informed consent. Patients were stratified based on pain intensity (i.e., low, medium, or high) and cancer treatment (i.e., chemotherapy or radiation therapy) to control for the confounding variables of pain intensity and the effects of cancer treatment. Patients and clinicians at the study sites were blinded to the patient's group assignment. At enrollment, patients completed a demographic questionnaire, Karnofsky Performance Status scale, Brief Pain Inventory, Barriers Questionnaire, 36-Item Short Form Health Survey, and Functional Assessment of Cancer Therapy–General. Patients and clinicians at the study sites were blinded to the patient's group assignment. The patients' medical records were reviewed for disease and treatment information. See procedure section for complete details. |
| **Intervention Fidelity** | Several strategies for treatment fidelity included study design, interventionist's training, and standardization of intervention across institutions. Subjects were screened and stratified by cancer therapy and were randomized to groups. |

excerpt from the abstract, introduction, literature review, theoretical framework literature, and methods and procedure section of a quantitative study (Thomas et al., 2012) (see Appendix A). Note that in this article there is both a literature review and a theoretical framework section that clearly support the study's objectives and purpose. Also note that parts of the text from the article were deleted to offer a number of examples within the text of this chapter.

### HELPFUL HINT

If you still have difficulty understanding a research study after using the strategies related to skimming and comprehensive reading, make a copy of your "marked-up" article, include your specific questions or area of difficulty, and ask your professor to read it. Comprehensive understanding and synthesis are necessary to analyze a study. Understanding the author's purpose and methods of a study reflects critical thinking and facilitates the evaluation of the study.

## STRATEGIES FOR CRITIQUING RESEARCH STUDIES

Evaluation of a research article requires a critique. The **critique** is the process of critical appraisal that objectively and critically evaluates a research report's content for scientific merit and application to practice. It requires some knowledge of the subject matter and knowledge of how to critically read and use critiquing criteria. You will find:

- Summarized examples of critiquing criteria for qualitative studies and an example of a qualitative critique in Chapter 7
- Summarized critiquing criteria and examples of a quantitative critique in Chapter 18
- An in-depth exploration of the criteria for evaluation required in quantitative research critiques in Chapters 8 through 18
- Criteria for qualitative research critiques presented in Chapters 5, 6, and 7
- Principles for qualitative and quantitative research in Chapters 1, 2, 3, and 4

Critiquing criteria are the standards, appraisal guides, or questions used to assess an article. In analyzing a research article, you must evaluate each step of the research process and ask questions about whether each step meets the criteria. For instance, the critiquing criteria in Chapter 3 ask if "the literature review identifies gaps and inconsistencies in the literature about a subject, concept, or problem," and if "all of the concepts and variables are included in the review." These two questions relate to critiquing the research question and the literature review components of the research process. Box 1-2 shows several places where the researchers in the study by Thomas and colleagues identified gaps in the literature, and how the study intended to fill these gaps by conducting a study for the stated objective and purpose (see Appendix A). Remember that when you are doing a critique, you are pointing out strengths as well as weaknesses. Developing critical reading skills will enable you to successfully complete a critique. The appraisal strategies that facilitate the understanding gained by reading for analysis are listed in Box 1-1. Standardized critical appraisal tools such as the Critical Appraisal Skills Programme—CASP Tools (www.phru. nhs.uk) can also be used by students and clinicians to systematically appraise the strength and quality of evidence provided in research articles (see Chapter 20).

Critiquing can be thought of as looking at a completed jigsaw puzzle. Does it form a comprehensive picture, or is there a piece out of place? What is the level of evidence provided by the study and its findings? What is the balance between the risks and benefits of the findings that contribute to clinical decisions? How can I apply the evidence to my patient, to my patient population, or in my setting? When reading several studies for synthesis, you must assess the interrelationship of the studies, as well as the overall strength and quality of evidence and its applicability to practice. Reading for synthesis is essential in critiquing research. Appraising a study helps with the development of an evidence table (see Chapter 20).

## OVERCOMING BARRIERS: USEFUL CRITIQUING STRATEGIES

Throughout the text, you will find features that will help refine the skills essential to developing your competence as a consumer of research (see Box 1-1). A Critical Thinking Decision Path related to each step of the research process will sharpen your decision-making skills as you critique research articles. Look for Internet resources in chapters that will enhance your consumer skills. Critical Thinking Challenges, which appear at the end of each chapter, are designed to reinforce your critical reading skills in relation to the steps of the research process. Helpful Hints, designed to reinforce your understanding, appear at various points throughout the chapters. Evidence-Based Practice Tips, which will help you apply evidence-based practice strategies in your clinical practice, are provided in each chapter.

When you complete your first critique, congratulate yourself; mastering these skills is not easy at the beginning, but we are confident that you can do it. Best of all, you can look forward to discussing the points of your appraisal because your critique will be based on objective data, not just personal opinion. As you continue to use and perfect critical analysis skills by critiquing studies, remember that these very skills are an expected clinical competency for delivering evidence-based and quality nursing care.

## EVIDENCE-BASED PRACTICE AND RESEARCH

Along with gaining comfort while reading and critiquing studies, there is one final step: deciding how, when, and if to apply the studies to your practice so that your practice is evidence based. Evidence-based practice allows you to systematically use the best available evidence with the integration of individual clinical expertise, as well as the patient's values and preferences, in making clinical decisions (Sackett et al., 2000). Evidence-based practice has processes and steps, as does the research process. These steps are presented throughout the text. Chapter 19 provides an overview of evidence-based practice steps and strategies.

When using evidence-based practice strategies, the first step is to be able to read a study and understand how each section is linked to the steps of the research process. The following section introduces you to the research process as presented in published articles. Once you read an article you must decide which level of evidence the research article provides and how well the study was designed and executed. Figure 1-1 illustrates a model for determining the levels of evidence associated with a study's design, ranging from systematic reviews of randomized clinical trials (RCTs) (see Chapters 9 and 10) to expert opinions. The rating system, or evidence hierarchy model, presented here is just one of many. Many hierarchies for assessing the relative worth of different types of research literature for both the qualitative and quantitative research literature are available. Early in the development

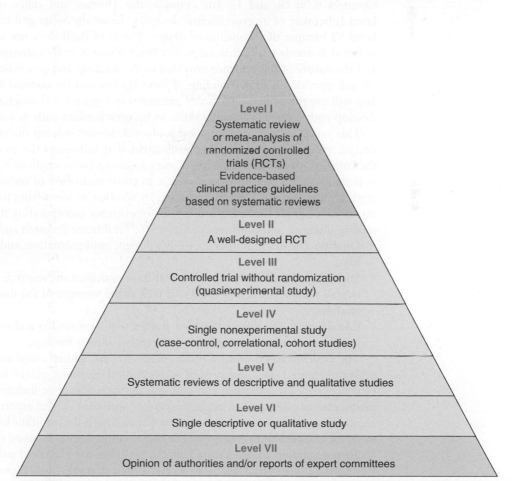

**FIGURE 1-1** Levels of evidence: evidence hierarchy for rating levels of evidence, associated with a study's design. Evidence is assessed at a level according to its source.

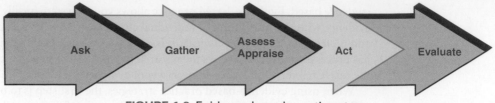

**FIGURE 1-2** Evidence-based practice steps.

of evidence-based practice, evidence hierarchies were thought to be very inflexible, with systematic reviews or meta-analyses at the top and qualitative research at the bottom. When assessing a clinical question that measures cause and effect this may be true; however, nursing and health care research is involved in a broader base of problem solving, and thus assessing the worth of a study within a broader context of applying evidence into practice requires a broader view.

The meaningfulness of an evidence rating system will become clearer as you read Chapters 8, 9, 10, and 11. For example, the Thomas and colleagues (2012) study is Level II because of its experimental design, whereas the Seiler and Moss (2012) study is Level VI because of its qualitative design. The level itself does not tell a study's worth; rather it is another tool that helps you think about a study's strengths and weaknesses and the nature of the evidence provided in the findings and conclusions. Chapters 7 and 18 will provide an understanding of how studies can be assessed for use in practice. You will use the evidence hierarchy presented in Figure 1-1 throughout the book as you develop your research consumer skills, so become familiar with its content.

This rating system represents levels of evidence for judging the strength of a study's design, which is just one level of assessment that influences the confidence one has in the conclusions the researcher has drawn. Assessing the strength of scientific evidence or potential research bias provides a vehicle to guide evaluation of research studies for their applicability in clinical decision making. In addition to identifying the level of evidence, one needs to grade the strength of a body of evidence incorporating the three domains of quality, quantity, and consistency (Agency for Healthcare Research and Quality, 2002).

- **Quality:** The extent to which a study's design, implementation, and analysis minimizes bias.
- **Quantity:** The number of studies that have evaluated the research question, including overall sample size across studies, as well as the strength of the findings from the data analyses.
- **Consistency:** The degree to which studies that have similar and different designs, but investigate the same research question, report similar findings.

The evidence-based practice process steps are: ask, gather, assess and appraise, act, and evaluate (Figure 1-2). These steps of *asking* clinical questions; identifying and *gathering* the evidence; critically *appraising* and synthesizing the evidence or literature; *acting* to change practice by coupling the best available evidence with your clinical expertise and patient preferences (e.g., values, setting, resources); and *evaluating* if the use of the best available research evidence is applicable to your patient or organization will be discussed throughout the text.

To maintain an evidence-based practice, studies are evaluated using specific criteria. Completed studies are evaluated in terms of their strength, quality, and consistency of evidence. Before one can proceed with an evidence-based project, it is necessary to understand the steps of the research process found in research studies.

## RESEARCH ARTICLES: FORMAT AND STYLE

Before you begin reading research articles, it is important to have a sense of their organization and format. Many journals publish research, either as the sole type of article, or in addition to clinical or theoretical articles. Although many journals have some common features, they also have unique characteristics. All journals have guidelines for manuscript preparation and submission. A review of these guidelines, which are found on a journal's Web site, will give you an idea of the format of articles that appear in specific journals.

Remember that even though each step of the research process is discussed at length in this text, you may find only a short paragraph or a sentence in an article that gives the details of the step. Because of a journal's publishing guidelines, the study that one reads in a journal is a shortened version of the researcher(s) completed work. You will also find that some researchers devote more space in an article to the results, whereas others present a longer discussion of the methods and procedures. Most authors give more emphasis to the method, results, and discussion of implications than to details of assumptions, hypotheses, or definitions of terms. Decisions about the amount of material presented for each step of the research process are bound by the following:

- A journal's space limitations
- A journal's author guidelines
- The type or nature of the study
- The researcher's decision regarding which component of the study is the most important.

The following discussion provides a brief overview of each step of the research process and how it might appear in an article. It is important to remember that a quantitative research article will differ from a qualitative research article. The components of qualitative research are discussed in Chapters 5 and 6, and are summarized in Chapter 7.

### Abstract

An **abstract** is a short, comprehensive synopsis or summary of a study at the beginning of an article. An abstract quickly focuses the reader on the main points of a study. A well-presented abstract is accurate, self-contained, concise, specific, nonevaluative, coherent, and readable. Abstracts vary in length from 50 to 250 words. The length and format of an abstract are dictated by the journal's style. Both quantitative and qualitative research studies have abstracts that provide a succinct overview of the study. An example of an abstract can be found at the beginning of the study by Thomas and colleagues (2012) (see Appendix A). Their abstract follows an outline format that highlights the major steps of the study. It partially reads as follows:

> Purpose/Objective: "To test the effectiveness of two interventions compared to usual care in decreasing attitudinal barriers to cancer pain management, decreasing pain intensity and improving functional status and quality of life."

Within this example, the authors provide a view of the study variables. The remainder of the abstract provides a synopsis of the background of the study and the methods, results, and conclusions. The studies in Appendices A through D all have abstracts.

## Introduction

Early in a research article, in a section that may or may not be labeled "Introduction," the researcher presents a background picture of the area researched and its significance to practice (see Chapter 2). In the Thomas and colleagues (2012) article, the basis of the research question is found early in the article (see Appendix A), as follows:

*"Despite important advances in its management, cancer pain remains a significant clinical problem. The effect of cancer pain on an individual's quality of life (QOL) can be significant and extend beyond disturbances in mood and physical function."*

Another example can be found in the Alhusen and colleagues (2012) study (see Appendix B), as follows:

*"Disparities in neonatal outcomes between African Americans and non-Latino white Americans are one of the most concerning and chronic health disparities affecting our nation (Alexander et al., 2008). Many of the health disparities in pre-term birth, low birth weight (LBW), and other adverse pregnancy outcomes are more prevalent in ethnic minority and low-income populations (Patrick & Bryan, 2005)."*

## Definition of the Purpose

The purpose of the study is defined either at the end of the researcher's initial introduction or at the end of the "Literature Review" or "Conceptual Framework" section. The study's purpose may or may not be labeled (see Chapters 2 and 3), or it may be referred to as the study's aim or objective. The studies in Appendices A, B, C, and D present specific purposes for each study in untitled sections that appear in the beginning of each article, as well as in the article's abstract.

## Literature Review and Theoretical Framework

Authors of studies present the literature review and theoretical framework in different ways. Many research articles merge the "Literature Review" and the "Theoretical Framework." This section includes the main concepts investigated and may be called "Review of the Literature," "Literature Review," "Theoretical Framework," "Related Literature," "Background," or "Conceptual Framework"; or it may not be labeled at all (see Chapters 2 and 3). By reviewing Appendices A through D, the reader will find differences in the headings used. Thomas and colleagues (2012) (see Appendix A) use no labels and present the literature review and a theoretical framework in the beginning of the article; the study in Appendix B has an untitled literature review and a theoretical model section; while the study in Appendix C has a literature review and a titled conceptual framework section. All three studies have literature reviews and a framework. One style is not better than another; the studies in the appendices contain all the critical elements but present the elements differently.

## Hypothesis/Research Question

A study's research questions or hypotheses can also be presented in different ways (see Chapter 2). Research articles often do not have separate headings for reporting the "Hypotheses" or "Research Question." They are often embedded in the "Introduction" or "Background" section, or not labeled at all (e.g., as in the studies in the appendices). If a study uses hypotheses, the researcher may report whether the hypotheses were or were not supported toward the end of the article in the "Results" or "Findings" section. Quantitative research studies have hypotheses or research questions. Qualitative research studies do not have hypotheses, but have research questions and purposes. The studies in Appendices A, B, and D have hypotheses. The study in Appendix C does not, since it is a qualitative study; rather it has a purpose statement.

## Research Design

The type of research design can be found in the abstract, within the purpose statement, or in the introduction to the "Procedures" or "Methods" section, or not stated at all (see Chapters 6, 9, and 10). For example, the studies in Appendices A, C, and D identify the design in the abstract.

One of your first objectives is to determine whether the study is qualitative (see Chapters 5 and 6) or quantitative (see Chapters 8, 9, and 10). Although the rigor of the critiquing criteria addressed do not substantially change, some of the terminology of the questions differs for qualitative and quantitative studies. Do not get discouraged if you cannot easily determine the design. One of the best strategies is to review the chapters that address designs, and to ask your professors for assistance. The following tips will help you determine whether the study you are reading employs a quantitative design:

- Hypotheses are stated or implied (see Chapter 2)
- The terms control and treatment group appear (see Chapter 9)
- The term survey, correlational, or ex post facto is used (see Chapter 10)
- The term random or convenience is mentioned in relation to the sample (see Chapter 12)
- Variables are measured by instruments or scales (see Chapter 14)
- Reliability and validity of instruments are discussed (see Chapter 15)
- Statistical analyses are used (see Chapter 16)

In contrast, qualitative studies generally do not focus on "numbers." Some qualitative studies may use standard quantitative terms (e.g., subjects) rather than qualitative terms (e.g., informants). Deciding on the type of qualitative design can be confusing; one of the best strategies is to review the qualitative chapters (see Chapters 5, 6, and 7). Begin trying to link the study's design with the level of evidence associated with that design as illustrated in Figure 1-1. This will give you a context for evaluating the strength and consistency of the findings and their applicability to practice. Chapters 8, 9, 10, and 11 will help you understand how to link the levels of evidence with quantitative designs. A study may not indicate the specific design used; however, all studies inform the reader of the methodology used, which can help you decide the type of design the authors used to guide the study.

## Sampling

The population from which the sample was drawn is discussed in the section "Methods" or "Methodology" under the subheadings of "Subjects" or "Sample" (see Chapter 12). Researchers should tell you both the population from which the sample was chosen and the number of subjects that participated in the study, as well as if they had subjects who dropped out of the study. The authors of the studies in the appendices discuss their samples in enough detail so that the reader is clear about who the subjects are and how they were selected.

## Reliability and Validity

The discussion of the instruments used to study the variables is usually included in a "Methods" section under the subheading of "Instruments" or "Measures" (see Chapter 14). Usually each instrument (or scale) used in the study is discussed, as well as its reliability and validity (see Chapter 15). The studies in Appendices A through D discuss each of the measures used in the "Methods" section under the subheading "Measures" or "Instruments." The reliability and validity of each measure is also presented.

In some cases, the reliability and validity of commonly used, established instruments in an article are not presented, and you are referred to other references. Ask assistance from your instructor if you are in doubt about the validity or reliability of a study's instruments.

## Procedures and Collection Methods

The data collection procedures, or the individual steps taken by the researcher to gather measurable data (usually with instruments or scales), are generally found in the "Procedures" section (see Chapter 14). In the studies in Appendices A through D, the researchers indicate how they conducted the study in detail under the subheading "Procedure" or "Instruments and Procedures." Notice that the researchers in each study included in the Appendices provided information that the studies were approved by an institutional review board (see Chapter 13), thereby ensuring that each study met ethical standards.

## Data Analysis/Results

The data-analysis procedures (i.e., the statistical tests used and the results of descriptive and/or inferential tests applied in quantitative studies) are presented in the section labeled "Results" or "Findings" (see Chapters 16 and 17). Although qualitative studies do not use statistical tests, the procedures for analyzing the themes, concepts, and/or observational or print data are usually described in the "Method" or "Data Collection" section and reported in the "Results," "Findings," or "Data Analysis" section (see Appendix D and Chapters 5 and 6).

## Discussion

The last section of a research study is the "Discussion" (see Chapter 17). In this section the researchers tie together all of the study's pieces and give a picture of the study as a whole. The researchers go back to the literature reviewed and discuss how their study is similar to, or different from, other studies. Researchers may report the results and discussion in one section, but usually report their results in separate "Results" and "Discussion" sections (see Appendices A, B, C, and D). One way is no better than another. Journal and space limitations determine how these sections will be handled. Any new or unexpected findings are usually described in the "Discussion" section.

## Recommendations and Implications

In some cases a researcher reports the implications and limitations based on the findings for practice and education, and recommends future studies in a separate section labeled "Conclusions"; in other cases, this appears in several sections labeled with such titles as "Discussion," "Limitations," "Nursing Implications," "Implications for Research and Practice," and "Summary." Again, one way is not better than the other—only different.

## References

All of the references cited are included at the end of the article. The main purpose of the reference list is to support the material presented by identifying the sources in a manner that allows for easy retrieval. Journals use various referencing styles.

## Communicating Results

Communicating a study's results can take the form of a research article, poster, or paper presentation. All are valid ways of providing data and have potential to effect high-quality patient care based on research findings. Evidence-based nursing care plans and QI practice protocols, guidelines, or standards are outcome measures that effectively indicate communicated research.

---

**HELPFUL HINT**

If you have to write a paper on a specific concept or topic that requires you to critique and synthesize the findings from several studies, you might find it useful to create an evidence table of the data (see Chapter 20). Include the following information: author, date, type of study, design, level of evidence, sample, data analysis, findings, and implications.

---

# SYSTEMATIC REVIEWS: META-ANALYSES, INTEGRATIVE REVIEWS, AND META-SYNTHESES

## Systematic Reviews

Other article types that are important to understand for evidence-based practice are systematic reviews, meta-analyses, integrative reviews (sometimes called narrative reviews), and meta-syntheses. A systematic review is a summation and assessment of a group of research studies that test a similar research question. If statistical techniques are used to summarize and assess more than one study, the systematic review is labeled as a meta-analysis. A meta-analysis is a summary of a number of studies focused on one question or topic, and uses a specific statistical methodology to synthesize the findings in order to draw conclusions about the area of focus. An integrative review is a focused review and synthesis of research or theoretical literature in a particular focus area, and includes specific steps of literature integration and synthesis without statistical analysis; it can include both quantitative and qualitative articles (Whittemore, 2005). At times such reviews use the terms systematic review and integrative review interchangeably. Both meta-synthesis and meta-summary are the synthesis of a number of qualitative research studies on a focused topic using specific qualitative methodology (Sandelowski & Barrosos, 2007).

The components of these reviews will be discussed in greater detail in Chapters 6, 11, and 20. These articles take a number of studies related to a clinical question and, using a specific set of criteria and methods, evaluate the studies as a whole. While they may vary somewhat in their approach, these reviews all help to better inform and develop evidence-based practice. The Cochrane Report in Appendix E is an example of a systematic review that is a meta-analysis.

## CLINICAL GUIDELINES

**Clinical guidelines** are systematically developed statements or recommendations that serve as a guide for practitioners. Two types of clinical guidelines will be discussed throughout this text: consensus, or expert-developed guidelines, and evidence-based guidelines. **Consensus guidelines**, or expert-based guidelines, are developed by an agreement of experts in the field. **Evidence-based guidelines** are those developed using published research findings. Guidelines are developed to assist in bridging practice and research, and are developed by professional organizations, government agencies, institutions, or convened expert panels. Clinical guidelines provide clinicians with an algorithm for clinical management or decision making for specific diseases (e.g., colon cancer) or treatments (e.g., pain management). Not all clinical guidelines are well developed and, like research, must be assessed before implementation. Though they are systematically developed and make explicit recommendations for practice, clinical guidelines may be formatted differently. Guidelines for practice are becoming more important as third party and government payers are requiring practice to be based on evidence. Guidelines should present scope and purpose of the practice, detail who the development group included, demonstrate scientific rigor, be clear in its presentation, demonstrate clinical applicability, and demonstrate editorial independence (See Chapter 11).

## QUALITY IMPROVEMENT

As a health care provider, you are responsible for continuously improving the quality and safety of health care for your patients and their families through systematic redesign of health care systems in which you work. The Institute of Medicine (2001) defined quality health care as care that is safe, effective, patient-centered, timely, efficient, and equitable. Therefore, the goal of QI is to bring about measurable changes across these six domains by applying specific methodologies within a care setting. While several QI methods exist, the core steps for improvement commonly include the following:
- Conducting an assessment
- Setting specific goals for improvement
- Identifying ideas for changing current practice
- Deciding how improvements in care will be measured
- Rapidly testing practice changes
- Measuring improvements in care
- Adopting the practice change as a new standard of care

Chapter 21 focuses on building your competence to participate in and lead QI projects by providing an overview of the evolution of QI in health care, including the nurse's role in meeting current regulatory requirements for patient care quality. Chapter 19 discusses QI models and tools such as cause-and-effect diagrams and process mapping, as well as skills for effective teamwork and leadership that are essential for successful QI projects.

As you venture through this textbook, you will be challenged to think not only about reading and understanding research studies, but also about applying the findings to your practice. Nursing has a rich legacy of research that has grown in depth and breadth. Producers of research and clinicians must engage in a joint effort to translate findings into practice that will make a difference in the care of patients and families.

## KEY POINTS

- Nursing research provides the basis for expanding the unique body of scientific evidence that forms the foundation of evidence-based nursing practice. Research links education, theory, and practice.
- As consumers of research, nurses must have a basic understanding of the research process and critical appraisal skills to evaluate research evidence before applying it to clinical practice.
- Critical appraisal is the process of evaluating the strengths and weaknesses of a research article for scientific merit and application to practice, theory, or education; the need for more research on the topic/clinical problem is also addressed at this stage.
- Critiquing criteria are the measures, standards, evaluation guides, or questions used to judge the worth of a research study.
- Critical reading skills will enable you to evaluate the appropriateness of the content of a research article, apply standards or critiquing criteria to assess the study's scientific merit for use in practice, or consider alternative ways of handling the same topic.
- Critical reading requires four stages of understanding: preliminary (skimming), comprehensive, analysis, and synthesis. Each stage includes strategies to increase your critical reading skills.
- A level of evidence model is a tool for evaluating the strength (quality, quantity, and consistency) of a research study and its findings.
- Each article should be evaluated for the study's strength and consistency of evidence as a means of judging the applicability of findings to practice.
- Research articles have different formats and styles depending on journal manuscript requirements and whether they are quantitative or qualitative studies.
- Evidence-based practice and QI begin with the careful reading and understanding of each article contributing to the practice of nursing, clinical expertise, and an understanding of patient values.
- QI processes are aimed at improving clinical care outcomes for patients and better methods of system performance.

## CRITICAL THINKING CHALLENGES

- How might nurses differentiate research from evidence-based practice for their colleagues?
- From your clinical practice, discuss several strategies nurses can undertake to promote evidence-based practice.
- What are some strategies you can use to develop a more comprehensive critique of an evidence-based practice article?
- A number of different components are usually identified in a research article. Discuss how these sections link with one another to ensure continuity.
- How can QI data be used to improve clinical practice?

## REFERENCES

Agency for Healthcare Research and Quality: Systems to rate the strength of scientific evidence. (2002). *File inventory, Evidence Report/Technology Assessment No. 47*, AHRQ Publication No. 02-E016.

Alhusen, J. L., Gross, D., Hayatt, M. J., et al. (2012). The influence of maternal-fetal attachment and health practices on neonatal outcomes in low-income women. *Research in Nursing & Health, 35*(2), 112–120.

American Association of Critical Care Nursing [AACN]: 2008.

American Nurses Association. (2004). *Code for nurses with interpretive statements*. Washington, DC: The Association.

Cronenwett, L., Sherwood, G., Barnsteiner, J., et al. (2007). Quality and safety education for nurses. *Nursing Outlook, 55*(3), 122–131.

Institute of Medicine Committee on Quality of Health Care in America. (2001). *Crossing the quality chasm: a new health system for the 21st century*. Washington, DC: National Academy Press.

Institute of Medicine [IOM]. (2011). *The Future of Nursing: Leading Change, Advancing Health*. Washington, DC: National Academic Press.

Murphy, F. A., Lipp, A., & Powles, D. L. (2012). Follow-up for improving psychological well-being for women after a miscarriage (Review). *The Cochrane Collaboration, 3*, 3.CD008679. doi:10.1002/14651858.CD008679.pub2.

Robert Wood Johnson Foundation. (2011). *Quality and Safety Education for Nurses (QSEN)* [Internet]. Retrieved from http://www.rwjf.org March 7, 2013

Sackett, D. L. , Straus, S., Richardson, S., et al. (2000). *Evidence-based medicine: How to practice and teach EBM* (2nd ed.). London: Churchill Livingstone.

Sandelowski, M., & Barroso, J. (2007). *Handbook of Qualitative Research,* New York, Springer Pub. Co.

Seiler, A.J., & Moss, V.A. (2012). The experiences of nurse practitioners providing health care to the homeless. *Journal of the American Academy of Nurse Practitioners, 24*, 303–312.

Thomas, M.L., Elliott, J.E., Rao, S.M., et al. (2012). A randomized clinical trial of education or motivational interviewing based coaching compared to usual care to improve cancer pain management. *Oncology Nursing, Forum, 39*(1), 39–49.

Whittemore, R. (2005). Combining evidence in nursing research. *Nursing Research, 54*(1), 56–62.

ꞓ∨olve WEBSITE

*Go to Evolve at http://evolve.elsevier.com/LoBiondo/ for review questions, critiquing exercises, and additional research articles for practice in reviewing and critiquing.*

# Research Questions, Hypotheses, and Clinical Questions

*Judith Haber*

**WEBSITE**

*Go to Evolve at http://evolve.elsevier.com/LoBiondo/ for review questions, critiquing exercises, and additional research articles for practice in reviewing and critiquing.*

## LEARNING OUTCOMES

*After reading this chapter, you should be able to do the following:*

- Describe how the research question and hypothesis relate to the other components of the research process.
- Describe the process of identifying and refining a research question or hypothesis.
- Discuss the appropriate use of research questions versus hypotheses in a research study.
- Identify the criteria for determining the significance of a research question or hypothesis.
- Discuss how the purpose, research question, and hypothesis suggest the level of evidence to be obtained from the findings of a research study.

- Discuss the purpose of developing a clinical question.
- Discuss the differences between a research question and a clinical question in relation to evidence-based practice.
- Apply critiquing criteria to the evaluation of a research question and hypothesis in a research report.

## KEY TERMS

| | | | |
|---|---|---|---|
| clinical question | hypothesis | population | statistical hypothesis |
| complex hypothesis | independent variable | purpose | testability |
| dependent variable | nondirectional | research hypothesis | theory |
| directional hypothesis | hypothesis | research question | variable |

At the beginning of this chapter you will learn about research questions and hypotheses from the perspective of the researcher, which, in the second part of this chapter, will help you to generate your own clinical questions that you will use to guide the development of evidence-based practice projects. From a clinician's perspective, you must understand the research question and hypothesis as it aligns with the rest of a study. As a practicing nurse, the clinical questions you will develop (see Chapters 19, 20, and 21) represent the first step of the evidence-based practice process for quality improvement programs such as those that decrease risk for development of decubitus ulcers.

When nurses ask questions such as, "Why are things done this way?" "I wonder what would happen if . . . ?" "What characteristics are associated with . . . ?" or "What is the effect of ____ on patient outcomes?", they are often well on their way to developing a research question or hypothesis. Research questions are usually generated by situations that emerge from practice, leading nurses to wonder about the effectiveness of one intervention versus another for a specific patient population.

For an investigator conducting a study, the research question or hypothesis is a key preliminary step in the research process. The **research question** (sometimes called the *problem statement*) presents the idea that is to be examined in the study and is the foundation of the research study. The **hypothesis** attempts to answer the research question.

Hypotheses can be considered intelligent hunches, guesses, or predictions that help researchers seek a solution or answer a research question. Hypotheses are a vehicle for testing the validity of the theoretical framework assumptions, and provide a bridge between **theory** (a set of interrelated concepts, definitions, and propositions) and the real world (see Chapter 4).

For a clinician making an evidence-informed decision about a patient care issue, a clinical question, such as whether chlorhexidine or povidone-iodine is more effective in preventing central line catheter infections, would guide the nurse in searching and retrieving the best available evidence. This evidence, combined with clinical expertise and patient preferences, would provide an answer on which to base the most effective decision about patient care for this population.

You will often find research questions or hypotheses at the beginning of a research article. However, because of space constraints or stylistic considerations in such publications, they may be embedded in the purpose, aims, goals, or even the results section of the research report. Nevertheless, it is equally important for both the consumer and the producer of research to understand the significance of research questions and hypotheses as the foundational elements of a study. This chapter provides a working knowledge of quantitative research questions and hypotheses, as well as the standards for writing and evaluating them based on a set of criteria. It also highlights the importance of clinical questions and how to develop them.

## DEVELOPING AND REFINING A RESEARCH QUESTION: STUDY PERSPECTIVE

A researcher spends a great deal of time refining a research idea into a testable research question. Research questions or topics are not pulled from thin air. As shown in Table 2-1, research questions should indicate that practical experience, critical appraisal of the scientific literature, or interest in an untested theory was the basis for the generation of a research idea. The research question should reflect a refinement of the researcher's initial

| TABLE 2-1 | HOW PRACTICAL EXPERIENCE, SCIENTIFIC LITERATURE, AND UNTESTED THEORY INFLUENCE THE DEVELOPMENT OF A RESEARCH IDEA | |
|---|---|---|
| **AREA** | **INFLUENCE** | **EXAMPLE** |
| **Practical Experience** | Clinical practice provides a wealth of experience from which research problems can be derived. The nurse may observe a particular event or pattern and become curious about why it occurs, as well as its relationship to other factors in the patient's environment. | Health professionals, including nurses and nurse midwives, frequently debate the benefit of psychological follow-up in preventing or reducing anxiety and depression following miscarriage. While such symptoms may be part of their grief following the loss, psychological follow-up might detect those women at risk for complications such as suicide. Evidence about physical management of women following miscarriage is well established, evidence on the psychological management is less well developed and represents a gap in the literature. Findings from a systematic review, "Follow-up for Improving Psychological Well-being for Women after a Miscarriage," that included six studies including >1000 women indicate there is insufficient evidence from randomized controlled trials to recommend any method of psychological follow-up (Murphy et al., 2012). |
| **Critical Appraisal of the Scientific Literature** | Critical appraisal of studies in journals may indirectly suggest a clinical problem by stimulating the reader's thinking. The nurse may observe the outcome data from a single study or a group of related studies that provide the basis for developing a pilot study, quality improvement project, or clinical practice guideline to determine the effectiveness of this intervention in their setting. | At a staff meeting, members of an interprofessional team at a hospital specializing in cancer treatment wanted to identify the most effective approaches for treating adult cancer pain by decreasing attitudinal barriers of patients to cancer pain management. Their search for, and critical appraisal of, existing research studies led the team to develop an interprofessional cancer pain guideline that was relevant to their patient population and clinical setting (MD Anderson Cancer Center, 2012). |
| **Gaps in the Literature** | A research idea may also be suggested by a critical appraisal of the literature that identifies gaps in the literature and suggests areas for future study. Research ideas also can be generated by research reports that suggest the value of replicating a particular study to extend or refine the existing scientific knowledge base. | Although advances in pain management can reduce cancer pain for a significant number of patients, attitudinal barriers held by patients can be a significant factor in the inadequate treatment of cancer pain. Those barriers need to be addressed if cancer pain management is to be improved. The majority of studies investigating the effectiveness of psychoeducational interventions were either not applicable in outpatient settings, or were labor intensive and not very feasible. However, use of motivational interviewing as a coaching intervention in decreasing patient attitudinal barriers to pain management had not been investigated, especially in an outpatient setting. The study focused on testing the effectiveness of an educational and a motivational interviewing coaching intervention in comparison to usual care in decreasing attitudinal barriers to cancer pain management, decreasing pain intensity, improving functional status, and improving quality of life (Thomas et al., 2012). |

*Continued*

| TABLE 2-1 | HOW PRACTICAL EXPERIENCE, SCIENTIFIC LITERATURE, AND UNTESTED THEORY INFLUENCE THE DEVELOPMENT OF A RESEARCH IDEA—cont'd | |
|---|---|---|
| **AREA** | **INFLUENCE** | **EXAMPLE** |
| **Interest in Untested Theory** | Verification of a theory and its concepts provides a relatively uncharted area from which research problems can be derived. Inasmuch as theories themselves are not tested, a researcher may consider investigating a concept or set of concepts related to a nursing theory or a theory from another discipline. The researcher would pose questions like, "If this theory is correct, what kind of behavior would I expect to observe in particular patients and under which conditions?" "If this theory is valid, what kind of supporting evidence will I find?" | The Roy Adaptation Model (RAM) (2009) was used by Fawcett and colleagues (2012) in a study examining womens' perceptions of Caesarean birth to test multiple relationships within the RAM as applied to the study population. |

thinking. The evaluator of a research study should be able to discern that the researcher has done the following:

• Defined a specific question area
• Reviewed the relevant literature
• Examined the question's potential significance to nursing
• Pragmatically examined the feasibility of studying the research question

## Defining the Research Question

Brainstorming with faculty or colleagues may provide valuable feedback that helps the researcher focus on a specific research question area. For example, suppose a researcher told a colleague that her area of interest was health disparities and how neonatal outcomes vary in ethnic minority, urban, and low-income populations. The colleague may have asked, "What is it about the topic that specifically interests you?" This conversation may have initiated a chain of thought that resulted in a decision to explore the relationship between maternal-fetal attachment and health practices on neonatal outcomes in low-income, urban women (Alhusen et al., 2012) (see Appendix B). Figure 2-1 illustrates how a broad area of interest (health disparities and neonatal outcomes) was narrowed to a specific research topic (maternal-fetal attachment and health practices on neonatal outcomes in low-income, urban women).

### EVIDENCE-BASED PRACTICE TIP

A well-developed research question guides a focused search for scientific evidence about assessing, diagnosing, treating, or assisting patients with understanding of their prognosis related to a specific health problem.

## Beginning the Literature Review

The literature review should reveal a relevant collection of studies and systematic reviews that have been critically examined. Concluding sections in such articles (i.e., the recommendations and implications for practice) often identify remaining gaps in the literature, the need for replication, or the need for extension of the knowledge base about a particular research focus (see Chapter 3). In the previous example about the influence of maternal-fetal attachment and

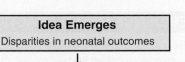

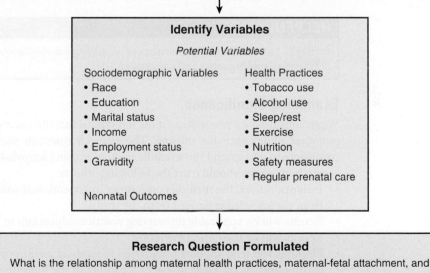

**Idea Emerges**
Disparities in neonatal outcomes

↓

**Brainstorming**
- What is the influence of maternal health practices during pregnancy on neonatal outcomes?
- What are positive health practices (e.g., obtaining regular prenatal care, abstaining from smoking, exercising regularly)?
- Are rates of preterm birth and low birth rate influenced by demographic variables?
- Does maternal-fetal attachment influence health practices during pregnancy?

↓

**Literature Review**
- Disparities in neonatal outcomes between African-Americans and non-Latino White Americans are one of the most concerning chronic health disparities in the United States.
- Poor and African-American women have twice the rates of pre-term births.
- Low birth weight is a major determinant of infant mortality.
- Health practices that a mother engages in during pregnancy are known to influence neonatal outcomes.
- Maternal-fetal attachment (MFA) is another factor influencing health practices during pregnancy. Higher levels of MFA correlate with high quality health practices.
- No longitudinal studies were found that examined these factors in relation to neonatal outcomes.

↓

**Identify Variables**
*Potential Variables*

Sociodemographic Variables
- Race
- Education
- Marital status
- Income
- Employment status
- Gravidity

Neonatal Outcomes

Health Practices
- Tobacco use
- Alcohol use
- Sleep/rest
- Exercise
- Nutrition
- Safety measures
- Regular prenatal care

↓

**Research Question Formulated**
What is the relationship among maternal health practices, maternal-fetal attachment, and adverse neonatal outcomes?

**FIGURE 2-1** Development of a research question.

health practices on neonatal outcomes in low-income, urban women, the researcher may have conducted a preliminary review of books and journals for theories and research studies on factors apparently critical to adverse pregnancy outcomes, such as pre-term birth and low birth weight and racial and/or ethnic differences in neonatal outcomes. These factors, called variables, should be potentially relevant, of interest, and measurable.

---

**EVIDENCE-BASED PRACTICE TIP**

The answers to questions generated by qualitative data reflect evidence that may provide the first insights about a phenomenon that has not been previously studied.

---

Possible relevant factors mentioned in the literature begin with an exploration of the relationship between maternal health practices during pregnancy, and neonatal outcomes. Another factor, maternal-fetal attachment, has been found to correlate with these high quality health practices. Other variables, called *demographic variables,* such as race, ethnicity, gender, age, income, education, and marital status, are also suggested as essential to consider. For example, are rates of pre-term birth and growth-restricted neonates higher in low-income women than in other women? This information can then be used to further define the research question and address a gap in the literature, as well as to extend the knowledge base related to relationships among maternal health practices, maternal-fetal attachment, race (black or white), and socio-economic status. At this point the researcher could write the tentative research question: "What are the relationships among maternal health practices, maternal-fetal attachment, and adverse neonatal outcomes?" Readers can envision the interrelatedness of the initial definition of the question area, the literature review, and the refined research question. Readers of research reports examine the end product of this process in the form of a research question and/or hypothesis, so it is important to have an appreciation of how the researcher gets to that point in constructing a study (Alhusen et al., 2012) (see Appendix B).

---

**HELPFUL HINT**

Reading the literature review or theoretical framework section of a research article helps you trace the development of the implied research question and/or hypothesis.

---

## Examining Significance

When considering a research question, it is crucial that the researcher examine the question's potential significance for nursing. The research question should have the potential to contribute to and extend the scientific body of nursing knowledge. Guidelines for selecting research questions should meet the following criteria:

- Patients, nurses, the medical community in general, and society will potentially benefit from the knowledge derived from the study.
- Results will be applicable for nursing practice, education, or administration.
- Results will be theoretically relevant.
- Findings will lend support to untested theoretical assumptions, extend or challenge an existing theory, fill a gap, or clarify a conflict in the literature.
- Findings will potentially provide evidence that supports developing, retaining, or revising nursing practices or policies.

If the research question has not met any of these criteria, it is wise to extensively revise the question or discard it. For example, in the previously cited research question, the significance of the question includes the following facts:

- Disparities in neonatal outcomes between African Americans and non-Latino white Americans are one of the most concerning chronic health disparities in the United States.

- Poor and African-American women have twice the rates of pre-term births.
- Low birth weight is a major determinant of infant mortality.
- Health practices that a mother engages in during pregnancy are known to influence neonatal outcomes.
- Maternal-fetal attachment (MFA) is another factor influencing health practices during pregnancy. Higher levels of MFA correlate with high quality health practices.
- No longitudinal studies were found that examined these factors in relation to neonatal outcomes.
- This study also sought to fill a gap in the related literature by extending research to focus on low income and ethnic minority women.

### EVIDENCE-BASED PRACTICE TIP

Without a well-developed research question, the researcher may search for wrong, irrelevant, or unnecessary information. This will be a barrier to identifying the potential significance of the study.

## Determining Feasibility

The feasibility of a research question must be pragmatically examined. Regardless of how significant or researchable a question may be, pragmatic considerations such as time; availability of subjects, facilities, equipment, and money; experience of the researcher; and any ethical considerations may cause the researcher to decide that the question is inappropriate because it lacks feasibility (see Chapters 4 and 8).

## THE FULLY DEVELOPED RESEARCH QUESTION

When a researcher finalizes a research question, the following characteristics should be evident:
- It clearly identifies the variables under consideration.
- It specifies the population being studied.
- It implies the possibility of empirical testing.

Because each element is crucial to the formulation of a satisfactory research question, the criteria will be discussed in greater detail. These elements can often be found in the introduction of the published article; they are not always stated in an explicit manner.

## Variables

Researchers call the properties that they study variables. Such properties take on different values. Thus a **variable**, as the name suggests, is something that varies. Properties that differ from each other, such as age, weight, height, religion, and ethnicity, are examples of variables. Researchers attempt to understand how and why differences in one variable relate to differences in another variable. For example, a researcher may be concerned about the variable of pneumonia in postoperative patients on ventilators in critical care units. It is a variable because not all critically ill postoperative patients on ventilators have pneumonia. A researcher may also be interested in what other factors can be linked to ventilator-acquired pneumonia (VAP). There is clinical evidence to suggest that elevation of the head of the bed is associated with decreasing risk for VAP. You can see that these factors are also variables that need to be considered in relation to the development of VAP in postoperative patients.

| TABLE 2-2 | **RESEARCH QUESTION FORMAT** | |
|---|---|---|
| **TYPE** | **FORMAT** | **EXAMPLE** |
| **Quantitative** | | |
| *Correlational* | Is there a relationship between **X** (independent variable) and **Y** (dependent variable) in the specified population? | Is there a relationship between maternal-fetal attachment and health practices and neonatal outcomes in low-income, urban women? (Alhusen et al., 2012) |
| *Comparative* | Is there a difference in **Y** (dependent variable) between people who have **X** characteristic (independent variable) and those who do not have **X** characteristic? | Do children with Type I Diabetes (TID) whose parents participate in coping skills training (CST) have better metabolic control (lower HbA1c) than children whose parents participate in an education program? (Grey et al., 2011) |
| *Experimental* | Is there a difference in **Y** (dependent variable) between Group A who received **X** (independent variable) and Group B who did not receive **X**? | What is the difference in attitudes to cancer pain management, pain intensity, pain relief, functional status, and quality of life in cancer patients who have received an educational intervention versus a coaching intervention versus usual care? (Thomas et al., 2012) |
| **Qualitative** | | |
| *Grounded theory* | What is/was it like to have **X**? | What is the meaning of survivorship for women with breast cancer? (Sherman et al., 2012) |

When speaking of variables, the researcher is essentially asking, "Is **X** related to **Y**? What is the effect of **X** on **Y**? How are $X_1$ and $X_2$ related to **Y**?" The researcher is asking a question about the relationship between one or more independent variables and a dependent variable. (*Note:* In cases in which multiple independent or dependent variables are present, subscripts are used to indicate the number of variables under consideration.)

An **independent variable**, usually symbolized by X, is the variable that has the presumed effect on the dependent variable. In experimental research studies, the researcher manipulates the independent variable (see Chapter 9). In nonexperimental research, the independent variable is not manipulated and is assumed to have occurred naturally before or during the study (see Chapter 10).

The **dependent variable**, represented by Y varies with a change in the independent variable. The dependent variable is not manipulated. It is observed and assumed to vary with changes in the independent variable. Predictions are made from the independent variable to the dependent variable. It is the dependent variable that the researcher is interested in understanding, explaining, or predicting. For example, it might be assumed that the perception of pain intensity (the dependent variable) will vary in relation to a person's gender (the independent variable). In this case we are trying to explain the perception of pain intensity in relation to gender (i.e., male or female). Although variability in the dependent variable is assumed to depend on changes in the independent variable, this does not imply that there is a causal relationship between X and Y, or that changes in variable X cause variable Y to change.

Table 2-2 presents a number of examples of research questions. Practice substituting other variables for the examples in Table 2-2. You will be surprised at the skill you develop in writing and critiquing research questions with greater ease.

Although one independent variable and one dependent variable are used in the examples, there is no restriction on the number of variables that can be included in a research question. Research questions that include more than one independent or dependent variable may be broken down into subquestions that are more concise.

Finally, it should be noted that variables are not inherently independent or dependent. A variable that is classified as independent in one study may be considered dependent in another study. For example, a nurse may review an article about sexual behaviors that are predictive of risk for human immunodeficiency virus (HIV)/acquired immunodeficiency syndrome (AIDS). In this case, HIV/AIDS is the dependent variable. When another article about the relationship between HIV/AIDS and maternal parenting practices is considered, HIV/AIDS status is the independent variable. Whether a variable is independent or dependent is a function of the role it plays in a particular study.

## Population

The **population** (a well-defined set that has certain properties) is either specified or implied in the research question. If the scope of the question has been narrowed to a specific focus and the variables have been clearly identified, the nature of the population will be evident to the reader of a research report. For example, a research question may ask, "Does an association exist among health literacy, memory performance, and performance-based functional ability in community-residing older adults?" This question suggests that the population under consideration includes community-residing older adults. It is also implied that the community-residing older adults were screened for cognitive impairment and presence of dementia, were divided into groups (impaired or normal), and participated in a memory training intervention or a health training intervention to determine its effect on affective and cognitive outcomes (McDougall et al., 2012). The researcher or reader will have an initial idea of the composition of the study population from the outset (see Chapter 12).

---

### EVIDENCE-BASED PRACTICE TIP

Make sure that the population of interest and the setting have been clearly described so that if you were going to replicate the study, you would know exactly who the study population needed to be.

---

## Testability

The research question must imply that it is **testable**; that is, measurable by either qualitative or quantitative methods. For example, the research question "Should postoperative patients control how much pain medication they receive?" is stated incorrectly for a variety of reasons. One reason is that it is not testable; it represents a value statement rather than a research question. A scientific research question must propose a relationship between an independent and a dependent variable, and do this in such a way that it indicates that the variables of the relationship can somehow be measured. Many interesting and important clinical questions are not valid research questions because they are not amenable to testing.

---

### HELPFUL HINT

Remember that research questions are used to guide all types of research studies, but are most often used in exploratory, descriptive, qualitative, or hypothesis-generating studies.

---

| TABLE 2-3 | COMPONENTS OF THE RESEARCH QUESTION AND RELATED CRITERIA | |
|---|---|---|
| **VARIABLES** | **POPULATION** | **TESTABILITY** |
| **Independent Variable**<br>• Maternal-fetal attachment<br>• Health practices<br>• Race<br>• Income<br>• Geographic setting: urban<br><br>**Dependent Variable**<br>• Neonatal outcomes | • African-American and non-Latino white women: pregnant | • Differential effect of maternal-fetal attachment and health practices, race and income on neonatal outcomes (birth weight and gestational age) |

The question "What are the relationships among maternal health practices, maternal fetal attachment, and adverse neonatal outcomes?" is a testable research question. It illustrates the relationship between the variables, identifies the independent and dependent variables, and implies the testability of the research question. Table 2-3 illustrates how this research question is congruent with the three research question criteria.

This research question was originally derived from a general area of interest: health disparities and neonatal outcomes (birth weight, gestational age), and maternal contributing factors (maternal-fetal attachment and health practices) as reflected in different racial and economic groups. The question crystallized further after a preliminary literature review (Althusen et al., 2012).

### HELPFUL HINT

- Remember that research questions are often not explicitly stated. The reader has to infer the research question from the title of the report, the abstract, the introduction, or the purpose.
- Using your focused question, search the literature for the best available answer to your clinical question.

## STUDY PURPOSE, AIMS, OR OBJECTIVES

Once the research question is developed and the literature review is critiqued in terms of the level, strength, and quality of evidence available for the particular research question, the purpose, aims, or objectives of the study become focused so that the researcher can decide whether a hypothesis should be tested or a research question answered.

The **purpose** of the study encompasses the aims or objectives the investigator hopes to achieve with the research, not the question to be answered. These three terms are synonymous with each other. The purpose communicates more than just the nature of the question. Through the researcher's selection of verbs, the purpose statement suggests the manner in which the researcher planned to study the question and the level of evidence to be obtained through the study findings. Verbs such as *discover, explore,* or *describe* suggest an investigation of an infrequently researched topic that might appropriately be guided by research questions rather than hypotheses. In contrast, verb statements indicating that the purpose is to test the effectiveness of an intervention or compare two alternative nursing strategies suggest a hypothesis-testing study for which there is an established knowledge base of the topic.

BOX 2-1     **EXAMPLES OF PURPOSE STATEMENTS**

- The purposes of this randomized clinical trial were to test the effectiveness of two interventions compared to usual care in decreasing attitudinal barriers to cancer pain management, pain intensity, and improving pain relief, functional status, and QOL (Thomas et al., 2012).
- The aim of this study was to compare a group educational intervention for parents of children with T1D to a coping skills training intervention (Grey et al., 2011).
- The purposes of this pilot study were to establish the feasibility of an intervention based on the Information-motivation-behavioral skills (IMB) model in this population (HIV) and begin to evaluate its effectiveness for improving medication adherence (Konkle-Parker et al., 2012).
- The aim of this study was to examine the extent to which the relationship between adverse stress and depression is mediated by university students' perceived ability to manage their stress (Sawatzky et al., 2012).

Remember that when the purpose of a study is to test the effectiveness of an intervention or compare the effectiveness of two or more interventions, the level of evidence is likely to have more strength and rigor than a study whose purpose is to explore or describe phenomena. Box 2-1 provides examples of purpose, aims, and objectives.

**EVIDENCE-BASED PRACTICE TIP**

The purpose, aims, or objectives often provide the most information about the intent of the research question and hypotheses, and suggest the level of evidence to be obtained from the findings of the study.

## DEVELOPING THE RESEARCH HYPOTHESIS

Like the research question, hypotheses are often not stated explicitly in a research article. You will often find that hypotheses are embedded in the data analysis, results, or discussion section of the research report. Similarly, the population may not be explicitly stated, but will have been identified in the background, significance, and literature review. It is then up to you to discern the nature of the hypotheses and population being tested. For example, in a study by Thomas and colleagues (2012) (see Appendix A), the hypotheses are embedded in the "Data Analysis" and "Results" sections of the article. You must interpret that the statement, "Analyses of covariance were performed to evaluate for differences in scores on average and worst pain intensity, pain relief, mean pain interference, functional status and quality of life among the three groups," represents the hypotheses that test the effect of the motivational-interviewing-based coaching compared to education or usual care on improving cancer pain management. In light of that stylistic reality, it is important for you to be acquainted with the components of hypotheses, how they are developed, and the standards for writing and evaluating them.

Hypotheses flow from the research question, literature review, and theoretical framework. Figure 2-2 illustrates this flow. A **hypothesis** is a declarative statement about the relationship between two or more variables that suggests an answer to the research question. A hypothesis predicts an expected outcome of a study. Hypotheses are formulated before the study is actually conducted because they provide direction for the collection, analysis, and interpretation of data.

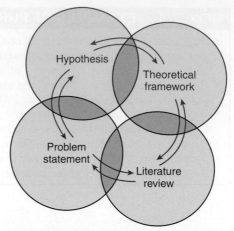

**FIGURE 2-2** Interrelationships of problem statement, literature review, theoretical framework, and hypothesis.

### HELPFUL HINT

When hypotheses are not explicitly stated by the author at the end of the introduction section or just before the methods section, they will be embedded or implied in the results or discussion section of a research article.

## Characteristics

Whether you are conducting research or critiquing published research studies, you need to know what constitutes a "good" hypothesis. Knowing the characteristics of hypotheses will enable you to have a standard for evaluating your own work or the work of others.

## Relationship Statement

The first characteristic of a hypothesis is that it is a declarative statement that identifies the predicted relationship between two or more variables; the independent variable ($X$) and a dependent variable ($Y$). The direction of the predicted relationship is also specified in this statement. Phrases such as *greater than; less than; positively, negatively,* or *curvilinearly related;* and *difference in* suggest the directionality that is proposed in the hypothesis. The following is an example of a directional hypothesis: "The rate of continuous smoking abstinence (dependent variable) at 6 months postpartum, based on self-report and biochemical validation, will be significantly higher in the treatment group (postpartum counseling intervention) than in the control group (independent variable)." The dependent and independent variables are explicitly identified, and the relational aspect of the prediction in the hypothesis is contained in the phrase *significantly higher in.*

The nature of the relationship, either causal or associative, is also implied by the hypothesis. A causal relationship is one in which the researcher can predict that the independent variable ($X$) causes a change in the dependent variable ($Y$). In research, it is rare that one is in a firm enough position to take a definitive stand about a cause-and-effect relationship. For example, a researcher might hypothesize higher maternal-fetal attachment will be related to improved health practices during pregnancy (Alhusen et al., 2012). It would be difficult for a researcher to predict a cause-and-effect relationship, however, because of the multiple intervening variables (e.g., income, pregnancy wantedness, age, pre-eclampsia, and diabetes) that might also influence the subject's health practices.

Variables are more commonly related in noncausal ways; that is, the variables are systematically related but in an associative way. This means that the variables change in relation to each other. For example, there is strong evidence that asbestos exposure is related to lung cancer. It is tempting to state that there is a causal relationship between asbestos exposure and lung cancer. Do not overlook the fact, however, that not all of those who have been exposed to asbestos will have lung cancer, and not all of those who have lung cancer have had asbestos exposure. Consequently, it would be scientifically unsound to take a position advocating the presence of a causal relationship between these two variables. Rather, one can say only that there is an associative relationship between the variables of asbestos exposure and lung cancer, a relationship in which there is a strong systematic association between the two phenomena.

## Testability

The second characteristic of a hypothesis is its testability. This means that the variables of the study must lend themselves to observation, measurement, and analysis. The hypothesis is either supported or not supported after the data have been collected and analyzed. The predicted outcome proposed by the hypothesis will or will not be congruent with the actual outcome when the hypothesis is tested.

Hypotheses may fail to meet the criteria of testability because the researcher has not made a prediction about the anticipated outcome, the variables are not observable or measurable, or the hypothesis is couched in terms that are value-laden.

---

**HELPFUL HINT**

When a hypothesis is complex (i.e., it contains more than one independent or dependent variable), it is difficult for the findings to indicate unequivocally that the hypothesis is supported or not supported. In such cases, the reader must infer which relationships are significant in the predicted direction from the findings or discussion section.

---

## Theory Base

A sound hypothesis is consistent with an existing body of theory and research findings. Whether a hypothesis is arrived at on the basis of a review of the literature or a clinical observation, it must be based on a sound scientific rationale. You should be able to identify the flow of ideas from the research idea to the literature review, to the theoretical framework, and through the research question(s) or hypotheses. For example, Thomas and colleagues (2012) (see Appendix A) investigated the effectiveness of a motivational–interviewing-based coaching intervention in comparison to education or usual care based on change theory, specifically the Transtheoretical Model of Change (Prochaska & DiClemente, 1984), which is a useful conceptual framework for coaching.

## Wording the Hypothesis

As you read the scientific literature and become more familiar with it, you will observe that there are a variety of ways to word a hypothesis. Regardless of the specific format used to state the hypothesis, the statement should be worded in clear, simple, and concise terms. If this criterion is met, the reader will understand the following:
- The variables of the hypothesis
- The population being studied
- The predicted outcome of the hypothesis

Information about hypotheses may be further clarified in the instruments, sample, or methods sections of a research report (see Chapters 12 and 14).

## TABLE 2-4    EXAMPLES OF HOW HYPOTHESES ARE WORDED

| VARIABLES* | HYPOTHESIS | TYPE OF DESIGN; LEVEL OF EVIDENCE SUGGESTED |
|---|---|---|
| **1. THERE ARE SIGNIFICANT DIFFERENCES IN SELF-REPORTED CANCER PAIN, SYMPTOMS ACCOMPANYING PAIN, AND FUNCTIONAL STATUS ACCORDING TO SELF-REPORTED ETHNIC IDENTITY.** | | |
| IV: Ethnic identity | Nondirectional, research | Nonexperimental; Level IV |
| DV: Self-reported cancer pain | | |
| DV: Symptoms accompanying pain | | |
| DV: Functional status | | |
| **2. INDIVIDUALS WHO PARTICIPATE IN USUAL CARE (UC) PLUS BLOOD PRESSURE (BP) TELEMONITORING (TM) WILL HAVE A GREATER REDUCTION IN BP FROM BASELINE TO 12-MONTH FOLLOW-UP THAN WOULD INDIVIDUALS WHO RECEIVE UC ONLY.** | | |
| IV: Telemonitoring (TM) | Directional, research | Experimental; Level II |
| IV: Usual care (UC) | | |
| DV: Blood pressure | | |
| **3. THERE WILL BE A GREATER DECREASE IN STATE ANXIETY SCORES FOR PATIENTS RECEIVING STRUCTURED INFORMATIONAL VIDEOS BEFORE ABDOMINAL OR CHEST TUBE REMOVAL THAN FOR PATIENTS RECEIVING STANDARD INFORMATION.** | | |
| IV: Preprocedure structured videotape information | Directional, research | Experimental; Level II |
| IV: Standard information | | |
| DV: State anxiety | | |
| **4. THE INCIDENCE AND DEGREE OF SEVERITY OF SUBJECT DISCOMFORT WILL BE LESS AFTER ADMINISTRATION OF MEDICATIONS BY THE Z-TRACK INTRAMUSCULAR INJECTION TECHNIQUE THAN AFTER ADMINISTRATION OF MEDICATIONS BY THE STANDARD INTRAMUSCULAR INJECTION TECHNIQUE.** | | |
| IV: Z-track intramuscular injection technique | Directional, research | Experimental; Level II |
| IV: Standard intramuscular injection technique | | |
| DV: Subject discomfort | | |
| **5. NURSES WITH HIGH SOCIAL SUPPORT FROM COWORKERS WILL HAVE LOWER PERCEIVED JOB STRESS.** | | |
| IV: Social support | Directional, research | Nonexperimental; Level IV |
| DV: Perceived job stress | | |
| **6. THERE WILL BE NO DIFFERENCE IN ANESTHETIC COMPLICATION RATES BETWEEN HOSPITALS THAT USE CERTIFIED NURSE ANESTHETISTS (CRNA) FOR OBSTETRICAL ANESTHESIA VERSUS THOSE THAT USE ANESTHESIOLOGISTS.** | | |
| IV: Type of anesthesia provider (CRNA or MD) | Null | Nonexperimental; Level IV |
| **7. THERE WILL BE NO SIGNIFICANT DIFFERENCE IN THE DURATION OF PATENCY OF A 24-GAUGE INTRAVENOUS LOCK IN A NEONATAL PATIENT WHEN FLUSHED WITH 0.5 mL OF HEPARINIZED SALINE (2 U/mL), COMPARED WITH 0.5 mL OF 0.9% OF NORMAL SALINE.** | | |
| IV: Heparinized saline | Null | Experimental; Level II |
| IV: Normal saline | | |
| DV: Duration of patency of intravenous lock | | |

*Abbreviations: *DV*, dependent variable; *IV*, independent variable.

## Statistical versus Research Hypotheses

You may observe that a hypothesis is further categorized as either a research or a statistical hypothesis. A **research hypothesis**, also known as a scientific hypothesis, consists of a statement about the expected relationship of the variables. A research hypothesis indicates what the outcome of the study is expected to be. A research hypothesis is also either directional or nondirectional. If the researcher obtains statistically significant findings for a research hypothesis, the hypothesis is supported. The examples in Table 2-4 represent research hypotheses.

| TABLE 2-5 | EXAMPLES OF STATISTICAL HYPOTHESES | | |
|---|---|---|---|
| **HYPOTHESIS** | **VARIABLES*** | **TYPE OF HYPOTHESIS** | **TYPE OF DESIGN SUGGESTED** |
| Oxygen inhalation by nasal cannula of up to 6 L/min does not affect oral temperature measurement taken with an electronic thermometer. | IV: Oxygen inhalation by nasal cannula<br>DV: Oral temperature | Statistical; null | Experimental |
| There will be no difference in the performance accuracy of adult nurse practitioners (ANPs) and family nurse practitioners (FNPs) in formulating accurate diagnoses and acceptable interventions for suspected cases of domestic violence. | IV: Nurse practitioner (ANP or FNP) category<br>DV: Diagnosis and intervention performance accuracy | Statistical; null | Nonexperimental |

*Abbreviations: *DV*, dependent variable; *IV*, independent variable.

A **statistical hypothesis**, also known as a null hypothesis, states that there is no relationship between the independent and dependent variables. The examples in Table 2-5 illustrate statistical hypotheses. If, in the data analysis, a statistically significant relationship emerges between the variables at a specified level of significance, the null hypothesis is rejected. Rejection of the statistical hypothesis is equivalent to acceptance of the research hypothesis.

### Directional versus Nondirectional Hypotheses

Hypotheses can be formulated directionally or nondirectionally. A **directional hypothesis** specificies the expected direction of the relationship between the independent and dependent variables. An example of a directional hypothesis is provided in a study by Grey and colleagues (2011) that investigated the effectiveness of a coping skills training (CST) intervention for parents of children with Type 1 Diabetes (T1D). The researchers hypothesized that "Parents of children with T1D who participate in CST will demonstrate fewer issues in coping, better family functioning (less parent responsibility and family conflict), and better quality of life (QOL) compared to parents of children with T1D who participate in an education program."

In contrast, a **nondirectional hypothesis** indicates the existence of a relationship between the variables, but does not specify the anticipated direction of the relationship. For example, Sawatzky and colleagues (2012) examined the extent to which the relationship between adverse stress and depression is mediated by university students' perceived ability to manage their stress. The study's nondirectional hypothesis is "When students experience stress that influences their academic performance, they are vulnerable to stress."

Nurses who are learning to critique research studies should be aware that both the directional and the nondirectional forms of hypothesis statements are acceptable. As you read research articles, you will note that directional hypotheses are much more commonly used than nondirectional hypotheses.

## RELATIONSHIP BETWEEN THE HYPOTHESIS, THE RESEARCH QUESTION, AND THE RESEARCH DESIGN

Regardless of whether the researcher uses a statistical or a research hypothesis, there is a suggested relationship between the hypothesis, the design of the study, and the level of evidence provided by the results of the study. The type of design, experimental or nonexperimental (see Chapters 9 and 10), will influence the wording of the hypothesis. For

## CRITICAL THINKING DECISION PATH

### *Determining the Type of Hypothesis or Readiness for Hypothesis Testing*

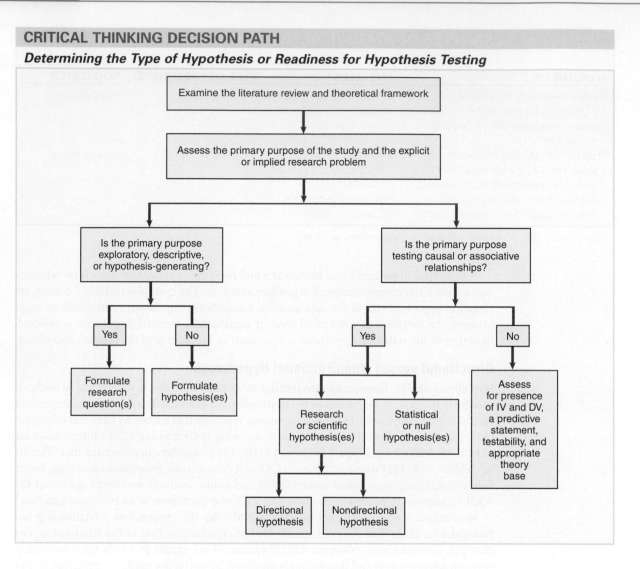

example, when an experimental design is used, you would expect to see hypotheses that reflect relationship statements, such as the following:

- $X_1$ is more effective than $X_2$ on $Y$.
- The effect of $X_1$ on $Y$ is greater than that of $X_2$ on $Y$.
- The incidence of $Y$ will not differ in subjects receiving $X_1$ and $X_2$ treatments.
- The incidence of $Y$ will be greater in subjects after $X_1$ than after $X_2$.

## EVIDENCE-BASED PRACTICE TIP

Think about the relationship between the wording of the hypothesis, the type of research design suggested, and the level of evidence provided by the findings of a study using each kind of hypothesis. You may want to consider which type of hypothesis potentially will yield the strongest results applicable to practice.

| TABLE 2-6 | ELEMENTS OF A CLINICAL QUESTION | | |
|---|---|---|---|
| **POPULATION** | **INTERVENTION** | **COMPARISON INTERVENTION** | **OUTCOME** |
| People with advanced cancer | Pain diaries | No pain diaries | Increased pain control |

Such hypotheses indicate that an experimental treatment (i.e., independent variable **X**) will be used and that two groups of subjects, experimental and control groups, are being used to test whether the difference in the outcome (i.e., dependent variable **Y**) predicted by the hypothesis actually exists. Hypotheses reflecting experimental designs also test the effect of the experimental treatment (i.e., independent variable **X**) on the outcome (i.e., dependent variable **Y**). This would suggest that the strength of the evidence provided by the results would be Level II (experimental design) or Level III (quasi-experimental design).

In contrast, hypotheses related to nonexperimental designs reflect associative relationship statements, such as the following:

- **X** will be negatively related to **Y**.
- There will be a positive relationship between **X** and **Y**.

This would suggest that the strength of the evidence provided by the results of a study that examined hypotheses with associative relationship statements would be at Level IV (nonexperimental design).

Table 2-6 provides an example of this concept. The Critical Thinking Decision Path will help you determine the type of hypothesis presented in a study, as well as the study's readiness for a hypothesis-testing design.

## DEVELOPING AND REFINING A CLINICAL QUESTION: A CONSUMER'S PERSPECTIVE

Practicing nurses, as well as students, are challenged to keep their practice up-to-date by searching for, retrieving, and critiquing research articles that apply to practice issues that are encountered in their clinical setting (Cullum, 2000). Practitioners strive to use the current best evidence from research when making clinical and health care decisions. As research consumers, you are not conducting research studies; however, your search for information from practice is converted into focused, structured clinical questions that are the foundation of evidence-based practice and quality improvement projects. Clinical questions often arise from clinical situations for which there are no ready answers. You have probably had the experience of asking, "What is the most effective treatment for . . . ?" or "Why do we still do it this way?"

Using similar criteria related to framing a research question, focused clinical questions form a basis for searching the literature to identify supporting evidence from research. Clinical questions have four components:

- Population
- Intervention
- Comparison
- Outcome

These components, known as PICO, provide an effective format for helping nurses develop searchable clinical questions. Box 2-2 presents each component of the clinical question.

> **BOX 2-2   COMPONENTS OF A CLINICAL QUESTION USING THE PICO FORMAT**
>
> **Population:** The individual patient or group of patients with a particular condition or health care problem (e.g., adolescents age 13 to 18 with type 1 insulin-dependent diabetes).
>
> **Intervention:** The particular aspect of health care that is of interest to the nurse or the health team (e.g., a therapeutic [inhaler or nebulizer for treatment of asthma], a preventive [pneumonia vaccine], a diagnostic [measurement of blood pressure], or an organizational [implementation of a bar coding system to reduce medication errors] intervention).
>
> **Comparison intervention:** Standard care or no intervention (e.g., antibiotic in comparison to ibuprofen for children with otitis media); a comparison of two treatment settings (e.g., rehabilitation center versus home care).
>
> **Outcome:** More effective outcome (e.g., improved glycemic control, decreased hospitalizations, decreased medication errors).

The significance of the clinical question becomes obvious as the research evidence from the literature is critiqued. The research evidence is used together with clinical expertise and the patient's perspective to develop or revise nursing standards, protocols, and policies that are used to plan and implement patient care (Cullum, 2000; Sackett et al., 2000; Thompson et al., 2004). Issues or questions can arise from multiple clinical and managerial situations. Using the example of pain, albeit from a different perspective, a nurse working in a palliative care setting wondered whether completing pain diaries was a useful thing in the palliative care of patients with advanced cancer. She wondered whether time was being spent developing something that had previously been shown to be useless or even harmful. After all, it is conceivable that monitoring one's pain in a diary actually heightens one's awareness and experience of pain. To focus the nurse's search of the literature, she developed the following question: *Does the use of pain diaries in the palliative care of patients with cancer lead to improved pain control?* Sometimes it is helpful for nurses who develop clinical questions from a consumer perspective to consider three elements as they frame their focused question: (1) the situation, (2) the intervention, and (3) the outcome.

- The situation is the patient or problem being addressed. This can be a single patient or a group of patients with a particular health problem (e.g., palliative care of patients with cancer).
- The intervention is the dimension of health care interest, and often asks whether a particular intervention is a useful treatment (e.g., pain diaries).
- The outcome addresses the effect of the treatment (e.g., intervention) for this patient or patient population in terms of quality and cost (e.g., decreased pain perception/low cost). It essentially answers whether the intervention makes a difference for the patient population.

The individual parts of the question are vital pieces of information to remember when it comes to searching for evidence in the literature. One of the easiest ways to do this is to use a table as illustrated in Table 2-6. Examples of clinical questions are highlighted in Box 2-3. Chapter 3 provides examples of how to effectively search the literature to find answers to questions posed by researchers and research consumers.

---

## BOX 2-3 EXAMPLES OF CLINICAL QUESTIONS

- Do children younger than 12 years pose a higher infection potential for immunosuppressed patients than visitors older than 12 years? (Falk et al., 2012)
- In a population of hospitalized older adults, is the onset of new urinary incontinence associated with the use of continence products (incontinence pads, urinary catheters, or independent toileting)? (Zisberg et al., 2011)
- In patients with chronic diseases like Type 2 diabetes, can nurse practitioners trained in diabetes management deliver care similar to that of primary care physicans? (Houweling et al., 2011)
- Does use of effective home safety devices reduce home injuries in children younger than 3 years? (Phelan et al., 2011)
- Does an immunization navigator program for urban adolescents increase immunization rates? (Szilagya et al., 2011)
- Is there a significant difference in the effect of a tailored nursing intervention (predischarge meeting and post-discharge telephone follow-up) on enrollment in a free cardiac rehabilitation program? (Cossette et al., 2012)
- Do residents, family members, and clinicians find a sensor data interface used to monitor activity levels of older adults useful in independent living settings? (Alexander et al., 2012)

---

## EVIDENCE-BASED PRACTICE TIP

You should be formulating clinical questions that arise from your clinical practice. Once you have developed a focused clinical question using the PICO format, you will search the literature for the best available evidence to answer your clinical question.

---

# APPRAISING THE EVIDENCE
## THE RESEARCH QUESTION AND HYPOTHESIS

The care that the researcher takes when developing the research question or hypothesis is often representative of the overall conceptualization and design of the study. In a quantitative research study, the remainder of a study revolves around answering the research question or testing the hypothesis. In a qualitative research study, the objective is to answer the research question. Because this text focuses on you as a research consumer, the following sections will primarily pertain to the evaluation of research questions and hypotheses in published research reports.

### Critiquing the Research Question

The following Critiquing Criteria box provides several criteria for evaluating the initial phase of the research process—the research question. Because the research question represents the basis for the study, it is usually introduced at the beginning of the research report to indicate the focus and direction of the study to the readers. You will then be in a position to evaluate whether the rest of the study logically flows from its foundation—the research question(s). The author will often begin by identifying the background and significance of the issue that led to crystallizing development of the unanswered question. The clinical and scientific background and/or significance will be summarized, and the purpose, aim, or objective of the study is identified. Finally, the research question and any related subquestions will be proposed before or after the literature review.

Sometimes you will find that the research question is not clearly stated at the conclusion of this section. In some cases it is only hinted at, and you are challenged to identify the research

**CRITIQUING CRITERIA**

*Developing Research Questions and Hypotheses*

**The Research Question**

1. Was the research question introduced promptly?
2. Is the research question stated clearly?
3. Does the research question express a relationship between two or more variables or at least between an independent and a dependent variable, implying empirical testability?
4. How does the research question specify the nature of the population being studied?
5. How has the research question been supported with adequate experiential and scientific background material?
6. How has the research question been placed within the context of an appropriate theoretical framework?
7. How has the significance of the research question been identified?
8. Have pragmatic issues, such as feasibility, been addressed?
9. How have the purpose, aims, or goals of the study been identified?
10. Are research questions appropriately used (i.e., exploratory, descriptive, or qualitative study)?

**The Hypothesis**

1. Is the hypothesis concisely stated in a declarative form?
2. Are the independent and dependent variables identified in the statement of the hypothesis?
3. Is each hypothesis specific to one relationship so that each hypothesis can be either supported or not supported?
4. Is the hypothesis stated in such a way that it is testable?
5. Is the hypothesis stated objectively, without value-laden words?
6. Is the direction of the relationship in each hypothesis clearly stated?
7. How is each hypothesis consistent with the literature review?
8. How is the theoretical rationale for the hypothesis made explicit?
9. Given the level of evidence suggested by the research question, hypothesis, and design, what is the potential applicability to practice?

**The Clinical Question**

1. Does the clinical question specify the patient population, intervention, comparison intervention, and outcome?

question. In other cases the research question is embedded in the introductory text or purpose statement. To some extent, this depends on the style of the journal. Nevertheless, you, the evaluator, must remember that the main research question should be implied if it is not clearly identified in the introductory section, even if the subquestions are not stated or implied.

If this process is clarified at the outset of a research study, all that follows in terms of the design can be logically developed. You will have a clear idea of what the report should convey and can knowledgeably evaluate the material that follows. When critically appraising clinical questions, think about the fact that they should be focused and specify the patient or problem being addressed, the intervention, and the outcome for a particular patient population. There should be evidence that the clinical question guided the literature search and suggests the design and level of evidence to be obtained from the study findings.

## Critiquing the Hypothesis

As illustrated in the Critiquing Criteria box, several criteria for critiquing the hypothesis should be used as a standard for evaluating the strengths and weaknesses of hypotheses in a research report.

1. When reading a study, you may find the hypotheses clearly delineated in a separate hypothesis section of the research article (e.g., after the literature review or theoretical framework section[s]). In many cases the hypotheses are not explicitly stated and are only implied in the results or discussion section of the article. In these cases, you must infer the hypotheses from the purpose statement and the type of analysis used.
2. You should not assume that if hypotheses do not appear at the beginning of the article, they do not exist in the study. Even when hypotheses are stated at the beginning of an article, they are re-examined in the results or discussion section as the findings are presented and discussed.
3. If a hypothesis or set of hypotheses is presented, the data analysis should directly answer it.
4. The hypotheses should be consistent with both the literature review and the theoretical framework.
5. Although a hypothesis can legitimately be nondirectional, it is preferable, and more common, for the researcher to indicate the direction of the relationship between the variables in the hypothesis. You will find that when there are a lack of data available for the literature review (i.e., the researcher has chosen to study a relatively undefined area of interest), a nondirectional hypothesis may be appropriate.
6. The notion of testability is central to the soundness of a hypothesis. One criterion related to testability is that the hypothesis should be stated in such a way that it can be clearly supported or not supported.
7. Hypotheses are never proven beyond the shadow of a doubt through hypothesis testing. Researchers who claim that their data have "proven" the validity of their hypothesis should be regarded with grave reservation. You should realize that, at best, findings that support a hypothesis are considered tentative. If repeated replication of a study yields the same results, more confidence can be placed in the conclusions advanced by the researchers.
8. Quantifiable words such as greater than; less than; decrease; increase; and positively, negatively, or related convey the idea of objectivity and testability. You should immediately be suspicious of hypotheses that are not stated objectively.
9. You should recognize that how the proposed relationship of the hypothesis is phrased suggests the type of research design that will be appropriate for the study, as well as the level of evidence to be derived from the findings. For example, if a hypothesis proposes that treatment $X_1$ will have a greater effect on $Y$ than treatment $X_2$, an experimental (Level II evidence) or quasi-experimental design (Level III evidence) is suggested (see Chapter 8). If a hypothesis proposes that there will be a positive relationship between variables $X$ and $Y$, a nonexperimental design (Level IV evidence) is suggested (see Chapter 9).

## KEY POINTS

- Formulation of the research question and stating the hypothesis are key preliminary steps in the research process.
- The research question is refined through a process that proceeds from the identification of a general idea of interest to the definition of a more specific and circumscribed topic.
- A preliminary literature review reveals related factors that appear critical to the research topic of interest and helps to further define the research question.
- The significance of the research question must be identified in terms of its potential contribution to patients, nurses, the medical community in general, and society. Applicability of the question for nursing practice, as well as its theoretical relevance, must be established. The findings should also have the potential for formulating or altering nursing practices or policies.
- The feasibility of a research question must be examined in light of pragmatic considerations (e.g., time); availability of subjects, money, facilities, and equipment; experience of the researcher; and ethical issues.
- The final research question consists of a statement about the relationship of two or more variables. It clearly identifies the relationship between the independent and dependent variables, specifies the nature of the population being studied, and implies the possibility of empirical testing.
- Focused clinical questions arise from clinical practice and guide the literature search for the best available evidence to answer the clinical question.
- A hypothesis is a declarative statement about the relationship between two or more variables that predicts an expected outcome. Characteristics of a hypothesis include a relationship statement, implications regarding testability, and consistency with a defined theory base.
- Hypotheses can be formulated in a directional or a nondirectional manner and further categorized as either research or statistical hypotheses.
- Research questions may be used instead of hypotheses in exploratory, descriptive, or qualitative research studies.
- The purpose, research question, or hypothesis provides information about the intent of the research question and hypothesis and suggests the level of evidence to be obtained from the study findings.
- The critiquer assesses the clarity of the research question for the specificity of the population, and the implications for testability.
- The interrelatedness of the research question, the literature review, the theoretical framework, and the hypotheses should be apparent.
- The appropriateness of the research design suggested by the research question is also evaluated.

## CRITICAL THINKING CHALLENGES

- Discuss how the wording of a research question or hypothesis suggests the type of research design and level of evidence that will be provided.
- Using the study by Melvin and colleagues (Appendix D), describe how the background, significance, and purpose of the study are linked to the hypotheses.
- The prevalence of falls on your hospital unit has increased by 10% in the last two quarters. As a member of the Quality Improvement committee on your unit, you want to propose

a QI action plan guided by a clinical question. Develop a clinical question to address this problem.
- A nurse is caring for patients in a clinical situation that produces a clinical question having no ready answer. The nurse wants to develop and refine this clinical question using the PICO approach so that it becomes the basis for an evidence-based practice project. How can the nurse accomplish that objective?

## REFERENCES

Alexander, G. L., Wakefield, B. J., Rantz, M., et al. (2012). Passive sensor technology interface to assess elder activity in independent living. *Nursing Research, 60*(5), 318–325.

Alhusen, J. L., Gross, D., Hayat, M. J., et al. (2012). The influence of maternal-fetal attachment and health practices on neonatal outcomes in low-income, urban women. *Research in Nursing and Health, 35*, 112–120.

Cossette, S., Frasure-Smith, N., Dupuis, J., et al. (2012). Randomized controlled trial of tailored nursing interventions to improve cardiac rehabilitation enrollment. *Nursing Research, 61*(2), 111–120.

Cullum, N. (2000). User's guides to the nursing literature: an introduction. *Evidence-Based Nurs, 3*(2), 71–72.

Falk, J., Wongsa, S., Dang, J., et al. (2012). Using an evidence-based practice process to change child visitation guidelines. *Clinical Journal of Oncology Nursing, 16*(1), 21–23.

Fawcett, J., Aber, C., Haussler, S., et al. (2012). Women's perceptions of caesarean birth: A Roy international study. *Nursing Science Quarterly, 24*(4), 352–362.

Grey, M., Jaser, S. S., Whittemore, R., et al. (2011). Coping skills training for parents of children with type I diabetes. *Nursing Research, 60*(3), 173–181.

Houweling, S. T., Kleefstra, N., van Hateren, K. J., et al. (2011). Can diabetes management be safely transferred to nurses in a primary care setting: A randomized controlled trial. *Journal of Clinical Nursing, 20*, 1264–1272.

Konkle-Parker, D. J., Erlen, J. A., Dubbert, P. M., & May, W. (2012). Pilot testing of an HIV medication adherence intervention in a public clinic in the Deep South. *Journal of the American Academy of Nurse Practitioners, 24*(8), 488–495.

McDougall, G. J., Mackert, M., & Becker, H. (2012). Memory, performance, health literacy, and instrumental activities of daily living of community residing older adults. *Nursing Research, 61*(1), 70–75.

MD Anderson Cancer Center. (2012). *Adult cancer pain interdisciplinary clinical practice guideline.* Houston: The Author.

Murphy, F. A., Lipp, X., & Powles D. L. (2012). Follow-up for improving psychological well being for women after a miscarriage (Review). *Cochrane Database of Systematic Reviews, 3*, CD008679. doi: 10.1002/14651858.CD008679.pub2.

Phelan, K. J., Khoury, J., & Xu, Y. (2011). A randomized controlled trial of home injury hazard reduction the HOME injury study. *Archives of Pediatric Adolescent Medicine, 165*, 339–345.

Prochaska, J. O., & DiClemente, C. C. (1984). *The transtheoretical approach: Crossing the traditional boundaries of therapy.* Malabar, Florida: Krieger Publishing.

Sackett, D., Richardson, W. S., Rosenberg, W., et al. (2000). *Evidence-based medicine: How to practice and teach EBM.* London: Churchill Livingstone.

Sawatzky, R. G., Ratner, P. A., Richardson, C. G., et al. (2012). Stress and depression in students: The medicating role of stress management self-efficacy. *Nursing Research, 61*(1), 13–21.

Sherman, D. W., Rosedale, M. T., & Haber, J. (2012). Reclaiming life on one's own terms: A grounded study of the process of breast cancer survivorship. *Oncology Nursing Forum, 39*(3), 258–268.

Szilagyi, P. G., Humiston, S. G., Gallivan, S., et al. (2011). Effectiveness of a citywide patient immunization navigator program on improving adolescent immunizations and preventive care visit rates. *Archives of Pediatric Adolescent Medicine, 165*, 547–553.

Thomas, M. L., Elliott, J. E., Rao, S. M., et al. (2012). A randomized, clinical trial of education or motivational-interviewing-based coaching compared to usual care to improve cancer pain management. *Oncology Nursing Forum*, *39*(1), 39–49.

Thompson, C., Cullum, N., McCaughan, D., et al. (2004). Nurses, information use, and clinical decision-making: The real world potential for evidence-based decisions in nursing. *Evidence-Based Nursing*, *7*(3), 68–72.

Zisberg, A., Gary, S., Gur-Yaish, N., et al. (2011). In-hospital use of continence aids and new-onset urinary incontinence in adults aged 70 and older. *Journal of the American Geriatric Society*, *59*, 1099–104.

# evolve WEBSITE

*Go to Evolve at http://evolve.elsevier.com/LoBiondo/ for review questions, critquing exercises, and additional research articles for practice in reviewing and critiquing.*

# Gathering and Appraising the Literature

*Stephanie Fulton and Barbara Krainovich-Miller*

## ℮volve WEBSITE

*Go to Evolve at http://evolve.elsevier.com/LoBiondo/ for review questions, critiquing exercises, and additional research articles for practice in reviewing and critiquing.*

## LEARNING OUTCOMES

*After reading this chapter, you should be able to do the following:*

- Discuss the relationship of the literature review to nursing theory, research, and practice.
- Differentiate the purposes of the literature review from the perspective of the research investigator and the research consumer.
- Discuss the use of the literature review for quantitative designs and qualitative methods.
- Discuss the purpose of reviewing the literature for developing evidence-based practice and quality improvement projects.
- Differentiate between primary and secondary sources.
- Compare the advantages and disadvantages of the most commonly used electronic databases for conducting a literature review.
- Identify the characteristics of an effective electronic search of the literature.
- Critically read, appraise, and synthesize sources used for the development of a literature review.
- Apply critiquing criteria for the evaluation of literature reviews in research studies.
- Discuss the role of the "6S" hierarchy of pre-appraised evidence for application to practice.

## KEY TERMS

| | | | |
|---|---|---|---|
| 6S hierarchy of pre-appraised evidence | controlled vocabulary | print indexes | secondary source |
| Boolean operator | electronic databases | refereed, or | Web browser |
| citation management software | literature review | peer-reviewed, | |
| | primary source | journals | |

You may wonder why an entire chapter of a research text is devoted to gathering and appraising the literature. The main reason is because searching for, retrieving, and critically appraising the literature are key steps in the research process for researchers and also for nurses implementing evidence-based practice. A question you might ask is: "Will knowing more about how to gather and critically appraise the literature really help me as a student or later as a practicing nurse?" The answer is that it most certainly will! Your ability to locate and retrieve research studies, critically appraise them, and decide that you have the best available evidence to inform your clinical decision making is a skill essential to your current role as a student and your future role as a nurse who is a competent consumer of research.

Your critical appraisal, also called a critique of the literature, is an organized, systematic approach to evaluating a research study or group of studies using a set of standardized, established critical appraisal criteria to objectively determine the strength, quality, quantity, and consistency of evidence provided by literature to determine its applicability to research, education, or practice. The literature review of a published study generally appears near the beginning of the report. It provides an abbreviated version of the complete literature review conducted by a researcher and represents the building blocks, or framework, of the study. Therefore, the **literature review**, a systematic and critical appraisal of the most important literature on a topic, is a key step in the research process that provides the basis of a research study. The links between theory, research, education, and practice are intricately connected; together they create the knowledge base for the nursing discipline as shown in Figure 3-1.

The purpose of this chapter is to introduce you to the literature review as it is used in research, evidence-based practice, and quality improvement projects. It provides you with the tools to (1) locate, search for, and retrieve individual research studies, systematic reviews (see Chapters 1, 9, 10, and 19), and other documents (e.g., clinical practice guidelines); (2) differentiate between a research article and a conceptual article or book; (3) critically appraise a research study or group of research studies; and (4) differentiate between a research article and a conceptual article or book. These tools will help you develop your research consumer competencies and prepare your academic papers and evidence-based practice and quality improvement projects.

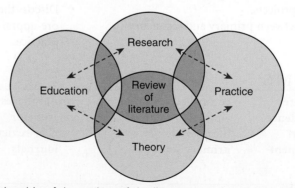

**FIGURE 3-1** Relationship of the review of the literature to theory, research, education, and practice.

---

**BOX 3-1    OVERALL PURPOSES OF A LITERATURE REVIEW**

**Major Goal**

To develop a strong knowledge base to conduct a research study or an evidence-based practice/quality improvement project

**Objectives**

A review of the literature does the following:

1. Determines what is known and unknown about a subject, concept, or problem
2. Determines gaps, consistencies, and inconsistencies in the literature about a subject, concept, or problem
3. Describes conceptual or theoretical frameworks used to examine problems
4. Generates useful research questions and hypotheses
5. Determines an appropriate research design, methodology, and analysis for answering the research question(s) or hypothesis(es) based on an assessment of the strengths and weaknesses of earlier works
6. Determines the need for replication or refinement of a study
7. Synthesizes the strengths and weaknesses and findings of available studies on a topic/problem
8. Uncovers a new practice intervention(s), or gains supporting evidence for revising or maintaining current intervention(s), protocols, and policies
9. Promotes revision and development of new practice protocols, policies, and projects/activities related to nursing practice based on evidence
10. Generates clinical questions that guide development of evidence-based practice and quality improvement projects

---

# REVIEW OF THE LITERATURE

## The Literature Review: The Researcher's Perspective

The overall purpose of the literature review in a research study is to present a strong knowledge base for the conduct of the study. It is important to understand when reading a research article that the researcher's main goal when developing the literature review is to develop the knowledge foundation for a sound study and to generate research questions and hypotheses. A literature review is essential to all steps of the quantitative and qualitative research processes. From this perspective, the review is broad and systematic, as well as in-depth. It is a critical collection and evaluation of the important literature in an area. From a researcher's perspective, the objectives in Box 3-1 (items 1-6) direct the questions the researcher asks while reading the literature to determine a useful research question(s) or hypothesis(es) and how best to design a study. Objectives 7 through 10 are applicable to the consumer of research perspective discussed later in the chapter.

The following overview about use of the literature review in relation to the steps of the quantitative and qualitative research process will help you to understand the researcher's focus. A critical review of relevant literature affects the steps of the quantitative research process as follows:

- Theoretical or conceptual framework: A literature review reveals concepts and/or theories or conceptual models from nursing and other disciplines that can be used to examine problems. The framework presents the context for studying the problem and can be viewed as a map for understanding the relationships between or among the variables in quantitative studies. The literature review provides rationale for the variables and explains concepts, definitions, and relationships between or among the independent and dependent variables used in the theoretical framework of the study (see Chapter 4). However, in

---

**TABLE 3-1    EXAMPLES OF PRIMARY AND SECONDARY SOURCES**

| PRIMARY: ESSENTIAL | SECONDARY: USEFUL |
|---|---|
| Material written by the person who conducted the study, developed the theory (model), or prepared the scholarly discussion on a concept, topic, or issue of interest (i.e., the original author). | Material written by a person(s) other than the person who conducted the research study or developed the theory. This material summarizes or critiques another author's original work and is usually in the form of a summary or critique (i.e., analysis and synthesis) of another's scholarly work or body of literature. Mainly used for Theoretical and Conceptual Framework. |
| Other primary sources include: autobiographies, diaries, films, letters, artifacts, periodicals, Internet communications on e-mail, listservs, interviews (e.g., oral histories, e-mail), photographs and tapes. | Other secondary sources include: response/commentary/critique of a research study, a theory paraphrased by others, or a work written by someone other than the original author (e.g., a biography or clinical article). |
| Can be published or unpublished. | Can be published or unpublished. |
| Primary source example: An investigator's report of their research study (e.g., articles in Appendices A-D) and the Cochrane report (Appendix E). | Secondary source example: An edited textbook (e.g., LoBiondo-Wood, G., & Haber, J. [2014]. *Nursing research: Methods and critical appraisal for evidence-based practice* [8th ed.], Philadelphia, Elsevier.) |
| Theoretical example: The following statement by Mercer (2004) cited from her original work is an example of a primary source of a theory. Mercer's conclusion states: "The argument is made to replace 'maternal role attainment' with becoming a mother to connote the initial transformation and continuing growth of the mother." (p. 231) | Theoretical example: Alhusen and colleague's 2012 description of the theoretical model for their study paraphrases a number of theoretical sources (Cranley, 1981; Rubin, 1967; Mercer, 2004) related to the relationship of the mother to the fetus and the role of mother (see Appendix B). |
| HINT: Critical appraisal of primary sources is essential to a thorough and relevant review of the literature. | HINT: Use secondary sources sparingly; however, secondary sources, especially a study's literature review that presents a critique of studies, is a valuable learning tool for a beginning research consumer. |

many research articles the literature review may not be labeled. For example, Thomas and colleagues (2012) did not label the literature review, yet the beginning section of the article is clearly the literature review (see Appendix A).

- Primary and secondary sources: The literature review should mainly use **primary sources**; that is, research articles and books by the original author. Sometimes it is appropriate to use **secondary sources**, which are published articles or books that are written by persons other than the individual who conducted the research study or developed the theory (Table 3-1).
- Research question and hypothesis: The literature review helps to determine what is known and not known; to uncover gaps, consistencies, or inconsistencies; and/or to disclose unanswered questions in the literature about a subject, concept, theory, or problem that generate, or allow for refinement of, research questions and/or hypotheses.
- Design and method: The literature review exposes the strengths and weaknesses of previous studies in terms of designs and methods and helps the researcher choose an appropriate design and method, including sampling strategy type and size, data collection

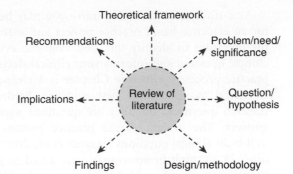

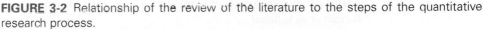

**FIGURE 3-2** Relationship of the review of the literature to the steps of the quantitative research process.

methods, setting, measurement instruments, and effective data analysis method. Often, because of journal space limitations, researchers include only abbreviated information about this in their article.

- Outcome of the analysis (i.e., findings, discussion, implications, recommendations): The literature review is used to help the researcher accurately interpret and discuss the results/findings of a study. In the discussion section of a research article, the researcher returns to the research studies, theoretical articles, or books presented earlier in the literature review and uses this literature to interpret and explain the study's findings (see Chapters 16 and 17). For example, Alhusen and colleagues' (2012) discussion section noted that "the findings of this study highlight the significance of MFA as predictor of neonatal health and wellbeing, and, potentially, health care costs" (see Appendix B). The literature review is also useful when considering implications of the research findings for making recommendations for practice, education, and further research. Alhusen and colleagues also stated in the discussion section that "future researchers should test culturally relevant interventions aimed at improving the maternal-fetal relationship." Figure 3-2 relates the literature review to all aspects of the quantitative research process.

In contrast to the styles of quantitative studies, literature reviews of qualitative studies are usually handled differently (see Chapters 5 to 7) but often, when published, will appear at the beginning of the article. In qualitative studies, often little is known about the topic under study, and thus literature reviews may appear abbreviated. Qualitative researchers use the literature review in the same manner as quantitative researchers to discuss the findings of the study.

## The Literature Review: The Consumer Perspective

From the perspective of the research consumer, you conduct an electronic database search of your clinical problem and appraise the studies to answer a clinical question or solve a clinical problem. Therefore, you search the literature widely and gather multiple resources to answer your question using an evidence-based practice approach. This search focuses you on the first three steps of the evidence-based practice process: asking clinical questions, identifying and gathering evidence, and critically appraising and synthesizing the evidence or literature. Objectives 7 through 10 in Box 3-1 specifically reflect the purposes of a literature review for these projects.

As a student or practicing nurse you may be asked to generate a clinical question for an evidence-based practice project and search for, retrieve, and critically appraise the literature to identify the "best available evidence" that provides the answer to a clinical question and informs your clinical decision making using the evidence-based practice process outlined in Chapter 1. A clear and precise articulation of a question is critical to finding the best evidence. Evidence-based questions may sound like research questions, but they are questions used to search the existing literature for answers. The evidence-based practice process uses the PICO format to generate well-built clinical questions (Haynes et al., 2006; Richardson, 1995). For example, students in an adult health course were asked to generate a clinical question related to health promotion for older women using the PICO format (see Chapter 2). The PICO format is as follows:

**P** Problem/patient population; specifically defined group
**I** Intervention; what intervention or event will be studied?
**C** Comparison of intervention; with what will the intervention be compared?
**O** Outcome; what is the effect of the intervention?

One group of students was interested in whether regular exercise prevented osteoporosis for postmenopausal women who had osteopenia. The PICO format for the clinical question that guided their search was as follows:

**P** Postmenopausal women with osteopenia (Age is part of the definition.)
**I** Regular exercise program (How often is regular? Weekly? Twice a week?)
**C** No regular exercise program
**O** Prevention of osteoporosis (How and when was this measured?)

Their assignment required that they do the following:

- Search the literature using electronic databases (e.g., Cumulative Index to Nursing and Allied Health Literature [CINAHL via EBSCO], MEDLINE, Cochrane Database of Systematic Reviews) for the background information that enabled them to identify the significance of osteopenia and osteoporosis as a women's health problem.
- Identify systematic reviews, practice guidelines, and individual research studies that provided the "best available evidence" related to the effectiveness of regular exercise programs on prevention of osteoporosis.
- Critically appraise the information gathered based on standardized critical appraisal criteria and tools (see Chapters 1, 11, 19, and 20).
- Synthesize the overall strengths and weaknesses of the evidence provided by the literature.
- Draw a conclusion about the strength, quality, and consistency of the evidence.
- Make recommendations about applicability of evidence to clinical nursing practice that guides development of a health promotion project about osteoporosis risk reduction for postmenopausal women with osteopenia.

As a practicing nurse, you will be called on to develop new EBP/QI projects and/or to update current EBP protocols, practice standards, or policies in your health care organization. This will require that you know how to retrieve and critically appraise research articles, practice guidelines, and systematic reviews to determine the degree of support or nonsupport found in the literature. A critical appraisal of the literature related to a specific clinical question uncovers data that contribute evidence to support or refute current practice, clinical decision making, and practice changes.

## Research Conduct and Consumer of Research Purposes: Differences and Similarities

How does the literature review differ when it is used for research purposes versus consumer of research purposes? The literature review in a research study is used to develop a sound research proposal for a study that will generate knowledge. From a consumer perspective, the major focus of reviewing the literature is to uncover the best available evidence on a given topic that has been generated by research studies that can potentially be used to improve clinical practice and patient outcomes. From a student perspective, the ability to critically appraise the literature is essential to acquiring a skill set for successfully completing scholarly papers, presentations, debates, and evidence-based practice projects. Both types of literature reviews are similar in that both should be framed in the context of previous research and background information and pertinent to the objectives presented in Box 3-1.

---

### HELPFUL HINT

Remember, the findings of one study on a topic do not provide sufficient evidence to support a change in practice; be cautious when a nurse colleague tells you to change your practice based on the results of one study.

---

### EVIDENCE-BASED PRACTICE TIP

For a research consumer, formulating a clinical question using the PICO format provides a focus that guides an efficient electronic search of the literature.

---

## SEARCHING FOR EVIDENCE

In your student role, when you are preparing an academic paper, you read the required course materials, as well as additional literature retrieved from your electronic search on your topic. Students often state, "I know how to do research." Perhaps you have thought the same thing because you "researched" a topic for a paper in the library. However, in this situation it would be more accurate for you to say that you have "searched" the literature to uncover research and conceptual information to prepare an academic paper on a topic. You will search for **primary sources**, which are articles, books, or other documents written by the person who conducted the study or developed the theory. You will also search for **secondary sources**, which are materials written by persons other than the those who conducted a research study or developed a particular theory. Table 3-1 provides definitions and examples of primary and secondary sources, and Table 3-2 shows steps and strategies for conducting a literature search.

In Chapter 1, the EBM hierarchy of evidence is introduced to help you determine the levels of evidence of sources and the quality, quantity, and consistency of the evidence located during a search. Here, the **"6S" hierarchy of pre-appraised evidence** (Figure 3-3) is introduced to help you find pre-appraised evidence or evidence that has previously undergone an evaluation process for your clinical questions. This model (DiCenso et al., 2009) was developed to assist clinicians in their search for the highest level of evidence. Therefore, the main use of the 6S hierarchy is for efficiently identifying the highest level of evidence to facilitate your search on your clinical question or problem. It is important to keep in mind that there are limitations to using pre-appraised sources because they might not address

| TABLE 3-2 | STEPS AND STRATEGIES FOR CONDUCTING A LITERATURE SEARCH |
| --- | --- |
| **STEPS OF LITERATURE REVIEW** | **STRATEGY** |
| **Step I:** Determine clinical question or research topic | Keep focused on the types of patients that you care for in your setting. Keep focused on the assignment's objective; if EBP project start with a PICO question. Use the literature to develop your ideas. |
| **Step II:** Identify key variables/terms | Ask your reference librarian for help, and read the online Help. Include the elements of your PICO and see if you can limit to research articles or use publication types to focus your results. |
| **Step III:** Conduct computer search using at least two recognized electronic databases | Conduct the search yourself or with the help of your librarian; it is essential to use at least two health-related databases, such as CINAHL via EBSCO, MEDLINE, PsycINFO, or ERIC. |
| **Step IV:** Review abstracts online and weed out irrelevant articles | Scan through your retrieved search, read the abstracts provided, and mark only those that fit your topic; select "references" as well as "search history" and "full-text articles" if available, before printing, saving, or e-mailing your search. |
| **Step V:** Retrieve relevant sources | Organize by article type or study design and year and reread the abstracts to determine if the articles chosen are relevant and worth retrieving. |
| **Step VI:** Store or print relevant articles; if unable to print directly from database order through interlibrary loan | Download the search to an online search management, writing and collaboration tool designed to help you (e.g., RefWorks, EndNote, Zotero). Using a system will ensure that you have the information for each citation (e.g., journal name, year, volume number, pages) and it will format the reference list—this can save an immense amount of time when composing your paper. Download PDF versions of articles as needed. |
| **Step VII:** Conduct preliminary reading and weed out irrelevant sources | Review critical reading strategies (e.g., read the abstract at the beginning of the articles [see Chapter 1]). |
| **Step VIII:** Critically read each source (summarize and critique each source) | Use critical appraisal strategies (e.g., use an evidence table [see Chapter 19] or a standardized critiquing tool), process each summary and critical appraisal (no more than one page long), include the references in APA style at the top or bottom of each abstract. |
| **Step IX:** Synthesize critical summaries of each article | Decide how you will present the synthesis of overall strengths and weaknesses of the reviewed articles (e.g., present chronologically and according to type: research as well as conceptual literature-so the reader can see the evidence's progression; or present similarities and differences between and among studies and or concepts). At the end summarize the findings of the literature review, draw a conclusion and make recommendations based on your conclusion. Include the reference list. |

your particular clinical question. This model suggests that, when searching the literature, you consider prioritizing your search strategy and begin your search by looking for the highest level information resource available.

The highest level of the pyramid is a *computerized decision support system (CDSS)* that integrates evidence-based clinical information into an electronic medical record.

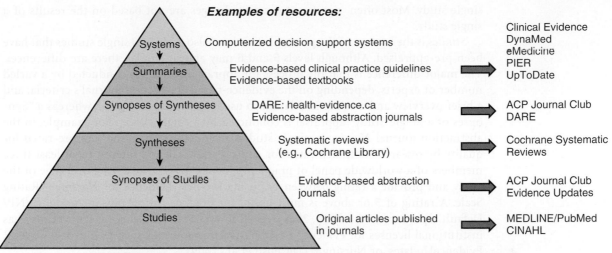

**Examples of resources:**

| | | |
|---|---|---|
| Systems | Computerized decision support systems | Clinical Evidence DynaMed eMedicine PIER UpToDate |
| Summaries | Evidence-based clinical practice guidelines Evidence-based textbooks | |
| Synopses of Syntheses | DARE: health-evidence.ca Evidence-based abstraction journals | ACP Journal Club DARE |
| Syntheses | Systematic reviews (e.g., Cochrane Library) | Cochrane Systematic Reviews |
| Synopses of Studies | Evidence-based abstraction journals | ACP Journal Club Evidence Updates |
| Studies | Original articles published in journals | MEDLINE/PubMed CINAHL |

**FIGURE 3-3** The 6S levels of organization of evidence from health care research.

In these systems, specific patient data can be entered and then matched against a knowledge base to generate patient-specific recommendations or assessments. More and more clinical settings are adding these CDSSs, although it is not a reality in most institutions.

The next level down is *Summaries,* which includes clinical practice guidelines and electronic evidence-based textbooks such as Clinical Evidence (www.clinicalevidence.com), Dynamed (http://dynamed.ebscohost.com/), the Physicians Information and Education Resource (PIER) (http://pier.acponline.org/overview.html), and UpToDate (http://www.uptodate.com). These summaries about specific conditions are updated regularly. Also included in Summaries are evidence-based guidelines that provide recommendations based on high quality evidence. Many organizations like the Oncology Nursing Society create evidence-based guidelines called Putting Evidence into Practice (http://www.ons.org/Research/PEP/).

The next level, *Synopses of Syntheses,* provides a pre-appraised summary of a systematic review. These can be found in journals such as *Evidence-Based Nursing* (http://ebn.bmj.com/) and *Evidence-Based Medicine* (http://ebm.bmj.com/) or in the Database of Abstracts of Reviews of Effects (http://www.crd.york.ac.uk/crdweb/AboutDare.asp). These synopses provide a synthesis of the review; some include a commentary related to strength of the evidence and applicability to a patient population.

*Syntheses* (Systematic Reviews) are the next type of information resource in the 6S pyramid. Systematic reviews (e.g., a Cochrane review) are a synthesis of research on a clinical topic. Systematic reviews use strict methods to search and appraise studies. They include quantitative summaries—meta-analysis (see Chapter 11).

*Synopses of Studies* is a synopsis of a single study that has been appraised by an expert who provides an overview and appraisal of the study, including a commentary on the study's context and practice implications. Examples of synopses of single studies can be found in journals such as *Evidence-Based Nursing* or *Evidence-Based Medicine.* Keep in mind that a synopsis of a single study, while critically pre-appraised, still remains a single study. Most often, significant practice changes are not based on the results of a single study.

*Studies* is the bottom of the pyramid. This level also addresses single studies that have been pre-appraised. Although levels 5 and 6 may appear similar, there are differences. The major difference is that the process for appraising level 5 is conducted by a varied number of experts, depending on the evidence-based abstraction journal's criteria, and a brief overview and a rating in relation to use in practice is included, whereas a "Synopses of a Single Study" appraisal is conducted by a single expert. For example, in the abstraction journal *Nursing+,* single studies included on their site "are pre-rated for quality by research staff, then rated for clinical relevance and interest by at least three members of a worldwide panel of practicing nurses" who write a brief overview of the study and provide a rating between 1-7 using the Best Evidence for *Nursing+* Rating Scale. A rating of 5 or above is most useful for practice (http://plus.mcmaster.ca/NP/Default.aspx, retrieved July 14, 2012). As with level 5, you must see if your library has institutional licenses for evidence-based abstraction journals such as Journalwise ACP, EvidenceUpdates, or Nursing+ (DiCenso et al., 2009).

The 6S model is a tool that can help guide your search for the strongest and most relevant evidence. This model, although an important tool to guide your search for evidence-based information, does not replace the importance of critically reading each piece of evidence and assessing its quality and applicability for current practice.

---

**HELPFUL HINT**

- Make an appointment with your institution's reference librarian so you can take advantage of his or her expertise in accessing electronic databases.
- Take the time to set up your computer for electronic library access.
- Learn how to use an online search management/writing tool such as RefWorks, EndNote, or Zotero.

---

## Performing an Electronic Search
### Why Use an Electronic Database?

Perhaps you are still not convinced that electronic database searches are the best way to acquire information for a review of the literature. Maybe you have searched using Google or Yahoo! and found relevant information. This is an understandable temptation, especially if your assignment requires you to use only five articles. Try to think about it from another perspective and ask yourself, "Is this the most appropriate and efficient way to find out the latest and strongest research on a topic that affects patient care?" Duncan and Holtslander (2012) looked at the information-seeking behaviors of senior nursing students and found that more time is needed to teach nursing students to use electronic resources, including CINAHL. This study specifically highlighted that students were frustrated with their ability to locate appropriate terms to use in their search. A way to decrease your frustration is to take the time to learn how to do a sound database search. Following the strategies and hints provided in this chapter will help you gain the essential competencies needed for your course assignments and career in nursing. The Critical Thinking Decision Path shows a way to locate evidence to support your research or clinical question (Kendall, 2008).

## CRITICAL THINKING DECISION PATH
### *Search for Evidence Thought Flow*

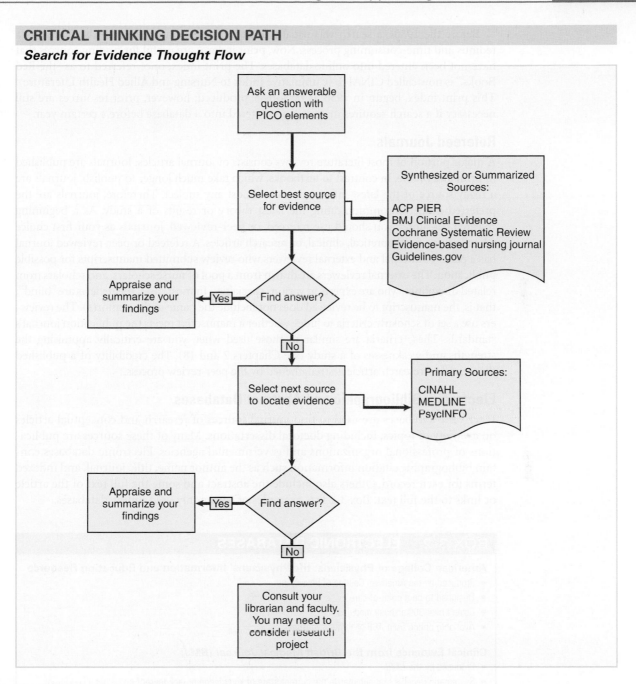

## TYPES OF RESOURCES

### Print and Electronic Indexes: Books and Journals

Most college/university libraries have an online card catalog to find print and online books, journals (by journal titles only), videos and other media items, scripts, monographs, conference proceedings, masters' theses, dissertations, archival materials, and more.

Before the 1980s, a search was usually done by hand using print indexes. This was a tedious and time-consuming process. Now, print indexes are useful for finding sources that have not been entered into online databases. The print index, once referred to as "the Red Books," is now called CINAHL (Cumulative Index to Nursing and Allied Health Literature). This print index, begun in 1956, is no longer produced; however, print resources are still necessary if a search requires materials not entered into a database before a certain year.

## Refereed Journals

A major portion of most literature reviews consists of journal articles. Journals are published in print and online. In contrast to textbooks, which take much longer to publish, journals are a ready source of the latest information on almost any subject. Therefore, journals are the preferred mode of communicating the latest theory or results of a study. As a beginning research consumer, you should use refereed, or peer-reviewed, journals as your first choice when looking for theoretical, clinical, or research articles. A refereed or peer-reviewed journal has a panel of internal and external reviewers who review submitted manuscripts for possible publication. The external reviewers are drawn from a pool of nurse scholars, and scholars from related disciplines, who are experts in various specialties. In most cases, the reviews are "blind"; that is, the manuscript to be reviewed does not include the name of the author(s). The reviewers use a set of scholarly criteria to judge whether a manuscript meets the publication journal's standards. These criteria are similar to those used when you are critically appraising the strengths and weaknesses of a study (see Chapters 7 and 18). The credibility of a published theoretical or research article is strengthened by the peer-review process.

## Electronic: Bibliographic and Abstract Databases

Electronic databases are used to find journal sources of research and conceptual articles on a variety of topics, including doctoral dissertations. Many of these sources are publications of professional organizations and governmental agencies. Electronic databases contain bibliographic citation information such as the author name, title, journal, and indexed terms for each record. Others also include the abstract and some the full text of the article or links to the full text. Box 3-2 lists examples of commonly used online databases.

---

### BOX 3-2    ELECTRONIC DATABASES

**American College of Physicians: the Physicians' Information and Education Resource**
- Produced by the American College of Physicians
- Designed to be a point-of-care evidence-based resource
- Covers over 300 disease modules
- Available online from ACP or through StatRef!

**Clinical Evidence from the *British Medical Journal (BMJ)***
- Produced by the *BMJ*
- Systematic reviews that summarize the current state of knowledge or lack thereof on medical conditions
- Provide evidence reviews for more than 250 conditions
- Available online from BMJ and Ovid Technologies, Inc.

**Cumulative Index to Nursing and Allied Health Literature (CINAHL)**
- Print version known as the "Red Books"
- Records date back to 1937
- Available as part of the EBSCO online service; includes more than 130 Evidence-Based Care Sheets

## BOX 3-2   ELECTRONIC DATABASES—cont'd

### Cumulative Index to Nursing and Allied Health Literature (CINAHL)—cont'd
- Over 5,000 journals indexed for inclusion in database
- Citations in CINAHL are assigned index terms from a controlled vocabulary

### The Cochrane Library
- Collection of six databases that contain high-quality evidence ranging from original articles to synopsis of synthesis
- Includes the Cochrane Database of Systematic Reviews
- Full Cochrane Library available from Wiley Online Library; other databases that make up the Cochrane Library are available from other vendors, including Ovid Technologies, Inc.
- Cochrane systematic reviews are indexed and searchable in both CINAHL and MEDLINE

### Education Resource Information Center (ERIC)
- Sponsored by the Institute of Education and the U.S. Department of Education
- Focuses on education research and information
- Currently indexes more than 600 journals and also includes references to books, conference papers, and technical reports
- Coverage begins in 1966
- ERIC is freely available from the ERIC web site and by subscription from EBSCO, OCLC, and Ovid Technologies, Inc.

### Embase
- A biomedical and pharmacological database provides access to over 7,000 journals dating back to 1947
- Indexes an additional 5 million records not covered on MEDLINE
- Covers many European journals not indexed in other sources
- Allows EMTREE subject heading and keyword searching
- Available via Ovid Technologies, Inc. and Elsevier

### MEDLINE
- Produced by the National Library of Medicine in the United States
- Premier bibliographic database for journal articles in life sciences
- Earliest records from the late 1800s and approximately 5,500 worldwide journals are indexed
- Indexed with MeSH (Medical Subject Headings)
- MEDLINE is available for free via PubMed and by subscription from EBSCO and Ovid Technologies, Inc.

### ProQuest Dissertations and Theses Database
- Produced ProQuest
- Earliest records from 1637
- Full text database covers over 2.7 million dissertations with over 1 million available for PDF download

### Psychinfo
- Produced by the American Psychological Association (APA)
- An abstract database of the psychosocial literature beginning with citations dating back to 1800
- Covers more than 2,500 journals
- 99% are peer-reviewed journals
- Also includes book chapters and dissertations
- Indexed with the Thesaurus of Psychological Index Terms
- Available via APA PsycNET, EBSCO, Ovid Technologies, Inc. and ProQuest

### Web of Science
- Multidisciplinary database that collects citation information from over 5,600 journals
- Allows you to search for the number of times a reference has been cited and where; allowing assessment of the impact of a specific paper
- Coverage begins in 1900

**TABLE 3-3 COMPARISON OF CINAHL AND MEDLINE (PUBMED)**

| | CINAHL | MEDLINE |
|---|---|---|
| **Producer and Vendors** | Owned and Produced by EBSCO | Produced by the National Library of Medicine and available via PubMed; Ovid Technologies, Inc.; EBSCO; Thomson Reuters Web of Knowledge |
| **Years of Coverage** | Dates back to 1937 | Dates back to 1947 |
| **Full Text** | Full text added for more than 770 journals but primarily citation and abstracts for most records and many libraries have enabled linking to full text and interlibrary loan | Links to PubMed Central (2.4 million articles) and many libraries have enabled linking to full text articles and interlibrary loan |
| **Journal Coverage** | More than 5,000 journals | More than 5,600 biomedical journals |
| **Database Size** | More than 3.2 million records | More than 21 million records |
| **Controlled Vocabulary** | CINAHL subject headings (12,714) have been applied to citations 1981 to the present | MeSH (Medical Subject Headings) tree consists of 16 branches (e.g., Diseases, Chemicals and Drugs) and over 26,000 terms |
| **Evidence-Based Practice Features** | More than 130 Evidence-Based Care Sheets | Clinical Queries tool to filter for systematic reviews |
| **Special Features** | Ability to exclude MEDLINE records from search; limit to research articles; research instruments limit | Premier biomedical database available free of charge |
| **Link to Tutorial** | support.epnet.com/cinahl/ | www.nlm.nih.gov/bsd/disted/pubmedtutorial/index.html |

Data from DiCenso et al. (2009). Accessing pre-appraised evidence: fine-tuning the 5S model into a 6S model. *Evidence-Based Nursing 12*(4): 99-101.

Your college/university most likely enables you to access such databases electronically whether on campus or not. The most relevant and frequently used source for nursing literature remains the Cumulative Index to Nursing and Allied Health Literature (CINAHL). Full text has been added to this database, so in many cases you will find the full article right at your fingertips. Another premier resource is MEDLINE, which is produced by the National Library of Medicine. MEDLINE focuses on the life sciences and dates back to the late 1800s for some records, with the majority being from 1966 forward. While there is a subscription cost for CINAHL, a free version of MEDLINE, PubMed, is available from the National Library of Medicine. See Table 3-3 for a comparison of these two online databases.

## Electronic: Secondary or Summary Databases

Some databases contain more than just journal article information. These resources contain either summaries or synopses of studies, as described in the 6S pyramid, overviews of diseases or conditions, or a summary of the latest evidence to support a particular treatment. American College of Physicians: The Physicians' Information and Education Resource is one such resource. Users can enter a disease name and find out what treatment is supported by graded evidence (see Chapter 1). Another excellent resource is the Cochrane Library, which consists of six databases, including the Cochrane Database of Systematic Reviews.

## Internet: Search Engines

You are probably familiar with accessing a **Web browser** (e.g., Internet Explorer, Mozilla Firefox, Chrome, Safari) to conduct searches for items such as music, and using search

| TABLE 3-4 | SELECTED EXAMPLES OF WEB SITES TO SUPPORT EVIDENCE-BASED PRACTICE | |
|---|---|---|
| **WEB SITE** | **SCOPE** | **NOTES** |
| Virginia Henderson International Nursing Library www.nursinglibrary.org | Access to the *Registry of Nursing Research* database, which contains nearly 30,000 abstracts of research studies and conference papers. | Service offered without charge; locate conference abstracts and research study abstracts. This library is supported by Sigma Theta Tau International, Honor Society of Nursing. |
| National Guideline Clearinghouse www.guidelines.gov | Public resource for evidence-based clinical practice guidelines. There are over 1,150 guidelines, including non-U.S. publications. | Offers a useful online feature of side-by-side comparison of guidelines and the ability to browse by disease/condition and treatment/intervention. |
| Joanna Briggs Institute www.joannabriggs.edu.au | An international not-for-profit, membership based research and development organization. | Although membership is required for access to their resources they provide Recommended Links worth reviewing as well as descriptions on their levels of evidence and grading scale. |
| Turning Research into Practice (TRIP) www.tripdatabase.com | Content from a wide variety of free online resources, including synopses, guidelines, medical images, e-textbooks, and systematic reviews, brought together under the TRIP search engine. | Check this site for a wide sampling of available evidence and the ability to filter by publication type such as evidence based synopses, systematic reviews, guidelines, textbooks, and primary research. |
| Agency for Health Research and Quality www.ahrq.gov | Over 200 evidence topic reports (including 159 archived), over 30 technical reports, as well as research reviews. | Free source of important government documents for both consumers and conductors of research; also searchable via PubMed. |
| Cochrane Collaboration www.cochrane.org | Provides access to abstracts from Cochrane Database of Systematic Reviews. Full text of reviews and access to the databases that are part of the Cochrane Library—Database of Abstracts of Reviews of Effeciveness, Cochrane Controlled Trials Register, Cochrane Methodology Register, Health Technology Assessment database (HTA), and NHS Economic Evaluation Database (NHS EED) are accessible via Wiley. | Abstracts of Cochrane Reviews, available free and can be browsed or searched; uses many databases in its reviews, including CINAHL via EBSCO and MEDLINE; some are primary sources (e.g., systematic reviews/meta-analyses); others (if commentaries of single studies) are a secondary source; important source for clinical evidence but limited as a provider of primary documents for literature reviews. |

engines such as Google or Google Scholar to find information or articles. However, "surfing" the Web is not a good use of your time for scholarly literature searches. Table 3-4 indicates sources of online information; all are free except Joanna Briggs Institute. Review information carefully to determine if it is a good source of primary research studies. Note that Table 3-4 includes government web sites such as www.hrsa.gov and www.nih.gov, which are sources of health information, and some clinical practice guidelines based on systematic reviews of the literature; however, most Web sites are not a primary source of research studies. Less common and less used sources of scholarly material are audio, video, personal communications (e.g., letters, telephone or in-person interviews), unpublished doctoral dissertations, masters' theses, and conference proceedings.

Most searches using electronic databases include not only citation information but also the abstract of the article and options for obtaining the full text. If the full text is not available, look for other options such as the *abstract* to learn more about the article. Reading the abstract (see Chapter 1) is critical to determine if you need to retrieve the article through another mechanism. Use both CINAHL and MEDLINE electronic databases; this will facilitate all steps of critically reviewing the literature, especially identifying the gaps.

---

**EVIDENCE-BASED PRACTICE TIP**

Reading systematic reviews, if available, on your clinical question/topic will enhance your ability to implement evidence-based nursing practice because they generally offer the strongest and most consistent level of evidence and can provide helpful search terms. A good first step for any question is to search the Cochrane Database of Systematic Reviews to see if someone has already researched your question.

---

### How Far Back Must the Search Go?

Students often ask questions such as, "How many articles do I need?" "How much is enough?" "How far back in the literature do I need to go?" When conducting a search, you should use a rigorous focusing process or you may end up with hundreds or thousands of citations. Retrieving too many citations is usually a sign that there was something wrong with your search technique, or you may not have sufficiently narrowed your clinical question.

Each electronic database offers an explanation of each feature; it is worth your time to click each icon and explore the explanations offered because this will increase your confidence. Also keep in mind the types of articles you are retrieving. Many electronic resources allow you to limit your search to randomized controlled trials or systematic reviews. In CINAHL there is a limit for "Research" that will restrict the citations you retrieve to research articles. Figure 3-4 is an example of using the Research limit to locate the articles on maternal-fetal attachment and health practices, such as Alhusen and colleague's study (see Appendix B).

A general timeline for most academic or evidence-based practice papers/projects is to go back in the literature at least 3 years, and preferably 5 years, although some research projects may warrant going back 10 or more years. Extensive literature reviews on particular topics or a concept clarification methodology study helps you to limit the length of your search.

As you scroll through and mark the citations you wish to include in your downloaded or printed search, make sure you include all relevant fields when you save or print. In addition to indicating which citations you want and choosing which fields to print or save, there is an opportunity to indicate if you want the "search history" included. It is always a good idea to include this information. It is especially helpful if your instructor suggests that some citations were missed, because then you can replicate your search and together determine which variable(s) you missed so that you do not make the same error again. This is also your opportunity to indicate if you want to e-mail the search to yourself. If you are writing a paper and need to produce a bibliography you can export your citations to **citation management software**, which formats and stores your citations so that they are available for electronic retrieval when they are needed to insert in a paper you are writing. Quite a few of these software programs are available; some are free, such as Zotero, and others you or your institution must purchase, including EndNote and RefWorks.

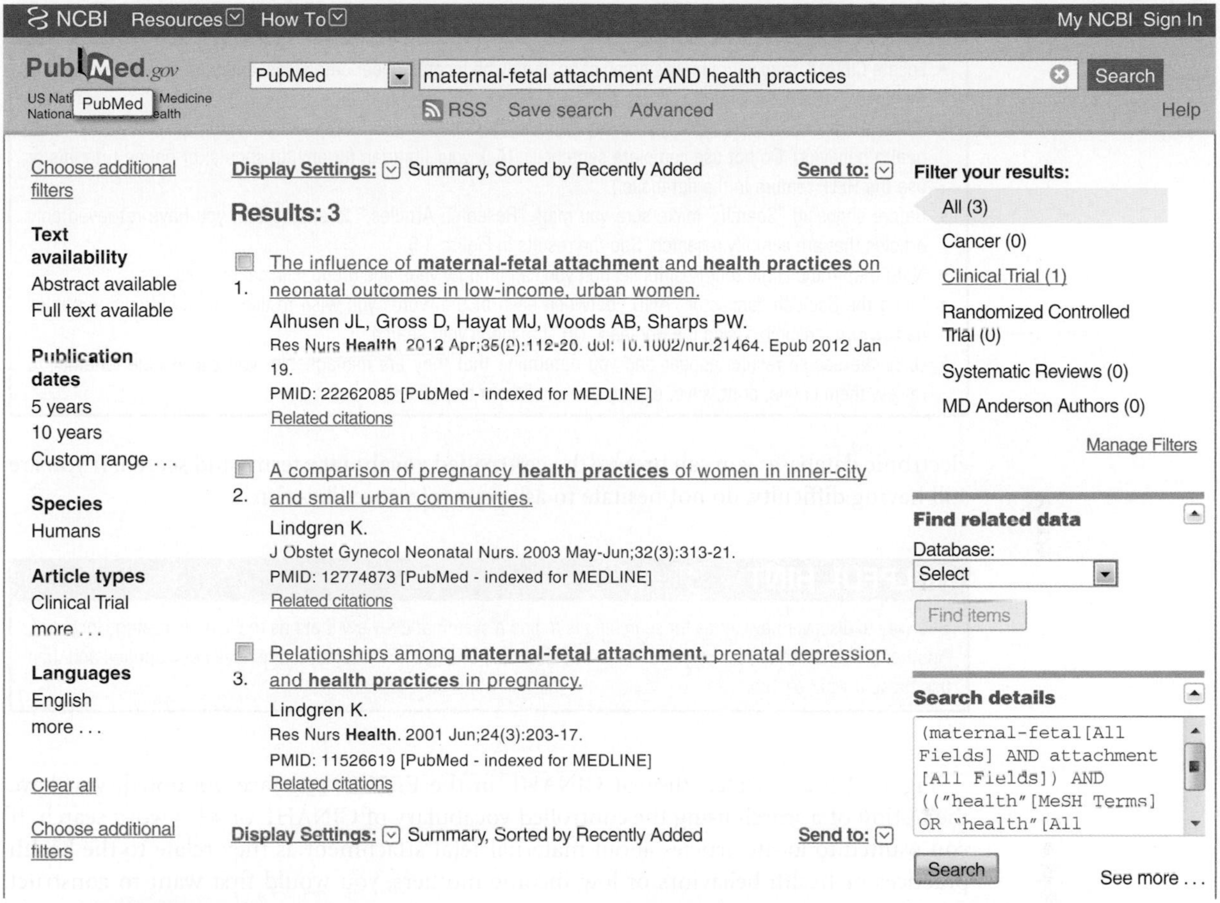

**FIGURE 3-4** Example from PubMed to locate articles on MFA and health practices. When you click on the title of the article you can see your options for locating the full text of the article. As with CINAHL, PubMed primarily has citations and abstracts about the articles with links to take you to the full article.

## HELPFUL HINT

Ask your instructor for guidance if you are uncertain how far back you need to conduct your search. If you come across a systematic review on your specific clinical topic, scan it to see what years the review covers; then begin your search from the last year forward to the present to fill in the gap.

### What Do I Need to Know?

Each database usually has a specific search guide that provides information on the organization of the entries and the terminology used. The suggestions and strategies in Box 3-3 incorporate general search strategies, as well as those related to CINAHL and MEDLINE. Finding the right terms to "plug in" as keywords for a computer search is an important aspect of conducting a search. When possible, you want to match the words that you use to describe your question with the terms that indexers have assigned to the articles. In many

---

**BOX 3-3     TIPS: USING CINAHL VIA EBSCO**

- Locate CINAHL from your library's home page. It may be located under databases, online resources, or nursing resources.
- In the Advanced Search, type in your key word, subject heading, or phrase (e.g., maternal-fetal attachment, health behavior). Do not use complete sentences. (Ask your librarian for any tip sheets, or online tutorials or use the HELP feature in the database.)
- Before choosing "Search," make sure you mark "Research Articles," to ensure that you have retrieved only articles that are actually research. See the results in Figure 3-5.
- Note that in the Limit Your Results section you can limit by year, age group, clinical queries, etc.
- Using the Boolean connector "AND" between each of the words you wish to use plus additional variables narrows your search. Using the Boolean "OR" broadens your search.
- Once the search results appear and you determine that they are manageable, you can decide whether to review them online, print, save, export, or e-mail them to yourself.

---

electronic databases you can browse the **controlled vocabulary** terms and search. If you are still having difficulty, do not hesitate to ask your reference librarian.

**HELPFUL HINT**

One way to discover new terms for searching is to find a systematic review that has the search strategy included. Another is to search for your keyword in the title field only and see how subject terms have been applied and then use those in your search.

Figure 3-5 is a screen shot of CINAHL in the EBSCO interface. As noted, you have the option of a search using the controlled vocabulary of CINAHL or a keyword search. If you wanted to locate articles about maternal-fetal attachment as they relate to the health practices or health behaviors of low-income mothers, you would first want to construct your PICO:

**P**  maternal-fetal attachment in low-income mothers (specifically defined group)
**I**  health behaviors or health practices (event to be studied)
**C**  none (comparison of intervention)
**O**  neonatal outcomes (outcome)

In this example, the two main concepts are maternal-fetal attachment and health practices and how these impact neonatal outcomes. Many times when conducting a search, you only enter in keywords or controlled vocabulary for the first two elements of your PICO—in this case, maternal-fetal attachment and health practices or behaviors. The other elements can be added if your list of results is overwhelming, but many times you can pick from the results you have by just combining the first two. Figure 3-6 shows a Venn diagram of this approach.

Maternal-fetal attachment should be part of your search as a keyword search, but "prenatal bonding" is the appropriate CINAHL subject heading. To be comprehensive, you should use "OR" to link these terms together. The second concept, of health practices OR health behavior, is accomplished in a similar manner. The subject heading or controlled vocabulary assigned by the indexers could be added in for completeness. (See Figure 3-5 for screen shots from CINAHL on how to build a multi-line search using both keywords and subject headings.)

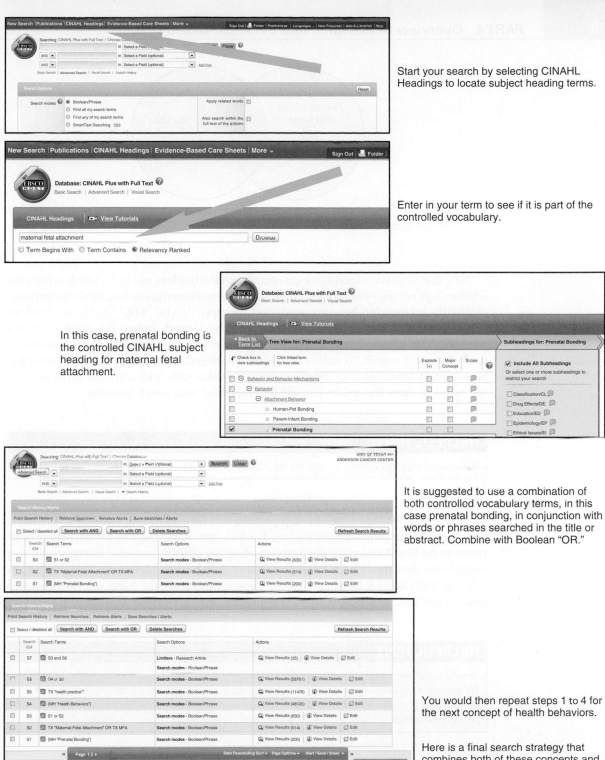

Start your search by selecting CINAHL Headings to locate subject heading terms.

Enter in your term to see if it is part of the controlled vocabulary.

In this case, prenatal bonding is the controlled CINAHL subject heading for maternal fetal attachment.

It is suggested to use a combination of both controlled vocabulary terms, in this case prenatal bonding, in conjunction with words or phrases searched in the title or abstract. Combine with Boolean "OR."

You would then repeat steps 1 to 4 for the next concept of health behaviors.

Here is a final search strategy that combines both of these concepts and applies the Research limit. Note that the Alhusen article is first on the list!

**FIGURE 3-5** Example from CINAHL to locate articles on MFA and health practices.

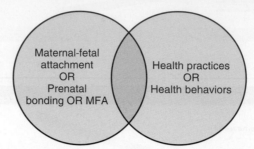

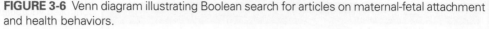

**FIGURE 3-6** Venn diagram illustrating Boolean search for articles on maternal-fetal attachment and health behaviors.

Note that these two concepts are connected with the **Boolean operator**, which defines the relationships between words or groups of words in your literature search. Boolean operators dictate the relationship between words and concepts. "AND," "OR," "NOT," are Boolean operators. "AND" requires that both concepts be located within the results that are returned. "OR" allows you to group together like terms or synonyms and "NOT" eliminates terms from your search. To restrict our retrieval to research, the "Research Article" limit has been applied. Searching is an iterative process and takes some trial and error to use the correct terms to locate the articles you will find useful for your search question.

### HELPFUL HINT

When combining synonyms for a concept, use the Boolean operator "OR"—OR is more!

Lawrence (2007) has a step-by-step presentation for conducting a search in CINAHL. She describes the controlled vocabulary, Boolean operators, and tips for narrowing your results in the EBSCO interface. For further reading, the series in *Journal of Emergency Nursing* outlines the steps for embarking on an evidence-based search (Bernardo, 2008; Engberg & Schlenk, 2007; Klem & Northcutt, 2008). These articles cover the stages of evidence-based practice and basic search hints.

### HELPFUL HINT

Look for useful tools within the search interfaces of electronic databases to make your searching more efficient. For example, when searching for a particular age-group, use the built-in limits of the database instead of relying on a keyword search. Other shortcuts include the Clinical Queries in CINAHL and MEDLINE that pull out therapy or diagnostic articles.

## How Do I Complete the Search?

Once you are confident in your search strategies for identifying key articles, it is time to critically read what you have found. Critically reading scholarly material, especially research articles, requires several readings and the use of critiquing criteria (see Chapters 1, 7, and 18). Do not be discouraged if all of the retrieved articles are not as useful as you first thought; this happens to the most experienced reviewer of literature. If most of the articles are not useful, be prepared to do another search, but discuss the search terms you will use next time with your instructor and/or the reference librarian; you may also want to add a third database. It is very helpful if you provide a printout of the search you have completed when consulting with your instructor or librarian. It is a good practice to always save your search history when conducting a search. In the example of maternal-fetal bonding and health behaviors in low-income women, the third database of choice may be PsycINFO (see Box 3-2).

### HELPFUL HINT

Read the abstract carefully to determine if it is a research article; you will usually see the use of level headings such as methodology and results in research articles. It is also a good idea to review the references of your articles; if any seem relevant, you can retrieve them.

## LITERATURE REVIEW FORMAT: WHAT TO EXPECT

Becoming familiar with the format of the literature review will help you use critiquing criteria to evaluate the review. To decide which style you will use so that your review is presented in a logical and organized manner, you must consider the following:

- The research or clinical question/topic
- The number of retrieved sources reviewed
- The number and type of research versus conceptual materials

Some reviews are written according to the variables being studied and presented chronologically under each variable. Others present the material chronologically with subcategories or variables discussed within each time period. Still others present the variables and include subcategories related to the study's type or designs or related variables.

Seiler and Moss (2012) logically present the concepts addressed by their qualitative study (see Appendix C). The researchers state that the purpose of the study was to "gain insight into the unique experiences of nurse practitioners who provide health care to the homeless." The authors have a specifically titled section called Literature Review on the second page of the article, where they review the aspects of their topic, including "Health status of the homeless," "Healthcare experiences of the homeless," and "The role of the NP." The authors' conclusion at the end of these three sections is that a study needs to be conducted to assess the health care provider's perceptions of providing health care to the homeless.

### EVIDENCE-BASED PRACTICE TIP

Sort the research articles you retrieve according to the levels of evidence model in Chapter 1. Remember that articles that are systematic reviews, especially meta-analyses, generally provide the strongest and most consistent evidence to include in a literature review.

## HELPFUL HINT

When writing your literature review you want to include enough information so that your professor or fellow students could re-create your search path and come up with the same results. This means including information regarding the databases searched, the date you searched, years of coverage, terms used, number of sources retrieved, and any limits or restrictions that you used to narrow the search. Also include any standardized tools you used to critically appraise your retrieved literature. Another important strategy is to make an outline which will become your level headings for your paper which will demonstrate your organization and the logic of the approach you used.

## APPRAISING THE EVIDENCE

Whether you were a researcher writing the literature review for a research study you planned to conduct, or a nurse or nursing student writing a literature review for an evidence-based practice or quality improvement project, you would need to critically appraise all research reports using appropriate criteria. If you are appraising an individual research study that is to be included in a literature review, it must be evaluated in terms of critical appraisal criteria that are related to each step of the research process (see the critical appraisal criteria at the end of Chapters 2, 3, 8 to 18 for quantitative studies and Chapters 5 to 7 for qualitative studies) so the strengths and weaknesses of each study can be identified. Standardized critical appraisal tools (see Chapters 1, 11, and 20) available for specific research designs (e.g., systematic reviews, clinical trials, cohort studies) can also be used to critically appraise research studies (see Chapters 1 and 18).

Critiquing the literature review of research or theoretical reports is a challenging task for seasoned consumers of research, so do not be surprised if you feel a little intimidated by the prospect of critiquing published research. The important issue is to determine the overall value of the literature review, including both research and theoretical materials. The purposes of a literature review (see Box 3-1) and the characteristics of a well-written literature review (Box 3-4) provide the framework for developing the evaluation criteria for a literature review.

The literature review should be presented in an organized manner. Theoretical and research literature can be presented chronologically from earliest work of the theorist or first studies on a topic to most recent; sometimes the theoretical literature that provided the foundation for the existing research will be presented first, followed by the research studies that were derived from this theoretical base. Other times, the literature can be clustered by concept, pro or con positions, or evidence that highlights differences in the theoretical and/or research findings. The overall question to be answered is, "Does the review of the literature develop and present a knowledge base for a research study, or does it provide sufficient evidence for an EBP or QI project?" (see Box 3-1).

However the literature review is organized, it should provide a strong knowledge base to carry out the research, educational, or clinical practice project. Questions related to the logical organization and presentation of the reviewed studies are somewhat more challenging for beginning research consumers. The more you read research studies, the more competent you become at differentiating a well-organized literature review from one that has a limited organizing framework.

Whenever possible, read both quantitative (meta-analyses) and qualitative (meta-syntheses) systematic reviews pertaining to a clinical question. "A quantitative systematic review is

> ## BOX 3-4 CHARACTERISTICS OF A WELL-WRITTEN REVIEW OF THE LITERATURE
>
> Each reviewed source of information reflects critical thinking and scholarly writing and is relevant to the study/topic/project, and the content meets the following criteria:
> - Identifies research questions and hypotheses or answers clinical questions
> - Consists of mainly primary sources; there are a sufficient number of research sources
> - Organizes the literature review using a systematic approach
> - Uses established critical appraisal criteria for specific study designs to evaluate the study for strengths, weaknesses, or limitations, as well as for conflicts or gaps in information that relate directly or indirectly to the area of interest
> - Provides evidence of a synthesis of the critiques that highlight the overall strengths and weaknesses of the studies reviewed and how they are similar or different between and among studies
> - Summarizes each research or conceptual article succinctly and with appropriate references
> - Concludes with a summary synthesis of the reviewed material and provides recommendations for implementing the study or EBP/QI project

considered a quantitative research methodology like a single study RCT or a cohort study. It is considered an original study which uses data from other studies as data sources. For citation purposes, it is a primary source" (D. Ciliska, personal communication, August 9, 2012). Well done meta-analyses uses a rigorous appraisal and synthesis of a group of like studies to answer a question. A systematic review would be considered a well done study and would represent the best available evidence on a particular clinical issue.

The systematic review on "follow-up for improving psychological well-being for women after miscarriage" (Murphy et al., 2012) is an example of a quantitative systematic review that critically appraises and synthesizes the evidence from research studies related to the whether follow-up affects the psychological well-being of women following miscarriages (see Appendix E).

The Critiquing Criteria box summarizes general critiquing criteria for a review of the literature. Other sets of critiquing criteria may phrase these questions differently or more broadly; for example, "Does the literature search seem adequate?" "Does the report demonstrate scholarly writing?" These may seem to be difficult questions for you to answer; one place to begin, however, is by determining whether the source is a refereed journal. It is reasonable to assume that a scholarly refereed journal publishes manuscripts that are adequately searched, use mainly primary sources, and are written in a scholarly manner. This does not mean, however, that every study reported in a refereed journal will meet all of the critiquing criteria for a literature review and other components of the study in an equal manner. Because of style differences and space constraints, each citation summarized is often very brief, or related citations may be summarized as a group and lack a critique. You still must answer the critiquing questions. Consultation with a faculty advisor may be necessary to develop skill in answering these questions.

The key to a strong literature review is a careful search of published and unpublished literature. Whether writing or critically appraising a literature review written for a published research study, it should reflect a synthesis or pulling together of the main points or value of all of the sources reviewed in relation to the study's research question or hypothesis (see Box 3-1). The relationship between and among these studies must be explained. The synthesis of a written review of the literature usually appears at the end of the review

## CRITIQUING CRITERIA

### Review of the Literature

1. Are all of the relevant concepts and variables included in the literature review?
2. Does the search strategy include an appropriate and adequate number of databases and other resources to identify key published and unpublished research and theoretical sources?
3. Are both theoretical literature and research literature included?
4. Is there an appropriate theoretical/conceptual framework to guide the development of the research study?
5. Are primary sources mainly used?
6. What gaps or inconsistencies in knowledge does the literature review uncover?
7. Does the literature review build on earlier studies?
8. Does the summary of each reviewed study reflect the essential components of the study design (e.g., type and size of sample, reliability and validity of instruments, consistency of data collection procedures, appropriate data analysis, identification of limitations)?
9. Does the critique of each reviewed study include strengths, weaknesses, or limitations of the design, conflicts, and gaps in information related to the area of interest?
10. Does the synthesis summary follow a logical sequence that presents the overall strengths and weaknesses of the reviewed studies and arrive at a logical conclusion?
11. Is the literature review presented in an organized format that flows logically (e.g., chronologically, clustered by concept or variables), enhancing the reader's ability to evaluate the need for the particular research study or evidence-based practice project?
12. Does the literature review follow the proposed purpose of the research study or evidence-based practice project?
13. Does the literature review generate research questions or hypotheses or answer a clinical question?

section before the research question or hypothesis reporting section and method section. If not labeled as such, it is usually evident in the last paragraph of the introduction and/or the end of the review of the literature.

Searching the literature, like critiquing the literature, is an acquired skill. Practicing your search and critical appraisal skills on a regular basis will make a huge difference. Seeking guidance from faculty is essential to developing critical appraisal skills. Synthesizing the body of literature you have critiqued is even more challenging. Critiquing the literature will help you apply new knowledge from your critical appraisal to practice. This process is vital to the "survival and growth of the nursing profession and is essential to evidence-based practice" (Pravikoff & Donaldson, 2001).

## HELPFUL HINT

- If you are doing an academic assignment make sure you check with your instructor as to whether or not unpublished material may be used and whether theoretical or conceptual articles are appropriate; if theoretical and conceptual articles are appropriate, secure critiquing criteria for this type of literature.
- Use standardized critical appraisal criteria to evaluate your research articles.
- Make a table to represent the components of your study and fill in your evaluation to help you see the big picture of your analysis (see Chapter 20 for an example of a summary table).
- Synthesize the results of your analysis to try and determine what was similar or different between and among these studies related to your topic/clinical question and then draw a conclusion.

## KEY POINTS

- Review of the literature is defined as a broad, comprehensive, in-depth, systematic critique and synthesis of scholarly publications, unpublished scholarly print and online materials, audiovisual materials, and personal communication.
- Review of the literature is used for development of research studies, as well as other consumer of research activities such as development of evidence-based practice and quality improvement projects.
- There are differences between use of the review of the literature for research and for EBP/QI projects. For an EBP/QI project, your search should focus on the highest level of primary source literature available per the hierarchy of evidence, and it should relate to the specific clinical problem.
- The main objectives for the consumer of research in relation to conducting and writing a literature review are to acquire the ability to (1) conduct an electronic research and/or print research search on a topic; (2) efficiently retrieve a sufficient amount of materials for a literature review in relation to the topic and scope of project; (3) critically appraise (i.e., critique) research and theoretical material based on accepted critiquing criteria; (4) critically evaluate published reviews of the literature based on accepted standardized critiquing criteria; (5) synthesize the findings of the critique materials for relevance to the purpose of the selected scholarly project; and (6) determine applicability to practice.
- Primary research and theoretical resources are essential for literature reviews.
- Secondary sources, such as commentaries on research articles from peer-reviewed journals, are part of a learning strategy for developing critical critiquing skills.
- It is more efficient to use electronic databases rather than print resources or general web search engines for retrieving materials.
- Strategies for efficiently retrieving literature for nursing include consulting the reference librarian and using at least two online sources (e.g., CINAHL, MEDLINE).
- Literature reviews are usually organized according to variables, as well as chronologically.
- Critiquing and synthesizing a number of research articles, including systematic reviews, is essential to implementing evidence-based nursing practice.

## CRITICAL THINKING CHALLENGES

- Using the PICO format, generate a clinical question related to health promotion for elementary school children.
- For an EBP project, why is it necessary to critically appraise studies that are published in a refereed journal?
- Who should be the main users of the 6S pyramid model?
- How does the 6S pyramid model develop your critical appraisal skills?
- A general guideline for a literature search is to use a timeline of 3 to 5 years. When would a nurse researcher or consumer of research need to search beyond this timeline?
- What is the relationship of the research article's literature review to the theoretical or conceptual framework?

# REFERENCES

Alhusen, J. L., Gross, D., Hayat, X., et al. (2012). The influence of maternal-fetal attachment and health practices on neonatal outcomes in low-income, urban women. *Research in Nursing & Health, 35*(2), 112–120.

Bernardo, L. M. (2008). Finding the best evidence, part 1: Understanding electronic databases. *Journal of Emergency Nursing, 34*(1), 59–60.

Ciliska, D. Personal communication, August 9, 2012.

DiCenso, A., Bayley, L., & Haynes, R. B. (2009). Accessing pre-appraised evidence: Fine-tuning the 5S model into a 6S model. *Evidence-Based Nursing, 12*(4), 99–101.

Duncan, V., & Holtslander, L. (2012). Utilizing grounded theory to explore the information-seeking behavior of senior nursing students. *Journal of the Medical Library Association, 100*(1), 20–27.

Engberg, S., & Schlenk, E. A. (2007). Asking the right question. *Journal of Emergency Nursing, 33*(6), 571–573.

Haynes, R. B., Sackett, D. L., Guyatt et al. (2006). *Clinical epidemiology: How to do clinical practice research* (3rd ed.). Philadelphia, PA: Lippincott, Williams & Wilkins.

Kendall, Sandra. (2008). Evidence-Based Resources Simplified, *Canadian Family Physician, 54*(2), 241–243.

Klem, M. L., & Northcutt, T. (2008). Finding the best evidence, part 2: The basics of literature searches. *Journal of Emergency Nursing, 34*(2), 151–153.

Lawrence, J. C. (2007). Techniques for searching the CINAHL database using the EBSCO interface. *Association of periOperative Registered Nurses (AORN) Journal, 85*(4), 779-780, 782–788, 790–771.

Mercer, R. T. (2004). Becoming a mother versus maternal role attainment. *Journal of Nursing Scholarship, 36*(3), 226–232.

Murphy, F. A., Lipp, A., & Powles, D. L. (2012). Follow-up for improving psychological well being for women after a miscarriage. *Cochrane Database of Systematic Reviews, 3*, CD008679.

National Library of Medicine. *PubMed Quick Start*[Internet]. Retrieved from http://www.ncbi.nlm.nih.gov/books/NBK3827/#pubmedhelp.PubMed_Quick_Start

Pravikoff, D., & Donaldson, N. (2001). The Online Journal of Clinical Innovations. *Online Journal of Issues in Nursing, 6*(1). Retrieved from www.nursingworld.org/MainMenuCategories/ANAMarketplace/ANAPeriodicals/OJIN/TableofContents/Volume62001/No2May01/ArticlePreviousTopic/ClinicalInnovations.asp

Richardson, W. S., Wilson, M. C., Nishikawa, J., & Hayward, R. S. (1995). The well-built clinical question: a key to evidence-based decisions. *ACP Journal Club, 123*(3), A12–13.

Seiler, A. J., & Moss, V. A. (2012). The experiences of nurse practitioners providing health care to the homeless. *Journal of the American Academy of Nurse Practitioners, 24*(5), 303–312.

Thomas, M., Elliott, J., Rao, S., et al. (2012). A randomized, clinical trial of education or motivational-interviewing-based coaching compared to usual care to improve cancer pain management. *Oncology Nursing Forum, 39*(1), 39–49.

# evolve WEBSITE

*Go to Evolve at http://evolve.elsevier.com/LoBiondo/ for review questions, critiquing exercises, and additional research articles for practice in reviewing and critiquing.*

# Theoretical Frameworks for Research

*Melanie McEwen*

WEBSITE

*Go to Evolve at http://evolve.elsevier.com/LoBiondo/ for review questions, critiquing exercises, and additional research articles for practice in reviewing and critiquing.*

## LEARNING OUTCOMES

*After reading this chapter, you should be able to do the following:*

- Identify the purpose of conceptual and theoretical frameworks for nursing research.
- Describe how a conceptual framework guides research.
- Differentiate between conceptual and operational definitions.
- Describe the relationship between theory, research, and practice.

- Describe the points of critical appraisal used to evaluate the appropriateness, cohesiveness, and consistency of a framework guiding research.
- Explain the ways in which theory is used in nursing research.

## KEY TERMS

| | | | |
|---|---|---|---|
| concept | deductive | middle range theory | situation-specific theory |
| conceptual definition | grand theory | model | theoretical framework |
| conceptual framework | inductive | operational definition | theory |
| construct | | | |

The author would like to acknowledge the contribution of Patricia Liehr, who contributed this chapter in a previous edition.

To introduce the discussion of the use of theoretical frameworks for nursing research, consider the example of Emily, a novice oncology nurse. From this case study, reflect on how nurses can understand the theoretical underpinnings of both nursing research and evidence-based nursing practice, and re-affirm how nurses should integrate research into practice.

Emily graduated with her BSN a little more than a year ago and recently changed positions to work on a pediatric oncology unit in a large hospital. She quickly learned that working with very ill, and often dying children is tremendously rewarding, even though it is frequently heartbreaking.

One of Emily's first patients was Benny, a 14-year-old boy admitted with a recurrence of leukemia. When she first cared for Benny, he was extremely ill. Benny's oncologist implemented the protocols for cases such as his, but the team was careful to explain to Benny and his family that his prognosis was guarded. In the early days of his hospitalization, Emily cried with his mother when they received his daily lab values and there was no apparent improvement. She observed that Benny was growing increasingly fatigued and had little appetite. Despite his worsening condition, however, Benny and his parents were unfailingly positive, making plans for a vacation to the mountains and the upcoming school year.

At the end of her shift one night before several days off, Emily hugged Benny's parents as she feared that Benny would die before her next scheduled work day. Several days later, when she listened to the report at the start of her shift, Emily was amazed to learn that Benny had been heartily eating a normal diet. He was fully ambulatory and had been cruising the halls with his baseball coach and playing video games with two of his cousins. When she entered Benny's room for her initial assessment, she saw the much-improved teenager dressed in shorts and a T-shirt, sitting up in bed using his iPad. A half-finished chocolate milkshake was on the table in easy reaching distance. He joked with Emily about *Angry Birds* as she performed her assessment. Benny steadily improved over the ensuing days and eventually went home with his leukemia again in remission.

As Emily became more comfortable in the role of oncology nurse, she continued to notice patterns among the children and adolescents on her floor. Many got better, even though their conditions were often critical. In contrast, some of the children who had better prognoses failed to improve as much, or as quickly, as anticipated. She realized that the kids who did better than expected seemed to have common attributes or characteristics, including positive attitudes, supportive family and friends, and strong determination to "beat" their cancer. Over lunch one day, Emily talked with her mentor, Marie, about her observations, commenting that on a number of occasions she had seen patients rebound when she thought that death was imminent.

Marie smiled. "Fortunately this is a pattern that we see quite frequently. Many of our kids are amazingly resilient." Marie told Emily about the work of several nursing researchers who studied the phenomenon of resilience and gave her a list of articles reporting on their findings. Emily followed up with Marie's prompting and learned about "psychosocial resilience in adolescents" (Tusaie et al., 2007) and "adolescent resilience" (Ahern, 2006; Ahern et al., 2008). These works led her to a "middle range theory of resilience" (Polk, 1997). From her readings, she gained insight into resilience, learning to recognize it in her patients. She also identified ways she might encourage and even promote resilience in children and teenagers. Eventually, she decided to enroll in a graduate nursing program to learn how to research different phenomena of concern to her patients and discover ways to apply the findings to improve nursing care and patient outcomes.

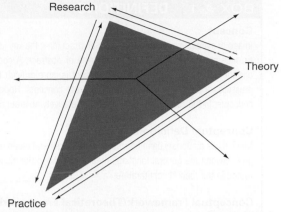

Research

Theory

Practice

**FIGURE 4-1** Discipline knowledge: theory-practice-research connection.

## PRACTICE-THEORY-RESEARCH LINKS

Several important aspects of how theory is used in nursing research are embedded in Emily's story. First, it is important to notice the links among practice, theory, and research. Each is intricately connected with the others to create the knowledge base for the discipline of nursing (Figure 4-1). In her practice, Emily recognized a pattern of characteristics in some patients that appeared to enhance their recovery. Her mentor directed her to research that other nurses had published on the phenomenon of "resilience." Emily was then able to apply the information on resilience and related research findings as she planned and implemented care. Her goal was to enhance each child's resilience as much as possible and thereby improve their outcomes.

Another key message from the case study is the importance of reflecting on an observed phenomenon and discussing it with colleagues. This promotes questioning and collaboration, as nurses seek ways to improve practice. Finally, Emily was encouraged to go to the literature to search out what had been published related to the phenomenon she had observed. Reviewing the research led her to a middle range theory on resilience and challenged her to consider how she might ultimately conduct her own research into the phenomenon.

## OVERVIEW OF THEORY

Theory is a set of interrelated concepts that provides a systematic view of a phenomenon. A theory allows relationships to be proposed and predictions made, which in turn can suggest potential actions. Beginning with a theory gives a researcher a logical way of collecting data to describe, explain, and predict nursing practice, making it critical in research.

In nursing, science is the result of the interchange between research and theory. The purpose of research is to build knowledge through the generation or testing of theory that can then be applied in practice. To build knowledge, research should develop within a theoretical structure or blueprint that facilitates analysis and interpretation of findings. The use of theory provides structure and organization to nursing knowledge. It is important that nurses understand that nursing practice is based on the theories that are generated and validated through research (McEwen & Wills, 2011).

## BOX 4-1   DEFINITIONS

**Concept**

Image or symbolic representation of an abstract idea; the key identified element of a phenomenon that is necessary to understand it. Concept can be concrete or abstract. A concrete concept can be easily identified, quantified, and measured; whereas an abstract concept is more difficult to quantify or measure. For example, weight, blood pressure, and body temperature are concrete concepts. Hope, uncertainty, and spiritual pain are more abstract concepts. In the case study, resilience is a relatively abstract concept.

**Conceptual Definition**

Much like a dictionary definition, conveying the general meaning of the concept. However, the conceptual definition goes beyond the general language meaning found in the dictionary by defining or explaining the concept as it is rooted in the theoretical literature.

**Conceptual Framework/Theoretical Framework**

A set of interrelated concepts that represents an image of a phenomenon. These two terms are often used interchangeably. The conceptual/theoretical framework refers to a structure that provides guidance for research or practice. The framework identifies the key concepts and describes their relationships to each other and to the phenomena (variables) of concern to nursing. It serves as the foundation on which a study can be developed or as a map to aid in the design of the study.

**Construct**

Complex concept; constructs usually comprise more than one concept and are built or "constructed" to fit a purpose. Health promotion, maternal-infant bonding, health-seeking behaviors, and health-related quality of life are examples of constructs.

**Model**

A graphic or symbolic representation of a phenomenon. A graphic model is empirical and can be readily represented. A model of an eye or a heart is an example. A symbolic or theoretical model depicts a phenomenon that is not directly observable and is expressed in language or symbols. Written music or Einstein's theory of relativity are examples of symbolic models. Theories used by nurses or developed by nurses frequently include symbolic models. Models are very helpful in allowing the reader to visualize the key concepts/constructs and their identified interrelationships.

**Operational Definition**

Specifies how the concept will be measured. That is, the operational definition defines what instruments will be used to assess the presence of the concept and will be used to describe the amount or degree to which the concept exists.

**Theory**

Set of interrelated concepts that provides a systematic view of a phenomenon.

In an integrated, reciprocal manner, theory guides research and practice; practice enables testing of theory and generates research questions; and research contributes to theory-building and establishing practice guidelines (see Figure 4-1). Therefore, what is learned through practice, theory, and research interweaves to create the knowledge fabric of nursing. From this perspective, like Emily in the case study, each nurse should be involved in the process of contributing to the knowledge or evidence-based practice of nursing.

Several key terms are often used when discussing theory. It is necessary to understand these terms when considering how to apply theory in practice and research. They include **concept, conceptual definition, conceptual/theoretical framework, construct, model, operational definition,** and **theory.** Each term is defined and summarized in Box 4-1.

| TABLE 4-1 | CONCEPTS AND VARIABLES: CONCEPTUAL AND OPERATIONAL DEFINITIONS | | |
|---|---|---|---|
| **CONCEPT** | **CONCEPTUAL DEFINITION** | **VARIABLE** | **OPERATIONAL DEFINITION** |
| Maternal-fetal attachment (Alhusen et al., 2012) | "The extent to which women engage in behaviors that represent an affiliation and interaction with their unborn child" | MFA | Total score on Maternal-Fetal Attachment Scale (a 24-item, Likert-type questionnaire) |
| Health practices (Alhusen et al., 2012) | Health practices that mother engages in during pregnancy | Health practices | Total score on the Health Practices in Pregnancy Questionnaire II (a 34-item, Likert-type questionnaire) |
| Neonatal outcomes | Compilation of birth weight and gestational age | Neonatal outcomes | Scores based on gestational age and scored against reference values of birth weight at 22-44 completed weeks of gestation |

Concepts and constructs are the major components of theories, and convey the essential ideas or elements of a theory. When a nurse researcher decides to study a concept/construct, the researcher must precisely and explicitly describe and explain the concept, devise a mechanism to identify and confirm the presence of the concept of interest, and determine a method to measure or quantify it. To illustrate, Table 4-1 shows the key concepts and conceptual and operational definitions provided by Alhusen and colleagues (2012) in their study on maternal fetal attachment and neonatal outcomes (see Appendix B).

## TYPES OF THEORIES USED BY NURSES

As stated previously, a theory is a set of interrelated concepts that provides a systematic view of a phenomenon. Theory provides a foundation and structure that may be used for the purpose of explaining or predicting another phenomenon. In this way, a theory is like a blueprint or a guide for modeling a structure. A blueprint depicts the elements of a structure and the relationships among the elements; similarly, a theory depicts the concepts that compose it and suggests how the concepts are related.

Nurses use a multitude of different theories as the foundation or structure for research and practice. Many have been developed by nurses and are explicitly related to nursing practice; others, however, come from other disciplines. Knowledge that draws upon both nursing and non-nursing theories is extremely important in order to provide excellent, evidence-based care.

### Theories from Related Disciplines used in Nursing Practice and Research

Like engineering, architecture, social work, and teaching, nursing is a practice discipline. That means that nurses use concepts, constructs, models, and theories from many

| TABLE 4-2 | THEORIES USED IN NURSING PRACTICE AND RESEARCH |
|---|---|
| **DISCIPLINE** | **EXAMPLES OF THEORIES/CONCEPTS USED BY NURSES** |
| Biomedical sciences | Germ theory (principles of infection), pain theories, immune function, genetics/genomics, pharmacotherapeutics |
| Sociologic sciences | Systems theory (e.g., VonBertalanffy), family theory (e.g., Bowen), role theory (e.g., Merton), critical social theory (e.g., Habermas), cultural diversity (e.g., Leininger) |
| Behavioral sciences | Developmental theories (e.g., Erikson), human needs theories (e.g., Maslow), personality theories (e.g., Freud), stress theories (e.g., Lazarus & Folkman), health belief model (e.g., Rosenstock) |
| Learning theories | Behavioral learning theories (e.g., Pavlov, Skinner), cognitive development/interaction theories (e.g., Piaget), adult learning theories (e.g., Knowles) |
| Leadership/management | Change theory (e.g., Lewin), conflict management (e.g., Rapaport), quality framework (e.g., Donabedian) |

disciplines in addition to nursing-specific theories. This is, to a large extent, the rationale for the "liberal arts" education that is required before entering a baccalaureate nursing (BSN) program. Exposure to knowledge and theories of basic and natural sciences (e.g., mathematics, chemistry, biology) and social sciences (e.g., psychology, sociology, political science) provides a fundamental understanding of those disciplines and allows for application of key principles, concepts, and theories from each, as appropriate.

Likewise, BSN-prepared nurses use principles of administration and management and learning theories in their patient-centered, holistic practices. Table 4-2 lists a few of the many theories and concepts from other disciplines that are commonly used by nurses in practice and research that become part of the foundational framework for nursing.

## Nursing Theories used in Practice and Research

In addition to the many theories and concepts from disciplines other than nursing, the nursing literature presents a number of theories that were developed specifically by and for nurses. Typically, nursing theories reflect concepts, relationships, and processes that contribute to the development of a body of knowledge specific to nursing's concerns. Understanding these interactions and relationships among the concepts and

### HELPFUL HINT

In research and practice, concepts often create descriptions or images that emerge from a conceptual definition. For instance, pain is a concept with different meanings based on what type or aspect of pain being referred to. As such, there are a number of methods and instruments to measure pain. So a nurse researching postoperative pain would conceptually define pain based on the patient's perceived discomfort associated with surgery, and then select a pain scale/instrument that allows the researcher to operationally define pain as the patient's score on that scale.

| BOX 4-2 | GRAND THEORY EXAMPLE |
|---|---|

Lavoie, Talbot, and Mathieu (2011) used Neuman's model (1995) as a guideline to identify primary, secondary, and tertiary prevention activities to prevent PTSD among nurses exposed to traumatic events in the workplace. The researchers used a qualitative study design consisting of semi-structured interviews and focus groups. They determined that support activities such as peer support systems, psycho-education, and emergency department simulations can and should be developed to address all three levels of prevention.

phenomena is essential to evidence-based nursing care. Further, theories unique to nursing help define how it is different from other disciplines.

Nursing theories are often described based on their scope or degree of abstraction. Typically, these are reported as "grand," "middle range," or "situation specific" (also called "micro-range") nursing theories. Each is described in this section.

## Grand Nursing Theories

Grand nursing theories are sometimes referred to as nursing conceptual models and include the theories/models that were developed to describe the discipline of nursing as a whole. This comprises the works of nurse theorists such as Florence Nightingale, Virginia Henderson, Martha Rogers, Dorthea Orem, and Betty Neuman. Grand nursing theories/models are all-inclusive conceptual structures that tend to include views on person, health, and environment to create a perspective of nursing. This most abstract level of theory has established a knowledge base for the discipline. These works are used as the conceptual basis for practice and research, and are tested in research studies.

One grand theory is not better than another with respect to nursing research. Rather, these varying perspectives allow a researcher to select a framework for research that best depicts the concepts and relationships of interest, and decide where and how they can be measured as study variables. What is most important about the use of grand nursing theoretical frameworks for research is the logical connection of the theory to the research question and the study design. Nursing literature contains excellent examples of research studies that examine concepts and constructs from grand nursing theories. See Box 4-2 for an example.

## Middle Range Nursing Theories

Beginning in the late 1980s, nurses recognized that grand theories were difficult to apply in research, and considerable attention moved to the development and research of "middle range" nursing theories. In contrast to grand theories, middle range nursing theories contain a limited number of concepts and are focused on a limited aspect of reality. As a result, they are more easily tested through research and more readily used as frameworks for research studies (McEwen & Wills, 2011).

A growing number of middle range nursing theories have been developed, tested through nursing research, and/or are used as frameworks for nursing research. Examples are Pender's Health Promotion Model (Pender et al., 2006); the Theory of Uncertainty in Illness (Mishel, 1988, 1990, 1999); and the Theory of Holistic Comfort (Kolcaba, 1994, 2009).

Examples of development, use, and testing of middle range theories are becoming increasingly common in the nursing literature. The Theory of Uncertainty in Illness, one fairly commonly used middle range nursing theory, was part of the theoretical framework

BOX 4-3    MIDDLE RANGE THEORY EXEMPLARS

An integrative research review was undertaken to evaluate the connection between symptom experience and illness-related uncertainty among patients diagnosed with brain tumors. The Theory of Uncertainty in Illness (Mishel, 1988, 1990, 1999) was the conceptual framework for interpretation of the review's findings. The researchers concluded that somatic symptoms are antecedent to uncertainty among brain tumor patients, and that nursing strategies should attempt to understand and manage symptoms to reduce anxiety and distress by mitigating illness-related uncertainty (Cahill et al., 2012).

Hurlbut et al. (2011) conducted a study that examined the relationship between spirituality and health-promoting behaviors among homeless women. This study was based on Pender's Health Promotion Model (HPM) (Pender, Murdough, & Parsons, 2006). Several variables for the study were operationalized and measured using the Health Promotion Lifestyle Profile II, a survey instrument that was developed to be used in studies that focus on HPM concepts.

in a research review that focused on symptom investigation and management in brain tumor patients (Cahill et al., 2012) (See Box 4-3).

## Situation-Specific Nursing Theories: Micro-Range, Practice, or Prescriptive Theories

Situation-specific nursing theories are sometimes referred to as micro-range, practice, or prescriptive theories. Situation-specific theories are more specific than middle range theories and are composed of a limited number of concepts. They are narrow in scope, explain a small aspect of phenomena and processes of interest to nurses, and are usually limited to specific populations or field of practice (Im, 2005; Peterson, 2008; Whall, 2005). Im and Chang (2012) observed that as nursing research began to require theoretical bases that are easily operationalized into nursing research, situation-specific theories provided closer links to research and practice. The idea and practice of identifying a work as a situation-specific theory is still fairly new. Often what is noted by an author as a middle range theory would more appropriately be termed situation specific. Most commonly, however, a theory is developed from a research study, and no designation (e.g., middle range, situation-specific) is attached to it.

Examples of self-designated, situation-specific theories include the theory of heart failure self-care (Riegel & Dickson, 2008) and a situation-specific theory of Asian immigrant women's menopausal symptom experiences (Im, 2010). Increasingly, qualitative research studies are being used by nurses to develop and support theories and models that can and should be expressly identified as situation specific. This will become progressively more common as more nurses seek graduate study and are involved in nursing research, and increasing attention is given to the importance of evidence-based practice (Im & Chang, 2012; McEwen & Wills, 2011).

Im and Chang (2012) conducted a comprehensive research review that examined how theory has been described in nursing literature for the last decade. They reported a dramatic increase in the number of grounded theory research studies, along with increases in studies using both middle range and situation-specific theories. In contrast, the number and percentage directly dealing with grand nursing theories has fluctuated. Table 4-3 provides examples of grand, middle range, and situation-specific nursing theories used in nursing research.

| | | |
|---|---|---|
| **TABLE 4-3** | **LEVELS OF NURSING THEORY: EXAMPLES OF GRAND, MIDDLE RANGE, AND SITUATION-SPECIFIC NURSING THEORIES** | |

| GRAND NURSING THEORIES | MIDDLE RANGE NURSING THEORIES | SITUATION-SPECIFIC (OR MICRO) NURSING THEORIES |
|---|---|---|
| Florence Nightingale: Notes on Nursing (1860) | Health promotion model (Pender, Murdaugh, & Parsons, 2006) | Theory of the peaceful end of life (Ruland & Moore, 1998) |
| Dorothy Johnson: The Behavioral Systems Model for Nursing (1990) | Uncertainty in illness theory (Mishel, 1988, 1990, 1999) | Theory of chronic sorrow (Eakes, Burke, & Hainsworth, 1998) |
| Martha Rogers: Nursing: A Science of Unitary Human Beings (1970; 1990) | Theory of unpleasant symptoms (Lenz et al., 2009) | Asian immigrant women's menopausal symptom experience in the U.S. (Im, 2010) |
| Betty Neuman: The Neuman Systems Model (1995) | Theory of holistic comfort/theory of comfort (Kolcaba, 1994; 2009) | Theory of caucasians' cancer pain experience (Im, 2006) |
| Dorthea Orem: The Self Care Deficit Nursing Theory (2001) | Theory of resilience (Polk, 1997) | Becoming a mother (Mercer, 2004) |
| Callista Roy: Roy Adaptation Model (2009) | Theory of health promotion in preterm infants (Mefford, 2004) | |
| | Theory of flight nursing expertise (Reimer & Moore, 2010) | |

# HOW THEORY IS USED IN NURSING RESEARCH

Nursing research is concerned with the study of individuals in interaction with their environments. The intent is to discover interventions that promote optimal functioning and self-care across the life-span; the goal is to foster maximum wellness (McEwen & Wills, 2011). In nursing research, theories are used in the research process in one of three ways:

- Theory is generated as the outcome of a research study (qualitative designs)
- Theory is used as a research framework, as the context for a study (qualitative or quantitative designs)
- Research is undertaken to test a theory (quantitative designs)

## Theory-Generating Nursing Research

When research is undertaken to create or generate theory, the idea is to examine a phenomenon within a particular context and identify and describe its major elements or events. Theory-generating research is focused on "What" and "How," but does not usually attempt to explain "Why." Theory-generating research is **inductive**; that is, it uses a process in which generalizations are developed from specific observations. Research methods used by nurses for theory generation include concept analysis, case studies, phenomenology, grounded theory, ethnography, and historical inquiry. Chapters 5, 6, and 7 describe these research methods. As you review qualitative methods and study examples in the literature, be attuned to the stated purpose(s) or outcomes of the research and note whether a situation-specific (practice or micro) theory or model or middle range theory is presented as a finding or outcome.

## Theory as Framework for Nursing Research

In nursing research, theory is most commonly used as the conceptual framework, theoretical framework, or conceptual model for a study. Frequently, correlational research designs attempt to discover and specify relationships between characteristics of individuals, groups, situations, or events. Correlational research studies often focus on one or more concepts, frameworks, or theories to collect data to measure dimensions or characteristics of phenomena and explain why and the extent to which one phenomenon is related to another. Data is typically gathered by observation or self-report instruments (see Chapter 10 for nonexperimental designs).

> **HELPFUL HINT**
>
> When researchers use conceptual frameworks to guide their studies, you can expect to find a system of ideas synthesized for the purpose of organizing, thinking, and providing study direction. Whether the researcher is using a conceptual or a theoretical framework, conceptual and then operational definitions will emerge from the framework.

Often in correlational (nonexperimental/quantitative) research, one or more theories will be used as the conceptual/theoretical framework for the study. In these cases, a theory is used as the context for the study and basis for interpretation of the findings. The theory helps guide the study and enhances the value of its findings by setting the findings within the context of the theory and previous works describing use of the theory in practice or research. When using a theory as a conceptual framework for research, the researcher will
- Identify an existing theory(ies) and designate and explain the study's theoretical framework
- Develop research questions/hypotheses consistent with the framework
- Provide conceptual definitions taken from the theory/framework
- Use data collection instrument(s) (and operational definitions) appropriate to the framework
- Interpret/explain findings based on the framework
- Determine support for the theory/framework based on the study findings
- Discuss implications for nursing and recommendations for future research to address the concepts and relationships designated by the framework

## Theory-Testing Nursing Research

Finally, nurses may use research to test a theory. Theory testing is **deductive**; that is, one in which hypotheses are derived from theory and tested, employing experimental research methods. In experimental research, the intent is to move beyond explanation to prediction of relationships between characteristics or phenomena among different groups or in various situations. Experimental research designs require manipulation of one or more phenomena to determine how the manipulation affects or changes the dimension or characteristics of other phenomena. In these cases, theoretical statements are written as research questions or hypotheses. Experimental research requires quantifiable data, and statistical analyses are used to measure differences (see Chapter 9).

In theory-testing research, the researcher (1) chooses a theory of interest and selects a propositional statement to be examined; (2) develops hypotheses that have measurable variables; (3) conducts the study; (4) interprets the findings considering the predictive ability of the theory; and (5) determines if there are implications for further use of the theory in nursing practice and/or whether further research could be beneficial.

**EVIDENCE-BASED PRACTICE TIP**

In practice, you can use observation and analysis to consider the nuances of situations that matter to patient health. This process often generates questions that are cogent for improving patient care. In turn, following the observations and questions into the literature can lead to published research that can be applied in practice.

## APPLICATION TO RESEARCH AND EVIDENCE-BASED PRACTICE

To build knowledge that promotes evidence-based practice, research should develop within a theoretical structure that facilitates analysis and interpretation of findings. When a study is placed within a theoretical context, the theory guides the research process, forms the questions, and aids in design, analysis, and interpretation. In that regard, a theory, conceptual model, or conceptual framework provides parameters for the research and enables the researcher to weave the facts together.

As a consumer of research, you should know how to recognize the theoretical foundation of a study. Whether evaluating a qualitative or a quantitative study, it is essential to understand where and how the research can be integrated within nursing science and applied in evidence-based practice. As a result, it is important to identify whether the intent is to (1) generate a theory, (2) use the theory as the framework that guides the study, or (3) test a theory. This section provides examples that illustrate different types of theory used in nursing research (e.g., non-nursing theories, middle range nursing theories) and examples from the literature highlighting the different ways that nurses can use theory in research (e.g., theory-generating study, theory testing, theory as a conceptual framework).

### Application of Theory in Qualitative Research

As discussed, in many instances, a theory, framework, or model is the outcome of nursing research. This is often the case in research employing qualitative methods such as grounded theory. From the study's findings, the researcher builds either an implicit or an explicit structure explaining or describing the findings of the research.

For example, Seiler and Moss (2012) (see Appendix C) reported findings from a study of nurse practitioners (NPs) who care for homeless persons. The researchers were interested in understanding the unique experiences of NPs to help healthcare providers gain insight into this very specialized population and to aid in improving care. Their findings were grouped into five "themes": why they do what they do; a unique population with unique needs; NP characteristics; how the relationship develops; and lessons learned. Multiple sub-themes and salient examples were discussed, which would be useful for any healthcare provider working with homeless persons. The researchers concluded that NPs "must take the entire context of their patients' lives into consideration in order to find the most compassionate and effective way to treat, diagnose, and provide education for each individual." Thus, the findings from this study can be used as part of a framework for future practitioners to use and researchers to expand on.

Generally, when the researcher is using qualitative methods and inductive reasoning, the critical reader will find the framework or theory at the end of the manuscript in the discussion section (see Chapters 5 to 7). The reader should be aware that the framework may be implicitly suggested rather than explicitly diagrammed (Box 4-4).

The nursing literature is full of similar examples in which inductive, qualitative research methods were used to develop theory. Banner and colleagues (2011) conducted a grounded

> ### BOX 4-4    RESEARCH
>
> Lasiter (2011) used grounded theory research methods to examine perceptions of "feeling safe" in an intensive care unit (ICU). In this study, 10 older adults were interviewed at three time points: in the ICU, after transferring to an intermediate care unit, and following discharge. Analysis of the data resulted in a theoretical model of older adults' perception of feeling safe in the ICU. In the theory, Lasiter identified "requisites" to feeling safe: initiative, oversight, predictability, and proximity. She determined that "feeling safe" in the ICU was a function of the ability to "initiate interaction" with a nurse (e.g., use the call button), oversight (knowing that the nurses were watching and monitoring them), predictability (believing the nurses had a high level of education and knew what to do), and proximity (feeling that the nurses were close enough to respond quickly). These requisites, coupled with the expected nurse-patient action and interaction, determined the patient's level of "feeling safe." She concluded that nurses can use the model to improve nursing care in the ICU.

theory study of 30 women designed to enhance understanding of the life adjustments made by women who have had cardiac surgery. They stated that there is a need to develop innovative, gender-sensitive health education and services for women undergoing coronary artery bypass surgery. Finally, Purtzer (2012) developed a theoretical model—the transformative decision-making process for mammography screening—based on a grounded theory study of low-income women. She concluded that nursing interventions can serve as catalysts to encourage women in their decision to have a mammogram.

## Examples of Theory as Research Framework

When the researcher uses quantitative methods, the framework is typically identified and explained at the beginning of the paper, before the discussion of study methods. For example, in their study examining the impact of post-traumatic stress symptoms (PTSS) on relationships among Army couples, Melvin and colleagues (2012) (see Appendix D) explained how the Couple Adaptation to Traumatic Stress (CATS) Model (developed by Nelson-Goff & Smith, 2005) was used as the conceptual framework for the study. Specifically, the research examined the effect of PTSS on and among the identified variables, specifically looking at resilience, moderating factors (e.g., age, gender, rank) and couple functioning factors (e.g., conflict resolution problems). The CATS model was used to form their hypotheses and interpret their findings. Their conclusions were interpreted with respect to the framework, suggesting that nurses and other health care professionals working with military couples should seek to understand the interaction of the model's variables and relationships when providing care.

The Transtheoretical Model (TTM) (Prochaska & DiClemente, 1984) is a behavioral change theory frequently used by nurse researchers. The TTM was the conceptual framework for an experimental study that compared motivational-interviewing coaching with standard treatment in managing cancer pain (Thomas et al., 2012) (see Appendix A). In another example, one of the works read by Emily from the case study dealt with resilience in adolescents (Tusaie et al., 2007). The researchers in this work used the Lazarus theory of stress and coping as part of the theoretical framework researching factors such as optimism, family support, age, and life events.

## Examples of Theory-Testing Research

Although many nursing studies that are experimental and quasi experimental (see Chapter 9) are frequently conducted to test interventions (see Appendix A), examples of research expressly conducted to test a theory are relatively rare in nursing literature. One such work is

## CRITERIA FOR CRITIQUING A THEORETICAL FRAMEWORK

1. Is the framework for research clearly identified?
2. Is the framework consistent with a nursing perspective?
3. Is the framework appropriate to guide research on the subject of interest?
4. Are the concepts and variables clearly and appropriately defined?
5. Was sufficient literature presented to support study of the selected concepts?
6. Is there a logical, consistent link between the framework, the concepts being studied, and the methods of measurement?
7. Are the study findings examined in relationship to the framework?

a multi-site, multi-methods study examining women's perceptions of caesarean birth (Fawcett et al., 2012). This work tested multiple relationships within the Roy Adaptation Model as applied to the study population.

## Critiquing the Use of Theory in Nursing Research

It is beneficial to seek out, identify, and follow the theoretical framework or source of the background of a study. The framework for research provides guidance for the researcher as study questions are fine-tuned, methods for measuring variables are selected, and analyses are planned. Once data are collected and analyzed, the framework is used as a base of comparison. Ideally, the research should explain: Did the findings coincide with the framework? Did the findings support or refute findings of other researchers who used the framework? If there were discrepancies, is there a way to explain them using the framework? The reader of research needs to know how to critically appraise a framework for research (see Critiquing Criteria box).

The first question posed is whether a framework is presented. Sometimes a structure may be guiding the research, but a diagrammed model is not included in the manuscript. You must then look for the theoretical framework in the narrative description of the study concepts. When the framework is identified, it is important to consider its relevance for nursing. The framework does not have to be one created by a nurse, but the importance of its content for nursing should be clear. The question of how the framework depicts a structure congruent with nursing should be addressed. For instance, although the Lazarus Transaction Model of Stress and Coping was not created by a nurse, it is clearly related to nursing practice when working with people facing stress. Sometimes frameworks from different disciplines, such as physics or art, may be relevant. It is the responsibility of the author to clearly articulate the meaning of the framework for the study and to link the framework to nursing.

Once the meaning and applicability of the theory (if the objective of the research was theory development) or the theoretical framework to nursing are articulated, you will be able to determine whether the framework is appropriate to guide the research. As you critically appraise a study you would identify a mismatch, for example, in which a researcher presents a study of students' responses to the stress of being in the clinical setting for the first time within a framework of stress related to recovery from chronic illness. You should look closely at the framework to determine if it is "on target" and the "best fit" for the research question and proposed study design.

Next, the reader should focus on the concepts being studied. Does the researcher clearly describe and explain concepts that are being studied and how they are defined and translated into measurable variables? Is there literature to support the choice of concepts? Concepts should clearly reflect the area of study. For example, using the concept of "anger," when "incivility" or "hostility" is more appropriate to the research focus creates difficulties in defining variables and determining methods of measurement. These issues have to do with the logical consistency between the framework, the concepts being studied, and the methods of measurement.

Throughout the entire critiquing process, from worldview to operational definitions, the reader is evaluating the fit. Finally, the reader will expect to find a discussion of the findings as they relate to the theory or framework. This final point enables evaluation of the framework for use in further research. It may suggest necessary changes to enhance the relevance of the framework for continuing study, and thus serves to let others know where one will go from here.

Evaluating frameworks for research requires skill that must be acquired through repeated critique and discussion with others who have critiqued the same work. As with other abilities and skills, you must practice and use the skills to develop them further. With continuing education and a broader knowledge of potential frameworks, you will build a repertoire of knowledge to assess the foundation of a research study and the framework for research, and/or to evaluate findings where theory was generated as the outcome of the study.

## KEY POINTS

- The interaction among theory, practice, and research is central to knowledge development in the discipline of nursing.
- The use of a framework for research is important as a guide to systematically identify concepts and to link appropriate study variables with each concept.
- Conceptual and operational definitions are critical to the evolution of a study.
- In developing or selecting a framework for research, knowledge may be acquired from other disciplines or directly from nursing. In either case, that knowledge is used to answer specific nursing questions.
- Theory is distinguished by its scope. Grand theories are broadest in scope and situation-specific theories are most narrow in scope and at the lowest level of abstraction; middle range theories are in the middle.
- In critiquing a framework for research, it is important to examine the logical, consistent link among the framework, the concepts for study, and the methods of measurement.

## CRITICAL THINKING CHALLENGES

- Search recent issues of a prominent nursing journal (e.g., *Nursing Research*, *Research in Nursing & Health*) for notations of conceptual frameworks of published studies. How many explicitly discussed the theoretical framework? How many did not mention any theoretical framework? What kinds of theories were mentioned (e.g., grand nursing theories, middle range nursing theories, non-nursing theories)? How many studies were theory generating? How many were theory testing?
- Identify a non-nursing theory that you would like to know more about. How could you find out information on its applicability to nursing research and nursing practice? How could you identify whether and how it has been used in nursing research?
- Select a nursing theory, concept, or phenomenon (e.g., resilience from the case study) that you are interested in and would like to know more about. Consider: How could you

find studies that have used that theory in research and practice? How could you locate published instruments and tools that reportedly measure concepts and constructs of the theory?

- Consider: How can middle range and situation-specific nursing theories be operationalized and turned into explicit guidelines for evidence-based practice?

## REFERENCES

Ahern, N. R. (2006). Adolescent resilience: an evolutionary concept analysis. *Journal of Pediatric Nursing, 21*(3), 175–185.

Ahern, N. R., Ark, P., & Byers, J. (2008). Resilience and coping strategies in adolescents. *Pediatric Nursing, 20*(10), 32–36.

Alhusen, J. L., Gross, D., Hayat, M. J., et al. (2012). The influence of maternal-fetal attachment and health practices on neonatal outcomes in low-income, urban women. *Research in Nursing & Health, 35*(2), 112–120.

Banner, D., Miers, M., Clarke, B., et al. (2011). Women's experiences of undergoing coronary artery bypass graft surgery. *Journal of Advanced Nursing, 68*(4), 919–930.

Cahill, J., LoBiondo-Wood, G., Bergstrom, N., et al. (2012). Brain tumor symptoms as antecedents to uncertainty: an integrative review. *Journal of Nursing Scholarship, 44*(2), 145–155.

Eakes, G., Burke, M. L., & Hainsworth, M. A. (1998). Middle rang theory of chronic sorrow. *Image: Journal of Nursing Scholarship, 30*(2), 179–185.

Fawcett, J., Abner, C., Haussler, S., et al. (2012). Women's perceptions of caesarean birth: a Roy international study. *Nursing Science Quarterly, 24*(40), 352–362.

Hurlbut, J. M., Robbins, L. K., & Hoke, M. M. (2011). Correlations between spirituality and health-promoting behaviors among sheltered homeless women. *Journal of Community Health Nursing, 28*(1), 81–91.

Im, E. (2005). Development of situation-specific theories: an integrative approach. *Advances in Nursing Science, 28*(2), 137–151.

Im, E. (2006). A situation-specific theory of Caucasian cancer patients' pain experience. *Advances in Nursing Science, 29*(3), 232–244.

Im, E. (2010). A situation-specific theory of Asian immigrant women's menopausal symptom experience in the United States. *Advances in Nursing Science (ANS),33*(20), 143–157.

Im, E., & Chang, S. J. (2012). Current trends in nursing theories. *Journal of Nursing Scholarship, 44*(2), 156–164.

Johnson, D. E. (1990). The behavioral system model for nursing. In M. E. Parker (Ed.), *Nursing theories in practice* (pp. 23–32). New York, NY: National League for Nursing Press.

Kolcaba, K. Y. (1994). A theory of holistic comfort for nursing. *Journal of Advanced Nursing, 19*(6), 1178–1184.

Kolcaba, K. Y. (2009). Comfort. In S. J. Peterson, & T. S. Bredow (Eds.), *Middle range theories: application to nursing research* (pp. 254–272). Philadelphia, PA: Lippincott Williams & Wilkins.

Lasiter, S. (2011). Older adults' perceptions of feeling safe in an intensive care unit. *Journal of Advanced Nursing, 67*(12), 2649–2657.

Lavoie, S, Talbot, L. R., & Mathieu, L. (2011). Post-traumatic stress disorder symptoms among emergency nurses: their perspective and a 'tailor-made' solution. *Journal of Advanced Nursing, 67*(7), 1514–1522.

Lenz, E. R., Pugh, L. C., Miligan, R. A., et al. (1997). The middle range theory of unpleasant symptoms: an update. *Advances in Nursing Science, 19*(3), 14–27.

McEwen, M., & Wills, E. (2011). *Theoretical basis for nursing* (3rd ed.). Philadelphia, PA: Lippincott.

Mefford, L. C. (2004). A theory of health promotion for preterm infants based on Levine's conservation model of nursing. *Nursing Science Quarterly, 17*(3), 260–266.

Melvin, K. C., Gross, D., Hayat, M. J., et al. (2012). Couple functioning and post-traumatic stress symptoms in U.S. army couples: the role of resilience. *Research in Nursing & Health, 35*(2), 164–177.

Mercer, R. T. (2004). Becoming a mother versus maternal role attainment. *Journal of Nursing Scholarship, 36*(3), 226–232.

Mishel, M. H. (1988). Uncertainty in illness. *Journal of Nursing Scholarship, 20*(4), 225–232.

Mishel, M. H. (1990). Reconceptualization of the uncertainty in illness theory. *Image: Journal of Nursing Scholarship, 22*(4), 256–262.

Mishel, M. H. (1999). Uncertainty in chronic illness. *Annual Review of Nursing Research, 17,* 269–294.

Nelson-Goff, B. S., & Smith, D. (2005). Systemic traumatic stress: the couple adaptation to traumatic stress model. *Journal of Marital and Family Therapy, 31,* 145–157.

Neuman, B. (1995). *The Neuman systems model* (3rd ed.). Stanford, CT: Appleton & Lange.

Nightingale, F. (1969). *Notes on nursing: what it is and what it is not.* New York, NY: Dover Publications (Original work published 1860).

Orem, D. E. (2001). *Nursing: concepts of practice* (6th ed.). St Louis, MO: Mosby.

Pender, N. J., Murdaugh, C., & Parsons, M. (2006). *Health promotion in nursing practice* (5th ed.). Upper Saddle River, NJ: Prentice Hall.

Peterson, S. J. (2008). Introduction to the nature of nursing knowledge. In S. J. Peterson & T. S. Bredow (Eds.), *Middle range theories: application to nursing research* (pp. 3–41). Philadelphia, PA: Lippincott, Williams & Wilkins.

Polk, L. V. (1997). Toward a middle range theory of resilience. *Advances in Nursing Science, 19*(3), 1–13.

Prochaska, J. O. & DiClemente, C. C. (1984). *The transtheoretical approach: Crossing traditional boundaries of therapy.* Homewood, IL: Dow Jones-Irwin.

Purtzer, M. A. (2012). A transformative decision-making process for mammography screening among rural, low-income women. *Public Health Nursing, 29*(3), 247–255.

Reimer, A. P., & Moore, S. M. (2010). Flight nursing expertise: towards a middle-range theory. *Journal of Advanced Nursing, 66*(5), 1183–1192.

Riegel, B., & Dickson, V. V. (2008). A situation-specific theory of heart failure self-care. *Journal of Cardiovascular Nursing, 23*(3), 190–196.

Rogers, M. E. (1970). *An introduction to the theoretical basis of nursing.* Philadelphia, PA: Davis.

Rogers, M. E. (1990). Nursing: the science of unitary, irreducible, human beings: update: 1990. In E. A. M. Barrett (ed.), *Visions of Rogers' science-based nursing* (pp. 5–11). New York, NY: National League for Nursing Press.

Roy, C. (2009). *The Roy adaptation model* (3rd ed.). Upper Saddle River, NJ: Pearson.

Ruland, C. M., & Moore, S. M. (1998). Theory construction based on standards of care: a proposed theory of the peaceful end of life. *Nursing Outlook, 46*(4), 169–175.

Seiler, A. J., & Moss, V. A. (2012). The experiences of nurse practitioners providing health care to the homeless. *Journal of the American Academy of Nurse Practitioners, 24*(5), 303–312.

Thomas, M. L., Elliott, J. E., Rao, S. M., et al. (2012). A randomized, clinical trial of education or motivational-interviewing-based coaching compared to usual care to improve cancer pain management. *Oncology Nursing Forum, 39*(1), 39–49.

Tusaie, K., Puskar, K., & Sereika, S. M. (2007). A predictive and moderating model of psychosocial resilience in adolescents. *Journal of Nursing Scholarship, 39*(1), 54–60.

Whall, A. L. (2005). The structure of nursing knowledge: analysis and evaluation of practice, middle range and grand theory. In J. J. Fitzpatrick & A. L. Whall (Eds.), *Conceptual models of nursing: analysis and application* (pp. 5–20). Upper Saddle River, NJ: Prentice-Hall.

# evolve WEBSITE

*Go to Evolve at http://evolve.elsevier.com/LoBiondo/ for review questions, critiquing exercises, and additional research articles for practice in reviewing and critiquing.*

# PART II

# Processes and Evidence Related to Qualitative Research

Research Vignette: *Marianne T. Marcus*

# RESEARCH VIGNETTE

## ▮PROGRAM OF RESEARCH ON SUBSTANCE USE DISORDERS

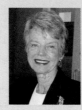

**Marianne T. Marcus, EdD, RN, FAAN**
**John P. McGovern Distinguished Professor of Addictions Nursing**
**University of Texas–Houston Health Science Center School of Nursing**
**Houston, Texas**

My career trajectory illustrates the evolution of nursing education, practice, and research, as well as the impact of a chance encounter with a group in a drug treatment facility where our school was conducting a primary care clinic in a long-term residential drug treatment program, a therapeutic community (TC). This was the beginning of my focus on substance use disorders. I realized I knew little about addictive disorders. I wondered, "What causes addiction and how does it affect health?" "What is a therapeutic community, and how does it work?" And perhaps most important, "What do nurses know about substance use disorders and how do they learn it?"

I explored ways to develop the skills for teaching and doing research in this field. This coincided with a federal initiative to increase health professional competence in meeting the challenge of substance use and abuse. Beginning in 1990, we obtained 3-year Faculty Development grants from the Substance Abuse Mental Health Services Administration, Center for Substance Abuse Prevention. Nursing and health professions faculty acquired knowledge and skills to enhance the curriculum and begin research in this area (Marcus, 1997; Marcus, 2000). We also were funded to create a nursing addictions graduate program (Marcus & Stafford, 2002).

My program of research related to TCs began with a grounded theory qualitative study to explore the lived experience of recovery in a TC. Residents of TCs participated. TCs provide a highly structured hierarchical environment in which the community is the key agent for behavior change. Participants likened the TC experience to making a career change, an arduous process that takes determination, commitment, readiness, and time. They indicated that the experience is one of translation rather than transformation, a redirection of skills to more constructive activities. The theory that emerged from this study defines four progressive steps, or stages of recovery in TC treatment, and the properties common to each (Marcus, 1998).

For individuals whose lives were characterized by impulsivity and lack of self-control, the rigor of a TC is restrictive and inherently stressful, and the dropout rate is high. Recognizing that successful outcomes are correlated with time in treatment led me to hypothesize that stress-reduction strategies might enhance progression and retention. Mindfulness-based stress reduction (MBSR) is a meditation program to help individuals bring nonreactive, nonjudgmental attention to their present moment experiences. MBSR is congruent with the goals of the TC to encourage self-regulation, awareness insight, problem-solving, and sense of well-being. Next, two feasibility studies of MBSR were conducted (Marcus, Fine, & Kouzekanani, 2001; Marcus et al., 2003). These studies positioned us for a National Institute of Drug Abuse-funded behavioral therapies trial of MBSR as an adjunct to TC treatment. Behavior change, from harmful substance use to sobriety, is important for the prevention and treatment of many conditions caused by deleterious lifestyles (Marcus et al., 2007). We developed a MBSR treatment protocol for TC treatment (MBTC), trained MBSR teachers, monitored treatment integrity, and conducted a pilot study. This study aimed to describe the stress response to TC treatment and determine the effect of MBSR on stress, self-change, impulsivity, and program progression and retention. Findings indicated that admission stress levels were associated with early dropout and that the intervention reduced stress significantly faster than TC treatment alone (Marcus et al., 2009). We also gathered data on self-change (Carroll et al., 2008; Liehr et al., 2010) and impulsivity (Bankston et al., 2009). Currently, we are adapting our MBTC protocol to an adolescent population and conducting a pilot study.

As I learn more, I realize there is an important role for prevention. My prevention approach has been through community-based participatory research, a method that involves community stakeholders in all study aspects with the ultimate goal of building capacity to improve the community's health. A chance encounter with a youth minister led to a fruitful collaboration. We responded to a call for studies in HIV/AIDS and substance abuse prevention studies in minorities, and were funded to design and implement an intervention to prevent these health problems for African-American adolescents in faith-based settings (Marcus et al., 2004). We continue to study the effects of a mentored afterschool program on promoting healthy lifestyles among youth in an underserved neighborhood. Community members are learning to provide an evidence-based curriculum, and health professions students are learning about community health needs (Marcus et al., 2011).

We have much to learn about this complex problem, and nursing research can contribute a great deal to finding the answers. I enjoy the daily challenge of research and I am pleased that my career took this unexpected turn. My research came about because of a need to respond to a major public health problem. I have focused on the best ways to educate health professionals to meet this challenge and on the development of prevention and treatment interventions.

## REFERENCES

Bankston, S., Moeller, F. G., Schmitz, J. M., et al. (2009). Substance abuser impulsivity decreases with a 9 month stay in a therapeutic community. *The American Journal of Drug and Alcohol Abuse, 35,* 417–420.

Carroll, D., Lange, B., Liehr, P., et al. (2008). Evaluating mindfulness-based stress reduction: analyzing stories of stress to formulate focus group questions. *Archives of Psychiatric Nursing, 22*(2), 107–109.

Liehr, P., Marcus, M. T., Carroll, D., et al. (2010). Linguistic analysis to assess the effect of a mindfulness intervention on self-change for adults in substance use recovery. *Substance Abuse, 31,* 79–85.

Marcus, M. T. (1997). Faculty development and curricular change: A process and outcomes model for substance abuse education. *Journal of Professional Nursing, 13*(3),168–177.

Marcus, M. T. (1998). Changing careers: becoming clean and sober in a therapeutic community. *Qualitative Health Research, 8*(4), 466–480.

Marcus, M. T. (2000). An interdisciplinary team model for substance abuse prevention in communities. *Journal of Professional Nursing, 16*(3),158–168.

Marcus, M. T., Fine, M., & Kouzekanani, K. (2001). Mindfulness-based meditation in a therapeutic community, *Journal of Substance Use, 5*(5), 305–311.

Marcus, M. T., Fine, M., Moeller, F. G., et al. (2003). Change in stress levels following mindfulness-based stress reduction in a therapeutic community. *Addictive Disorders and Their Treatment, 2*(3), 63–68.

Marcus, M. T., Liehr, P., Schmit, J., et al. (2007). Behavioral therapies trials: a case example. *Nursing Research, 56*(6), 210–216.

Marcus, M. T., Schmitz, J., Moeller, F. G., et al. (2009). Mindfulness-based stress reduction in therapeutic community treatment: a stage 1 trial. *The American Journal of Drug and Alcohol Abuse*, *35*(2), 103–108.

Marcus, M. T., & Stafford, L. (2002). A model for preparing nurses for the challenge of substance use disorders. *Drug and Alcohol Professional*, *2*(3), 23–30.

Marcus, M. T., Taylor, W. C., Hormann, M. D., et al. (2011). Linking service-learning with community-based participatory research: an interprofessional course for health professional students. *Nursing Outlook*, *59*(1), 47–54.

Marcus, M. T., Walker, T., Swint, J. M., et al. (2004). Community-based participatory research to prevent substance abuse and HIV/AIDS in African American adolescents. *Journal of Interprofessional Care*, *18*(4), 347–359.

# Introduction to Qualitative Research

*Mark Toles and Julie Barroso*

## evolve WEBSITE

*Go to Evolve at http://evolve.elsevier.com/LoBiondo/ for review questions, critiquing exercises, and additional research articles for practice in reviewing and critiquing.*

## LEARNING OUTCOMES

*After reading this chapter, the student should be able to do the following:*

- Describe the components of a qualitative research report.
- Describe the beliefs generally held by qualitative researchers.
- Identify four ways qualitative findings can be used in evidence-based practice.

## KEY TERMS

| | | | |
|---|---|---|---|
| context dependent | inclusion and exclusion | naturalistic setting | qualitative research |
| data saturation | criteria | paradigm | theme |
| grand tour question | inductive | | |

Let's say that you are reading an article that reports findings that HIV-infected men are more adherent to their antiretroviral regimens than HIV-infected women. You wonder, "Why is that? Why would women be less adherent in taking their medications? Certainly, it is not solely due to the fact that they are women." Or you are working in a postpartum unit and have just discharged a new mother who has debilitating rheumatoid arthritis. You wonder, "What is the process by which disabled women decide to have children? How do they go about making that decision?" These, like so many other questions we have as nurses, can be best answered through research conducted using qualitative methods. Qualitative research gives us the answers to those difficult "why?" questions.

Although qualitative research can be used at many different places in a program of research, you can most often find it answering questions we have when we understand very little about some phenomenon in nursing.

## WHAT IS QUALITATIVE RESEARCH?

Qualitative research is a broad term that encompasses several different methodologies that share many similarities. Qualitative studies help us formulate an understanding of a phenomenon. While qualitative research has a long history in the social sciences, it is only within the past two decades that it has become more accepted in nursing research. For many years, nursing students in doctoral programs were dissuaded from conducting qualitative studies; the push was for the traditional quantitative approach, which was viewed by many as being more prestigious to those in the "hard" sciences. So as nursing gained its foothold in academics, doctoral students were urged to study using the quantitative paradigm, or worldview, to help nursing research gain legitimacy in academe. Today there is a new generation of nurse scholars who are trained in qualitative methods, and who encourage students to use methods that best answer their research questions, as opposed to ones that might add a veneer of scientific legitimacy to its conduct, but do not answer the research question at hand.

Qualitative research is discovery oriented; that is, it is explanatory, descriptive, and inductive in nature. It uses words, as opposed to numbers, to explain a phenomenon. Qualitative research lets us see the world through the eyes of another—the woman who struggles to take her antiretroviral medication, or the woman who has carefully thought through what it might be like to have a baby despite a debilitating illness. Qualitative researchers assume that we can only understand these things if we consider the context in which they take place, and this is why most qualitative research takes place in naturalistic settings. Qualitative studies make the world of an individual visible to the rest of us. Qualitative research involves an "interpretative, naturalistic approach to the world; meaning that qualitative researchers study things in their natural settings, attempting to make sense of or interpret phenomena in terms of the meaning people bring to them" (Denzin & Lincoln, 2011, p. 3).

## WHAT DO QUALITATIVE RESEARCHERS BELIEVE?

Qualitative researchers believe that there are multiple realities that can be understood by carefully studying what people can tell us or what we can observe as we spend time with them. For example, the experience of having a baby, while it has some shared characteristics, is not the same for any two women, and is definitely different for a disabled mother. Thus, qualitative researchers believe that reality is socially constructed and context dependent. Even the experience of reading this book is different for any two students; one may be completely engrossed by the content, while another is reading, but is worrying about whether or not her financial aid will be approved soon (Fig. 5-1).

Because qualitative researchers believe that the discovery of meaning is the basis for knowledge, their research questions, approaches, and activities are often quite different from quantitative researchers (see the Critical Thinking Decision Path). Qualitative researchers, for example, seek to understand the "lived experience" of the research participants. They might use interviews or observations to gather new data, and use new data

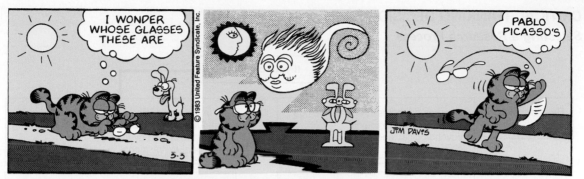

**FIGURE 5-1** Shifting perspectives: seeing the world as others see it. (GARFIELD, © 1983 Paws, Inc. Reprinted with permission of Universal Press Syndicate. All rights reserved.)

to create narratives about research phenomena. Thus, qualitative researchers know that there is a very strong imperative to clearly describe the phenomenon under study. Ideally, the reader of a qualitative research report, if even slightly acquainted with the phenomenon, would have an "aha!" moment in reading a well-written qualitative report.

So, you may now be saying, "Wow! This sounds great! Qualitative research is for me!" Many nurses feel very comfortable with this approach because we are educated with regard to how to talk to people about the health issues concerning them; we are used to listening, and listening well. But the most important consideration for any research study is whether or not the methodology fits the question. This means that qualitative researchers must select an approach for exploring phenomena that will actually answer their research questions. Thus, as you read studies and are considering them as evidence on which to base your practice, you should ask yourself, "Does the methodology fit with the research question under study?"

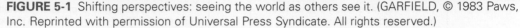

## HELPFUL HINT

All research is based on a paradigm, but this is seldom specifically stated in a research report.

## DOES THE METHODOLOGY FIT WITH THE RESEARCH QUESTION BEING ASKED?

As we said before, qualitative methods are often best for helping us to determine the nature of a phenomenon and the meaning of experience. Sometimes, authors will state that they are using qualitative methods because little is known about a phenomenon; that alone is not a good reason for conducting a study. Little may be known about a phenomenon because it does not matter! For researchers to ask people to participate in a study, to open themselves and their lives to us, they should be asking about things that will help to make a difference in people's lives or in how to provide more effective nursing care. You should be able to articulate a valid reason for conducting a study, beyond "little is known. . . ."

In the examples at the start of this chapter, we would want to know why HIV-infected women are less adherent to their medication regimens, so we can work to change these barriers and anticipate them when our patients are ready to start taking these pills. Similarly, we need to understand the decision-making processes women use to decide whether

**CRITICAL THINKING DECISION PATH**

*Selecting a Research Process*

**If your beliefs are**

| Researcher beliefs | Humans are biopsychosocial beings, known by their biological, psychological, and social characteristics. | **or** | Humans are complex beings who attribute unique meaning to their life situations. They are known by their personal expressions. |
|---|---|---|---|
| | Truth is objective reality that can be experienced with the senses and measured by the researcher. | | Truth is the subjective expression of reality as perceived by the participant and shared with the researcher. Truth is context laden. |

**then you'll ask questions, such as**

| Example questions | What is the difference in blood pressure and heart rate for adolescents who are angry compared to those who are not angry? | **or** | What is the structure of the lived experience of anger for adolescents? |
|---|---|---|---|

**and select approaches**

| Approaches | QUANTITATIVE | **or** | QUALITATIVE |
|---|---|---|---|

**leading to research activities**

| Research activities | Researcher selects a representative (of population) sample and determines size before collecting data. | **or** | Researcher selects participants who are experiencing the phenomenon of interest and collects data until saturation is reached. |
|---|---|---|---|
| | Researcher uses an extensive approach to collect data. | | Researcher uses an intensive approach to collect data. |
| | Questionnaires and measurement devices are preferably administered in one setting by an unbiased individual to control for extraneous variables. | | Researcher conducts interviews and participant or nonparticipant observation in environments where participants usually spend their time. Researcher bias is acknowledged and set aside. |
| | Primarily deductive analysis is used, generating a numerical summary that allows the researcher to reject or accept the null hypothesis. | | Primarily inductive analysis is used, leading to a narrative summary, which synthesizes participant information, creating a description of human experience. |

> **BOX 5-1    STEPS IN THE RESEARCH PROCESS**
>
> - Review of the literature
> - Study design
> - Sample
> - Setting: recruitment and data collection
> - Data collection
> - Data analysis
> - Findings
> - Conclusions

or not to have a child when they are disabled, so we can guide or advise the next woman who is going through this process. To summarize, we say a qualitative approach "fits" a research question when the researchers seek to understand the nature or experience of phenomena by attending to personal accounts of those with direct experiences related to the phenomena. Next, let's discuss the parts of a qualitative research study.

## COMPONENTS OF A QUALITATIVE RESEARCH STUDY

The components of a qualitative research study include the review of literature, study design, study setting and sample, approaches for data collection and analysis, study findings, and conclusions with implications for practice and research. As we reflect on these parts of qualitative studies, we will see how nurses use the qualitative research process to develop new knowledge for practice (Box 5-1).

### Review of the Literature

When researchers are clear that a qualitative approach is the best way to answer the research question, their first step is to review the relevant literature and describe what is already known about the phenomena of interest. This may require creativity on the researcher's part, because there may not be any published research on the phenomenon in question. Usually, there are studies on similar subjects, or with the same patient population, or on a closely related concept. For example, researchers may want to study how women who have a disabling illness make decisions about becoming pregnant. While there may be no other studies in this particular area, there may be some on decision-making in pregnancy when a woman does not have a disabling illness. These studies would be important in the review of the literature because they identify concepts and relationships that can be used to guide the research process. For example, findings from the review can show us the precise needs for new research, what participants should be in the study sample, and what kinds of questions should be used to collect the data.

Let's consider an example. Say a group of researchers wanted to examine HIV-infected women's adherence to antiretroviral therapy. If there was no research on this exact topic, the researcher might examine studies on adherence to therapy in other illnesses, such as diabetes or hypertension. They might include studies that examine gender differences in medication adherence. Or they might examine the literature on adherence in a stigmatizing illness, or look at appointment adherence for women, to see what facilitates or acts as a barrier to attending health care appointments. The major point here is that even though there may be no literature on the phenomena of interest, the review of the literature will identify existing related data that are useful for exploring the new questions. At the conclusion of an effective review, you should be able to easily identify the strengths and weaknesses in prior research; you should also have a clear understanding of the new research questions as well as the significance of studying them.

## Study Design

The study design is a description of how the qualitative researcher plans to go about answering the research questions. In qualitative research, there may simply be a descriptive or naturalistic design in which the researchers adhere to the general tenets of qualitative research, but do not commit to a particular methodology. There are many different qualitative methods used to answer the research questions. Some of these methods will be discussed in the next chapter. What is important, as you read from this point forward, is that the study design must be congruent with the philosophical beliefs that qualitative researchers hold. You would not expect to see a qualitative researcher use methods common to quantitative studies, such as a random sample or battery of questionnaires administered in a hospital outpatient clinic or a multiple regression analysis. Rather, you would expect to see a design that includes participant interviews or observation, strategies for inductive analysis, and plans for using data to develop narrative summaries with rich description of the details from participants' experiences (see Fig. 5-1). You may also read about a pilot study in the description of a study design; this is work the researchers did before undertaking the main study to make sure that the logistics of the proposed study were reasonable. For example, pilot data may describe whether the investigators were able to recruit participants and whether the research design led them to information they needed.

## Sample

The study sample refers to the group of people that the researcher will interview or observe in the process of collecting data to answer the research questions. In most qualitative studies, the researchers are looking for a purposeful or purposively selected sample (see Chapter 10). This means that they are searching for a particular kind of person who can illuminate the phenomenon they want to study. For example, the researchers may want to interview women with multiple sclerosis, or rheumatoid arthritis. There may be other parameters—called **inclusion** and **exclusion criteria**—that the researchers impose as well, such as requiring that participants be older than 18 years, or not using illicit drugs, or deciding about a first pregnancy (as opposed to subsequent pregnancies). When researchers are clear about these criteria, they are able to identify and recruit study participants with experiences needed to shed light on the phenomenon in question. Often the researchers make decisions such as determining who might be a "long-term survivor" of a certain illness. In this case, they must clearly understand why and how they decided who would fit into this category. Is a long-term survivor someone who has had an illness for 5 years? Ten years? What is the median survival time for people with this diagnosis? Thus, as a reader of nursing research, you are looking for evidence of sound scientific reasoning behind the sampling plan.

When the researchers have identified the type of person to include in the research sample, the next step is to develop a strategy for recruiting participants, which means locating and engaging them in the research. Recruitment materials are usually very specific. For example, if the researchers want to talk to HIV-infected women about adherence, they may distribute flyers or advertise their interest in recruiting women who are adherent, as well as those who are not. Or, they may want to talk to women who fit into only one of those categories. Similarly, the researchers who are examining decision making in pregnancy among women with disabling conditions would develop recruitment strategies that identify subjects with the conditions or characteristics they want to study.

In a research report, the researcher may include a description of the study sample in the findings (it can also be reported in the description of the sample). In any event, besides a demographic description of the study participants, a qualitative researcher should also report on key axes of difference in the sample. For example, in a sample of HIV-infected women, there should be information about stage of illness, what kind/how many pills they must take, how many children they have, and so on. This information helps you place the findings into some context.

## Setting: Recruitment and Data Collection

The study setting refers to the places where participants are recruited and the data are collected. Settings for recruitment are usually a point of contact for people of common social, medical, or other individual traits. In the example of finding HIV-infected women who are having difficulties with adherence, researchers might distribute flyers describing the study at AIDS service organizations, support groups for HIV-infected women, clinics, on-line support groups, and other places people with HIV may seek services. The settings for data collection are another critical area of difference between quantitative and qualitative studies. Data collection in a qualitative study is usually done in a naturalistic setting, such as someone's home, not in a clinic interview room or researcher's office. This is important in qualitative research because the researcher's observations can inform the data collection. To be in someone else's home, for example, is a great advantage as it helps the researcher to understand what that participant values. An entire wall in a participant's living room might contain many pictures of a loved one, so anyone who enters the home would immediately understand the centrality of that person in the participant's life. In the home of someone who is ill, many household objects may be clustered around a favorite chair: perhaps an oxygen tank, a glass of water, medications, a telephone, *TV Guide,* tissues, and so on. A good qualitative researcher will use clues like these, in the study setting, to complete the complex, rich drawing that is being rendered in the study.

## Data Collection

The procedures for data collection differ significantly in qualitative and quantitative studies. Where quantitative researchers focus on statistics and numbers, qualitative researchers are usually concerned with words, or what people can tell them and narratives about meaning or experience. Qualitative researchers interview their participants; they may interview an individual or any group of people in what is called a focus group. They may observe individuals as they go about daily tasks, such as sorting medications into a pill minder or caring for a child. But in all cases, the data collected are expressed in words. Most qualitative researchers use voice recorders so that they can be sure that they have captured what the participant says. This reduces the need to write things down and frees researchers up to listen fully. Interview recordings are usually transcribed verbatim and then listened to for accuracy. In a research report, investigators describe their procedures for collecting the data, such as obtaining informed consent, all the steps from inital contact to the end of the study visit, and how long each interview or focus group lasted or how much time the researcher spent "in the field" collecting data.

A very important consideration in qualitative data collection is the researchers' decision that they have a sufficient sample and that data collection is complete. Researchers generally continue to recruit participants until they have reached data saturation, which means that nothing new is emerging from the interviews. There usually is *not* a predetermined number of participants to be selected as there is in quantitative studies; rather, the researcher keeps recruiting until they have all of the data they need. One important exception to this is if the researcher is very interested in getting different types of people in the study. For example, in the study of HIV-infected women and medication adherence, the researchers may want some women who were very adherent in the beginning but then became less so over time, or they may want women who were not adherent in the beginning but then became adherent, or they may want to interview women with children and women without children to determine the influence of having children on adherence. Whatever the specific questions may be, sample sizes tend to be fairly small (fewer than 30 participants) because of the enormous amounts of written text that will need to be analyzed by the researcher.

Investigators use great care to design the interview questions because they must be crafted to help study participants describe their personal experiences and perceptions. Interview questions are different from research questions. Research questions are typically broad, encompassing, and written in scientific language. The interview questions may also be broad, like the overview or grand tour questions that seek the "big picture." For example, researchers might ask, "Tell me about taking your medications—the things that make it easier, and the things that make it harder," or "Tell me what you were thinking about when you decided to get pregnant." Along with overview questions, there are usually a series of prompts (additional questions) that were derived from the literature. These are areas that the researcher believes are important to cover (and that the participant will likely cover), but the prompts are there to remind the researcher in case the material is not mentioned. For example, with regard to medication adherence, the researcher may have read in other studies that motherhood can influence adherence in two very different ways: children can become a reason to live, which would facilitate taking antiretroviral medication; and children can be all-demanding, leaving the mother with little to no time to take care of herself. Thus, a neutrally worded question about the influence of children would be a prompt if the participants do not mention it spontaneously. In a research report, you should expect to find the primary interview questions identified verbatim; without them, it is impossible to know how the data were collected and how the researcher shaped what was discovered in the interviews.

### EVIDENCE-BASED PRACTICE TIP

Qualitative researchers use more flexible procedures than quantitative researchers. While collecting data for a project, they consider all of the experiences that may occur.

## Data Analysis

Next is the description of data analysis. Here, researchers tell you how they handled the raw data, which, in a qualitative study, are usually transcripts of recorded interviews. The goal of qualitative analysis is to find commonalities and differences in the interviews, and then to group these into broader, more abstract, overarching categories of meaning, sometimes called themes, that capture much of the data. In the example we have been using about decision-making regarding pregnancy for disabled women, one woman might talk about discussing the need for assistance with her friends if she became pregnant, and found that they were willing and able to help her with the baby. Another woman might talk about how she discussed the decision with her parents and siblings, and found them to be a ready source of aid. And yet a third woman may say that she talked about this with her church study group, and they told her that they could arrange to bring meals and help with housework during the pregnancy and afterward. On a more abstract level, these women are all talking about social support. So an effective analysis would be one that identifies this pattern in social support and, perhaps, goes further by also describing how social support influences some other concept in the data; for example, the women's decision-making about having a baby. In an ideal situation, written reports about the data will give you an example like the one you just read, but the page limitations of most journals limit the level of detail that researchers usually wish to present.

Many qualitative researchers use computer-assisted qualitative data analysis programs to find patterns in the interviews and field notes, which, in many studies, can seem overwhelming due to the sheer quantity of data to be dealt with. With Atlas.ti, a computer-assisted data analysis program, researchers from multiple sites can simultaneously code and analyze data from hundreds of files without using a single piece of paper. The software is a tool for managing and remembering steps in analysis; however, it does not replace the thoughtful work of the researcher who must apply the program to guide the analysis of the data. In research reports, you should see a description of the way data were managed and analyzed, whether the researchers used software or 3×5 index cards with handwritten notes.

## Findings

Then, at last, we come to the results! Findings in qualitative reports, as we have suggested already, are words—the findings are patterns of any kind in the data, such as the ways that participants talked, the things that they talked about, even their behaviors associated with where the researcher spent time with them. When researchers describe patterns in the data, they may describe a process (such as the way decision-making occurs); they may identify a list of things that are functioning in some way (such as a list of barriers and facilitators to taking medications for HIV-positive women); they may specify a set of conditions that must be present for something to occur (such as what parents state they need to care for a ventilator-dependent child at home); they may even describe what it is like to go through some health-related transition (such as what it is like to become the caretaker of a parent with dementia). This is by no means an all-inclusive list; rather, it is a range of examples to help you recognize what types of findings might be possible. Think of the findings as discoveries. The qualitative researcher has explored a phenomenon and the findings are a report on what he or she "found"; that is, what was discovered in the interviews and observations.

When researchers describe their results, they usually break the data down into units of meaning that help the data cohere and tell a story. Effective research reports will describe the logic that was used for breaking down the units of data. For example, are the themes—a means of describing a large quantity of data in a condensed format—identified from the most prevalent to the least prevalent? Are the researchers describing a process in temporal (time ordered) terms? Are they starting with things that were most important to the subject, then moving to less important? As a report on the findings unfolds, the researchers should proceed with a thorough description of the phenomenon, defining each of the themes for you, and fleshing out each of the themes with a thorough explanation of the role that it plays in the question under study. The author should also provide quotations that support each of their themes. Ideally, they will stage the quote, giving you some information about the subject from whom it came; for example, was the subject a newly diagnosed HIV-infected

African-American woman without children? Or was it a disabled woman who has chosen to become pregnant, but who has suffered two miscarriages? Staging of quotes is important because it allows you to put the information into some social context.

In a well-written report of qualitative research, some of the quotes will give you an "aha!" feeling. You will have a sense that the researcher has done an excellent job of getting to the core of the problem. Quotes are as critical to qualitative reports as numbers are to a quantitative study; you would not have a great deal of confidence in a quantitative or qualitative report in which the author asks you to believe the conclusion without also giving concrete, verifiable findings to back it up.

> **HELPFUL HINT**
>
> Values are involved in all research. It is important, however, that they not influence the results of the research.

## DISCUSSION OF THE RESULTS AND IMPLICATIONS FOR EVIDENCE-BASED PRACTICE

When the researchers are satisfied that their findings answer the research questions, they should summarize the results for you, and should compare their findings to the existing literature. Researchers usually explain how these findings are similar to or different from the existing literature. This is one of the great contributions of qualitative research: using findings to open up new venues of discovery that were not anticipated when the study was designed. For example, the researchers can use findings to develop new concepts or new conceptual models to explain broader phenomena. The conceptual work also identifies implications for how findings can be used in practice and can direct future research. Another alternative is for researchers to use their findings to extend or refine existing theoretical models. For example, a researcher may learn something new about stigma that has not been described in the literature, and in writing about these findings, the researcher may refer to an existing stigma theory, pointing out how his/her work extends that theory.

Nursing is a practice discipline, and the goal of nursing research is to use research findings to improve patient care. Qualitative methods are the best way to start to answer clinical and research questions that have not been addressed or when a new perspective is needed in practice. The qualitative answers to these questions provide important evidence that offers the first systematic insights into phenomena previously not well understood and often lead to new perspectives in nursing practice and improved patient care outcomes.

Kearney (2001) developed a typology of levels and applications of qualitative research evidence that helps us see how new evidence can be applied to practice (Table 5-1). She described five categories of qualitative findings that are distinguished from one another in their levels of complexity and discovery: those restricted by a priori frameworks, descriptive categories, shared pathway or meaning, depiction of experiential variation, and dense explanatory description. She argued that the greater the complexity and discovery within qualitative findings, the stronger the potential for clinical application.

Findings developed with only a priori frameworks provide little or no evidence for changing practice because the researchers have prematurely limited what they are able to learn from participants or describe in their analysis. Findings that identify descriptive categories portray a higher level of discovery when a phenomenon is vividly portrayed

| TABLE 5-1 | KEARNEY'S CATEGORIES OF QUALITATIVE FINDINGS, FROM LEAST TO MOST COMPLEX | |
|---|---|---|
| **CATEGORY** | **DEFINITION** | **EXAMPLE** |
| Restricted by a priori frameworks | Discovery aborted because researcher has obscured the findings with an existing theory | Use of the theory of "relatedness" to describe women's relationships without substantiation in the data, or when there may be an alternative explanation to describe how women exist in relationship to others; the data seem to point to an explanation other than "relatedness" |
| Descriptive categories | Phenomenon is vividly portrayed from a new perspective; provides a map into previously uncharted territory in the human experience of health and illness | Children's descriptions of pain, including descriptors, attributed causes, and what constitutes good care during a painful episode |
| Shared pathway or meaning | Synthesis of a shared experience or process; integration of concepts that provides a complex picture of a phenomenon | Description of women's process of recovery from depression; each category was fully described, and the conditions for progression were laid out; able to see the origins of a phase in the previous phase |
| Depiction of experiential variation | Describes the main essence of an experience, but also shows how the experience varies, depending on the individual or context | Description of how pregnant women recovering from cocaine addiction might or might not move forward to create a new life, depending on the amount of structure they imposed on their behavior and their desire to give up drugs and change their lives |
| Dense explanatory description | Rich, situated understanding of a multifaceted and varied human phenomenon in a unique situation; portray the full range and depth of complex influences; densely woven structure to findings | Unique cultural conditions and familial breakdown and hopelessness led young people to deliberately expose themselves to HIV infection in order to find meaning and purpose in life; describes loss of social structure and demands of adolescents caring for their diseased or drugged parents who were unable to function as adults |

from a new perspective. For nursing practice, these findings serve as maps of previously uncharted territory in human experience. Findings in Kearney's third category, shared pathway or meaning, are more complex. In this type of finding, there is an integration of concepts or themes that result in a synthesis of a shared process or experience that lead to a logical, complex portrayal of the phenomenon. The researcher's ideas at this level reveal how discrete bits of data come together in a meaningful whole. For nursing practice, it allows us to reflect on the bigger picture and what it means for the human experience (Kearney, 2001). Findings that depict experiential variation describe the essence of an experience and how this experience varies, depending on the individual or context. For nursing practice, this type of finding helps us see a variety of viewpoints, realizations of a human experience, and the contextual sources of that variety. In nursing practice, these findings explain how different variables can produce different consequences in different people or settings. Finally, findings that are presented as a dense explanatory description are at the highest level of complexity and discovery. They provide a rich, situated understanding of a multifaceted and varied human phenomenon in a unique

| TABLE 5-2 | KEARNEY'S MODES OF CLINICAL APPLICATION FOR QUALITATIVE RESEARCH |
|---|---|
| **MODE OF CLINICAL APPLICATION** | **EXAMPLE** |
| Insight or empathy: We can better understand our patients and offer more sensitive support | Nurse is better able to understand the behaviors of the patient, who is a woman recovering from depression |
| Assessment of status or progress: Descriptions of trajectories of illness | Nurse is able to describe trajectory of recovery from depression and can assess how the patient is moving through this trajectory |
| Anticipatory guidance: Sharing of qualitative findings with the patient | Nurse is able to explain the phases of recovery from depression to the patient and to reassure her that she is not alone, that others have made it through a similar experience |
| Coaching: Advising patients of steps they can take to reduce distress or improve adjustment to an illness, according to the evidence in the study | Nurse describes the six stages of recovery from depression to the patient, and, in ongoing contact, points out how the patient is moving through the stages, coaching her to recognize signs that she is improving and moving through the stages |

situation. These types of findings portray the full depth and range of complex influences that propel people to make decisions. Physical and social context are fully accounted for. There is a densely woven structure of findings in these studies that provide a rich fund of clinically and theoretically useful information for nursing practice. The layers of detail work together in the findings to increase understanding of human choices and responses in particular contexts (Kearney, 2001).

**EVIDENCE-BASED PRACTICE TIP**

Qualitative research findings can be used in many ways, including improving ways clinicians communicate with patients and with each other.

So how can we further use qualitative evidence in nursing? The evidence provided by qualitative studies is used conceptually by the nurse: qualitative studies let nurses gain access to the experiences of patients, and help nurses expand their ability to understand their patients, which should lead to more helpful approaches to care (Table 5-2).

Kearney proposed four modes of clinical application: insight or empathy, assessment of status or progress, anticipatory guidance, and coaching. The simplest mode, according to Kearney, is to use the information to better understand the experiences of our patients, which in turn helps us to offer more sensitive support. Qualitative findings can also help us assess the patient's status or progress through descriptions of trajectories of illness or by offering a different perspective on a health condition. They allow us to consider a range of possible responses from patients. We can then determine the fit of a category to a particular client, or try to locate them on an illness trajectory. Anticipatory guidance includes sharing of qualitative findings directly with patients. The patient can learn about others with a similar condition, and can learn what to anticipate. This allows them to better garner resources for what might lie ahead, or look for markers of improvement. Anticipatory guidance can also be tremendously comforting in that the sharing of research results can help patients realize they are not alone, that there are others who have been through a similar experience with an illness. Finally, Kearney argues that coaching is a way of using qualitative findings; in this instance, nurses can advise patients of steps they can take to reduce distress, improve symptoms, or monitor trajectories of illness (Kearney, 2001).

Unfortunately, qualitative research studies do not fare well in the typical systematic reviews upon which evidence-based practice recommendations are based. Randomized clinical trials and other types of intervention studies traditionally have been the major focus of evidence-based practice. Typically, the selection of studies to be included in systematic reviews is guided by levels of evidence models that focus on the effectiveness of interventions according to their strength and consistency of their predictive power. Given that the levels of evidence models are hierarchical in nature, which perpetuate intervention studies as the "gold standard" of research design, the value of qualitative studies and the evidence offered by their results have remained unclear. Qualitative studies historically have been ranked lower in a hierarchy of evidence, as a "weaker" form of research design.

Remember, however, that qualitative research is not designed to test hypotheses or make predictions about causal effects. As we use qualitative methods, these findings become more and more valuable as they help us discover unmet patient needs, entire groups of patients that have been neglected, and new processes for delivering care to a population. Though qualitative research uses different methodologies and has different goals, it is important to explore how and when to use the evidence provided by findings of qualitative studies in practice.

## APPRAISING THE EVIDENCE FOUNDATION OF QUALITATIVE RESEARCH

A final example illustrates the differences in the methods discussed in this chapter and provides you with the beginning skills of how to critique qualitative research. The information in this chapter, coupled with information presented in Chapter 7, provide the underpinnings of critical appraisal of qualitative research (see Critiquing Criteria box, Chapter 7). Consider the question of nursing students learning how to conduct research. The empirical analytical approach (quantitative research) might be used in an experiment to see if one teaching method led to better learning outcomes than another. The students' knowledge might be tested with a pretest, the teaching conducted, and then a posttest of knowledge obtained. Scores on these tests would be analyzed statistically to see if the different methods produced a difference in the results.

In contrast, a qualitative researcher may be interested in the process of learning research. The researcher might attend the class to see what occurs and then interview students to ask them to describe how their learning changed over time. They might be asked to describe the experience of becoming researchers or becoming more knowledgeable about research. The goal would be to describe the stages or process of this learning. Or a qualitative researcher might consider the class as a culture and could join to observe and interview students. Questions would be directed at the students' values, behaviors, and beliefs in learning research. The goal would be to understand and describe the group members' shared meanings. Either of these examples are ways of viewing a question with a qualitative perspective. The specific qualitative methodologies are described in Chapter 6.

Many other research methods exist. Although it is important to be aware of the basis of the qualitative research methods used, it is most important that the method chosen is the one that will provide the best approach to answering the question being asked. This idea provides an important point for qualitative research. One research method does not rank higher than another; rather, a variety of methods based on different paradigms are essential for the development of a well informed and comprehensive approach to evidence-based nursing practice.

## KEY POINTS

- All research is based on philosophical beliefs, a worldview, or a paradigm.
- Qualitative research encompasses different methodologies.
- Qualitative researchers believe that reality is socially constructed and is context dependent.
- Values should be kept as separate as possible from the conduct of research.
- Qualitative research like quantitative research follows a process but the components of the process vary.
- Qualitative research contributes to evidence-based practice.

## CRITICAL THINKING CHALLENGES

- Discuss how a researcher's values could influence the results of a study. Include an example in your answer.
- Can the expression, "We do not always get closer to the truth as we slice and homogenize and isolate [it]" be applied to both qualitative and quantitative methods? Justify your answer.
- What is the value of qualitative research in evidence-based practice? Give an example.
- Discuss how you could apply the findings of a qualitative research study about coping with a miscarriage.

## REFERENCES

Denzin, N. K., & Lincoln, Y. S. (2011). *The SAGE handbook of qualitative research* (4th ed.). Thousand Oaks, CA: Sage.

Kearney, M. H. (2001). Levels and applications of qualitative research evidence. *Research in Nursing and Health, 24*, 145–153.

# evolve WEBSITE

*Go to Evolve at http://evolve.elsevier.com/LoBiondo/ for review questions, critiquing exercises, and additional research articles for practice in reviewing and critiquing.*

# Qualitative Approaches to Research

*Mark Toles and Julie Barroso*

## e volve WEBSITE

*Go to Evolve at http://evolve.elsevier.com/LoBiondo/ for review questions, critquing exercises, and additional research articles for practice in reviewing and critiquing.*

## LEARNING OUTCOMES

*After reading this chapter, you should be able to do the following:*

- Identify the processes of phenomenological, grounded theory, ethnographic, and case study methods.
- Recognize appropriate use of community-based participatory research methods.

- Discuss significant issues that arise in conducting qualitative research in relation to such topics as ethics, criteria for judging scientific rigor, and combination of research methods.
- Apply critiquing criteria to evaluate a report of qualitative research.

## KEY TERMS

| | | | |
|---|---|---|---|
| auditability | credibility | fittingness | meta-summary |
| bracketing | culture | grounded theory | meta-synthesis |
| case study method | data saturation | method | phenomenological |
| community-based par- | domains | instrumental case study | method |
| ticipatory research | emic view | intrinsic case study | theoretical sampling |
| constant comparative | ethnographic method | key informants | triangulation |
| method | etic view | lived experience | |

Qualitative research combines the science and art of nursing to enhance the understanding of human health experience. This chapter focuses on four commonly used qualitative research methods: phenomenology, grounded theory, ethnography, and case study. Community-based participatory research is also presented. Each of these methods, although distinct from the others, shares characteristics that identify it as a method within the qualitative research tradition.

Traditional hierarchies of research evaluation and how they categorize evidence from strongest to weakest, with emphasis on support for the effectiveness of interventions, is presented in Chapter 1. This perspective is limited, however, because it does not take into account the ways that qualitative research can support practice, as discussed in Chapter 5. There is no doubt about the merit of qualitative studies; the problem is that no one has developed a satisfactory method for including them in the evidence hierarchies. In addition, qualitative studies can answer the critical "why" questions that result from many evidence-based practice summaries; such summaries may report the answer to a research question, but they do not explain *how* it operates in the landscape of caring for people.

As a research consumer, you should know that qualitative methods are the best way to start to answer clinical and research questions when little is known or a new perspective is needed for practice. The very fact that qualitative research studies have increased exponentially in nursing and other social sciences speaks to the urgent need of clinicians to answer these "why" questions and to deepen our understanding of experiences of illness. Thousands of reports of well-conducted qualitative studies exist on topics such as the following:

- Personal and cultural constructions of disease, prevention, treatment, and risk
- Living with disease and managing the physical, psychological, and social effects of multiple diseases and their treatment
- Decision-making experiences with beginning and end-of-life, as well as assistive and life-extending, technological interventions
- Contextual factors favoring and mitigating against quality care, health promotion, prevention of disease, and reduction of health disparities (Sandelowski, 2004; Sandelowski & Barroso, 2007)

Findings from qualitative studies such as these provide valuable insights about unique phenomena, patient populations, or clinical situations. In doing so, they provide nurses with data needed to guide and change practice.

In this chapter, you are invited to look through the lens of human experience to learn about phenomenological, grounded theory, ethnographic, community-based participatory research, and case study methods. You are encouraged to put yourself in the researcher's shoes and imagine how it would be to study an issue of interest from the perspective of each of these methods. No matter which method a researcher uses, there is a demand to embrace the wholeness of humans, focusing on the human experience in natural settings.

The researcher using these methods believes that each unique human being attributes meaning to his or her experience and that experience evolves from his or her social and historical context. Thus, one person's experience of pain is distinct from another's and can be elucidated by the individual's subjective description of it. For example, researchers interested in studying the lived experience of pain for the adolescent with rheumatoid arthritis will spend time in the adolescents' natural settings, perhaps in their homes and schools (see Chapter 5). Research efforts will focus on uncovering the meaning of pain as it extends beyond the number of medications taken or a rating on a pain scale. Qualitative methods are grounded in the belief that objective data do not capture the whole of the human experience. Rather, the meaning of the adolescent's pain emerges within the

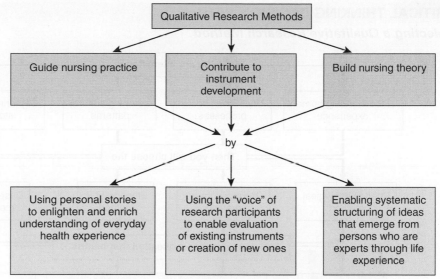

**FIGURE 6-1** Qualitative approach and nursing science.

context of personal history, current relationships, and future plans as the adolescent lives daily life in dynamic interaction with the environment.

## QUALITATIVE APPROACH AND NURSING SCIENCE

Qualitative research is particularly well suited to study the human experience of health, a central concern of nursing science. Because qualitative methods focus on the whole of human experience and the meaning ascribed by individuals living the experience, these methods extend understanding of health beyond traditional measures of isolated concepts to include the complexity of the human health experience as it is occurring in everyday living. The evidence provided by qualitative studies that consider the unique perspectives, concerns, preferences, and expectations each patient brings to a clinical encounter offers in-depth understanding of human experience and the contexts in which they occur. Qualitative research, in addition to providing unique perspectives, has the ability to guide nursing practice, contribute to instrument development (see Chapter 15), and develop nursing theory (Figure 6-1).

## QUALITATIVE RESEARCH METHODS

Thus far you have studied an overview of the qualitative research approach (see Chapter 5). Recognizing how the choice to use a qualitative approach reflects one's worldview and the nature of some research questions, you have the necessary foundation for exploring selected qualitative methodologies. Now, as you review the Critical Thinking Decision Path and study the remainder of Chapter 6, note how different qualitative methods are appropriate for distinct areas of interest and also note how unique research questions might be studied with each method. In this chapter, we will explore several qualitative research

**CRITICAL THINKING DECISION PATH**

*Selecting a Qualitative Research Method*

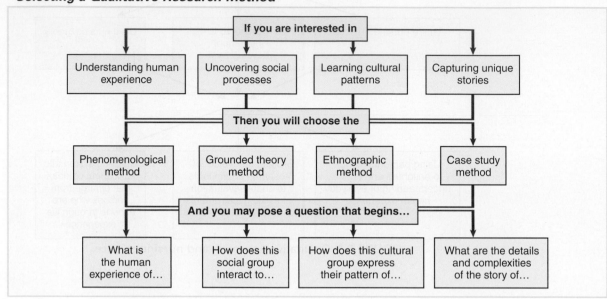

methods in depth, including phenomenological, grounded theory, ethnographic, case study, and community-based participatory research methods.

## Phenomenological Method

The **phenomenological method** is a process of learning and constructing the meaning of human experience through intensive dialogue with persons who are living the experience. It rests on the assumption that there is a structure and essence to shared experiences that can be narrated (Marshall & Rossman, 2011). The researcher's goal is to understand the meaning of the experience as it is lived by the participant. Phenomenological studies usually incorporate data about the lived space, or spatiality; the lived body, or corporeality; lived time, or temporality; and lived human relations, or relationality. Meaning is pursued through a dialogic process, which extends beyond a simple interview and requires thoughtful presence on the part of the researcher. There are many schools of phenomenological research, and each school of thought uses slight differences in research methods. For example, Husserl belonged to the group of transcendental phenomenologists, who saw phenomenology as an interpretive, as opposed to an objective, mode of description. Using vivid and detailed attentiveness to description, researchers in this school explore the way knowledge comes into being. They seek to understand knowledge that is based on insights rather than objective characteristics (Richards & Morse, 2007). In contrast, Heidegger was an existential phenomenologist, who believed that the observer cannot separate him/herself from the lived world. Researchers in this school study how being in the world is a reality that is perceived; they study a reciprocal relationship between observers and the phenomenon of interest (Richards & Morse, 2007). In all forms of phenomenological research, you will find researchers asking a question about the lived experience and using methods that explore phenomena as they are embedded in people's lives and environments.

## Identifying the Phenomenon

Because the focus of the phenomenological method is the lived experience, the researcher is likely to choose this method when studying some dimension of day-to-day existence for a particular group of people. See below for an example of this, in which Moules and colleagues' (2012) study the lived experience of being a grandparent whose grandchild has cancer.

## Structuring the Study

When thinking about methods, we say the methodological approach "structures the study." This phrase means that the method shapes the way we think about the phenomenon of interest and the way we would go about answering a research question. For the purpose of describing structuring, the following topics are addressed: the research question, the researcher's perspective, and sample selection.

*Research Question.* The question that guides phenomenological research always asks about some human experience. It guides the researcher to ask the participant about some past or present experience. In most cases, the research question is not exactly the same as the question used to initiate dialogue with study participants. In fact, the research question and the interview questions are very similar; however, the difference is important. For example, Moules and colleagues (2012) state that the objective of their study was to understand, from the perspectives of the grandparents, the complexity and unique character of experiences of having a grandchild diagnosed, treated, and living with childhood cancer. Their ultimate goal was to guide the initiation of a network of support to the eldest of three generations of family members who are touched by cancer as they care for their own children (parents of the child with cancer) while loving, grieving, and worrying for their grandchildren (Moules et al., 2012).

*Researcher's Perspective.* When using the phenomenological method, the researcher's perspective is bracketed. This means that the researcher identifies their own personal biases about the phenomenon of interest to clarify how personal experience and beliefs may color what is heard and reported. Further, the phenomenological researcher is expected to set aside their personal biases—to bracket them—when engaged with the participants. By becoming aware of personal biases, the researcher is more likely to be able to pursue issues of importance as introduced by the participant, rather than leading the participant to issues the researcher deems important (Richards & Morse, 2007).

---

### HELPFUL HINT

Although the research question may not always be explicitly reported, it may be identified by evaluating the study's purpose or the question/statement posed to the participants.

---

Using phenomenological methods, researchers strive to identify personal biases and hold them in abeyance while querying the participant. Readers of phenomenological articles may find it difficult to identify bracketing strategies because they are seldom explicitly identified in a research manuscript. Sometimes, a researcher's worldview or assumptions provide insight into biases that have been considered and bracketed. In the Moules study, bracketing was not discussed. This does not detract from the quality of the report. Usually, you will only find something about bracketing if there was a significant issue to report.

*Sample Selection.* As you read a report of a phenomenological study you will find that the participants were selected purposively and that members of the sample either are living the experience the researcher studies or have lived the experience in their past. Because phenomenologists believe that each individual's history is a dimension of the present, a past experience exists in the present moment. For the phenomenologist, it is a matter of asking the right questions and listening. Even when a participant is describing a past experience, remembered information is being gathered in the present at the time of the interview.

**HELPFUL HINT**

Qualitative studies often use purposive sampling (see Chapter 12).

### Data Gathering

Written or oral data may be collected when using the phenomenological method. The researcher may pose the query in writing and ask for a written response, or may schedule a time to interview the participant and record the interaction. In either case, the researcher may return to ask for clarification of written or recorded transcripts. To some extent, the particular data collection procedure is guided by the choice of a specific analysis technique. Different analysis techniques require different numbers of interviews. A concept known as "data saturation" usually guides decisions regarding how many interviews are enough. **Data saturation** is the situation of obtaining the full range of themes from the participants, so that in interviewing additional participants, no new data are emerging (Marshall & Rossman, 2011).

### Data Analysis

Several techniques are available for data analysis when using the phenomenological method. Although the techniques are slightly different from each other, there is a general pattern of moving from the participant's description to the researcher's synthesis of all participants' descriptions. Colaizzi (1978) suggests a series of seven steps:

1. Read the participants' narratives to acquire a feeling for their ideas in order to understand them fully.
2. Extract significant statements to identify key words and sentences relating to the phenomenon under study.
3. Formulate meanings for each of these significant statements.
4. Repeat this process across participants' stories and cluster recurrent meaningful themes. Validate these themes by returning to the informants to check interpretation.
5. Integrate the resulting themes into a rich description of the phenomenon under study.
6. Reduce these themes to an essential structure that offers an explanation of the behavior.
7. Return to the participants to conduct further interviews or elicit their opinions on the analysis in order to cross-check interpretation.

Moules and colleagues (2012) do not cite a reference for data analysis; however, they do describe their methodology as having entered the hermeneutic circle as an engaged participant. They state that the hermeneutic circle is the generative recursion between the whole and part; an immersion into a dynamic and evolving interaction with the data both as a whole and in part through extensive readings and re-readings, reflection, dialogue, and by challenging assumptions, all of which help the researcher move toward an understanding that opens up new possibilities.

It is important to note here that giving verbatim transcripts to participants can have unanticipated consequences. It is not unusual for people to deny that they said something in a certain way, or that they said it at all. Even when the actual recording is played for them, they may have difficulty believing it. This is one of the more challenging aspects of any qualitative method: every time a story is told, it changes for the participant. The participant may sincerely feel that the story as it was recorded is not the story as it is now.

## EVIDENCE-BASED PRACTICE TIP

Phenomenological research is an important approach for accumulating evidence when studying a new topic about which little is known.

## Describing the Findings

When using the phenomenological method, the nurse researcher provides you with a path of information leading from the research question, through samples of participants' words and the researcher's interpretation, to the final synthesis that elaborates the lived experience as a narrative. When reading the report of a phenomenological study, the reader should find that detailed descriptive language is used to convey the complex meaning of the lived experience that offers the evidence for this qualitative method (Richards & Morse, 2007). Moules and colleagues (2012) listed the following as their interpretive findings:

1. Speed at which your life changes: The phone call that heralds a shaking of a universe
2. Out of sync, unfair, and trading places
3. A knowing silence
4. Lives on hold while a view of the world changes: Holding one's breath
5. The quest for normalcy: A new kind of normal
6. Helplessness: Nothing you can do
7. Criticism, blame, and guilt
8. Grandparents' needs
9. The reemergence of sibling rivalry in adults
10. Pride of their children

The respondents also gave advice as grandparents to other grandparents:

1. Pay attention to the whole family.
2. Be prepared for the ride.
3. Keep perspective and take care of yourself so that you do not become a burden.
4. Keep optimism and hope; be available and step in even at times when not invited.
5. Be prepared for the curves that happen without warning.

These themes described the emotions, vulnerability, challenges, and issues experienced by these grandparents. Moreover, by using direct participant quotes, researchers enable readers to evaluate the connections between what individual participants said and how the researcher labeled or interpreted what they said.

## Grounded Theory Method

The **grounded theory method** is an inductive approach involving a systematic set of procedures to arrive at a theory about basic social processes (Silverman & Marvasti, 2008). The emergent theory is based on observations and perceptions of the social scene and evolves during data collection and analysis, as a product of the actual research process (Corbin & Strauss, 2008). Grounded theory is widely used by social scientists today, largely because it describes a research approach to construct theory where no theory exists, or in situations where existing theory fails to provide evidence to explain a set of circumstances.

Developed originally as a sociologist's tool to investigate interactions in social settings (Glaser & Strauss, 1967), the grounded theory method is used in many disciplines; in fact, investigators from different disciplines use grounded theory to study the same phenomenon from their varying perspectives (Corbin & Strauss, 2008; Denzin & Lincoln, 1998; Marshall & Rossman, 2011; Strauss & Corbin, 1994, 1997). For example, in an area of study such as chronic illness, a nurse might be interested in coping patterns within families, a psychologist might be interested in personal adjustment, and a sociologist might focus on group behavior in health care settings. Theories generated by each discipline will reflect the discipline and serve to help explain the phenomenon of interest within the discipline (Liehr & Marcus, 2002). In grounded theory, the usefulness of the study stems from the transferability of theories; that is, a theory derived from one study is applicable to another. Thus, the key objective of grounded theory is the development of formal theories spanning many disciplines that accurately reflect the cases from which they were derived (Sandelowski, 2004).

### Identifying the Phenomenon

Researchers typically use the grounded theory method when they are interested in social processes from the perspective of human interactions or patterns of action and interaction between and among various types of social units (Denzin & Lincoln, 1998). The basic social process is sometimes expressed in the form of a gerund (i.e., the -ing form of a verb when functioning as a noun), which is designed to indicate change occurring over time as social reality gets negotiated. For example, McCloskey (2012) describes the basic social process of women negotiating menopause as "changing focus."

### Structuring the Study

*Research Question.*  Research questions appropriate for the grounded theory method are those that address basic social processes that shape human behavior. In a grounded theory study, the research question can be a statement or a broad question that permits in-depth explanation of the phenomenon. McCloskey's (2012) study question was, "How do women move through the transition from menstrual to postmenstrual life?"

*Researcher's Perspective.*  In a grounded theory study, the researcher brings some knowledge of the literature to the study, but an exhaustive literature review may not be done. This allows theory to emerge directly from data and to reflect the contextual values that are integral to the social processes being studied. In this way, the new theory that emerges from the research is "grounded in" the data (Richards & Morse, 2007).

*Sample Selection.*  Sample selection involves choosing participants who are experiencing the circumstance and selecting events and incidents related to the social process under investigation. (To read about a purposive sample, see Chapter 12.) McCloskey (2012) used community-based recruiting for her study; since perimenopausal women can be found in many places, she put notices in suburban and rural newspapers, a community center, a women's shelter, and advertised by word of mouth.

## Data Gathering

In the grounded theory method, you will find that data are collected through interviews and through skilled observations of individuals interacting in a social setting. Interviews are recorded and transcribed, and observations are recorded as field notes. Open-ended questions are used initially to identify concepts for further focus. At her first data collection point, McCloskey (2012) interviewed 15 women; this was followed by a focus group with the same women. Then, to revisit the study question, she reinterviewed 4 of the original 15 and added 4 new participants, for a study total of 19. She also collected data from journals in which the women reflected on and expanded their responses to the interview questions.

## Data Analysis

A major feature of the grounded theory method is that data collection and analysis occur simultaneously. The process requires systematic data collection and documentation using field notes and transcribed interviews. Hunches about emerging patterns in the data are noted in memos that the researcher uses to direct activities in fieldwork. This technique, called **theoretical sampling**, is used to select experiences that will help the researcher to test hunches and ideas and to gather complete information about developing concepts. The researcher begins by noting indicators or actual events, actions, or words in the data. As data are concurrently collected and analyzed, new concepts, or abstractions, are developed from the indicators (Charmaz, 2000; Strauss, 1987).

The initial analytical process is called *open coding* (Strauss, 1987). Data are examined carefully line by line, broken down into discrete parts, then compared for similarities and differences (Corbin & Strauss, 2008). Coded data are continuously compared with new data as they are acquired during research. This is a process called the **constant comparative method**. When data collection is complete, codes in the data are clustered to form categories. The categories are expanded and developed or they are collapsed into one another, and relationships between the categories are used to develop new "grounded" theory. As a result, data collection, analysis, and theory generation have the direct, reciprocal relationship which grounds new theory in the perspectives of the research participants (Charmaz, 2000; Richards & Morse, 2007; Strauss & Corbin, 1990).

---

**HELPFUL HINT**

In a report of research using the grounded theory method, you can expect to find a diagrammed model of a theory that synthesizes the researcher's findings in a systematic way.

---

## Describing the Findings

Grounded theory studies are reported in detail that permit readers to follow the exact steps in the research process. Descriptive language and diagrams of the research process are used as evidence to document the researchers' procedures for moving from the raw data to the new theory. McCloskey (2012) found the basic social process of moving through menopause was "changing focus." During this process, women noted changes in all aspects of their lives. The most significant change was that of perspective and priority. Women changed focus from attending to the needs and distractions of other people and other things to a focus on themselves. They accomplished this through the following:

1. Monitoring the voice of the woman within: Detecting changes and identifying influences
2. Listening to the voices of others: Checking it out and seeking women's wisdom
3. Integrating the wisdom: Putting a name to it and just knowing
4. Nourishing the woman within: Focusing on self and taking time for me
5. Becoming a wise woman: Putting the pieces together and discovering new dimensions of me

---

**EVIDENCE-BASED PRACTICE TIP**

When thinking about the evidence generated by the grounded theory method, consider whether the theory is useful in explaining, interpreting, or predicting the study phenomenon of interest.

---

## Ethnographic Method

Derived from the Greek term ethnos, meaning people, race, or cultural group, the **ethnographic method** focuses on scientific description and interpretation of cultural or social groups and systems (Creswell, 1998). The goal of the ethnographer is to understand the research participants' views of their world, or the emic view. The **emic** (insiders') **view** is contrasted to the **etic** (outsiders') **view**, which is obtained when the researcher uses quantitative analyses of behavior. The ethnographic approach requires that the researcher enter the world of the study participants to watch what happens, listen to what is said, ask questions, and collect whatever data are available. It is important to note that the term ethnography is used to mean both the research technique and the product of that technique; that is, the study itself (Creswell, 1998; Richards & Morse, 2007; Tedlock, 2000). Vidick and Lyman (1998) trace the history of ethnography, with roots in the disciplines of sociology and anthropology, as a method born out of the need to understand "other" and "self." Nurses use the method to study cultural variations in health and patient groups as subcultures within larger social contexts (Liehr & Marcus, 2002).

## Identifying the Phenomenon

The phenomenon under investigation in an ethnographic study varies in scope from a long-term study of a very complex culture, such as that of the Aborigines (Mead, 1949), to a short-term study of a phenomenon within subunits of cultures. Kleinman (1992) notes the clinical utility of ethnography in describing the "local world" of groups of patients who are experiencing a particular phenomenon, such as suffering. The local worlds of patients have cultural, political, economic, institutional, and social-relational dimensions in much the same way as larger complex societies. An example of ethnography is found in MacKinnon's (2011) study of the safeguarding work of rural nurses who provide maternity care in small acute care hospitals. MacKinnon used institutional ethnography, which focuses on textual forms that replicate discourse, and the power relations that underpin discourse, over separations of space and time. Institutional ethnography traces the social and institutional determinants of experience; it is oriented to uncover oppressive power relations (MacKinnon, 2011).

## Structuring the Study

*Research Question.* In ethnographic studies, notice that questions are asked about "lifeways" or particular patterns of behavior within the social context of a culture or subculture. In this type of research, **culture** is viewed as the system of knowledge and linguistic expressions used by social groups that allows the researcher to interpret or make sense of the world (Aamodt, 1991; Richards & Morse, 2007). Thus, ethnographic nursing studies address questions that concern how cultural knowledge, norms, values, and other contextual variables influence people's health experiences. For example, MacKinnon's (2011) research question is implied in her purpose statement: "To explore the nature and social organization of rural nurses' work of providing maternity care." MacKinnon provides a detailed exploration of the safeguarding activities that rural nurses described when they shared chronological accounts of what they do every day and reflecting on what it was like for them to provide maternity care in a small rural hospital. Remember that ethnographers have a broader definition of culture, where a particular social context is conceptualized as a culture. In this case, rural nurses who provide maternity care in a small rural hospital are seen as a cultural entity that is appropriate for ethnographic study.

*Researcher's Perspective.* When using the ethnographic method, the researcher's perspective is that of an interpreter entering an alien world and attempting to make sense of that world from the insider's point of view (Richards & Morse, 2007). Like phenomenologists and grounded theorists, ethnographers make their own beliefs explicit and bracket, or set aside, their personal biases as they seek to understand the worldview of others.

*Sample Selection.* The ethnographer selects a cultural group that is living the phenomenon under investigation. The researcher gathers information from general informants and from key informants. **Key informants** are individuals who have special knowledge, status, or communication skills, and who are willing to teach the ethnographer about the phenomenon (Richards & Morse, 2007). For example, MacKinnon's (2011) research took place in a geographically large and relatively isolated eastern region of British Columbia. She described the setting in detail, allowing the reader to see just how isolated it is. Thirty registered nurses who worked in four rural acute care hospitals participated; 12 of them were new graduates.

---

### HELPFUL HINT

Managing personal bias is an expectation of researchers using all of the methods discussed in this chapter.

---

## Data Gathering

Ethnographic data gathering involves immersion in the study setting and the use of participant observation, interviews of informants, and interpretation by the researcher of cultural patterns (Richards & Morse, 2007). Ethnographic research in nursing, as in other disciplines, involves face-to-face interviewing with data collection and analysis taking place in the natural setting. Thus fieldwork is a major focus of the method. Other techniques may include obtaining life histories and collecting material items reflective of the culture. For example, photographs and films of the informants in their world can be used as data sources. In her study, MacKinnon (2011) observed the nurses as they went about their routine work; interviewed nurses, other health care providers, and front-line managers; and collected and analyzed texts that the nurses used or referred to during their work and/or interviews.

## Data Analysis

Like the grounded theory method, ethnographic data are collected and analyzed simultaneously. Data analysis proceeds through several levels as the researcher looks for the meaning of cultural symbols in the informant's language. Analysis begins with a search for domains or symbolic categories that include smaller categories. Language is analyzed for semantic relationships, and structural questions are formulated to expand and verify data. Analysis proceeds through increasing levels of complexity until the data, grounded in the informant's reality, are synthesized by the researcher (Richards & Morse, 2007). MacKinnon (2011) described analysis of data as beginning with an embodied experience; that is, through the informant's stories and descriptions the researcher begins to identify some of the translocal relations, discourses, and institutional work processes that shape the informant's everyday work. Institutional ethnography, which is specific to the workplace, provides a way to learn about how the various experiences as women and nurses are organized by things outside of their everyday experiences (MacKinnon, 2011).

## Describing the Findings

Ethnographic studies yield large quantities of data that reflect a wide array of evidence amassed as field notes of observations, interview transcriptions, and sometimes other artifacts such as photographs. The first level description is the description of the scene, the parameters or boundaries of the research group, and the overt characteristics of group members (Richards & Morse, 2007). Strategies that enhance first level description include maps/floor plans of the setting, organizational charts, and documents. Researchers may report item-level analysis, followed by pattern and structure level of analysis. Ethnographic research articles usually provide examples from data, thorough descriptions of the analytical process, and statements of the hypothetical propositions and their relationship to the ethnographer's frame of reference, which can be rather detailed and lengthy. MacKinnon (2011) found that nurses in rural hospitals working in maternity care engaged in safeguarding work. This included anticipating problems and emergencies and being prepared; careful watching, surveillance, and vigilance; negotiating safety; being able to react in emergency situations; and mobilizing emergency transport systems.

### EVIDENCE-BASED PRACTICE TIP

Evidence generated by ethnographic studies will answer questions about how cultural knowledge, norms, values, and other contextual variables influence the health experience of a particular patient population in a specific setting.

## Case Study

Case study research, which is rooted in sociology, has a complex history and many definitions (Aita & McIlvain, 1999). As noted by Stake (2000), a case study design is not a methodological choice; rather, it is a choice of what to study. Thus the case study method is about studying the peculiarities and the commonalities of a specific case, irrespective of the actual strategies for data collection and analysis that are used to explore the research questions. Case studies include quantitative and/or qualitative data, but are defined by their focus on uncovering an individual case and, in some instances, identifying patterns in variables that are consistent across a set of cases. Stake (2000) distinguishes intrinsic from instrumental case study. **Intrinsic case study** is undertaken to have a better understanding of the case; for example, one child with chicken pox, as opposed to a group or all children with chicken pox. The researcher at least temporarily subordinates other curiosities so that the stories of those "living the case" will be teased out (Stake, 2000). **Instrumental case study** is used when researchers are pursuing insight into an issue or want to challenge some generalization; for example, the qualities of sleep and restfulness in a set of four children with chicken pox. Very often, in case studies, there is an emphasis on holism, which means that researchers are searching for global understanding of a case within a spatially or temporally defined context.

## Identifying the Phenomenon

Although some definitions of case study demand that the focus of research be contemporary, Stake's (1995, 2000) defining criterion of attention to the single case broadens the scope of phenomenon for study. By a single case, Stake is designating a focus on an individual, a family, a community, an organization—some complex phenomenon that demands close scrutiny for understanding. Colón-Emeric and colleagues (2010) used a case study design to examine the influence of government regulations on mindful staff behavior in nursing homes as it related to resident health outcomes, and to explore how regulations sometimes increased mindfulness and other times limited it. To explore the way regulations influence mindful work in nursing homes, they used purposive sampling to choose high- and low-performing cases (nursing homes) for study and comparison.

## Structuring the Study

**Research Question.** Stake (2000) suggests that research questions be developed around issues that serve as a foundation to uncover complexity and pursue understanding. Although researchers pose questions to begin discussion, the initial questions are never all-inclusive; rather, the researcher uses an iterative process of "growing questions" in the field. That is, as data are collected to address these questions, it is expected that other questions will emerge and serve as guides to the researcher to untangle the complex, context-laden story within the case. For example, in Colón-Emeric and colleagues' study (2010), data were collected with semi-structured interviews, observations of staff members at work, and informal interviews with staff members to clarify or expand on data gathered with observation. By using multiple ways of identifying mindful behaviors, describing the experiences with government regulations, and registering the effects of regulations on mindful behaviors, the researchers were able to describe the phenomenon of interest at the level of entire cases. They were also able to compare the influence of regulations and mindful work practices on resident outcomes between nursing homes in their sample.

**Researcher's Perspective.** When the researcher begins with questions developed around suspected *issues* of importance, they are said to have an "etic" focus, which means the research is focused on the perspective of the researcher. As case study researchers engage the phenomenon of interest in individual cases, the uniqueness of individual stories unfold and shift from an etic (researcher orientation) to an emic (participant orientation) focus (Stake, 2000). Ideally, the case study researcher will develop an insider view which permits narration of the way things happen in the case.

**Sample Selection.** This is one of the areas where scholars in the field present differing views, ranging from only choosing the most common cases to only choosing the most unusual cases (Aita & McIlvain, 1999). Stake (2000) advocates selecting cases that may offer the best opportunities for learning. In some instances, the convenience of studying the case may even be a factor. For instance, if there are several patients who have undergone heart transplantation from which to choose, practical factors may influence who offers the best opportunity for learning. Persons who live in the area and can be easily visited at home or in the medical center might be better choices than those living much further away (where multiple contacts over time might be impossible). Similarly, the researcher may choose to study a case in which a potential participant has an actively involved family, because understanding the family context of transplant patients may shed important new light on their healing. It can safely be said that no choice is perfect when selecting a case; however, selecting cases for their contextual features fosters the strength of data that can be learned at the level of the individual case. For example, in Colón-Emeric and colleagues' (2010) study, the selection of eight nursing homes, chosen for the purpose of exploring mindful behavior in a setting, permitted the detailed data collection necessary for complete description of each case.

## Data Gathering

Case study data are gathered using interviews, field observations, document reviews, and any other methods that accumulate evidence for describing or explaining the complexity of the case. Stake (1995) advocates development of a data gathering plan to guide the progress of the study from definition of the case through decisions regarding data collection involving multiple methods, at multiple time points, and sometimes with multiple participants within the case. In the Colón-Emeric and colleagues' study (2010), multiple methods for collecting data were used, such as daily observations of staff at work and informal interviews to clarify observations. In addition, on multiple occasions during each case, research team members interviewed nursing home staff members for 45 to 60 minutes.

## Data Analysis/Describing Findings

Data analysis is often concurrent with data gathering and description of findings as the narrative in the case develops. Qualitative case study is characterized by researchers spending extended time on site, personally in contact with activities and operations of the case, and reflecting and revising meanings of what transpires (Stake, 2000). Reflecting and revising meanings are the work of the case study researcher, who records data, searches for patterns, links data from multiple sources, and develops preliminary thoughts regarding the meaning of collected data. This reflective and iterative process for writing the case narrative produces a unique form of evidence. Many times case study research reports do not list all of the research activities. However, reported findings are usually embedded in the following: (1) a chronological development of the case; (2) the researcher's story of coming to know the case; (3) the one-by-one description of case dimensions; and (4) vignettes that highlight case qualities (Stake, 1995). For example, Colón-Emeric and colleagues (2010) analyzed mindful behaviors in staff work, with an appraisal of trends in government regulations and nursing home resident health outcomes. Analysis consisted of the search for patterns in raw data, variation in the patterns within and between cases, and identification of themes that described common patterns within and between the cases. The researchers learned that a shared nursing home mission shaped staff perceptions of the purpose and utility of regulations. In nursing homes that tended to focus on individual resident needs and preferences, regulations increased mindful behavior; however, in facilities that focused on the cost of providing care, regulations reduced mindful care practices. These findings offered organizational tools that nursing home managers can use to create more mindful or attentive resident care in nursing homes.

---

**EVIDENCE-BASED PRACTICE TIP**

Case studies are a way of providing in-depth evidence-based discussion of clinical topics that can be used to guide practice.

---

## Community-Based Participatory Research

Community-based participatory research (CBPR) is a research method that systematically accesses the voice of a community to plan context-appropriate action. CBPR provides an alternative to traditional research approaches that assume a phenomenon may be separated from its context for purposes of study. Investigators who use CBPR recognize that engaging members of a study population as active and equal participants, in all phases of the research, is crucial for the research process to be a means of facilitating change (Holkup et al., 2004). Change or action is the intended "end-product" of CBPR, and "action research" is a term related to CBPR. Many scholars consider CBPR to be a type of action research and group them within the tradition of critical science (Fontana, 2004).

In his book Action Research, Stringer (1999) distilled the research process into three phases: look, think, act. In the look phase Stringer (1999) describes "building the picture" by getting to know stakeholders so that the problem is defined in their terms and the problem definition is reflective of the community context. He characterizes the think phase as interpretation and analysis of what was learned in the look phase. As investigators "think," the researcher is charged with connecting the ideas of the stakeholders so that they provide evidence that is understandable to the larger community group (Stringer, 1999). Finally, in the act phase, Stringer (1999) advocates planning, implementation, and evaluation based on information collected and interpreted in the other phases of research.

DiStefano and colleagues (2012) used focus groups and key informant interviews to identify and contextualize factors that shape HPV and HIV prevention and risk among Pacific Islander young adults. Their findings contextualized risk at the macro and micro levels of physical, social, economic, and policy environments, and led them to add a further cultural environment to the model. These researchers felt that risk and prevention interventions should focus on applying individual and community agency at the micro level for this group. Their nine themes included misinformation and otherization; dominant concerns regarding premarital pregnancy; restricted intergenerational communication; family shame and privacy; gendered manifestations of religio-cultural norms; barriers impeding access to sexual health resources; parents' role in prevention; community versus individual responsibility; and family and ethnic pride (DiStefano et al., 2012).

---

**EVIDENCE-BASED PRACTICE TIP**

Although qualitative in its approach to research, community-based participatory research leads to an action component in which a nursing intervention is implemented and evaluated for its effectiveness in a specific patient population.

TABLE 6-1 **CHARACTERISTICS OF QUALITATIVE RESEARCH GENERATING ETHICAL CONCERNS**

| CHARACTERISTICS | ETHICAL CONCERNS |
| --- | --- |
| Naturalistic setting | Some researchers using methods that rely on participant observation may believe that consent is not always possible or necessary. |
| Emergent nature of design | Planning for questioning and observation emerges over the time of the study. Thus it is difficult to inform the participant precisely of all potential threats before he or she agrees to participate. |
| Researcher-participant interaction | Relationships developed between the researcher and participant may blur the focus of the interaction. |
| Researcher as instrument | The researcher is the study instrument, collecting data and interpreting the participant's reality. |

## ISSUES IN QUALITATIVE RESEARCH

### Ethics

Protection of human subjects is always the most important aspect of any scientific investigation. This demand exists for both quantitative and qualitative research approaches. Human subjects' protection in quantitative approaches is discussed in Chapter 13. These basic tenets hold true for the qualitative approach. However, several characteristics of the qualitative methodologies outlined in Table 6-1 generate unique concerns and require an expanded view of protecting human subjects.

### Naturalistic Setting

The central concern that arises when research is conducted in naturalistic settings focuses on the need to gain informed consent. The need to acquire informed consent is a basic researcher responsibility, but is not always easy to obtain in naturalistic settings. For instance, when research methods include observing groups of people interacting over time, the complexity of gaining consent becomes apparent: Have all parties consented for all periods of time? Have all parties been consented? What have all parties consented to doing? These complexities generate controversy and debate among qualitative researchers. The balance between respect for human participants and efforts to collect meaningful data must be continuously negotiated. The reader should look for information that the researcher has addressed this issue of balance by recording attention to human participant protection.

### Emergent Nature of Design

The emergent nature of the research design in qualitative research underscores the need for ongoing negotiation of consent with participants. In the course of a study, situations change, and what was agreeable at the beginning may become intrusive. Sometimes, as data collection proceeds and new information emerges, the study shifts direction in a way that is not acceptable to participants. For instance, if the researcher were present in a family's home during a time when marital discord arose, the family may choose to renegotiate the consent. From another perspective, Morse (1998) discussed the increasing involvement of participants in the research process, sometimes resulting in their request to have their name published in the findings or be included as a coauthor. If the participant originally signed a consent form and then chose an active identified role, Morse (1998) suggests that the participant then sign a "release for publication" form to address this request. The emergent qualitative research process demands ongoing negotiation of researcher-participant relationships, including the consent relationship. The opportunity to renegotiate consent establishes a relationship of trust and respect characteristic of the ethical conduct of research.

## Researcher-Participant Interaction

The nature of the researcher-participant interaction over time introduces the possibility that the research experience will become a therapeutic one. It is a case of research becoming practice. It is important to recognize that there are basic differences between the intent of nurses when engaging in practice and when conducting research (Smith & Liehr, 2003). In practice, the nurse has caring-healing intentions. In research, the nurse intends to "get the picture" from the perspective of the participant. The process of "getting the picture" may be a therapeutic experience for the participant. Talking to a caring listener about things that matter promotes healing, even though it was not intended. From an ethical perspective, the qualitative researcher is promising only to listen and to encourage the other's story. If this experience is therapeutic for the participant, it becomes an unplanned benefit of the research. If it becomes harmful, the ethics of continuing the research becomes an issue and the study design will require revision.

## Researcher as Instrument

The responsibility to establish rigor in data collection and analysis requires that the researcher acknowledge any personal bias and strive to interpret data in a way that accurately reflects the participant's point of view. This serious ethical obligation may require that researchers return to the subjects at critical interpretive points and ask for clarification or validation.

## Credibility, Auditability, and Fittingness

Quantitative studies are concerned with reliability and validity of instruments, as well as internal and external validity criteria as measures of scientific rigor (see the Critical Thinking Decision Path), but these are not appropriate for qualitative work. The rigor of qualitative methodology is judged by unique criteria appropriate to the research approach. Credibility, auditability, and fittingness were scientific criteria proposed for qualitative research studies by Guba and Lincoln in 1981. Although these criteria were proposed decades ago, they still capture the rigorous spirit of qualitative inquiry and persist as reasonable criteria for appraisal of scientific rigor in the research. The meanings of credibility, auditability, and fittingness are briefly explained in Table 6-2.

## Triangulation

Triangulation is a term used in surveying and navigation. Triangulation has grown in popularity over the past several years and refers to the combination of several methods. Triangulation can be defined as using two pieces of information to locate a third, unique finding. Marshall and Rossman (2011) define it as the act of bringing more than one source of data to bear on a single point. Data from different sources can be used to corroborate, elaborate, or illuminate the phenomenon in question. For example, we might interview a patient and his nurse to triangulate and learn a broader conception of the

| TABLE 6-2 | CRITERIA FOR JUDGING SCIENTIFIC RIGOR: CREDIBILITY, AUDITABILITY, FITTINGNESS |
|---|---|
| **CRITERIA** | **CRITERIA CHARACTERISTICS** |
| Credibility | Truth of findings as judged by participants and others within the discipline. For instance, you may find the researcher returning to the participants to share interpretation of findings and query accuracy from the perspective of the persons living the experience. |
| Auditabililty | Accountability as judged by the adequacy of information leading the reader from the research question and raw data through various steps of analysis to the interpretation of findings. For instance, you should be able to follow the reasoning of the researcher step-by-step through explicit examples of data, interpretations, and syntheses. |
| Fittingness | Faithfulness to everyday reality of the participants, described in enough detail so that others in the discipline can evaluate importance for their own practice, research, and theory development. For instance, you will know enough about the human experience being reported that you can decide whether it "rings true" and is useful for guiding your practice. |

patient's recovery. Silverman and Marvasti (2008) advocate for beginning from a theoretical perspective or model when using triangulation, and for choosing methods and data that will give an account of structure and meaning from within that perspective. As you read nursing research, you will quickly discover that approaches and methods, such as triangulation, are being combined to contribute to theory building, guide practice, and facilitate instrument development.

Although certain kinds of questions may be answered effectively by combining qualitative and quantitative methods in a single study (e.g., triangulating research methods), this does not necessarily make the findings and related evidence stronger. In fact, if a researcher inappropriately combines methods in a single study, the findings could be weaker and less credible. As a nurse, you need to determine why researchers chose a particular approach for their study and whether this was an appropriate choice. You are encouraged to follow the ongoing debate about combining methods as nurse researchers strive to determine which research combinations foster understanding and contributions to nursing science.

## EVIDENCE-BASED PRACTICE TIP

- Triangulation offers an opportunity for researchers to increase the strength and consistency of evidence provided by the use of both qualitative and quantitative research methods.
- The combination of stories with numbers (qualitative and quantitative research approaches) through use of triangulation may provide the most complete picture of the phenomenon being studied and, therefore, the best evidence for guiding practice.

## Synthesizing Qualitative Evidence: Meta-Synthesis

The depth and breadth of qualitative research has grown over the years, and it has become important to qualitative researchers to synthesize critical masses of qualitative findings.

The terms most commonly used to describe this activity are qualitative meta-summary and qualitative meta-synthesis. Qualitative **meta-summary** is a quantitatively-oriented aggregation of qualitative findings that are topical or thematic summaries or surveys of data. Meta-summaries are integrations that are approximately equal to the sum of parts, or the sum of findings across reports in a target domain of research. They address the manifest content in findings and reflect a quantitative logic: to discern the frequency of each finding and to find in higher frequency findings the evidence of replication foundational to validity in most quantitative research. Qualitative meta-summary involves the extraction and further abstraction of findings, and the calculation of manifest frequency effect sizes (Sandelowski & Barroso, 2003a). Qualitative meta-synthesis is an interpretive integration of qualitative findings that are interpretive syntheses of data, including the phenomenologies, ethnographies, grounded theories, and other integrated and coherent descriptions or explanations of phenomena, events, or cases that are the hallmarks of qualitative research. Meta-syntheses are integrations that are more than the sum of parts in that they offer novel interpretations of findings. These interpretations will not be found in any one research report; rather, they are inferences derived from taking all of the reports in a sample as a whole. Meta-syntheses offer a coherent description or explanation of a target event or experience, instead of a summary view of unlinked features of that event or experience. Such interpretive integrations require researchers to piece the individual syntheses constituting the findings in individual research reports together to craft one or more meta-syntheses. Their validity does not reside in a replication logic, but in an inclusive logic whereby all findings are accommodated and the accumulative analysis displayed in the final product. Meta-synthesis methods include constant comparison, taxonomic analysis, the reciprocal translation of in vivo concepts, and the use of imported concepts to frame data (Sandelowski & Barroso, 2003b). Meta-synthesis integrates qualitative research findings on a topic and is based on comparative analysis and interpretative synthesis of qualitative research findings that seeks to retain the essence and unique contribution of each study (Sandelowski & Barroso, 2007).

Sandelowski and Barroso (2005) reported the results of a qualitative meta-synthesis and meta-summary that integrated the findings of qualitative studies of expectant parents who experienced a positive prenatal diagnosis. Using the methods of qualitative research synthesis (e.g., meta-analysis and meta-summary), Sandelowski and Barroso (2007) reviewed and synthesized findings from 17 qualitative studies retrieved from multiple databases. This meta-synthesis provided a way to describe findings across a set of qualitative studies and create knowledge that is relevant to clinical practice. Sandelowski (2004) cautions that the use of qualitative meta-synthesis is laudable and necessary, but requires careful application of qualitative meta-synthesis methods. There are a number of meta-synethesis studies being conducted by nurse scientists. It will be interesting for research consumers to follow the progress of researchers who seek to develop criteria for appraising a set of qualitative studies and using those criteria to guide the incorporation of these studies into systematic literature reviews.

# APPRAISING THE EVIDENCE
## QUALITATIVE RESEARCH

General criteria for critiquing qualitative research are proposed in the following Critiquing Criteria box. Each qualitative method has unique characteristics that influence what the research consumer may expect in the published research report, and journals often have page restrictions that penalize qualitative research. The criteria for critiquing are formatted

## CRITIQUING CRITERIA
### *Qualitative Approaches*

**Identifying the Phenomenon**
1. Is the phenomenon focused on human experience within a natural setting?
2. Is the phenomenon relevant to nursing and/or health?

**Structuring the Study**
*Research Question*
3. Does the question specify a distinct process to be studied?
4. Does the question identify the context (participant group/place) of the process that will be studied?
5. Does the choice of a specific qualitative method fit with the research question?

*Researcher's Perspective*
6. Are the biases of the researcher reported?
7. Do the researchers provide a structure of ideas that reflect their beliefs?

*Sample Selection*
8. Is it clear that the selected sample is living the phenomenon of interest?

**Data Gathering**
9. Are data sources and methods for gathering data specified?
10. Is there evidence that participant consent is an integral part of the data-gathering process?

**Data Analysis**
11. Can the dimensions of data analysis be identified and logically followed?
12. Does the researcher paint a clear picture of the participant's reality?
13. Is there evidence that the researcher's interpretation captured the participant's meaning?
14. Have other professionals confirmed the researcher's interpretation?

**Describing the Findings**
15. Are examples provided to guide the reader from the raw data to the researcher's synthesis?
16. Does the researcher link the findings to existing theory or literature, or is a new theory generated?

to evaluate the selection of the phenomenon, the structure of the study, data gathering, data analysis, and description of the findings. Each question of the criteria focuses on factors discussed throughout the chapter. Appraising qualitative research is a useful activity for learning the nuances of this research approach. You are encouraged to identify a qualitative study of interest and apply the criteria for critiquing. Keep in mind that qualitative methods are the best way to start to answer clinical and/or research questions that previously have not been addressed in research studies or that do not lend themselves to a quantitative approach. The answers provided by qualitative data reflect important evidence that may provide the first insights about a patient population or clinical phenomenon.

In summary, the term **qualitative research** is an overriding description of multiple methods with distinct origins and procedures. In spite of distinctions, each method shares a common nature that guides data collection from the perspective of the participants to create a story that synthesizes disparate pieces of data into a comprehensible whole that provides evidence and promises direction for building nursing knowledge.

### KEY POINTS

- Qualitative research is the investigation of human experiences in naturalistic settings, pursuing meanings that inform theory, practice, instrument development, and further research.
- Qualitative research studies are guided by research questions.
- Data saturation occurs when the information being shared with the researcher becomes repetitive.
- Qualitative research methods include five basic elements: identifying the phenomenon, structuring the study, gathering the data, analyzing the data, and describing the findings.
- The phenomenological method is a process of learning and constructing the meaning of human experience through intensive dialogue with persons who are living the experience.
- The grounded theory method is an inductive approach that implements a systematic set of procedures to arrive at theory about basic social processes.
- The ethnographic method focuses on scientific descriptions of cultural groups.
- The case study method focuses on a selected phenomenon over a short or long time period to provide an in-depth description of its essential dimensions and processes.
- Community-based participatory research is a method that systematically accesses the voice of a community to plan context-appropriate action.
- Ethical issues in qualitative research involve issues related to the naturalistic setting, emergent nature of the design, researcher-participant interaction, and researcher as instrument.
- Credibility, auditability, and fittingness are criteria for judging the scientific rigor of a qualitative research study.
- Triangulation has shifted from a strategy for combining research methods to assess accuracy to expansion of research methods in a single study or multiple studies to enhance diversity, enrich understanding, and accomplish specific goals. A better term may be crystallization.
- Multimethod approaches to research are promising.

### CRITICAL THINKING CHALLENGES

- How can triangulation increase the effectiveness of qualitative research?
- How can a nurse researcher select a qualitative research method when he or she is attempting to accumulate evidence regarding a new topic about which little is known?
- How can the case study approach to research be applied to evidence-based practice?
- Describe characteristics of qualitative research that can generate ethical concerns.

## REFERENCES

Aamodt, A. A. (1991). Ethnography and epistemology: generating nursing knowledge. In J. M. Morse (Ed.), *Qualitative nursing research: a contemporary dialogue.* Newbury Park, CA: Sage.

Aita, V. A., & McIlvain, H.E. (1999). An armchair adventure in case study research. In B. Crabtree, & W. L. Miller (Eds.), *Doing qualitative research.* Thousand Oaks, CA: Sage.

Charmaz, K. (2000). Grounded theory: Objectivist and constructivist methods. In N. K. Denzin, & Y. S. Lincoln (Eds.), *Handbook of qualitative research*. Thousand Oaks, CA: Sage.

Colaizzi, P. (1978). Psychological research as a phenomenologist views it. In R. S. Valle, & M. King (Eds.), *Existential phenomenological alternatives for psychology*. New York, NY: Oxford University Press.

Colón-Emeric C. S., Plowman D., Bailey, D., et al. (2010). Regulation and mindful resident care in nursing homes. *Qualitative Health Research*, *20*, 1283–1294.

Corbin, J., & Strauss, A. (2008). *Basics of qualitative research*. Los Angeles, CA: Sage.

Creswell, J. W. (1998). *Qualitative inquiry and research design: Choosing among five traditions*. Thousand Oaks, CA: Sage.

Denzin, N. K., & Lincoln, Y. S. (1998). *The landscape of qualitative research*. Thousand Oaks, CA: Sage.

DiStefano, A. S., Hui, B., Barrera-Ng, A., et al. (2012). Contextualization of HIV and HPV risk and prevention among Pacific Islander young adults in Southern California. *Social Science and Medicine*, *75*, 699–708.

Fontana, J.S. (2004). A methodology for critical science in nursing. *Adv Nurs Sci*, *27*(2), 93–101.

Glaser, B. G., & Strauss, A.L. (1967). *The discovery of grounded theory: Strategies for qualitative research*. Chicago, IL: Aldine.

Guba, E., & Lincoln, Y. (1981). *Effective evaluation*. San Francisco: Jossey-Bass.

Holkup, PA, Tripp-Reimer, T., Salois, EM, Weinert, C. (2004). Community-based participatory research: An approach to intervention research with a Native American community. *ANS Advance Nurs Science*, July-Sept; *27*(3), 162–175.

Kleinman, A. (1992). Local worlds of suffering: An interpersonal focus for ethnographies of illness experience. *Qual Health Res*, *2*(2), 127–134.

Liehr, P., & Marcus, M. T. (2002). Qualitative approaches to research. In G. LoBiondo-Wood, & J. Haber (Eds.), *Nursing research: Methods, critical appraisal, and utilization* (5th ed.) (pp. 139–164). St Louis, MO: Mosby.

MacKinnon, K. (2011). Rural nurses' safeguarding work: Reembodying patient safety. *Adv Nurs Sci*, *34*(2), 119–129.

Marshall, C., & Rossman, G. B. (2011). *Designing qualitative research* (5th ed.). Los Angeles, CA: Sage.

McCloskey, C. R. (2012). Changing focus: Women's perimenopausal journey. *Health Care Women International*, *33*(6), 540–559.

Mead, M. (1949). *Coming of age in Samoa*. New York, NY: New American Library, Mentor Books.

Morse, J. M. (1998). The contracted relationship: ensuring protection of anonymity and confidentiality. *Qual Health Res*, *8*(3), 301–303.

Moules, N. J., Laing, C. M., McCaffrey, G., et al. (2012).Grandparents' experiences of childhood cancer, part 1: Doubled and silenced. *J Ped Onc Nurs*, *29*(3), 119–132.

Richards, L., & Morse, J. M. (2007). *Read me first for a user's guide to qualitative methods* (2nd ed.). Los Angeles, CA: Sage.

Sandelowski, M. (2004). Using qualitative research. *Qual Health Res*, *14*(10), 1366–1386.

Sandelowski, M., & Barroso, J. (2003a). Creating metasummaries of qualitative findings. *Nursing Research*, *52*, 226–33.

Sandelowski, M., & Barroso, J. (2003b). Toward a metasynthesis of qualitative findings on motherhood in HIV-positive women. *Research in Nursing & Health*, *26*, 153–170.

Sandelowski, M., & Barroso, J. (2005). The travesty of choosing after positive prenatal diagnosis. *J Obstet Gynecol Neonatal Nursing*, *34*(4), 307–318.

Sandelowski, M., & Barroso, J. (2007). *Handbook for synthesizing qualitative research*. Philadelphia, PA: Springer.

Silverman, D., & Marvasti, A. (2008). *Doing qualitative research*. Los Angeles, CA: Sage.

Smith, M. J., & Liehr, P. (2003). The theory of attentively embracing story. In M. J. Smith, & P. Liehr (Eds.), *Middle range theory for nursing*. New York, NY: Springer.

Stake, R. E. (1995). *The art of case study research*. Thousand Oaks, CA: Sage.

Stake, R. E. (2000). Case studies. In N. K. Denzin, & Y. S. Lincoln (Eds.), *Handbook of qualitative research* (2nd ed.). Thousand Oaks, CA: Sage.

Strauss, A. L. (1987). *Qualitative analysis for social scientists*. New York, NY: Cambridge University Press.

Strauss, A., & Corbin, J. (1990). *Basics of qualitative research: grounded theory procedures and techniques.* Newbury Park, CA: Sage.

Strauss, A., & Corbin, J. (1994). Grounded theory methodology. In N. K. Denzin, & Y. S. Lincoln (Eds.), *Handbook of qualitative research*. Thousand Oaks, CA: Sage.

Strauss, A., & Corbin, J. (Eds.), (1997). *Grounded theory in practice*. Thousand Oaks, CA: Sage.

Stringer, E. T. (1999). *Action research* (2nd ed.). Thousand Oaks, CA: Sage.

Tedlock, B. (2000). Ethnography and ethnographic representation. In N. K. Denzin, & Y. S. Lincoln (Eds.), *Handbook of qualitative research*. Thousand Oaks, CA: Sage.

Vidick, A. J., & Lyman, S. M. (1998). Qualitative methods: their history in sociology and anthropology. In N. K. Denzin, & Y. S. Lincoln (Eds.), *The landscape of qualitative research: theories and issues.* Thousand Oaks, CA: Sage.

# ⊖volve WEBSITE

*Go to Evolve at http://evolve.elsevier.com/LoBiondo/ for review questions, critquing exercises, and additional research articles for practice in reviewing and critiquing.*

# 7

# Appraising Qualitative Research

*Helen J. Streubert*

## ⊝volve WEBSITE

*Go to Evolve at http://evolve.elsevier.com/LoBiondo/ for review questions, critiquing exercises, and additional research articles for practice in reviewing and critiquing.*

## LEARNING OUTCOMES

*After reading this chapter, you should be able to do the following:*

- Identify the influence of stylistic considerations on the presentation of a qualitative research report.
- Identify the criteria for critiquing a qualitative research report.
- Evaluate the strengths and weaknesses of a qualitative research report.
- Describe the applicability of the findings of a qualitative research report.
- Construct a critique of a qualitative research report.

## KEY TERMS

| | | | |
|---|---|---|---|
| auditability | grounded theory | saturation | transferability |
| credibility | phenomena | theme | trustworthiness |
| emic view | | | |

Nurses contribute significantly to the growing body of health care research. Specifically, the influence of their work can be found in nursing, medical, health care, and business journals. Nurse researchers continue to partner with other health care professionals to develop, implement, and evaluate a variety of evidence-based interventions to improve client outcomes. The methods used to develop evidence-based practice include quantitative, qualitative, and mixed research approaches. In addition to the increase in the number of research studies and publications, there is also a significant record of externally funded research by nurses adding to the credibility of the work. The willingness of private and publicly funded organizations to invest in nursing research attests to its quality and potential for affecting health care outcomes of individuals, families, groups, and communities. Quantitative, qualitative, and mixed research methods are all important to the ongoing development of a sound evidence-based practice. As a result of this increased focus, this chapter will help the reader to understand how to assess the quality of qualitative research studies.

Qualitative and quantitative research methods are derived from strong traditions in the physical and social sciences. The two types of research are different in their purpose, approach, analysis, and conclusions. Therefore the use of each requires an understanding of the traditions on which the methods are based. The historical development of the methods identified as qualitative or quantitative can be discovered in this and other texts. This chapter aims to demonstrate a set of criteria that can be used to determine the quality of a qualitative research report. Nurses must fully understand how to assess the value of qualitative research, particularly in light of the requirement that nursing practice be evidence-based. According to Straus and Sackett (2005), evidence-based practice requires that patient values, clinical expertise, and the best evidence from published research be used in combination.

Leeman and Sandelowski (2012) attest to the value of patient outcomes-based qualitative research, but also challenge qualitative researchers to consider the value of these methods by learning about the evidence base that supports the adoption of evidence-based practice in the clinical setting. They contend that it is important to study the "culture and networks of social systems" (p. 172) in which evidence-based practice exists in order to better understand the context which empowers the adoption of particular practices. Mantzoukas (2007) argues that it is the reflection by practitioners that leads to an appropriate contextual application of evidence-based interventions. This supports the ideas posited by Leeman and Sandelowski. Qualitative methodology provides nurses an opportunity to study the processes and relationships that lead to the acceptance of evidence-based practice, an understanding of which can be used as a foundation to provide improved patient care.

As a framework for understanding how the appraisal of qualitative research can support evidence-based practice, a published research report and critiquing criteria will be presented. The critiquing criteria will be used to demonstrate the process of appraising a qualitative research report.

## STYLISTIC CONSIDERATIONS

Qualitative research differs from quantitative research in some very fundamental ways. Qualitative researchers represent a basic level of inquiry that seeks to discover and understand concepts, phenomena, or cultures. Jackson and colleagues (2007) state the primary focus of qualitative research is to understand human beings' experiences in a humanistic and interpretive way (p. 21). In a qualitative study you should not expect to find hypotheses; theoretical frameworks; dependent and independent variables; large, random samples; complex statistical procedures; scaled instruments; or definitive conclusions about how to use the findings. Because the intent of qualitative research is to describe, explain, or understand phenomena or cultures, the report is generally written in a narrative that is meant to convey the full meaning and richness of the phenomena or cultures being studied. This narrative includes subjective comments that are intended to provide the depth and richness of the phenomena under study.

The goal of a qualitative research report is to describe in as much detail as possible the "insider's" or emic view of the phenomenon being studied. The emic view is the view of the person experiencing the phenomenon reflective of his or her culture, values, beliefs, and experiences. What the qualitative researcher hopes to produce in the report is an understanding of what it is like to experience a particular phenomenon or be part of a specific culture.

One of the most effective ways to help the reader understand the emic view is to use quotes reflecting the phenomenon as experienced. For this reason the qualitative research report has a more conversational tone than a quantitative report. In addition, data are frequently reported using concepts or phrases that are called themes (see Chapters 5 and 6). A **theme** is a label. Themes represent a way of describing large quantities of data in a condensed format. To illustrate the application of a theme and how it helps the reader understand the emic view, the following is offered from a report published by Seiler and Moss (2012, Appendix C). The authors' purpose is to "gain insights into the unique experiences of nurse practitioners (NPs) who provide health care to the homeless." The following quote is used by Seiler and Moss to demonstrate the theme of "making a difference." Using the informant's words, the researchers share how working with the homeless makes a difference:

> *"There's so much need and so much difference that we can make, so I feel like my efforts reap so much reward, so it makes it the best job ever though I'm exhausted at the end of the day because it is hard."*

The richness of the narrative provided in a qualitative research study cannot be shared in its entirety in a journal publication. Page limitations imposed by journals frequently limit research reports to 15 pages. Despite this limitation, it is the qualitative researcher's responsibility to illustrate the richness of the data and to convey to the audience the relationship between the themes identified and the quotes shared. This is essential in order to document the rigor of the research, which is called **trustworthiness** in a qualitative research study. It is challenging to convey the depth and richness of the findings of a qualitative study in a published research report. A perusal of the nursing and health care literature will demonstrate a commitment by qualitative researchers and journal editors to publish qualitative research findings. Regardless of the page limit, Jackson and colleagues (2007) offer that it is the researcher's responsibility to ensure objectivity, ethical diligence, and rigor regardless of the method selected to conduct the study. Fully sharing the depth and richness of the data will also help practitioners to decide on the appropriateness of applying the findings to their practice.

There are some journals that by virtue of their readership are committed to publication of more lengthy reports. Qualitative Health Research is an example of a journal that provides the opportunity for longer research reports. Guidelines for publication of research reports are generally listed in each nursing journal or are available from the journal editor. It is important to note that criteria for publication of research reports are not based on a specific type of research method (i.e., quantitative or qualitative). The primary goal of journal editors is to provide their readers with high quality, informative, timely, and interesting articles. To meet this goal, regardless of the type of research report, editors prefer to publish manuscripts that have scientific merit, present new knowledge, support the current state of the science, and engage their readership. The challenge for the qualitative researcher is to meet these editorial requirements within the page limit imposed by the journal of interest.

Nursing journals do not generally offer their reviewers specific guidelines for evaluating qualitative and quantitative research reports. The editors make every attempt to see that reviewers are knowledgeable in the method and subject matter of the study. This determination is often made, however, based on the reviewer's self-identified area of interest. Research reports are often evaluated based on the ideas or philosophical viewpoints held by the reviewer. The reviewer may have strong feelings about particular types of qualitative or quantitative research methods. Therefore it is important to clearly state the qualitative approach used and, where appropriate, its philosophical base.

Fundamentally, principles for evaluating research are the same. Reviewers are concerned with the plausibility and trustworthiness of the researcher's account of the research and its potential and/or actual relevance to current or future theory and practice (Horsburgh, 2003, p. 308). The Critiquing Criteria: Qualitative Research box below provides general guidelines for reviewing qualitative research. For information on specific guidelines for appraisal of phenomenology, ethnography, grounded theory, historical, and action research, see Streubert and Carpenter (2011). If you are interested in additional information on the specifics of qualitative research design, see Chapters 5 and 6.

## CRITIQUING CRITERIA

### *Qualitative Research*

**Statement of the Phenomenon of Interest**
1. What is the phenomenon of interest and is it clearly stated for the reader?
2. What is the justification for using a qualitative method?
3. What are the philosophical underpinnings of the research method?

**Purpose**
1. What is the purpose of the study?
2. What is the projected significance of the work to nursing?

**Method**
1. Is the method used to collect data compatible with the purpose of the research?
2. Is the method adequate to address the phenomenon of interest?
3. If a particular approach is used to guide the inquiry, does the researcher complete the study according to the processes described?

**Sampling**
1. What type of sampling is used? Is it appropriate given the particular method?
2. Are the informants who were chosen appropriate to inform the research?

**Data Collection**
1. Is data collection focused on human experience?
2. Does the researcher describe data collection strategies (i.e., interview, observation, field notes)?
3. Is protection of human participants addressed?
4. Is saturation of the data described?
5. What are the procedures for collecting data?

**Data Analysis**
1. What strategies are used to analyze the data?
2. Has the researcher remained true to the data?
3. Does the reader follow the steps described for data analysis?
4. Does the researcher address the credibility, auditability, and fittingness of the data?

*Continued*

*Credibility*

a. Do the participants recognize the experience as their own?

b. Has adequate time been allowed to fully understand the phenomenon?

*Auditability*

a. Can the reader follow the researcher's thinking?

b. Does the researcher document the research process?

*Fittingness*

a. Are the findings applicable outside of the study situation?

b. Are the results meaningful to individuals not involved in the research?

c. Is the strategy used for analysis compatible with the purpose of the study?

*Findings*

1. Are the findings presented within a context?

2. Is the reader able to apprehend the essence of the experience from the report of the findings?

3. Are the researcher's conceptualizations true to the data?

4. Does the researcher place the report in the context of what is already known about the phenomenon? Was the existing literature on the topic related to the findings?

*Conclusions, Implications, and Recommendations*

1. Do the conclusions, implications, and recommendations give the reader a context in which to use the findings?

2. How do the conclusions reflect the study findings?

3. What are the recommendations for future study? Do they reflect the findings?

4. How has the researcher made explicit the significance of the study to nursing theory, research, or practice?

# APPLICATION OF QUALITATIVE RESEARCH FINDINGS IN PRACTICE

The purpose of qualitative research is to describe, understand, or explain phenomena or cultures. **Phenomena** are those things that are perceived by our senses. For example, pain and losing a loved one are considered phenomena. Unlike quantitative research, prediction and control of phenomena are not the aim of the qualitative inquiry. Therefore, qualitative results are applied differently than more traditional quantitative research findings. Barbour and Barbour (2003, p. 185) state that

> *"rather than seeking to import and impose templates and methods devised for another purpose, qualitative researchers and reviewers should look . . . for inspiration from their own modes of working and collaborating and seek to incorporate these, forging new and creative solutions to perennial problems, rather than hoping that these will simply disappear in the face of application of pre-existing sets of procedures."*

Further, Barbour and Barbour (2003) offer that qualitative research can provide the opportunity to give voice to those who have been disenfranchised and have no history. Therefore the application of qualitative findings will necessarily be context-bound (Russell & Gregory, 2003). This means that if a qualitative researcher studies, for example, professional dignity in nursing, the application of these findings is confined to individuals who are similar to those who informed the research.

Qualitative research findings can be used to create solutions to practical problems (Glesne, 1999). Qualitative research also has the ability to contribute to the evidenced-based practice literature (Cesario et al., 2002; Gibson & Martin, 2003; Walsh & Downe, 2005). For instance, in the development of a grounded theory study of the emotional process of stroke recovery, Gallagher (2011) shares how critical it is for care providers to let their patients set goals despite practitioners' level of knowledge and experience. As the author in this research report points out, those recovering from stroke at times feel a dissonance from their provider. Once stroke victims have their basic needs met, they report an incongruity between the goals they set for themselves and what their therapists see as priorities.

It is important to view research findings within context, whether quantitative or qualitative. For instance, a quantitative study of survivorship in female breast cancer survivors (Meneses et al., 2007) should not be viewed as applicable to survivors of another "survivor" situation such as an epidemic or mass casualty. The findings must be used within context, or additional studies must be conducted to validate the applicability of the findings across situations and patient populations. This is true in qualitative research, as well. Nurses who wish to use the findings of qualitative research in their practice must validate them, through thorough examination and synthesis of the literature on the topic, through their own observations, or through interaction with groups similar to the study participants, to determine whether the findings accurately reflect the experience.

Morse and colleagues (2000) offer "qualitative outcome analysis (QOA) [as a] systematic means to confirm the applicability of clinical strategies developed from a single qualitative project, to extend the repertoire of clinical interventions, and evaluate clinical outcomes" (p. 125). Using this process, the researcher employs the findings of a qualitative study to develop interventions and then to test those selected. Qualitative outcome analysis allows the researcher/clinician to implement interventions based on the client's expressed experience of a particular clinical phenomenon. Further, Morse and colleagues (2000) state, "QOA may be considered a form of participant action research" (p. 129). Application of knowledge discovered during qualitative data collection adds to our understanding of clinical phenomena by using interventions that are based on the client's experience. QOA is considered a form of evaluation research and as such has the potential to add to evidence-based practice literature either at Level V or at Level VI depending on how the study is designed.

Another use of qualitative research findings is to initiate examination of important concepts in nursing practice, education, or administration. For example, surgical consent as a concept has been studied using both qualitative and quantitative methods. It is considered a significant responsibility in nursing. Therefore studying its multiple dimensions is important. In a study by Cole (2012), the author examined implied consent as it relates to patient autonomy. The informants were nurses in a one day surgical unit. The outcome of her research was a richer understanding of how nurses view implied consent and the dimensions of the relationship necessary for the patient to exercise his or her autonomy. The study adds to the existing body of knowledge on patient consent and extends the current state of the science by examining a specific area of nursing practice and the experience of practicing nurses. This type of study is at Level V or VI, which includes either systematic reviews or single studies that are descriptive or qualitative in their design (see Chapter 1).

Meta-synthesis is also a widely accepted method of synthesizing findings from a number of qualitative research studies in an attempt to further validate the conceptualizations found among individual qualitative studies. According to Finfgeld-Connett

(2010) meta-synthesis is a way of integrating findings from a number of disparate investigations to increase their utilization in practice and in policy formation. Further, when these evidentiary-based generalizations are made, they add to the generalizability and transferability of the research (p. 252).

Finally, qualitative research can be used to discover evidence about phenomena of interest that can lead to instrument development. When qualitative methods are used to direct the development of structured measurement instruments, it is usually part of a larger empirical research project. Instrument development from qualitative research studies is useful to practicing nurses because it is grounded in the reality of human experience with a particular phenomenon and informs item development. A study completed by Richards (2008) illustrates the use of both qualitative and quantitative methods to develop, revise, and test a pain assessment instrument.

## CRITIQUE OF A QUALITATIVE RESEARCH STUDY

## THE RESEARCH STUDY

The study "Becoming Normal: A Grounded Theory Study on the Emotional Process of Stroke Recovery" by Patti Gallagher (2011), published in *Canadian Journal of Neuroscience Nursing*, is critiqued. The article is presented in its entirety and followed by the critique on p. 153.

## Becoming Normal: a Grounded Theory Study on the Emotional Process of Stroke Recovery

*By Patti Gallagher, RN, MN, CNS*

### Abstract

*The purpose of this grounded theory study was to examine the emotional process of stroke recovery, personally experienced by stroke survivors. Nine stroke survivors living in Atlantic Canada participated in this study. Data collection came from formal unstructured interviews and one group interview.*

*The central problem experienced by these stroke survivors was being less than 100%. The basic social process used to address this problem was becoming normal, which is composed of three stages: recognizing stroke will not go away, choosing to work on recovery, and working on being normal. Each stage has several phases.*

*Being less than 100% is the emotional result of being unable to do certain things that serve to form individuals' identities. A critical finding was that physical and emotional recovery is inseparable, and recovery is directed towards regaining the ability to perform these certain things. Becoming normal was influenced both positively and negatively by the following conditions: personal strengths and attributes, past history, family support, professional support, faith and comparing self to peers.*

*The results of this study have implications for nursing practice, nursing education and nursing research. It adds to nursing knowledge by illuminating the close relationship between physical and emotional recovery, the duration of the stroke recovery process, and the necessity for survivors to make a deliberate choice to recover.*

### INTRODUCTION

Stroke, a sudden and catastrophic event, can instantly change the life of the affected individuals and those close to them. Considerable investigation has focused on the physical effects of stroke and functional recovery patterns. Unfortunately, the same is not true about the emotional effects of stroke. Indeed, very little is written about emotional recovery from acute stroke. At the same time, what is written is often not supported by the use of scientific tools or sound research methods, which could enhance the significance of the findings (Kelly-Hayes, et al., 1998; Kirkevold, 1997; Roberts & Counsell, 1998). Understanding emotional effects and, more specifically, the process of emotional recovery after a stroke can be important to enhancing stroke recovery work. This includes work performed by health care professionals who interact with people who experience stroke, as well as with their families.

Often, health care professionals who care for stroke survivors note that many people work hard to recover from stroke and regain their life. However, there are others who do not seem to be able to motivate themselves to undergo similar work (Doolittle, 1991; 1992; MacLean, Pound, Wolfe, & Rudd, 2002). As a clinician who works with stroke survivors,

I wanted to examine stroke survival work from the perspective of persons who considered themselves stroke survivors. I hoped to gain an understanding of what drives a stroke survivor to work on recovery.

The purpose of this grounded theory study was to examine the process of emotional recovery after stroke from the perspective of stroke survivors. The resulting substantive theory of "becoming normal" adds to nursing knowledge with a new framework of stroke recovery that is grounded in the stroke survivors' experiences. Some of these theoretical findings are supported by previous research by others. "Becoming normal" illuminates the close relationship between physical and emotional recovery, the duration of the stroke recovery process, and the necessity of making a deliberate choice to recover.

### *LITERATURE REVIEW*

When using grounded theory, the initial literature review is conducted to sensitize the researcher to the phenomenon of interest without biasing or blinding the researcher to emerging concepts. Upon analysis of the research data and the emergence of relevant concepts, a more in-depth literature review is conducted. This process facilitates researcher openness to emerging concepts, as revealed by the participants (Chenitz & Swanson, 1986; Glaser, 1978; Morse & Field, 1995; Streubert & Carpenter, 1999). Others may argue that an initial literature review may bias the researchers and blind them to emerging concepts (Glaser, 1978).

For the purpose of this research, an initial sampling of the literature related to the topic of emotional issues in stroke was undertaken to provide an overview of the current state of the knowledge. The following concepts were identified as being of particular concern in the examination of emotional recovery following stroke: post-stroke depression, self-worth, hope, crisis and chronic illness. Indeed, there has been research conducted that examined the importance of depression, self-worth, hope and crisis on the emotional recovery from chronic illness. However, emotional recovery post-stroke is still not clearly understood, although feelings that were identified as important, such as depression (Robinson & Price, 1982; Robinson, Starr, Kubos, & Price, 1983; Robinson & Bolla-Wilson, 1986), self-esteem (Chang & Mackenzie, 1998; Doolittle, 1991; 1992; Hafsteinsdottir & Grypdonck, 1997), hope (Hafsteinsdottir & Grypdonck, 1997; Popovich, 1991), and crisis (Backe, Larrson, & Fridlund, 1996; Nilsson, Jannson, & Norberg, 1997), were examined individually within separate studies. There was no evidence of inter-relationship, or of their essential significance in emotional stroke recovery (Bennet, 1996; Kelly-Hayes, et al., 1998). There was sparse literature available concerning the process of emotional recovery from the stroke-survivor's perspective (Doolittle, 1991), although many authors noted that the perspective of the stroke survivor was critical to nurses' understanding of and aiding emotional recovery from stroke (Bays, 2001; Bennett, 1996; Hafsteinsdottir & Grypdonck, 1997; Kirkevold, 1997). It is also evident that stroke is multifaceted and can be viewed from different lenses, such as stroke as a crisis or stroke within a chronic illness trajectory. However, no evidence of substantial work from these perspectives was found.

The process of emotional recovery from stroke is poorly understood and under-researched. As such, it would be premature to force the information gained from a study of emotional recovery into an existing theoretical framework. The potential to lose important information related to stroke recovery while trying to fit research findings within an inappropriate framework could be significant (Glaser, 1978).

### ETHICS APPROVAL

Ethics approval was obtained from the local university, as well as the provincial branch of the Heart and Stroke Foundation of Canada. Research did not begin until written approval was received. The executive director of the Heart and Stroke Foundation received a copy of the research proposal for their board to review as the initial sample for this study was a convenience sample of stroke survivors recruited from a list of participants in a stroke recovery program. The facilitators for the program sent letters of invitation to past participants of the program. Those who agreed to be interviewed mailed a letter of intent, they were contacted and, following a full explanation of the study with an opportunity for questions, arrangements were made to meet in person and obtain consent.

### STUDY PARTICIPANTS

Nine stroke survivors ranging in age from 42 to 82 years and living in Atlantic Canada participated in this study, conducted in 2004, and were representative of a variety of stroke types, ages, marital and family circumstances. One had been locked in, three aphasic, four had right-sided weakness and four left side. All were highly motivated people who were eager to do whatever it took to recover from their stroke, as well as to share their experiences.

Data collection came from individual formal unstructured interviews and one focus group session where the emerging theory was presented for discussion and confirmation. All participants were invited to attend a group session when the analysis was approaching completion and the substantive grounded theory developed. The focus group interview was held in order to provide a test of credibility (did the emerging theory resonate with the group and explain their response to stroke). Five stroke survivors and their families attended the focus group, which was held six months after the final interview.

Each person was interviewed at least once. Subsequent interviews to clarify content obtained in the first interview occurred. Participants were informed of this prior to obtaining consent, and the formal consent contained a statement that indicated the researcher might wish to speak with the participant more than once. Participants were encouraged to contact the researcher in the event they had something further to ask or had questions or concerns. In addition, provisions were in place to provide participants with an opportunity to receive support if they had concerns or problems at any time during the project. The researcher agreed to contact each participant following the interview to ensure there were no problems or issues.

Four participants contacted the researcher following their interviews, as they felt they had something further to contribute and gave information that added to clarification of the process of "becoming normal." Participants were informed that the aim was to hear the story from their perspective and that the interview should preferably take place in a quiet, private setting. Four participants had family present during their interviews. At times family members interjected but, for the most part, were silent observers.

Stroke survivors who participated in the study sustained a stroke that left them with a level of physical impairment that required admission to a rehabilitation unit following admission to an acute stroke unit. Each was living at home at the time of the interview. The period of time from their stroke event to interview ranged from as recent as six months to four years for one participant. The median time was one year post stroke.

Half of the participants had some degree of aphasia during their initial acute stroke period, but all were able to communicate during the time of the interview. It was interesting to note that participants who experienced aphasia reported significant events and turning points unique to their stroke recovery where they recognized their inability to communicate, but were fully present and aware. They shared their reactions and impact on recovery.

## METHODOLOGY

The process of emotional recovery post-stroke is under-explored, particularly from the stroke survivors' perspective and, therefore, poorly understood. Grounded theory is considered an ideal research method to employ when examining a relatively unstudied process related to a social psychological problem. The goals for this study were 1) to determine the central issues for stroke survivors' emotional recovery, 2) identify the basic social process that accounts for stroke survivors' emotional recovery, and 3) to consider implications of this emergent theory for nursing education, practice, and research.

For the purpose of this study, grounded theory, as defined by Glaser (1978), was utilized. Grounded theory is a qualitative, inductive methodology that serves to explore how people manage problems (Glaser, 1978). Grounded theory is based on symbolic interactionism (Blumer, as cited in Annells, 1996), which has three premises: 1) Human beings act towards things on the basis of the meanings those things have for them, 2) Such meanings arise out of the interaction of the individual with others, and 3) An interpretative process is used by the person in each instance in which he must deal with things in his environment.

Within that structural context, the purpose of the method is to generate a theory that explains the basic problem, what is going on around that problem, what factors are present, how they relate, and how participants process that problem. The stroke survivor population is very large. It is estimated that in Canada there are 300,000 stroke survivors (Hakim, Silver, & Hodgson, 1998; Lindsay et al., 2008), and little has been examined regarding the emotional experiences of recovery from the perspective of the survivor. Therefore, the initial study findings may have limited applicability. Furthermore, the theory that arises from this study may be modified as other future studies are conducted and, therefore, can be useful as a starting point for generating further theoretical support (Wuest, 2000).

In grounded theory methodology, data collection and data analysis occur concomitantly. The analysis is often referred to as circular and the search for emerging concepts and themes begins from the moment data collection begins (Glaser, 1978; Morse & Field, 1995; Polit & Hungler, 1999). Data analysis consists of concept formation, concept development, identification of a core variable and formation of a grounded theory (Glaser, 1978). In this study, all interviews were coded line by line with three levels of coding utilized: Level I (open coding), Level II (categorizing), and Level III (Basic Social-Psychological Process Identification (Glaser, 1978).

In qualitative research, researchers pursue rigour through establishing the trustworthiness of their interpretations (Guba & Lincoln, 1985). Trustworthiness is evaluated using the criteria of credibility: dependability and confirmability, and transferability (Guba & Lincoln, 1985). Glaser (1978) describes credibility as having fit, grab and work. This means that a theory "should be able to explain what happened, predict what will happen and interpret what is happening in the area of substantive or formal inquiry" (Glaser, p. 4). The final test of credibility lies with the subject groups. If the theory fits, the group will give evidence of the theory's acceptability (Glaser, 1978), hence the need for the focus group session to test the emerging theory.

An audit trail was maintained so that others could examine the assumptions made by the researcher and attest to their trustworthiness. The audit trail allows for the traits of dependability of the data over time (stability) and confirmability of data (objectivity) to be measured (Polit & Hungler, 1999).

Transferability is a feature related to providing enough description to allow for determining if the findings from the data can be transferred to other groups in similar situations (Glaser, 1978; Polit & Hungler, 1999; Streubert & Carpenter, 1995). As identified by Glaser (1978), thick description is a hallmark of grounded theory methodology utilized to ensure transferability of data. In a brief journal article it is often difficult when working within content restrictions to include significant thick description.

### FINDINGS
See Figure 1 and Table 1.

### CENTRAL PROBLEM
The central problem experienced by these stroke survivors was being less than 100%. This refers to a change in personal identity rooted in physical changes that prevent survivors from carrying out activities that they see as self-defining. It is not about losses but about *being less*. The effects of their stroke changes who they are and affects what is central to their individuality and what makes them feel worthwhile. They feel less than 100%. Their personal identity is inextricably tied to being able to do certain things. These tasks are important to the roles they perform in what they identify as normal life and being normal; recovery of these personally critical skills is vital for emotional recovery. In this sense, both physical and emotional recovery is intertwined.

> *Mr. E.: I guess I'm not very good at explaining things, but I began to feel that these things that I had all these years were being taken away from me, I didn't have any control over it. Then you mean to tell me that the disease doesn't take over? Well, it takes over up here (pointing to his head). You are conscious enough to know that something is being taken away from you.*

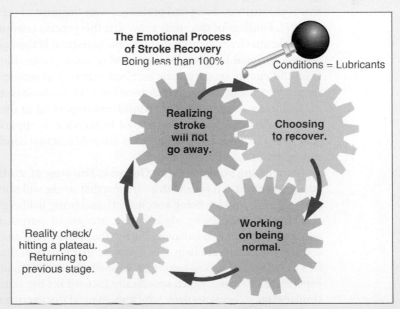

**The Emotional Process of Stroke Recovery**
Being less than 100%

Conditions = Lubricants

Realizing stroke will not go away.

Choosing to recover.

Working on being normal.

Reality check/hitting a plateau. Returning to previous stage.

**FIGURE 1** Model of becoming normal.

| TABLE 1 | STAGES OF BECOMING NORMAL AND STEPS WITHIN EACH STAGE | |
|---|---|---|

**Central Problem: Being Less than 100%**
**Social Process: Becoming Normal**

| STAGES AND PHASES (THEMES AND SUBTHEMES) | | |
|---|---|---|
| **REALIZING STROKE WILL NOT GO AWAY** | **CHOOSING TO RECOVER** | **WORKING ON BEING NORMAL** |
| • Being vigilant | • Identifying losses | • Making the list |
| • Being knocked off | • Looking at options | • Rehabbing self/taking risks |
| • Being flabbergasted | • Choosing to work on recovery | • Having success and moving on |
| • Becoming aware | | • Getting a reality check/hitting a plateau |

Being less than 100% is similar to the loss of self-concept identified by Ellis-Hill and Horn (2000) and Dowswell et al. (2000), as participants described this aspect as "lives turned upside down" and related to past and present self-concepts.

## BASIC SOCIAL PROCESS

The basic social process used to address this central problem of *being less than 100%* is "becoming normal", which is composed of three stages: recognizing stroke will not go away, choosing to work on recovery, and working on being normal (see Figure 1). Each stage has several phases (see Table 1). Becoming normal is influenced both positively and negatively by the following conditions: personal strengths and attributes, past history of stroke or adverse events, family support, professional support, faith, and comparing self to peers.

Stroke survivors work long and hard on stroke recovery. Similarly, Kirkevold (2002) in her "unfolding illness trajectory of stroke" study noted: "Adjustment to stroke is a process that is gradually evolving and prolonged over the most of the first year following the stroke" (p. 887). Findings of this study show that this process continued far beyond the first year.

Stroke survivors identify that becoming normal is their goal and they continue to work toward this goal long after their period of acute stroke. Indeed, they are willing to invest time and energy on personally ascribed meaningful recovery, which speaks to the critical nature of collaborative goal identification with stroke survivors.

A number of conditions are considered important to the process of becoming normal. Personal strengths and attributes, past history, family support, professional support, spiritual faith and comparing self to peers are instrumental conditions for the process, but will not be discussed in this article.

**Recognizing Stroke Will Not Go Away.** This stage of stroke recovery begins with the first stroke symptom and ends with awareness that stroke will not go away. It takes place in three phases: being vigilant, being knocked off, and being flabbergasted and becoming aware.

**Being Vigilant.** Being vigilant is a process of purposefully observing one's feelings and how one's body is behaving during the stroke event and relating these observations to someone who can seek help. It is a process that is in operation until personal safety, identified as receiving medical help is established. Eaves (2000), in her study of stroke survivors' experience of stroke, which specifically focused on the initial impact of stroke, defined a similar stage to being vigilant, which she named discovering stroke and delaying treatment.

*Mr. H.: I came indoors and very soon after, I felt peculiarity in the right hand and arm . . . it was not normal and then my lips began to tingle. Then I realized; I knew it was a stroke. So, as soon as my family got home from work, we got in the car and went to the hospital.*

**Being Knocked off.** Being knocked off is a state of relinquishing control to others while barely being able to take in what is happening. This phase begins with admission to the emergency department and ends when stroke survivors become completely aware of what has happened. The paradox is that while patients were so vigilant during the initial phase of the stroke, they were distanced from subsequent events for a period of time.

*Mrs. D.: Well, then they took me down for an ultrasound and then they did a CAT scan and one thing or another like that, but uh, I don't know, I just seemed to be a party to it, but in the distance like. It wasn't really real to me.*

White and Johnstone (2000) describe a passive stage early on in stroke recovery. They surmise that the survivors want to put their faith in experienced and trusted experts who will help them make sense of the event. The survivors in this study reported being unaware of events at this time and, thus, were not looking at experts to help them make sense of this event.

**Being Flabbergasted.** Being flabbergasted (an in vivo phrase one stroke survivor used that eloquently described to others how they too felt) is a process of being astonished and dismayed by functional changes that stroke causes. It is characterized by distress and fear, which intensifies with the recognition that one's independence has been compromised. This is different from being vigilant. They are now looking at what they cannot do versus observing their weakness.

*Mrs. D.: I realized by then that this wasn't game time, just things that you take for granted that you are doing for yourself and you just can't. It is a low blow.*

Ellis-Hill et al. (2000), in their life narrative study of eight couples noted a similar phase, which they called self-body split. In their study, stroke survivors who experienced dysphasia were excluded, as the first interview occurred in the immediate acute stroke interval. In this present study, conducted in the postacute phase of stroke recovery, being flabbergasted was present and could last longer in those who initially experienced dysphasia.

**Becoming Aware.** This is an extension or continuation of being flabbergasted. This is the time when stroke survivors recognize stroke effects. This includes both internal acknowledgement of existing stroke effects and awareness of the potential permanence of these effects. Becoming aware often occurs simultaneously with being flabbergasted.

*Mr. C.: When I was at the centre (rehabilitation centre), maybe about two weeks or so, it certainly hit me like a bolt of lightning, the reality of what I had. I am locked in! It certainly got through to my brain, when I suddenly realized that I might even stay this way.*

Similarly, other researchers have discovered that awareness of the consequences of stroke is critical for recovery and this confrontation had to occur before patients could be ready for rehabilitation (Lewinter & Mikkelsen, 1995; Kirkevold, 2002). Until there was awareness that the stroke would not go away, there was no movement to the next stage, which is choosing to recover.

**Choosing to Recover.** Choosing to recover is a process of purposefully making a decision to engage in stroke recovery work. It is a turning point in "becoming normal" and a deliberate thoughtful decision antecedent to stroke work. This was a finding unique to this study. The decision to recover is a personal decision, although family support influences the choices stroke survivors make. It takes place in three phases: identifying losses, looking at options, and choosing to work on recovery.

**Identifying Losses.** Identifying losses is a process of detailing functional losses that occur as a result of stroke and threaten to change stroke survivor's identities. Stroke survivors reflect on who they are, what is important to them, and how functional losses can affect that identify. It is a process of internal personal reflection.

> *Mr. A.: I have a workshop in the basement and I do home repairs and so on. I would sure miss being able to go down to the workshop and cut up a piece of wood. If I was unable to do that, it would be a real pain.*

Similarly, identifying losses is reported frequently in the literature and that stroke survivors tally losses in relation to what is important to them, as persons (Boynton De Sepulveda & Chang, 1994; Doolittle, 1992; Dowswell et al., 2000). As in this study, they noted that health professionals often did not question stroke survivors about their feelings regarding stroke effects and what was most disturbing to them. Stroke survivors felt this information would be helpful for appropriate professional support.

**Looking at Options.** Looking at options is a process of examining various courses of action and their consequences. Stroke survivors identified three possible courses of action as being: doing nothing, contemplating suicide, and working on recovery. According to other researchers, stroke survivors who did nothing, in effect waited for the stroke to pass, did not do well in overall recovery (Boynton De Sepulveda & Chang, 1994; White & Johnston, 2000). All stroke survivors in this study rejected this option.

**Choosing to Work on Recovery.** In this study, deciding to work on recovery was noted to be a specific decision unto itself. It was described as an epiphanylike event and all participants could identify when they personally arrived at this decision. It is possible that goal-setting by stroke survivors, which has been identified elsewhere, implicitly includes deciding to work on recovery. However, in this study it seemed to be a separate juncture and all participants made this decision.

> *Mr. H.: This is one of the experiences of life where you've got to learn to deal with and that's not easy to deal with. You did, you operated in a certain way and at a certain level and, for me, I don't willingly accept the idea that I am going to live at a lower level.*

The phenomenon of stroke survivors making a conscious decision to recover is a new finding that adds to our understanding of the stroke recovery process. It is possible that goal-setting by stroke survivors, which has been identified elsewhere, implicitly includes deciding to work on recovery. However, in this study, deciding to work on recovery was a very specific decision.

**Working on Being Normal.** Working on being normal is the process of engaging in stroke work to become normal and is a sustained process that goes on for a long time. Stroke survivors define what "being normal" will be for them. Although some may accept a lower level of recovery or less than 100% recovery, for the majority of stroke survivors, being normal is being the same person as before the stroke. For the most part, stroke survivors were intent on achieving 100% recovery and many were working towards that goal beyond one year post-stroke.

> *Mrs. D.: (talking about finally being able to shower independently) I had the stroke three years ago this March, about this time. It took a long time, so I just had to give it a try one day because I had tried it many times. So, now I lean against the wall and haul my bad leg up and over.*

The stroke survivors' goal of becoming 100%, as discovered in this study, has been supported by other researchers (Burton, 2000; Dowswell et al, 2000). Conversely, other researchers report finding stroke survivors adapt to stroke losses and accept a lower level of functioning (Eaves, 2000; Lewinter & Mikkelsen, 1995). Still others have reported this goal lasted for only one year (Dowswell et al, 2000; Lawlor et al., 1999). These reported findings of acceptance of lower levels of recovery contrast with the process of becoming normal discovered in this study.

Stroke work is both physical and emotional. Emotional work is related to determining what level of recovery is acceptable and pushing oneself to go on over a significant length of time. It is an iterative process that consists of three phases: making the list, rehabbing self, and having success and moving on.

**Making the List.** Making the list is the process of naming what skills are important for personal identity and then prioritizing the list. It is composed of taking inventory and determining what is important. There is a tallying of losses that need to be overcome in order to regain identity and become normal. The purpose of this inventory is to look at losses in order to develop priorities for recovery work.

Determining what is important is the process of establishing priorities among the losses listed for regaining identity. Emotionally, this is a critical stage. What was identified as being important was as diverse as the individuals who participated in this study. Whatever was deemed most important to recover was worked on more diligently and at the expense of other gains. Doolittle's (1992) longitudinal descriptive ethnographic account of the experience of stroke recovery noted that, as in this study, participants expended energy on restoring function to areas of their bodies that performed functions that mattered to them and that gave them their identity.

Stroke survivors treasured health care professionals who identified what was important to them and their need to start on these tasks. It should be stated that being able to participate in basic ADL skills were often initial goals and that personal priorities followed as next goals. However, once basic needs are met, there is often incongruence between what therapists set as goals and what stroke survivors set as priorities. Depending on the degree of incongruence, the outcome for stroke survivors is frustration with the team focusing on what are, to the survivor, unimportant goals (Burton, 2000; Doolittle, 1992; Dowswell et al, 2000; Lawler et al., 1999; Hafsteinsdottir & Grypdonck, 1997). Conflict also arises when stroke survivors hold unrealistic expectations for recovery due to their comparative inexperience with the stroke recovery trajectory and require support from the team to help determine priorities.

> *Mr. F.: I had set goals for myself, as far as the recovery, some of which I never met. But, in time, I found, I discovered, they were realistic. I kind of broke down one day in Physio . . . So, finally, my physiotherapist helped me through it and said "Look, you are doing very very well, don't set unrealistic expectations." Well, I stopped beating myself up about that I think, mentally and set a more realistic expectation.*

Similarly, Lawlor et al. (1999) identified the critical role nurses can play in working with stroke survivors in mutual goal-setting. They found that when stroke survivors set goals that were not realistic, nurses did not intervene to help set more realistic goals due to the concern that they might discourage survivors and set them back. In this study, there were nurses who diligently worked with stroke survivors to assist them with setting realistic goals that were meaningful to the survivor. These nurses were treasured by the stroke survivors.

**Rehabbing Self.** Rehabbing self is the process of taking the list and working purposefully on achieving the tasks according to priority. This process continued until "being normal" was accomplished. Rehabbing self is also a process of moving from a passive dependent recipient of therapy to becoming totally independent in rehabbing self. Being independent in "rehabbing self" often marked the true beginning of this phase. Stroke survivors became, for the most part, independent in self-care and activities of daily living. They began to work on tasks on that list that were truly important and critical to their self-identity. Problem-solving skills and strengths were important conditions in this phase.

Taking risks: One aspect of rehabbing self that was reported by several participants was taking risks. This was a strategy employed in the phase of rehabbing self. It was identified as trying something without a guarantee that it was possible or would work. Often the risk was related to trying something that was important to the survivor and, for the most part, risks were thoughtfully taken. Stroke survivors relate that when they were restricted from taking risks they felt devalued and depressed. They truly appreciated individuals who would strategize with them and support their efforts. It was also noted that even when these attempts met with failure, for the most part they resolved to try again at a later time. Risk taking was often described as a personal triumph and a feeling of taking control in recovery.

*Mr. H.: She realized it was important to me and she backed off and kept an eye on me. That was fine, she kept an eye on me, but she let me do things. I was willing to be careful, but I needed to be able to do what lay within my power, and if it wasn't within my power, I needed to be allowed to fail.*

Doolittle (1992) named taking risks "experiencing the possibilities" and noted, "What was so amazing about these risk-taking endeavours was the tremendous world of possibilities these situations opened up for the individuals" (p. 123). As in this study, it was reported that risk taking was often performed in secret, hidden from families or hospital staff. Reluctance to be reprimanded was the leading reason for these covert activities.

**Having Success and Moving on.** Having success and moving on is described as meeting one goal or accomplishing one task and then going back to the list and moving on to the next task. Like a cogwheel that moves one notch at a time, it is perpetual motion. Little time is spent on pausing, reflecting, or celebrating successes. Praise and recognition of accomplishments comes from family and professionals and is important to stroke survivors.

*Mr. J.: She was very encouraging that way, and she didn't see me every day, and she would see me once a week and she would see the difference . . . those things are helpful and encouraging. I would think of different things the therapists here would say because they were a better yardstick than we are towards ourselves.*

Stroke survivors need to have success and be recognized for it, even if they do not take the time themselves to pause and reflect (Lawlor et al., 1999; Pilkington, 1999). Having success and moving on is the most complex phase of the process and at times stroke survivors may fail to accomplish a task. Thus, getting a reality check and/or hitting a plateau can occur.

**Getting a Reality Check.** Failure to accomplish a task or the sudden realization that something the stroke survivor hoped to accomplish will not happen was another epiphany-like event. At that time, work on being normal halted. Some participants regressed to the stage of realizing stroke would not go away and it took time to move through the stages again. It was a devastating experience, but did not occur to all participants; indeed, often only to those who had experienced very devastating strokes.

> Mr.C.: *I remember going to the cafeteria for lunch and everyone was laughing. I wanted to holler out to them "don't you know I may never walk again!" My world stopped. After a while I realized I will walk again, just not now. I have other things to do now.*

Getting a reality check is similar to being flabbergasted, but with a subtle difference. It is often time-oriented where the stroke survivor is not realistic on how much time and work is involved and is expecting success too soon. Getting a reality check has not been reported in the literature as a specific event, rather as part of having unrealistic goals. In this study it was a specific event. Those who experienced it recalled the instant when they recognized they were not going to be successful and described the circumstances, the setting and the people involved. It was an epiphany-like occurrence.

When they became aware they were not going to meet their goals, some participants regressed, necessitating they work through the stages of realizing the stroke will not go away, making the decision to recover and working on being normal again. A reordering of what was important occurred and, for some, getting this reality check was devastating; it took time to move through the stages again. Others were able to handle this philosophically and changed the yardstick they used to measure their progress.

> Mr. J.: *I guess my attitude is I will try it later. I would just have to lay it aside and come back to it later.*

**Hitting a Plateau.** Hitting a plateau is a phase in "working on recovery" where progress with completing the tasks on the list stalls, or the speed of progress slows. Some called it hitting a wall. They found that being forewarned that this may occur was what helped them keep things in perspective. In other words, they were expecting it to happen at some point. Those who were not prepared experienced increased anxiety and worried that their recovery had stopped. Looking back and looking forward were strategies used to overcome this period. Health care professionals and family members would identify where they were and how far they had progressed, and that allowed them to recognize accomplishments and gather strength to move forward.

Hitting a plateau is common in stroke recovery and, yet, many stroke survivors are not prepared for this and can become depressed when it happens (Burton, 2000; Doolittle, 1992; Dowswell et al., 2000). Doolittle stated: "We live in a culture where there is pressure for continuous progress. If this was not so, plateaus might be viewed in a more positive context as periods of stabilization where the body replenishes itself" (p. 123).

## IMPLICATIONS

This substantive theory of becoming normal adds to nursing knowledge with a new framework of stroke recovery that is grounded in survivors' experiences. Some of these theoretical findings are supported by previous research. "Becoming normal" adds to nursing knowledge by illuminating the close relationship between physical and emotional recovery, the duration of the stroke recovery process, and the necessity for survivors of making a deliberate choice to recover.

The process of becoming normal expands nursing knowledge by explicitly revealing how emotional recovery from stroke is grounded in regaining self-defining physical abilities, as opposed to functional capacities. The framework reveals areas where nursing practice may be tailored to support survivor priorities, leading to a more positive impact on stroke recovery. As well, findings reveal that stroke survivors' progress toward becoming normal is adversely affected by those who believe that stroke recovery is limited to time and discourage survivors in trying new things and setting long-term goals.

At times, nurses were viewed as being domineering, restrictive and detrimental to recovery. They felt that nurses would not allow them to try things and would restrict their independence. Often they recognized it was for safety reasons, but they felt nurses were over-cautious. According to Kirkevold (1997) nurses have the potential to be positive influences on stroke recovery. By virtue of their continuous presence, nurses should be perceived as being essential. They are present for 24 hours of the day, as compared to therapists and physicians who spend brief intervals with stroke survivors (Kirkevold, 1997).

Recognition of the stage stroke survivors are in and the key tasks they accomplish in each stage can be helpful to nurses in identifying critical strategies for supporting stroke survivors in their recovery process. For example, an important finding is that during most of the stage of *recognizing the stroke will not go away,* stroke survivors are unable to take in new information. *Being knocked off* is a phase where there is little recognition of stroke effects and what is going on. These findings suggest that this is not the time to focus nursing interventions on patient education. Rather, nurses need to be vigilant for patient cues that identify when the survivor is moving into the phase of *becoming aware.* At that time, nurses can provide support, information and hope for recovery.

As noted, *choosing to recover* is a deliberate thoughtful step and is a personal decision of the stroke survivor. The theory generated in this research suggests that rehabilitation efforts made by health professionals are ineffective if stroke survivors have not made this decision. Stroke survivors in this study stated they made a deliberate choice to work on recovery and were able to tell others, if asked.

The majority of the stroke recovery work that was most meaningful to stroke survivors for becoming normal, occurred post discharge and with limited resources, and study participants noted that community reintegration and community resources are sorely lacking in helping them over the long term. Health policy initiatives should be developed to address this need.

Often hitting a plateau occurred after discharge. Stroke survivors who were prepared prior to discharge were able to anticipate its occurrence and were able to cope and move on.

## LIMITATIONS

As with any grounded theory study there is opportunity for others to modify or extend the theory in further studies. The participants in this study were self-identified survivors who stated they wanted to recover and chose to work hard on recovery. It would be valuable to examine the perspective of those who did not choose to work. Recruiting from this population, however, may prove difficult. The study population in this research was recruited from an urban setting where rehabilitation units, as well as outpatient therapy were accessible. All stroke survivors were able to return to their own home. Stroke survivors who do not have access to therapy or who do not return home may also provide another view.

### CONCLUSIONS

At the completion of the study, each survivor was continuing on "working on being normal" and identified that he/she had not reached the goal of becoming 100%. The role of the health professional in developing a meaningful therapeutic relationship is inextricably linked to recognizing what is important to the individual stroke survivor and their specific stage of recovery. For the most part, stroke survivors in this study did not identify nurses as essential players in the professional network supporting their work in becoming normal. Those nurses who shared their professional recovery experiences and supported stroke survivors in achieving goals that were important and encouraged them in risk taking as an exhilarating recovery action, were valued; indeed, treasured.

> Mr. H.: I valued him (one rehabilitation nurse). He knew I needed to try and he let me. He said I know you are going to do it, let's figure a way to try it in a safe way.

## REFERENCES

Annells, M. (1996). Grounded Theory method: Philosophical perspective, paradigm of inquiry, and postmodernism. *Qualitative Health Research, 6,* 379–393.

Backe, M., Larrson, K., & Fridlund, B. (1996). Patients' conceptions of their life situation within the first week after a stroke event: A qualitative analysis. *Intensive Critical Care Nursing, 5,* 285–294.

Bays, C. (2001). Older adult's description of hope after a stroke. *Rehabilitation Nursing, 26,* 18–27.

Bennett, B. (1996). How nurses in a stroke rehabilitation unit attempt to meet the psychological needs of patients who become depressed following a stroke. *Journal of Advanced Nursing, 23,* 314–321.

Boynton De Sepulveda, L., & Chang, B. (1994). Effective coping with stroke disability in a community setting: The development of a causal model. *Journal of Neuroscience Nursing, 26,* 193–201.

Burton, C. (2000). Living with stroke: a phenomenological study. *Journal of Advanced Nursing, 32,* 301–309.

Chang, A.M., & Mackenzie, A.E. (1998). State self-esteem following stroke. *Stroke, 29,* 2325–2328.

Chenitz, W.C., & Swanson, J.M. (1986). *From practice to Grounded Theory. Qualitative research in nursing. Don Mills, ON:* Addison-Wesley Publishing.

Doolittle, N. (1991). Clinical ethnography of lacunar stroke: Implications for acute care. *Journal of Neuroscience Nursing, 23,* 235–240.

Doolittle, N. (1992). The experience of recovery following lacunar stroke. *Rehabilitation Nursing, 17,* 122–125.

Dowswell, G., Lawlor, J., Dowswell, T., Young, J., Forster, A., & Hearn, J. (2000). Investigating recovery from stroke: A qualitative study. *Journal of Clinical Nursing, 9,* 507–515.

Eaves, Y. (2000). "What happened to me": Rural African American elder's experiences of stroke. *Journal of Neuroscience Nursing, 32,* 37–48.

Ellis-Hill, C.S., & Horn, S. (2000). Change in identity and self-concept: A new theoretical approach to recovery following a stroke. *Clinical Rehabilitation, 14,* 279–287.

Ellis-Hill, C.S., Payne, S., & Ward, C. (2000). Self-body split: Issues of identity in physical recovery following a stroke. *Disability & Rehabilitation, 22,* 725–733.

Glaser, B. (1978). *Theoretical sensitivity.* San Francisco, CA: Sociology Press.

Guba, E.G., & Lincoln, Y.S. (1985). Naturalistic Inquiry. Beverly Hills, CA: Sage.

Hafsteinsdottir, T., & Grypdonck, M. (1997). Being a stroke patient: A review of the literature. *Journal of Advanced Nursing, 26,* 590–598.

Hakim, A., Silver, F., & Hodgson, C. (1998). Organized stroke care: A new era in stroke prevention and treatment. *Canadian Medical Association Journal, 159(6 Supp.),* S1.

Kelly-Hayes, M., Robertson, J., Broderick, J.P., Duncan, P., Hershey, L., Roth, E., et al. (1998). The American Heart Association stroke outcome classification. *Stroke, 29,* 1274–1280.

Kirkevold, M. (1997). The role of nursing in the rehabilitation of acute stroke patients: Toward a unified theoretical perspective. *Advances in Nursing Science, 19(4),* 55–64.

Kirkevold, M. (2002). The unfolding illness trajectory of stroke. *Disability & Rehabilitation,* 24, 877–899.

Lawlor, J., Dowswell, G., Hearn, J., Forster, A., & Young, J. (1999). Recovering from stroke: A qualitative investigation of the role of goal setting in late stroke recovery. *Journal of Advanced Nursing, 30(2),* 109–409.

Lewinter, M., & Mikkelsen, S. (1995). Patient's experience of rehabilitation after stroke. *Disability & Rehabilitation,* 17, 3–9.

Lindsay, P., Bayley, M., Helling, C., Hill, M., Woodbury, E., & Phillips, S. (2008). Canadian Stroke Strategy Best Practices and Standards Writing Group on behalf of the Canadian Stroke Strategy, a joint initiative of the Canadian Stroke Network and the Heart and Stroke Foundation of Canada. Canadian best practice recommendations for stroke care (updated 2008). *CMAJ, 179*(12), SI–S25.

MacLean, N., Pound, P., Wolfe, C., & Rudd, A. (2002). The concept of patient motivation. *Stroke, 33,* 444–448.

Morse, J., & Field, P.A. (1995). *Qualitative research methods for health professionals.* Thousand Oaks, CA. Sage Publications.

Nilsson, I., Jansson, L., & Norberg, A. (1997). To meet with a stroke: Patient's experiences and aspects seen through a screen of crises. *Journal of Advanced Nursing, 25,* 953–963.

Pilkington, EB. (1999). A qualitative study of life after stroke. *Journal of Neurosciences Nursing, 31*(6), 336–347.

Polit, D.E, & Hungler, B.P. (1999). *Nursing research principles and methods.* Philadelphia, PA. Lippincott.

Popovich, J.M. (1991) *Hope, coping, and rehabilitation outcomes in stroke patients.* Unpublished doctoral dissertation, Rush University, College of Nursing, Illinois.

Roberts, 1. & Counsell, C. (1998). Assessment of clinical outcomes in acute stroke trials. *Stroke, 29,* 986–991.

Robinson, R.G., & Bolla-Wilson, K. (1986). Depression influences intellectual impairment in stroke patients. *Stroke, 14,* 541–547.

Robinson, R.G., & Price, T.R. (1982). Post-stroke depressive disorders: A follow-up of 103 patients. *Stroke, 13,* 635–641.

Robinson, R.G., Starr, L., Kubos, K.L., & Price, T.R. (1983). A two year longitudinal study of post-stroke mood disorders: Findings during the initial evaluation. *Stroke, 14*(5), 736–741.

Robinson-Smith, G. (2002). Self-efficacy and quality oflife after stroke. *Journal of Neuroscience Nursing, 34,* 91–102.

Streubert, H., & Carpenter, D. (1995). *Qualitative research in nursing.* New York, NY. Lippincott.

White, M.A., & Johnstone, A.S. (2000). Recovery from stroke: Does rehabilitation counseling have a role to play? *Disability & Rehabilitation, 22*(3), 140–143.

Wuest, J. (2000). Negotiation with helping systems: An example of Grounded Theory evolving through emergent fit. *Qualitative Health Research, 10,* 51–71.

# THE CRITIQUE

"Becoming normal" is the grounded theory, basic psychosocial process described by Gallagher (2011) in her research report on stroke recovery. In the article, "Becoming normal: A grounded theory study on the emotional process of stroke recovery," the researcher helps us understand the psychosocial process of emotional recovery from the perspective of stroke survivors. This research report will be analyzed using the criteria found in the Critiquing Criteria box on pp. 135-136. The critique comments will be offered to help the reader understand the important questions to ask when considering the rigor of qualitative research. The critiquing criteria are not specific to the method, but provide general questions important to understanding the quality and applicability of the research report. Streubert and Carpenter (2011) provide methodology-specific critiquing questions in their text titled *Qualitative Nursing Research: Advancing the Humanistic Imperative.*

## STATEMENT OF THE PHENOMENON OF INTEREST

A phenomenon is a fact, occurrence, or experience that is observed or observable. In this research study, the phenomenon of interest is stroke recovery. Gallagher clearly states her intent to study this phenomenon and why it is justified: "Very little is written about emotional recovery from acute stroke" (p. 24). She offers "understanding emotional effects and, more specifically, the process of emotional recovery after stroke can be important to enhancing stroke recovery work. This includes work performed by health care professionals who interact with people who experience stroke, as well as with their families" (p. 24). In addition to sharing the relevance to nursing practice, the researcher also tells her audience that one of her three goals is to consider the implications of the research and how they relate to nursing education and research.

Gallagher helps her audience understand the philosophical underpinnings, or the frame in which the research is conducted, by explaining the utility of grounded theory in phenomenal sense-making. Additionally, she offers a description of grounded theory according to Barney Glaser, who is a highly regarded grounded theorist. The critical difference between grounded theory and other qualitative research methods is the focus on *process.* Researchers who use grounded theory are most interested in identifying the process elements of a phenomenon, not just describing the phenomenon.

The researcher's statement of the phenomenon using the critiquing criteria is clear. Gallagher names the phenomenon of interest, tells you why it is important to study it using grounded theory as a particular type of qualitative research methodology, and frames the reasons why grounded theory is the correct method for understanding the *process* of stroke recovery.

## PURPOSE

Gallagher tells the reader in the first line of the research abstract, which precedes the article, that the purpose of the study is "to examine the emotional process of stroke recovery, personally experienced by stroke survivors" (p. 24). The reader is able to see immediately the phenomenon of interest and what her purpose is in studying it. In addition to having a purpose for conducting research, nurse researchers have a responsibility to share their perceptions on why what they are studying has significance to the field. In this case, Gallagher tells us in the introduction that studying the emotional process of stroke recovery is important because it will assist nurses to help stroke survivors do the recovery work so essential to their "becoming normal." Additionally, in the methodology portion of the report, she states that one of her three goals is "to consider implications of this emergent theory for nursing education, practice and research" (p. 26).

## *METHOD*

Grounded theory is a different type of qualitative research method in that it goes beyond the traditional methods of phenomenology and ethnography, which focus on pure description of phenomena. In grounded theory research, the researcher describes the process that is at the heart of the inquiry. This process is psychosocial. According to Glaser (1978), a basic psychosocial process is characterized by stages that are pervasive, variable, and occur over time (Carpenter, 2011). Describing the process is at the heart of grounded theory methodology. The outcome of describing the process is the development of a theory; one that is grounded or emerges from the description of the social psychological process that develops from pure description by the participants. Thus the name, grounded theory.

Gallagher chooses grounded theory because "grounded theory is considered an ideal research method to employ when examining a relatively unstudied process related to a social psychological problem" (p. 26). The problem identified is the emotional process of stroke recovery. Given the stated problem, the research methodology is ideal.

The researcher uses grounded theory methodology to develop a theory for understanding the emotional recovery of stroke survivors. The primary responsibility of the researcher is to uncover the basic social psychological (BSP) at work. Another term for this is the core variable. The core variable is the essential, recurring theme in the description of what the participants are experiencing. In this research, Gallagher identifies the core variable as "being normal."

The research method requires the use of coding and memos. These are described in detail in the works of Glaser (1978, 1992), Strauss and Corbin (1998), and Strauss (1987). It is difficult to determine from the research report whether the researcher used the process completely as described by Glaser (1978). This is not unusual in published research reports because of the page constraints imposed on the researcher. Gallagher clearly describes the basic social process in detail and provides a table summarizing the stages and phases of emotional recovery. Further, she includes the trustworthiness of her data, which can be one indicator of her proper execution of the methodology.

## *SAMPLING*

Convenience sampling is reported by Gallagher as the method used to obtain her informants. This term is more frequently associated with quantitative research. The more frequently used terminology in qualitative research is purposive or purposeful sampling. Purposive sampling is selecting the sample based on the informants' knowledge of the phenomenon of interest (Field & Morse, 1985). Using this definition, Gallagher uses a purposive sample because all of her informants were stroke survivors. Thus, they are the appropriate individuals to describe the emotional process of stroke recovery. Glaser (1978), however, discusses theoretical sampling as the appropriate sampling technique to use in grounded theory studies. Specifically, Glaser describes theoretical sampling as "the process of data collection for generating theory whereby the analyst jointly collects, codes, and analyzes data, and decides what data to collect next and where to find them in order to develop a theory as it emerges" (p. 36). It is unclear why Gallagher did not use theoretical sampling.

The sample is appropriate to provide a description of the process of emotional recovery from stroke since all informants were stroke survivors. Gallagher notes her concerns about the participants who were not volunteers and suggests that future research might include participants who did not volunteer. There is a caution in seeing the sample as a limitation. Those who did not volunteer to participate may not be actively engaged in the "emotional process of stroke recovery" which was the phenomenon of interest in this research.

## DATA COLLECTION

The first critique question regarding data collection is whether the data collection is focused on human experience. Gallagher's research is clearly focused on how individuals deal with the emotional recovery from a stroke. Her data collection strategies include individual formal unstructured interviews and a focus group session. She reports that each participant was interviewed at least one time. In instances where clarity was not attained from review of the transcript, she reports returning to the informants for additional information.

Gallagher's report of protection of human subjects includes statements that reference university approval as well as the Heart and Stroke Foundation of Canada, which provided funding for her study. It is not typical for funding agencies to conduct a formal review of human subject's protection. However, it is typical for researchers health care agencies and universities to require independent review of research studies.

Saturation is not specifically addressed in the research report. Saturation refers to the repeating nature of data that leads the researcher to conclude that little or no new data will emerge regardless of the number of new subjects interviewed on the phenomenon under study. For instance, Gallagher reports the phases of emotional recovery from stroke include realizing stroke will not go away, choosing to recover, and working on being normal. Although the researcher does not specifically report that saturation was achieved, there is some level of confidence that this occurred because the study participants were given the opportunity to review the theory and determine whether it reflected their experiences. Indeed, those who reviewed the theory agreed the researcher had captured their experience.

## DATA ANALYSIS

Data analysis as reported by Gallagher includes the steps identified by Glaser (1978): concept formation, concept development, identification of the core variable, and formation of the grounded theory. She further reports using open coding, categorizing, and BSP identification. Assuming that the researcher followed the steps included in the report, the process outlined by Glaser was followed.

The validation of staying true to the data is often evident in reviewing the criteria for attaining trustworthiness of the data. Gallagher describes these steps in detail.

Credibility requires that the informants recognize the experience to be their own. Gallagher uses a focus group session to review the theory, thereby establishing credibility of the findings.

Auditability requires that others, not engaged in the research, be able to follow the *audit trail* of the primary researcher(s). This is very challenging to determine in a published research report. The proof of auditability would be achieved by reviewing the original work to see if similar conclusions were drawn. In the absence of this, the reader will need to ask whether he or she can follow the thinking of the researcher based on what is presented. In this case, there is evidence in the form of quotes that appears to support the concepts/themes included in the research report. Gallagher states that within the constraints of a "brief journal article it is often difficult . . . to include significant thick description" (p. 26). The thick description would provide the reader with a much richer report from which to decide whether the auditability criterion has been achieved.

Fittingness or **transferability** is the criterion that provides the reader with an opportunity to determine the usefulness of the data outside of the study. There are several relevant questions that help to guide the determination of fittingness: Do the participants' recognize the experiences as their own? Are the strategies used in the study compatible with the purpose of the study? Can the findings be used by others? Gallagher's use of a participant focus group to critique the theory supports the idea that study participants recognized the experiences, which were stated in the report, as their own. Gallagher's report implies that she used the processes described by Glaser (1978), which are compatible with the purpose of her research. The final question has to do with whether consumers of the work can use the research in their practice. As reported by Gallagher, the concepts/themes identified support the work completed by other researchers. This is painstakingly reported by the researcher. Given the answers to these questions, the reader can conclude that the research has fit or is transferable.

### EMPIRICAL GROUNDINGS OF THE STUDY: FINDINGS

In this section of the critique, the reader must ask whether the conceptualizations offered are true to the data. Does the report offer enough clarity and use of the participant's responses to make the reader comfortable with the findings? How is existing literature supportive of the findings?

---

**EVIDENCE-BASED PRACTICE TIP**

Qualitative studies are helpful in answering research questions about a concept or phenomenon that is not well understood or adequately covered in the literature.

---

Gallagher provides the reader with a view of the participants' lived experiences by sharing categorizations or naming of aspects of the raw data and then providing the actual statements made by informants to support the concepts or names. For example, there is a subcategory called "getting a reality check." The raw data to support the categorization is as follows:

*"I remember going to the cafeteria for lunch and everyone was laughing. I wanted to holler out to them 'don't you know I may never walk again!' My world stopped. After a while I realized I will walk again, just not now. I have other things to do now" (p. 30).*

Although limited in presentation, the reader is charged with identifying whether this statement is reflective of an individual "getting a reality check." In the absence of this, are there other ways the reader can determine whether the researcher is true to the data? In her report, Gallagher states that she returned to her participants and they validated that her conceptualizations were accurate. In light of this action, the reader has evidence that the researcher's findings represent the experiences of the informants.

Each conceptualization or theme category includes references to current literature. Gallagher clearly tells her readers when her data are similar to those discovered by other researchers and when they aren't. Returning to the example above, Gallagher reports that Ellis-Hill and Horn (2000) report a similar category in a life narrative study called self-body split. This is a good way of helping the audience determine whether the findings fit within the context of what is already known.

### CONCLUSIONS, IMPLICATIONS, AND RECOMMENDATIONS

The conclusions, implications, and recommendations of Gallagher's study are provided in a realistic context. Her primary conclusion is that "the role of the health professional in developing a meaningful therapeutic relationship is inextricably linked to recognizing what is important to the individual stroke survivor and their specific stage of recovery" (p. 31). Gallagher has provided the consumer of this work with a guidepost for understanding the emotional recovery of stroke survivors. She further states that her substantive theory provides a new framework for viewing stroke victim's recovery. Historically, stroke has been examined predominantly as a physical process. In this report, she is asking that nurses stay tuned to patient's plans, goals, and aspirations. She notes that practitioners sometimes decide goals for patients when, based on her research, patients don't want their hopes doused or their decision-making taken away. Understanding the emotional stage of stroke recovery is important and she believes that her model provides a lense to view these stages that are based in patients' experiences.

Her theory is offered as a contribution to nursing education and practice. And while she does not go far enough in explaining the application to nursing education, the reader can surmise that teaching her theory can help neophyte practitioners better understand the emotional work essential to stroke recovery. Gallagher states that her findings may have limited applicability; however, the study can serve as the starting point for generating further theoretical support, and the theory may be modified as future studies are conducted.

Gallagher's study is a well-written report on use of grounded theory methodology. The conclusions, implication, and recommendations are appropriate and are not overstated. The findings provide important insights into the process of stroke recovery. It adds to the body of nursing knowledge and, as such, is valuable to practitioners. As offered earlier in the critique, ultimately, meta-sythesis of similar studies will provide a stronger frame for applying the findings in an evidence-based practice environment.

## ■ CRITICAL THINKING CHALLENGES

- Discuss the similarities and differences between the stylistic considerations of reporting a qualitative study as opposed to a quantitative study in a professional journal.
- Discuss how one would go about incorporating qualitative research in evidence-based practice. Give an example.

## REFERENCES

Barbour, R. S., & Barbour, M. (2003). Evaluating and synthesizing qualitative research: The need to develop a distinctive approach. *Journal of Evaluation in Clinical Practice, 9*(2), 179–186.

Carpenter, D. R. (2011). Grounded theory as method. In Streubert, H. J. & Carpenter, D. R. (Eds.), *Qualitative nursing research: Advancing the humanistic imperative* (pp. 123–153). Philadelphia: Wolters Klower Health.

Cesario, S., Morin, K., & Santa-Donato, A. (2002). Evaluating the level of evidence of qualitative research. *Journal of Obstetric, Gynecologic and Neonatal Nursing, 31*(6), 708–714.

Cole, C. A. (2012). Implied consent and nursing practice: Ethical or convenient? *Nursing Ethics, 19*(4), 550–557.

Ellis-Hill, C. S., & Horn, S. (2000). Change in identity and self-concept: A new theoretical approach to recovery following a stroke. *Disability & Rehabilitation, 22,* 725–733.

Field, P. A., & Morse, J. M. (1985). *Nursing research: The application of qualitative approaches.* Rockville, MD: Aspen.

Finfgeld-Connett, D. (2010). Generalizability and transferability of meta-synthesis research findings. *Journal of Advanced Nursing, 66*(2), 246–254.

Gallagher, P. (2011). Becoming normal: A grounded theory study on the emotional process of stroke recovery. *Canadian Journal of Neuroscience Nursing, 33*(3), 24–32.

Gibson, B. E., & Martin, D. K. (2003).Qualitative research and evidence-based physiotherapy practice. *Physiotherapy, 89*(6), 350–358.

Glaser, B. G. (1978). *Theoretical sensitivity.* Mill Valley, CA: Sociology Press.

Glaser, B. G. (1992). *Emergence vs. forcing: Basics of grounded theory analysis.* Mill Valley, CA: Sociology Press.

Glesne, C. (1999). *Becoming qualitative researchers: An introduction* (2nd ed.). New York, NY: Longman.

Horsburgh, D. (2003). Evaluation of qualitative research, *Journal of Clinical Nursing, 12,* 307–312.

Jackson, R. L., Drummond, D. K., & Camara, S. (2007). What is qualitative research? *Qualitative Research Reports in Communication, 8*(1), 21–28.

Leeman, J., & Sandelowski, M. (2012). Practice-based evidence and qualitative inquiry. *Journal of Nursing Scholarship, 44*(2), 171–179.

Mantzoukas, S. (2007). A review of evidence-based practice, nursing research and reflection: levelling the hierarchy. *Journal of Clinical Nursing, 17,* 214–223.

Meneses, K. D., McNees, P., Loerzel, V. W., et al. (2007). Transition from treatment to survivorship: effects of a psychoeducational intervention on quality of life in breast cancer survivors. *Oncology Nursing Forum, 34*(5), 1007–1016.

Morse, J. M., Penrod, J., & Hupcey, J. E. (2000). Qualitative outcome analysis: evaluating nursing interventions for complex clinical phenomena. *Journal of Nursing Scholarship, 32*(2), 125–130.

Richards, K. M. (2008). RAP project: an instrument development study to determine common attributes for pain assessment among men and women who represent multiple pain-related diagnoses. *Pain Management Nursing, 9*(10), 33–43.

Russell, C. K., & Gregory, D. M. (2003). Evaluation of qualitative research studies. *Evidence-Based Nursing, 6*(2), 36–40.

Seiler, A. J., & Moss, V. A. (2012). The experience of nurse practitioners providing health care to the homeless. *Journal of the Academy of Nurse Practitioners, 24,* 301–312.

Straus, S. E., & Sackett, D. L. (2005). Evidence based medicine: how to practice and teach EBM (3rd ed.). Edinburgh, United Kingdom: Churchill Livingstone.

Strauss, A. (1987). *Qualitative analysis for social scientists.* New York, NY: Cambridge University Press.

Strauss, A., & Corbin, J. (1998). Basics of qualitative research: grounded theory procedures and techniques. Newbury Park, CA: Sage.

Streubert, H. J., & Carpenter, D. R. (2011). Qualitative nursing research: Advancing the humanistic imperative. Philadelphia, PA: Wolters Klower Health.

Walsh, D., & Downe, S. (2005). Meta-synthesis method of qualitative research: a literature review. *Journal of Advanced Nursing, 50*(2), 204–211.

# ℮volve WEBSITE

*Go to Evolve at http://evolve.elsevier.com/LoBiondo/ for review questions, critiquing exercises, and additional research articles for practice in reviewing and critiquing.*

# PART III

# Processes and Evidence Related to Quantitative Research

**Research Vignette:** *Nancy Bergstrom*

# RESEARCH VIGNETTE

## FROM PRESSURE ULCER PREDICTION TO PREVENTIVE INTERVENTIONS

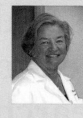

Nancy Bergstrom, RN, PhD, FAAN
Theodore J. and Mary E. Trumble Professor of Aging Research
Director, Center on Aging
Associate Dean for Research (interim)
School of Nursing
University of Texas Health Science Center–Houston
Houston, Texas

The Braden Scale for Predicting Pressure Sore Risk® was developed, tested for reliability and validity in a variety of settings, and introduced as a clinical tool in the 1980s and 1990s (Bergstrom et al., 1987; Bergstrom & Braden, 1992; Bergstrom et al., 1998). The tool was then tested for reliability, validity, and clinical utility in settings in the U.S. and abroad, was found to facilitate risk prediction in clinical settings, and was included in a number of practice guidelines (Bergstrom et al., 1992; National Pressure Ulcer Advisory Panel, 2009).

Since then, the Braden Scale has been translated into many languages (see www.bradenscale. com for selected translations known to use WHO or other approaches to translation). The Braden Scale has garnered widespread support in clinical settings such as hospitals and nursing and long-term care facilities.

Nevertheless, investigators have tried to improve on the Braden Scale through (1) efforts to make it more specific for unique settings (e.g., perioperative, acute care, rehabilitation); (2) creation of new tools, including additional risk factors and efforts to look at risk in different ways; (3) comparison of the Braden Scale with other tools to determine the "best" or "most appropriate" tool; and (4) more comprehensive approaches to risk assessment, such as creating a list of risk factors that have predicted risk in observational studies and retrospective reviews of large data sets. (More than 120 risk factors have been identified.) These studies consistently demonstrate that the Braden Scale is as good as, or better than, the comparison tools. The list of risk factors remains a popular option for risk prediction and theoretical assessment. These efforts to create a better tool continue.

Examination of the original conceptual framework (Braden & Bergstrom, 1987) reflects our efforts to simplify the list of risk factors by relating specific risk factors to more conceptual areas of risk. For instance, the Braden Scale subscales are based on risk factors such as mobility. Conceptually, issues of limited mobility are seen in medical diagnoses such as para-or quadriplegia, Parkinson's disease, multiple sclerosis, hip fracture/hip replacement, and various other fractures or surgeries. The commonality of these risk factors is limited mobility. Limited mobility tends to increase exposure to pressure because at-risk persons are generally unable to move enough to relieve pressure, which decreases blood flow to exposed tissue. The advantage of considering mobility conceptually, rather than by diagnosis only, is that the degree of individual mobility, and therefore pressure exposure, can be assessed more accurately. With a brief assessment of the individual, it is possible to gauge risk from length of exposure to pressure. Thus, the Braden Scale represents, for the most part, a conceptual assessment of the most important risk factors. It is a clinically useful way to assess risk efficiently. The added benefit of this tool is that it guides the selection and intensity of preventive measures. For instance, a person who is not limited in mobility, regardless of diagnosis, does not need to be repositioned.

The preponderance of research aiming to prevent pressure ulcers in the last 20 years has focused on developing a more precise tool to predict pressure ulcer risk. Yet, that objective does not appear to have been achieved. Prediction studies continue and, while this is good, *my biggest disappointment is that few studies to date have tested interventions related to preventing pressure ulcers based on risk assessment or specific risk factors.* Fortunately, the industry has provided us with new tools for prevention, especially in the areas of support surfaces and incontinence care.

Several investigators, mostly international, have undertaken studies to assess the effectiveness of support surfaces in the prevention of pressure ulcers. Clinical investigations are expensive, labor intensive, and fraught with pitfalls, yet several good studies using combinations of support surfaces and repositioning frequency have been reported (Defloor et al., 2009; Vanderwee et al, 2007; Moore et al., 2011). Still, it is not clear if these findings can be generalized to patients at all risk levels, and since many subjects in these studies may have been at lower risk, it may be possible that pressure ulcers in these patients would not have developed, even without intervention. For these reasons, the *need* to do one more study was more compelling to me than taking early retirement, and with wonderful colleagues and the financial support of the National Institutes of Health (NIH) and the Ontario Ministry of Health, The TURN Study was conducted.

One of the most widely accepted practices for the prevention of pressure ulcers is turning or repositioning patients at 2-hour intervals. Many potential reasons are cited when providing evidence for this practice. Because there was no evidence that other intervals were acceptable and there was some evidence for 2-hour turning, the practice was encouraged in the first guideline for the Prevention of Pressure Ulcer (guideline #3) by the Agency for Health Care Policy and Research, and the practice continued to be recommended in a number of guidelines.

Personally, I *really believed* this was necessary. Although I had conducted some small studies of support surface efficacy in prevention and reported that high-density foam replacement mattresses were superior to other mattresses and overlays, I still believed turning was necessary. I began to question this when something very personal occurred. My mother was hospitalized. I stayed with my mother all day, and before leaving for the night, I positioned her on her left side. When I returned the next morning, she was in the same position! However, she did not have a single red area on her skin! I found repeated evidence that she was not turned, but no evidence of pressure ulcers. As a result, I began to think that high-density foam mattresses were probably more effective in prevention of pressure ulcers than originally thought.

Pilot work began to determine appropriate turning intervals for "at risk" patients cared for on high-density foam mattresses. I did not want to do this study if there was a chance anyone would develop a serious ulcer. Our pilot work showed us that mild-risk patients (Braden Scores of 15-18) would not agree to participate in a turning study because they were independent in mobility and activity, needed to be in a position to see the TV, and didn't want to be bothered. We completed several pilot tests and a pilot test of our research protocol, submitted a comprehensive proposal, and received funding from NIH. Thus, the TURN Study began.

The TURN Study is a Phase 3 Clinical Trial (Clinical Trials.com, NCT00665535) to determine the optimal frequency of turning long-term–care residents cared for on high-density foam mattresses, stratified by risk (moderate: scores 13 and 14, or high: scores 10-12) for pressure ulcers according to the Braden Scale, for the purpose of preventing pressure ulcers. Twenty-seven long-term–care facilities in the U.S. and Canada agreed to participate. Subjects were older than 65 years, at risk for pressure sores, cared for on a high-density foam mattress, and were without pressure ulcers at the beginning of the study.

Subjects were randomly assigned by level of risk to turning at 2-, 3-, or 4-hour intervals while in bed. Repositioning and brief changes were done according to the assigned turning interval while in bed, and subjects received facility-based preventive care while out of bed. Certified nursing assistants turned participants according to the assigned interval and recorded observations on a safety documentation form that included prompts for elevating heels and reporting skin changes at each turn. The outcome of the study was blinded; that is, nurses performing the skin assessment each week were from a different unit and did not know to which turning schedule the resident was assigned.

Nine hundred forty two participants completed the study. While only 2% of the subjects (19 of 942) developed pressure ulcers, any changes that occur in turning protocols in the future must only be attempted when residents are at moderate or high risk, on a high-density foam mattress, and being monitored for safety. The results providing data on the turning frequencies will be published in research journals.

It is likely, based on the TURN Study and work by Defloor, that protocol changes will be recommended. There will be many opportunities for translational research focused on effectiveness of protocol changes, and testing recommendations for ensuring patient safety. Hopefully this will be the first of many studies of interventions based on risk levels.

## REFERENCES

Bergstrom, N., Braden, B. J., Laguzza, A., & Holman, V. (1987). The Braden scale for predicting pressure sore risk. *Nursing Research, 36(4),* 205–210.

Bergstrom, N., & Braden, B. (1992). A prospective study of pressure sore risk among institutionalized elderly. *Journal of the American Geriatrics Society, 40(8),* 747–758.

Bergstrom, N., Braden, B., Kemp, M., et al. (1998). Predicting pressure ulcer risk: a multi-site study of the predictive validity of the Braden scale. *Nursing Research, 47(5),* 261–269.

Bergstrom, N., Allman, R. M., Carlson, C. E., et al. (1992). Pressure ulcers in adults: prediction and prevention. *Clinical Practice Guideline, Number 3.* AHCPR Publication No. 92-0047.

Braden, B., & Bergstrom, N. (1987). A conceptual schema for the study of the etiology of pressure ulcers. *Rehabilitation Nursing, 12(1),* 8–12.

Defloor, T., Bacquer, D. D., & Grypdonck, M. H. (2005). The effect of various combinations of turning and pressure reducing devices on the incidence of pressure ulcers. *International Journal of Nursing Studies, 42(1),* 37–46.

Moore, Z., Cowman, S., & Conroy, R. M. (2011). A randomised controlled clinical trial of repositioning, using the 30 degrees tilt, for the prevention of pressure ulcers. *Journal of Clinical Nursing, 20(17-18),* 2633–2644. doi: 10.1111/j.1365-2702.2011.03736.x; 10.1111/j.1365-2702.2011.03736.x.

National Pressure Ulcer Advisory Panel (NPUAP), & European Pressure Ulcer Advisory Panel (EPUAP) (Eds.), (2009). *Pressure ulcer prevention: quick reference guide.* Washington, DC: National Pressure Ulcer Advisory Panel.

Vanderwee, K., Grypdonck, M. H., De Bacquer, D., & Defloor, T. (2007). Effectiveness of turning with unequal time intervals on the incidence of pressure ulcer lesions. *Journal of Advanced Nursing, 57(1),* 59–68.

# Introduction to Quantitative Research

*Geri LoBiondo-Wood*

## evolve WEBSITE

*Go to Evolve at http://evolve.elsevier.com/LoBiondo/ for review questions, critiquing exercises, and additional research articles for practice in reviewing and critiquing.*

## LEARNING OUTCOMES

*After reading this chapter, you should be able to do the following:*

- Define research design.
- Identify the purpose of research design.
- Define control and fidelity as it affects research design and the outcomes of a study.
- Compare and contrast the elements that affect fidelity and control.
- Begin to evaluate what degree of control should be exercised in a study.

- Define internal validity.
- Identify the threats to internal validity.
- Define external validity.
- Identify the conditions that affect external validity.
- Identify the links between study design and evidence-based practice.
- Evaluate research design using critiquing questions.

## KEY TERMS

| | | | |
|---|---|---|---|
| bias | extraneous or mediating | internal validity | randomization |
| constancy | variable | intervening variable | reactivity |
| control | generalizability | intervention fidelity | selection |
| control group | history | maturation | selection bias |
| dependent variable | homogeneity | measurement effects | testing |
| experimental group | independent variable | mortality | |
| external validity | instrumentation | pilot study | |

The word *design* implies the organization of elements into a masterful work of art. In the world of art and fashion, design conjures up images that are used to express a total concept. When an individual creates a structure such as a dress pattern or blueprints for the design of a house, the type of structure depends on the aims of the creator. The same can be said of the research process. The research process does not need to be a sterile procedure, but one where the researcher develops a masterful work within the limits of a research question or hypothesis and the related theoretical basis. The framework that the researcher creates is the **design.** When reading a study, you should be able to recognize that the research question, purpose, literature review, theoretical framework, and hypothesis all interrelate with, complement, and assist in the operationalization of the design (Figure 8-1). The degree to which there is a fit between these elements and the steps of the research process strengthens the study and also your confidence in the evidence provided by the findings and their potential applicability to practice.

Nursing is concerned with a variety of structures such as the provision of high quality and safe patient care, responses of patients to illness, and factors that affect caregivers. When patient care is administered, the nursing process is used. Previous chapters stress the importance of a clear research question or hypothesis, literature review, conceptual framework, and subject matter knowledge. How a researcher structures, implements, or designs a study affects the results of a study and ultimately its application to practice.

For you to understand the implications and usefulness of a study for evidence-based practice, the key issues of research design must be understood. This chapter provides an overview of the meaning, purpose, and issues related to quantitative research design, and Chapters 9 and 10 present specific types of quantitative designs.

## PURPOSE OF RESEARCH DESIGN

The research design in quantitative research has overlapping yet unique purposes. The design
- Provides the plan or blueprint
- Is the vehicle for systematically testing research questions and hypotheses
- Provides the structure for maintaining the **control** in the study

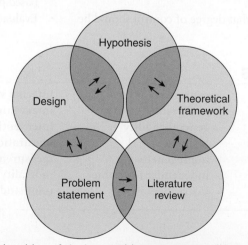

**FIGURE 8-1** Interrelationships of design, problem statement, literature review, theoretical framework, and hypothesis.

These design concepts guide a researcher in developing and conducting research. All research attempts to answer questions. The design coupled with the methods and analysis is the mechanism for finding solutions to research questions or hypotheses. Control is defined as the measures that the researcher uses to hold the conditions of the study uniform and avoid possible potential of bias on the dependent variable or outcome variable. Control measures help to avoid bias or threats to the internal validity of the study.

A research example that demonstrates how the design can aid in the solution of a research question and maintain control is the study by Thomas and colleagues (2012; see Appendix A), whose aim was to evaluate the effectiveness of education, motivational-interviewing–based coaching and usual care on the improvement of cancer pain management. Subjects who fit the study's inclusion criteria were randomly assigned to one of the three groups. The interventions were clearly defined. The authors also discuss how they maintained intervention fidelity or constancy of interventionists, data-collector training and supervision, and follow-up throughout the study. By establishing the specific sample criteria and subject eligibility (inclusion criteria; see Chapter 12) and by clearly describing and designing the experimental intervention, the researchers demonstrated that they had a well-developed plan and structure and were able to consistently maintain the study's conditions. A variety of considerations, including the type of design chosen, affect a study's successful completion. These considerations include the following:

- Objectivity in conceptualizing the research question or hypothesis
- Accuracy
- Feasibility
- Control and intervention fidelity
- Validity—internal
- Validity—external

There are statistical principles behind the forms of control, but it is more important that you have a clear conceptual understanding. The forms of control are important not only to assess the quality of the study but also application to a practice that is evidence based.

The next two chapters present different experimental, quasi-experimental, and nonexperimental designs. As you will recall from Chapter 1, a study's type of design is linked to the level of evidence. As you critically appraise the design, you must also take into account other aspects of a study's design and conduct. These aspects are reviewed in this chapter. How they are applied depends on the type of design (see Chapters 9 and 10).

## OBJECTIVITY IN THE RESEARCH QUESTION CONCEPTUALIZATION

Objectivity in the conceptualization of the research question is derived from a review of the literature and development of a theoretical framework (see Figure 8-1). Using the literature, the researcher assesses the depth and breadth of available knowledge on the question. The literature review and theoretical framework should demonstrate that the researcher reviewed the literature critically and objectively (see Chapters 3 and 4) because this affects the design chosen. For example, a research question about the length of a breast-feeding teaching program in relation to adherence to breast-feeding may suggest either a correlational or an experimental design (see Chapters 9 and 10), whereas a question related to fatigue levels and amount of sleep at different points in cancer treatment may suggest a survey or correlational study (see Chapter 10). Therefore the literature review should reflect the following:

- When the question was studied
- What aspects of the question were studied
- Where it was investigated and with what populations
- By whom it was investigated
- The gaps or inconsistencies in the literature

**HELPFUL HINT**

A literature review that incorporates all aspects of the question allows you to judge the objectivity of the research question and therefore whether the design chosen matches the question.

## ACCURACY

Accuracy in determining the appropriate design is also accomplished through the theoretical framework and literature review (see Chapters 3 and 4). Accuracy means that all aspects of a study systematically and logically follow from the research question or hypothesis. The simplicity of a research project does not render it useless or of less value. If the scope of a study is limited or focused, the researchers should demonstrate how accuracy was maintained. You should feel that the researcher chose a design that was consistent with the question and offered the maximum amount of control. The issues of control are discussed later in this chapter.

Also, many research questions have not yet been researched. Therefore a preliminary or **pilot study** is also a wise approach. A pilot study can be thought of as a beginning study in an area conducted to test and refine a study's data collection methods, and it helps to determine the sample size needed for a larger study. For example, Crane-Okada and colleagues (2012) published a report of their study which pilot tested the feasibility of the short-term effects of a 12-week Mindful Movement Program intervention for women age 50 years and older. The key is the accuracy, validity, and objectivity used by the researcher in attempting to answer the question. Accordingly, when reading research you should read various types of studies and assess how and if the criteria for each step of the research process were followed. Many journals publish not only randomized controlled studies (see Chapter 9), but also pilot studies.

## FEASIBILITY

When critiquing the research design, one also needs to be aware of the pragmatic consideration of feasibility. Sometimes feasibility issues do not truly sink in until one does research. It is important to consider feasibility when reviewing a study, including subject availability, time required for subjects to participate, costs, and data analysis (Table 8-1).

Before conducting a large experimental or a randomized controlled trial, it is helpful for researchers to conduct a pilot study with a small number of subjects to determine the feasibility of subject recruitment, the intervention, the data-collection protocol, the likelihood that subjects will complete the study, the reliability and validity of measurement instruments, and the study's costs. These pragmatic considerations are not presented as a step in

| TABLE 8-1 | PRAGMATIC CONSIDERATIONS IN DETERMINING THE FEASIBILITY OF A RESEARCH QUESTION |
|---|---|
| **FACTOR** | **PRAGMATIC CONSIDERATIONS** |
| Time | The research question must be one that can be studied within a realistic period. All research has completion deadlines. A study must be well circumscribed to provide ample completion time. |
| Subject Availability | A researcher must determine whether a sufficient number of subjects will be available and willing to participate. If one has a captive audience (e.g., students in a classroom), it may be relatively easy to enlist subjects. If a study involves subjects' independent time and effort, they may be unwilling to participate when there is no apparent reward. Potential subjects may have fears about harm or confidentiality and be suspicious of the research process. Subjects with unusual characteristics may be difficult to locate. People are generally cooperative about participating, but a researcher should consider enlisting more subjects than actually needed to prepare for subject attrition. At times, a research report may note how the inclusion criteria were liberalized or the number of subjects altered, as a result of some unforeseen recruitment or attrition consideration. |
| Facility and Equipment Availability | All research requires some equipment such as questionnaires, telephones, computers, or other apparatus. Most research requires availability of some facility type for data collection (e.g., a hospital unit or laboratory space). |
| Money | Research requires expenditure of money. Before starting a study the researcher itemizes expenses and projects the total study costs. A budget provides a picture of the monetary needs for items such as books, postage, printing, technical equipment, computer charges, and salaries. Expenses can range from about $1,000 for a small-scale project to hundreds of thousands of dollars per year for a large federally funded project. |
| Researcher Experience | Selection of a research problem should be based on the nurse's experience and knowledge because it is more prudent to develop a study related to a topic that is theoretically or experientially familiar. |
| Ethics | Research that place unethical demands on subjects may not be feasible for study. Researchers take ethical considerations seriously. Ethics considerations affect the design and methodology choice. |

the research process as are the theoretical framework or methods, but they do affect every step of the process and, as such, should be considered when assessing a study. When critiquing a study, note the credentials of the author and whether the study was part of a student project or part of a fully funded grant project. Finally, the pragmatic issues raised affect the scope and breadth of a study and the strength of evidence generated, and therefore its generalizability.

## CONTROL AND INTERVENTION FIDELITY

A researcher chooses a design to maximize the degree of **control**, fidelity or uniformity over the tested variables. Control is maximized by a well-planned study that considers each step of the research process and the potential threats to internal and external validity. In a study that tests interventions (randomized controlled trial; see Chapter 9), **intervention fidelity** (also referred to as **treatment fidelity**) is a key concept. *Fidelity* means trustworthiness or faithfulness. In a study, intervention fidelity means that the researcher actively standardized the intervention and planned how to administer the intervention to each subject in the same manner under the same conditions. An efficient design can maximize results, decrease bias, and control preexisting conditions that may affect outcomes. To accomplish these tasks, the research design and methods should demonstrate the researcher's efforts to maintain fidelity. Control is important in all designs. But the elements of control and fidelity differ based on the type of design. Thus, when various research designs are critiqued, the issue of control is always raised but with varying levels of flexibility. The issues discussed here will become clearer as you review the various designs types discussed in later chapters (see Chapters 9 and 10). Control is accomplished by ruling out extraneous or mediating variables that compete with the independent variables as an explanation for a study's outcome. An intervening, extraneous, or mediating variable is one that interferes with the operations of the variables being studied. An example would be the type of breast cancer treatment patients experienced (Thomas et al., 2012). Means of controlling extraneous variables include the following:

- Use of a homogeneous sample
- Use of consistent data-collection procedures
- Training and supervision of data collectors and interventionists
- Manipulation of the independent variable
- Randomization

> **EVIDENCE-BASED PRACTICE TIP**
>
> As you read studies, it is important to assess if the study includes a tested intervention and whether the report contains a clear description of the intervention and how it was controlled. If the details are not clear, it should make you think that the intervention may have been administered differently among the subjects, therefore affecting the interpretation of the results.

## Homogeneous Sampling

In a stop-smoking study, extraneous variables may affect the dependent (outcome) variable. The characteristics of a study's subjects are common extraneous variables. Age, gender, length of time smoked, amount smoked, and even smoking rules may affect the outcome in the stop-smoking example. These variables may therefore affect the outcome, even though they are extraneous or outside of the study's design. As a control for these and other similar problems, the researcher's subjects should demonstrate homogeneity or similarity with respect to the extraneous variables relevant to the particular study (see Chapter 12). Extraneous variables are not fixed but must be reviewed and decided on, based on the study's purpose and theoretical base. By using a sample of homogeneous subjects, based on inclusion and exclusion criteria, the researcher has used a straightforward step of control.

For example, in the study by Alhusen and colleagues (2012; see Appendix B), the researchers ensured homogeneity of the sample based on age and demographics. This step limits the generalizability or application of the outcomes to other populations when analyzing and discussing the outcomes (see Chapter 17). As you read studies, you will often see the research-ers limit the generalizability of the findings to like samples. Results can then be generalized only to a similar population of individuals. You may say that this is limiting. This is not necessarily so because no treatment or program can be applicable to all populations, nor is it feasible to examine a large number of different populations in one study. Thus as you appraise the findings of studies, you must take the differences in populations into consideration.

---

**HELPFUL HINT**

When reviewing studies, remember that it is better to have a "clean" study that can be used to make generalizations about a specific population than a "messy" one that can generalize little or nothing.

---

If the researcher feels that an extraneous variable is important, it may be included in the design. In the smoking example, if individuals are working in an area where smoking is not allowed and this is considered to be important, the researcher could build it into the design and set up a control for it. This can be done by comparing two different work areas: one where smoking is allowed and one where it is not. The important idea to keep in mind is that before the data are collected, the researcher should have identified, planned for, or controlled the important extraneous variables. Homogenity is important in all quantitative designs.

## Constancy in Data Collection

A basic, yet critical, component of control is constancy in data-collection. Constancy refers to the notion that the data-collection procedures should reflect to the consumer a cookbook-like recipe of how the researcher controlled the study's conditions. This means that environmental conditions, timing of data collection, data-collection instruments, and data-collection procedures used to collect the data are the same for each subject (see Chapter 14). Constancy in data collection is also referred to as **intervention fidelity.** The elements of intervention fidelity (Bellg et al., 2004; Resnick et al., 2005; Santacroce et al., 2004) are as follows:

- *Design*: The study is designed to allow an adequate testing of the hypothesis(es) in relation to the underlying theory and clinical processes
- *Training*: Ongoing training and supervision of the data collectors (interventionists) to assure that the intervention is being delivered as planned and in a similar manner with all the subjects
- *Delivery*: Assessing that the intervention is delivered as intended, including that the "dose" (as measured by the number, frequency and length of contact) is well de-scribed for all subjects and that the dose is the same in each group, and that there is a plan for possible problems
- *Receipt*: Assurance that the treatment has been received and understood by the subject
- *Enactment*: Assessment that the performance of the intervention skills that the subject performs are performed as intended.

The Thomas and colleagues article (Appendix A; see Procedures section) is an example of how intervention fidelity was maintained. A review of this study shows that data were collected from each subject in the same manner and under the same conditions by trained data collectors. This type of control aided the investigators' ability to draw conclusions, discuss limitations, and cite the need for further research. It also demonstrates a clear, consistent, and specific means of data collection. When interventions are implemented, researchers will often describe the training of and supervision of interventionists and/or data collectors that took place to ensure constancy. All study designs should demonstrate constancy (fidelity) of data collection, but studies that test an intervention require the highest level of intervention fidelity.

## Manipulation of Independent Variable

A third means of control is manipulation of the **independent variable**. This refers to the administration of a program, treatment, or intervention to only one group within the study and not to the other subjects in the study. The first group is known as the **experimental group** or **intervention,** and the other group is known as the **control group**. In a control group the variables under study are held at a constant or comparison level. For example, Thomas and colleagues (2012; see Appendix A) manipulated the provision of two interventions compared to usual care for breast cancer survivors using an experimental design.

Experimental and quasi-experimental designs use manipulation. These designs are used to test whether a treatment or intervention affects patient outcomes. Nonexperimental designs do not manipulate the independent variable. Lack of variable manipulation does not decrease the usefulness of a nonexperimental design, but the use of a control group in an experimental or quasi-experimental design is related to the level of the research question or hypothesis. For example, Melvin and colleagues (2012; see Appendix D) used a nonexperimental study to investigate combat-related post-traumatic stress symptoms (PTSS) in U.S. Army couples. This study did not manipulate post-traumatic symptoms (that would be unethical) but studied the relationship of couple functioning and PTSS.

> ### HELPFUL HINT
>
> Be aware that the lack of manipulation of the independent variable does not mean a weaker study. The level of the question, the amount of theoretical development, and the research that has preceded the project all affect the researcher's choice of the design. If the question is amenable to a design that manipulates the independent variable, it increases the power of a researcher to draw conclusions; that is, if all of the considerations of control are equally addressed.

## Randomization

Researchers may also choose other forms of control, such as randomization. **Randomization** is used when the required number of subjects from the population is obtained in such a manner that each subject in a population has an equal chance of being selected. Randomization eliminates bias, aids in the attainment of a representative sample, and can be used in various designs (see Chapter 12). Thomas and colleagues (2012; see Appendix A) randomized subjects to an intervention or control group.

Randomization can also be done with questionnaires. By randomly ordering items on the questionnaires, the investigator can assess if there is a difference in responses that can be related to the order of the items. This may be especially important in longitudinal studies where bias from giving the same questionnaire to the same subjects on a number of occasions can be a problem.

## QUANTITATIVE CONTROL AND FLEXIBILITY

The same level of control or elimination of bias *cannot* be exercised equally in all design types. When a researcher wants to explore an area in which little or no literature and/or research on the concept exists, the researcher may use a qualitative study or a non-experimental study (see Chapters 5 through 7 and 10). In these types of study the researcher is interested in describing a phenomenon in a group of individuals.

If it is determined from a review of a study that the researcher intended to conduct a correlational study, or a study that looks at the relationship between or among the variables, the issue of control takes on a different importance (see Chapter 10). Control must be exercised as strictly as possible. All studies should be evaluated for potential extraneous variables that may affect the outcomes; however, all studies, based on their design, exercise different levels of control. All aspects of control are strictly applied to studies that use an experimental design (see Chapter 9). You should be able to locate in the research report how the researcher maintained control in accordance with its design.

---

### EVIDENCE-BASED PRACTICE TIP

Remember that establishing evidence for practice is determined by assessing the validity of each step of the study, assessing if the evidence assists in planning patient care, and assessing if patients respond to the evidence-based care.

---

## INTERNAL AND EXTERNAL VALIDITY

When reading research, you must be convinced that the results of a study are valid, based on precision, and faithful to what the researcher wanted to measure. For a study to form the basis of further research, practice, and theory development, it must be credible and reflect how the researcher avoided bias. Bias can occur at any step of the research process. Bias can be a result of what questions are asked (see Chapter 2), what hypotheses are tested (see Chapter 2), how data are collected or observations made (see Chapter 14), number of subjects and how subjects are recruited and included (see Chapter 12), how groups are conceptualized in an experimental study (see Chapter 9), and how data are reported and analyzed (see Chapter 16). When bias occurs it is not that the researcher was careless or intended to cause bias, but as studies evolve and are carried out, problems can occur that need to be considered before studies are used to change practice. There are two important criteria for evaluating bias, credibility, and dependability of the results: internal validity and external validity. An understanding of the threats to internal validity and external validity is necessary for reading research and considering whether it is applicable to practice. Threats to validity are listed in Box 8-1, and discussion follows.

### Internal Validity

**Internal validity** asks whether the independent variable really made the difference or the change in the dependent variable. To establish internal validity the researcher rules out other factors or threats as rival explanations of the relationship between the variables.

---

**BOX 8-1 THREATS TO VALIDITY**

| **Internal Validity** | **External Validity** |
|---|---|
| • History | • Selection effects |
| • Maturation | • Reactive effects |
| • Testing | • Measurement effects |
| • Instrumentation | |
| • Mortality | |
| • Selection bias | |

---

There are a number of threats to internal validity, and these are considered by researchers in planning a study and by clinicians before implementing the results in practice (Campbell & Stanley, 1966). You should note that the threats to internal validity are most clearly applicable to experimental designs, but attention to factors that can compromise outcomes for all studies, and thereby the overall strength and quality of evidence of a study's findings, should be considered to some degree in all quantitative designs. If these threats are not considered as potential sources of bias, they could negate the results of the study. How these threats may affect specific designs are addressed in Chapters 9 and 10. Threats to internal validity include history, maturation, testing, instrumentation, mortality, and selection bias. Table 8-2 provides examples of the threats to internal validity. Generally, researchers will note the threats to validity that they encountered in the discussion and or limitations section of a research article.

## History

In addition to the independent variable, another specific event that may have an effect on the dependent variable may occur either inside or outside the experimental setting; this is referred to as **history**. An example may be that of an investigator testing the effects of an educational program for young adults on completion of organ donation card designations. During the course of the educational program, an ad featuring a known public figure is released on Facebook about the importance of organ donation and becoming an organ donor. The occurrence of this information on social media with a public figure engenders a great deal of media and press attention. In the course of the media attention, medical experts are interviewed widely and the importance of organ donation is supported. If the researcher finds an increase in the number of young adults who sign their organ donation cards, the researcher may not be able to conclude that the change in behavior is the result of the teaching program because it may have been influenced by the result of the information on social media and the resultant media coverage. See Table 8-2 for another example.

## Maturation

**Maturation** refers to the developmental, biological, or psychological processes that operate within an individual as a function of time and are external to the events of the study. For example, suppose one wishes to evaluate the effect of a teaching method on baccalaureate students' achievements on a skills test. The investigator would record the students' abilities before and after the teaching method. Between the pretest and posttest, the students have grown older and wiser. The growth or change is unrelated to the study and may explain the differences between the two testing periods rather than the experimental treatment. See Table 8-2 for another example. It is important to remember that maturation is more than

| TABLE 8-2 | EXAMPLES OF INTERNAL VALIDITY THREATS |
|---|---|
| **THREAT** | **EXAMPLE** |
| History | A study tested a teaching intervention in one hospital and compared outcomes to those of another hospital in which usual care was given. During the final months of data collection, the control hospital implemented a congestive heart failure critical pathway; as a result, data from the control hospital (cohort) was not included in the analysis. |
| Maturation | Breitenstein et al. (2012) evaluated the 1-year efficacy outcomes of a parenting program to promote parenting competency. Though the program had significant positive outcomes in parental self-efficacy, the authors noted that the children's maturation may have accounted for observed behavior problems in the children. |
| Testing | Thomas and colleagues (2012) had difficulty maintaining the subjects' attention-control techniques as subjects wished to discuss issues other than the intended topics of the study (Appendix A). |
| Instrumentation | Li et al. (2012) discussed issues that possibly affected instrumentation such as the reliance on chart reviews, family caregiver self-reports, perceptions of patient status as data collection strategies, and spacing of data collection time points. |
| Mortality | Thomas and colleagues (2012) noted that they had subject losses in all three of their groups and that the lack of statistical significance in their findings may have been related to an inadequate sample size even though the intervention had a positive outcome (Appendix A). |
| Selection bias | Thomas and colleagues (2012) controlled for selection bias by establishing inclusion and exclusion participation criteria for participation. Subjects were also stratified using a specific procedure that ensured balance across the three treatment groups. Sarna et al. (2012). "This study has many limitations common to self-reports surveys including the bias of self-selection of the sample (p. 261)." |

change resulting from an age-related developmental process, but could be related to physical changes as well. For example, in a study of new products to stimulate wound healing, one might ask whether the healing that occurred was related to the product or to the natural occurrence of wound healing.

## Testing

Taking the same test repeatedly could influence subjects' responses the next time the test is completed. For example, the effect of taking a pretest on the subject's posttest score is known as **testing**. The effect of taking a pretest may sensitize an individual and improve the score of the posttest. Individuals generally score higher when they take a test a second time, regardless of the treatment. The differences between posttest and pretest scores may not be a result of the independent variable but rather of the experience gained through the testing. Table 8-2 provides an example.

## Instrumentation

Instrumentation threats are changes in the measurement of the variables or observational techniques that may account for changes in the obtained measurement. For example, a researcher may wish to study types of thermometers (e.g., tympanic, digital, electronic) to compare the accuracy of using a tympanic thermometer to other temperature-taking methods. To prevent instrumentation threat, a researcher must check the calibration of the thermometers according to the manufacturer's specifications before and after data collection.

Another example that fits into this area is related to techniques of observation or data collection. If a researcher has several raters collecting observational data, all must be trained in a similar manner so that they collect data using a standardized approach, thereby ensuring interrater reliability (see Chapter 13) and intervention fidelity (see Table 8-2). At times, even though the researcher takes steps to prevent instrumentation problems, this threat may still occur and should be evaluated within the total context of the study.

## Mortality

**Mortality** is the loss of study subjects from the first data-collection point (pretest) to the second data-collection point (posttest). If the subjects who remain in the study are not similar to those who dropped out, the results could be affected. The loss of subjects may be from the sample as a whole or, in a study that has both an experimental and a control group, there may be differential loss of subjects. Differential loss of subjects means that more of the subjects in one group dropped out than the other group. See Table 8-2 for an example.

## Selection Bias

If the precautions are not used to gain a representative sample, **selection bias** could result from the way the subjects were chosen. Selection effects are a problem in studies in which the individuals themselves decide whether to participate in a study. Suppose an investigator wishes to assess if a new stop-smoking program contributes to smoking cessation. If the new program is offered to all, chances are only individuals who are more motivated to learn about how to stop smoking will take part in the program. Assessment of the effectiveness of the program is problematic, because the investigator cannot be sure if the new program encouraged smoking-cessation behaviors or if only highly motivated individuals joined the program. To avoid selection bias, the researcher could randomly assign subjects to groups. See Table 8-2 for an example of selection bias. In a nonexperimental study even with inclusion and exclusion selection criteria, selection bias is difficult to avoid completely.

---

### HELPFUL HINT

The list of internal validity threats is not exhaustive. More than one threat can be found in a study, depending on the type of study design. Finding a threat to internal validity in a study does not invalidate the results and is usually acknowledged by the investigator in the "Results" or "Discussion" or "Limitations" section of the study.

---

### EVIDENCE-BASED PRACTICE TIP

Avoiding threats to internal validity when conducting clinical research can be quite difficult at times. Yet this reality does not render studies that have threats useless. Take them into consideration and weigh the total evidence of a study for not only its statistical meaningfulness but also its clinical meaningfulness.

---

## External Validity

**External validity** deals with possible problems of generalizability of the study's findings to additional populations and to other environmental conditions. External validity questions under what conditions and with what types of subjects the same results can be expected to occur. The goal of the researcher is to select a design that maximizes both internal and external validity.

## CRITICAL THINKING DECISION PATH

### *Potential Threats to a Study's Validity*

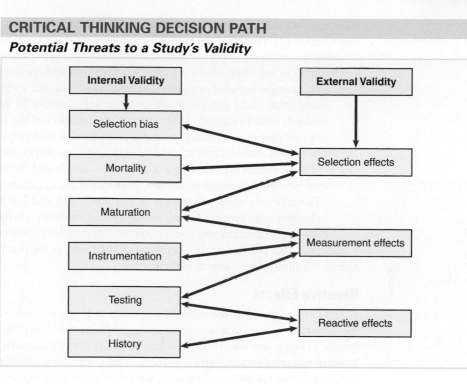

The factors that may affect external validity are related to selection of subjects, study conditions, and type of observations. These factors are termed *effects of selection, reactive effects,* and *effects of testing.* You will notice the similarity in the names of the factors of selection and testing to those of the threats to internal validity. When considering factors as internal threats, you should assess them as they relate to the testing of *independent* and *dependent* variables within the study. When assessing them as external threats, you should consider them in terms of the *generalizability* or use outside of the study to other populations and settings. The Critical Thinking Decision Path for threats to validity displays the way threats to internal and external validity can interact with each other. It is important to remember that this decision path is not exhaustive of the type of threats and their interaction. Problems of internal validity are generally easier to control. Generalizability issues are more difficult to deal with because it means that the researcher is assuming that other populations are similar to the one being tested.

## EVIDENCE-BASED PRACTICE TIP

Generalizability depends on who actually participates in a study. Not everyone who is approached actually participates, and not everyone who agrees to participate completes a study. As you review studies, think about how well this group reflects the population of interest.

## Selection Effects

Selection refers to the generalizability of the results to other populations. An example of the effects of selection occurs when the researcher cannot attain the ideal sample population. At times, the numbers of available subjects may be low or not accessible and the researcher may then need to choose a nonprobability method of sampling over a probability method (see Chapter 12). Therefore the type of sampling method used and how subjects are assigned to research conditions affect the generalizability to other groups, the external validity.

Examples of selection effects are reported when researchers note any of the following:

- "This sample included primarily Caucasian, non-Hispanic volunteer couples. Inferences about other racial groups should be made with caution. In addition, the recruitment methods which required consent from both members of the couple may have favored married couples with strong marital relationships, as evidenced by high scores in couple satisfaction and adjustment" (Melvin et al., 2012; see Appendix D).
- "[T]hese results are based on a convenience sample and therefore cannot be generalized beyond this group of women" (Alhusen et al., 2012; see Appendix B).
- "The relatively small sample size of Chinese youth and low variability of peer risky behaviors may account for the nonsignificant findings" (Wilgerodt, 2008).

These remarks caution you about potentially generalizing beyond the type of sample in a study, but also points out the usefulness of the findings for practice and future research aimed at building the research in these areas.

## Reactive Effects

Reactivity is defined as the subjects' responses to being studied. Subjects may respond to the investigator not because of the study procedures but merely as an independent response to being studied. This is also known as the Hawthorne effect, which is named after Western Electric Corporation's Hawthorne plant, where a study of working conditions was conducted. The researchers developed several different working conditions (i.e., turning up the lights, piping in music loudly or softly, and changing work hours). They found that no matter what was done, the workers' productivity increased. They concluded that production increased as a result of the workers' realization that they were being studied rather than because of the experimental conditions.

For example, in a study that compared daytime physical activity levels in children with and without asthma and the relationships among asthma, physical activity and body mass index, and child report of symptoms, the researchers noted "Children may change their behaviors due to the Hawthorne effect" (Tsai et al., 2012, p. 258). The researchers made recommendations for future studies to avoid such threats.

## Measurement Effects

Administration of a pretest in a study affects the generalizability of the findings to other populations and is known as measurement effects. As pretesting affects the posttest results within a study, pretesting affects the posttest results and generalizability outside the study. For example, suppose a researcher wants to conduct a study with the aim of changing attitudes toward acquired immunodeficiency syndrome (AIDS). To accomplish this, an education program on the risk factors for AIDS is incorporated. To test whether the education program changes attitudes toward AIDS, tests are given before and after the teaching intervention. The pretest on attitudes allows the subjects to examine their attitudes regarding AIDS. The subjects' responses on follow-up testing may differ from those of individuals who were given the education program and did not see the pretest. Therefore when a study is conducted and a pretest is given, it may "prime" the subjects and affect the researcher's ability to generalize to other situations. An example from a well done study that tested the feasibility and benefits of a program for adolescents with asthma (Staying Healthy—Asthma Responsible and Prepared

[SHARP]) is as follows: "We acknowledge the inherent limitations of self-report data. In addition, we caution about generalizing findings from this pilot study to large populations. Evaluating efficacy, effectiveness and impact of the SHARP program requires larger and more diverse students with asthma" (Kitner et al., 2012, p.10).

---

**HELPFUL HINT**

When reviewing a study, be aware of the internal and external validity threats.. These threats do not make a study useless—but actually more useful—to you. Recognition of the threats allows researchers to build on data, and allows you to think through what part of the study can be applied to practice. Specific threats to validity depend on the type of design and generalizations the researcher hopes to make.

---

There are other threats to external validity that depend on the type of design and methods of sampling used by the researcher, but these are beyond the scope of this text. Campbell and Stanley (1966) offer detailed coverage of the issues related to internal and external validity.

# APPRAISING THE EVIDENCE
## QUANTITATIVE RESEARCH

Critiquing the design of a study requires you to first have knowledge of the overall implications that the choice of a particular design may have for the study as a whole (see Critiquing Criteria box). When reading a study, first consider the level of evidence provided by the design and how the potential strength and quality of findings can be used to improve or change practice. When researchers design a study, but before the study begins, they decide how they will collect data, what instruments will be used, what the inclusion and exclusion criteria will be, and who and how large the sample will be to diminish bias or threats to the study's validity. These choices are based on the nature of the research question or hypothesis. Minimizing threats to internal and external validity of a study enhances the strength of evidence for any quantitative design. The concept of the research design is an all-inclusive one that parallels the concept of the theoretical framework. The research design is similar to the study's theoretical framework in that it deals with a piece of the study that affects the whole. For you to knowledgeably appraise the design in light of the entire study, it is important to understand the factors that influence the choice and the implications of the design. In this chapter, the meaning, purpose, and important factors of design choice, as well as the vocabulary that accompanies these factors, have been introduced.

Several criteria for evaluating the design related to maximizing control, minimizing threats to internal and external validity and, as a result, sources of bias can be drawn from this chapter. You should remember that the criteria are applied differently with various designs. Different application does not mean that you will find a haphazard approach to design. It means that each design has particular criteria that allow you to classify the design by type (e.g., experimental or nonexperimental). These criteria must be met and addressed in conducting a study. The particulars of specific designs are addressed in Chapters 9 and 10. The following discussion primarily pertains to the overall appraisal of a quantitative research design.

The research design should reflect that an objective review of the literature and establishment of a theoretical framework guided the development of the research question and

## CRITIQUING CRITERIA

### *Quantitative Research*

1. Is the type of design used appropriate?
2. Are the various concepts of control consistent with the type of design chosen?
3. Does the design used seem to reflect consideration of feasibility issues?
4. Does the design used seem to flow from the proposed research question, theoretical framework, literature review, and hypothesis?
5. What are the threats to internal validity or sources of bias?
6. What are the controls for the threats to internal validity?
7. What are the threats to external validity or generalizability?
8. What are the controls for the threats to external validity?
9. Is the design appropriately linked to the evidence hierarchy?

hypothesis and the choice of the design. When reading a study there is no explicit statement regarding how the design was chosen, but the literature reviewed will provide clues as to why the researcher chose the design of the study. You can evaluate this by critiquing the study's framework and literature review (see Chapters 3 and 4). Is the question new and not extensively researched? Has a great deal been done on the question, or is it a new or different way of looking at an old question? Depending on the level of the question, the investigators make certain choices. For example, in the Thomas and colleagues (2012) study, the researchers wanted to test a controlled intervention; thus they developed a randomized controlled trial (Level II design). However, the purpose of the Alhusen and colleagues (2012) study was much different. The Alhusen study examined the relationship between and among variables. The study did not test an intervention but explored how variables related to each other in a specific population (Level IV design). The choice of question and design allowed the researchers to assess different types of questions that are a part of nursing practice.

You should be alert for the means investigators use to maintain control (i.e., homogeneity in the sample, consistent data-collection procedures, how or if the independent variable was manipulated, and whether randomization was used). As you can see in Chapter 9, all of these criteria must be met for an experimental design. As you begin to understand the types of designs (i.e., experimental, quasi-experimental, and nonexperimental designs such as survey and relationship designs), you will find that control is applied in varying degrees, or—as in the case of a survey study—the independent variable is not manipulated at all (see Chapter 10). The level of control and its applications presented in Chapters 9 and 10 provide the remaining knowledge to fully critique the aspects of a study's design.

Once it has been established whether the necessary control or uniformity of conditions has been maintained, you must determine whether the study is feasible and the findings valid. You should ask whether the findings are the result of the variables tested—and thus internally valid—or whether there could be another explanation. To assess this aspect, the threats to internal validity should be reviewed. If the investigator's study was systematic, well grounded in theory, and followed the criteria for each of the processes, you will probably conclude that the study is internally valid. No study is perfect; there is always the potential for bias or threats to validity. This is not because the research was poorly conducted or the researcher did not think through the process completely; rather, it is that when conducting research with human subjects there is always some potential for error. Subjects can drop out of studies, and data collectors can make errors and be inconsistent. Sometimes errors cannot be controlled by the researcher. If there are policy changes during a study an intervention can be affected. As you read studies, note how every facet of the study was conducted, what potential errors could have arisen, and how the researcher addressed the sources of bias in the limitations section of the study. As nurses build a body of science, it is important that we learn from each other to avoid potential pitfalls in future research and its application to practice.

In addition, you must know whether a study has external validity or generalizability to other populations or environmental conditions. External validity can be claimed only after internal validity has been established. If the credibility of a study (internal validity) has not been established, a study cannot be generalized (external validity) to other populations. Determination of external validity of the findings goes hand-in-hand with the sampling frame (see Chapter 12). If the study is not representative of any one group or one phenomenon of interest, external validity may be limited or not present at all. You will find that establishment of internal and external validity requires not only knowledge of the threats to internal and external validity but also knowledge of the phenomenon being studied. Knowledge of the phenomenon being studied allows critical judgments to be made about the linkage of theories and variables for testing. As you appraise studies you should find that the design follows from the theoretical framework, literature review, research question, and hypotheses. You should feel, on the basis of clinical knowledge and knowledge of the research process, that the investigators are not comparing apples to oranges.

## KEY POINTS

- The purpose of the design is to provide the master plan for a study.
- There are many types of designs. No matter which type of design the researcher uses, the purpose always remains the same.
- You should be able to locate within the study a sense of the question that the researcher wished to answer. The question should be proposed with a plan for the accomplishment of the study. Depending on the question, you should be able to recognize the steps taken by the investigator to ensure control, eliminate bias, and increase generalizability.
- The choice of the specific design depends on the nature of the question. Specification of the nature of the research question requires that the design reflects the investigator's attempts to maintain objectivity, accuracy, pragmatic considerations, and, most important, control.
- Control affects not only the outcome of a study but also its future use. The design should also reflect how the investigator attempted to control threats to both internal and external validity.
- Internal validity must be established before external validity can be established.
- No matter which design the researcher chooses, it should be evident to the reader that the choice was based on a thorough examination of the research question within a theoretical framework.
- The design, research question, literature review, theoretical framework, and hypothesis should all interrelate to demonstrate a woven pattern.

- The choice of the design is affected by pragmatic issues. At times, two different designs may be equally valid for the same question.
- The choice of design affects the study's level of evidence.

## CRITICAL THINKING CHALLENGES

- How do the three criteria for an experimental design, manipulation, randomization, and control, minimize bias and decrease threats to internal validity?
- Argue your case for supporting or not supporting the following claim: "A study that does not use an experimental design does not decrease the value of the study even though it may influence the applicability of the findings in practice." Include examples to support your rationale.
- Why do researchers state that randomized clinical trials provide the strongest evidence for an individual study when using an evidence-based practice model?
- As you critically appraise a study that uses an experimental or quasi-experimental design, why is it important for you to look for evidence of intervention fidelity? How does intervention fidelity increase the strength and quality of the evidence provided by the findings of a study using these types of designs?

## REFERENCES

Alhusen, J. L., Gross, D., Hayatt, M. J., et al. (2012). The influence of maternal-fetal attachment and health practices on neonatal outcomes in low-income women. *Research in Nursing & Health*, 35, 112–120.

Bellg, A. J., Resnick, B., Minicucci, D. S., et al. (2004). Enhancing treatment fidelity in health care change studies: best practices and recommendations from the NIH Behavior Change Consortium. *Health Psychology*, 23(5), 443–451.

Braden, B., Bergstrom, N. A. (1987). Conceptual schema for the study of the etiology of pressure ulcers, *Rehabil Nurs*, 12(1):8–12.

Breitenstein, S. M., Gross, D., Fogg, L., et al. (2012). The Chicago parent program: comparing 1-year outcomes for African American and Latino parents of young children. *Research in Nursing & Health*, 5, 475-489,

Campbell, D., & Stanley, J. (1966). *Experimental and quasi-experimental designs for research*. Chicago, IL: Rand-McNally.

Crane-Okada, R., Kiger, H., Uman, GC., et al. (2012). Mindful movement program for older breast cancer survivors: A pilot study. *Cancer Nursing*, 35(4), E1–E13.

Kitner, E., Cook, G., Allen, A., et al. (2012). Feasibility and benefits of a school-based academic and counseling program for older school-age students with asthma. *Research in Nursing & Health*. In press. Epub ahead of print retrieved Oct, 35(5) 507–517.

Li, H., Powers, B. A., Melnyk, B. M., et al. (2012). Randomized controlled trial of CARE: an intervention to improve outcomes of hospitalized elders and family caregivers. *Research in Nursing & Health*. In press. Epub ahead of print retrieved 35(5), 533–549.

Melvin, K. C., Gross, D., Hayat, M. J., et al. (2012). Couple functioning and post-traumatic stress symptoms in US army couples: the role of resilence. *Research in Nursing & Health*, 35, 164–177.

Resnick, B., Bellg., A. J., Borrelli, B., et al. (2005). Examples of implementation and evaluation of treatment fidelity in the BCC studies: where are we and where we need to go. *Annuals of Behavioral Medicine*, Apr 29(Suppl), 46–54.

Santacroce, S. J., Maccarelli, L. M., & Grey, M. (2004). Intervention fidelity. *Nursing Research*, 53(1), 63–66.

Sarna, L., Bialous, S., Ong, M., et al. (2012). Nurses' treatment of tobacco dependence in hospitalized smokers in three states. *Research in Nursing & Health*, 35, 250–264.

Thomas, M. L., Elliott, J. E., Rao, S. M., et al. (2012). A randomized clinical trial of education or motivational-interviewing–based coaching compared to usual care to improve cancer pain management. *Oncology Nursing Forum*, 39(1), 39–49.

Tsai, S. Y., Ward, T., Lentz, M., & Kieckhefer, G. M. (2012). Daytime physical activity levels in school-age children with and without asthma. *Nursing Research*, 61(4), 252–159.

Wilgerodt, M. A. (2008). Family and peer influences on adjustment among Chinese, Filipino and white youth. *Nursing Research*, 57(6), 395–405.

## ℮volve WEBSITE

*Go to Evolve at http://evolve.elsevier.com/LoBiondo/ for review questions, critiquing exercises, and additional research articles for practice in reviewing and critiquing.*

# Experimental and Quasi-Experimental Designs

*Susan Sullivan-Bolyai and Carol Bova*

## ⊖volve WEBSITE

*Go to Evolve at http://evolve.elsevier.com/LoBiondo/ for review questions, critiquing exercises, and additional research articles for practice in reviewing and critiquing.*

## LEARNING OUTCOMES

*After reading this chapter, you should be able to do the following:*

- Describe the purpose of experimental and quasi-experimental research.
- Describe the characteristics of experimental and quasi-experimental studies.
- Distinguish the differences between experimental and quasi-experimental designs.
- List the strengths and weaknesses of experimental and quasi-experimental designs.
- Identify the types of experimental and quasi-experimental designs.

- List the criteria necessary for inferring cause-and-effect relationships.
- Identify potential validity issues associated with experimental and quasi-experimental designs.
- Critically evaluate the findings of experimental and quasi-experimental studies.
- Identify the contribution of experimental and quasi-experimental designs to evidence-based practice.

## KEY TERMS

| | | | |
|---|---|---|---|
| a priori | effect size | nonequivalent control group design | randomized controlled trial |
| after-only design | experimental design | one-group (pretest-posttest) design | Solomon four-group design |
| after-only nonequivalent control group design | extraneous variable | power analysis | testing |
| antecedent variable | independent variable | quasi-experimental design | time series design |
| attention control | intervening variable | randomization (random assignment) | treatment effect |
| control | intervention fidelity | | true or classic experiment |
| dependent variable | manipulation | | |
| design | mortality | | |

> **BOX 9-1**    **SUMMARY OF EXPERIMENTAL AND QUASI-EXPERIMENTAL RESEARCH DESIGNS**
>
> **Experimental Designs**
> - True experiment (pretest-posttest control group) design
> - Solomon four-group design
> - After-only design
>
> **Quasi-Experimental Designs**
> - Nonequivalent control group design
> - After-only nonequivalent control group design
> - One group (pretest-posttest) design
> - Time series design

## RESEARCH PROCESS

One purpose of scientific research is to determine cause-and-effect relationships. In nursing practice, we are concerned with identifying interventions to maintain or improve patient outcomes, and we base practice on evidence. We test the effectiveness of nursing interventions by using **experimental** and **quasi-experimental designs.** These **designs** differ from nonexperimental designs in one important way: the researcher does not observe behaviors and actions, but actively intervenes by manipulating study variables to bring about a desired effect. By manipulating an independent variable, the researcher can measure change in behaviors or actions, which is the dependent variable. Experimental and quasi-experimental studies are important to consider in relation to evidence-based practice because they provide the two highest levels of evidence (Level II and Level III) for a single study (see Chapter 1).

Experimental designs are particularly suitable for testing cause-and-effect relationships because they help eliminate potential threats to internal validity (see Chapter 8). To infer causality requires that these three criteria be met:

- The causal (independent) and effect (dependent) variables must be associated with each other.
- The cause must precede the effect.
- The relationship must not be explainable by another variable.

When critiquing experimental and/or quasi-experimental design studies, the primary focus is on the validity that the experimental treatment, or **independent variable,** caused the desired effect on the outcome, or **dependent variable.** The validity of the conclusion depends on how well other extraneous study variables were controlled that may have influenced or contributed to the findings.

The purpose of this chapter is to acquaint you with the issues involved in interpreting and applying to practice the findings of studies that use experimental and quasi-experimental designs (Box 9-1). The Critical Thinking Decision Path shows an algorithm that influences a researcher's choice of experimental or quasi-experimental design. In the literature, these types of studies are often referred to as *therapy* or *intervention* articles.

## CRITICAL THINKING DECISION PATH

*Experimental and Quasi-Experimental Designs*

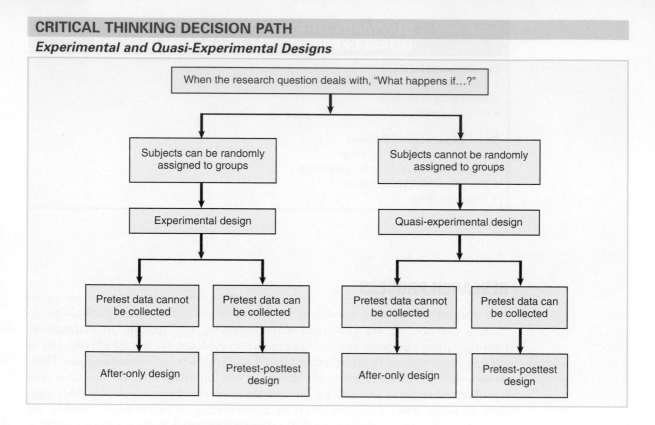

## TRUE EXPERIMENTAL DESIGN

A true **experimental design** has three identifying properties:

- **Randomization**
- **Control**
- **Manipulation**

A research study using a true experimental design is commonly called a **randomized controlled trial (RCT).** In hospital and clinic settings, it may be referred to as a "clinical trial" and is commonly used in drug trials. An RCT is considered the "gold standard" for providing information about cause-and-effect relationships. An individual RCT generates Level II evidence (see Chapter 1) because of reduced bias provided by randomization, control, and manipulation. A well-controlled design using these properties provides more confidence that the intervention will be effective and produce the same results over time (see Chapters 1 and 8). Box 9-2 shows examples of how these properties were used in the study in Appendix A.

### Randomization

Randomization, or **random assignment**, is required for a study to be considered a true experimental design with the distribution of subjects to either the experimental or the control

BOX 9-2    **EXPERIMENTAL DESIGN EXEMPLAR: RANDOMIZED CLINICAL TRIAL OF EDUCATION OR MOTIVATIONAL-INTERVIEWING–BASED COACHING COMPARED WITH USUAL CARE TO IMPROVE CANCER PAIN MANAGEMENT**

- This RCT reported 3 groups to compare differences: (1) A control group or usual care, where participants viewed a video on cancer developed by the American Cancer Society; (2) An education group that viewed a video on managing cancer pain and attitudinal barriers along with a pamphlet; and (3) A coaching group that received the information described in 2 **plus** four 30-minute nurse interventionist individualized phone sessions discussing pain management with participants to decrease pain intensity and attitudinal barriers to pain management, and improve their functional status and quality of life (dependent variables).
- Although no detailed power analysis for sample size is shared, the authors reported a medium effect size (difference between groups) was sought.
- Figure 1 in Appendix A illustrates how patients were stratified by pain level (low, medium, high) and cancer treatment (chemotherapy or radiation) to control for confounding variables and to ensure balance across groups.
- Next, subjects were randomly assigned to one of three groups (Control = 109, Education = 103, Coaching = 105). All participants who met the study criteria had an equal and known chance of being assigned to one of the three groups (*Note, the total is 317, not reported 318).
- The researchers also checked statistically whether random assignment produced groups that were similar; the Results section states that no significant differences were found among the three groups except for performance status scores (KPS) (i.e., those in the education group had lower performance status scores, meaning they were more disabled).
- For **attention-control** purposes (all groups receiving same amount of "attention"), all subjects in the usual care and education groups received an equivalent amount of time and the same number of nurse-driven telephone calls.
- There were no differences among groups on attitudinal barriers; however, patients in the coaching group reported improvement in pain interfering in daily life. The authors identify several limitations that could have attributed to the findings. Several other issues may explain why limited differences were seen among groups: the authors didn't report the reliability results of the instruments in this particular sample, especially the attitudinal barrier instrument that they reported had only 'adequate' reliability in other samples; the intervention fidelity plan was described but there were issues in maintaining fidelity as reported in the discussion section (additional calls and interactions with health care providers specific to treatment problems). Qualitative interviews with patients assigned to all 3 groups might also be beneficial to explore the nuances, benefits, and barriers with each of the described group treatment.

Thomas, M, Elliott, J.E., Rao, S.M., et al. (2012). A randomized clinical trial of education, or motivational-interviewing–based coaching compared to usual care to improve cancer pain management (see Appendix A).

group on a purely random basis. As shown in Box 9-2, each subject has an equal chance of being assigned to either group, which ensures that other variables that could affect change in the dependent variable will be equally distributed between the groups, reducing systematic bias. It also minimizes variance and decreases selection bias. Randomization may be done individually or by groups. Several procedures are used to randomize subjects to groups, such as a table of random numbers or computer-generated number sequences (Suresh, 2011). Whatever method is used, it is important that the process be truly random, that it be tamperproof, and that the group assignment is concealed. Note that random assignment to groups is different from random sampling as discussed in Chapter 12.

## Control

Control refers to the process (described in Chapter 8) by which the investigator holds certain conditions constant to limit bias that could influence the dependent variable(s). Control is acquired by manipulating the independent variable, by randomly assigning subjects to a group, by using a control group, and by preparing intervention and data collection protocols to maintain consistency for all study participants (see Chapter 14). Box 9-2 illustrates how a control group was used by Thomas and colleagues (2012; see Appendix A). In experimental research, the control group receives the usual treatment or a placebo (an inert pill in drug trials).

## Manipulation

Manipulation is the process of "doing something," a different dose of "something," or comparing different types of treatment by manipulating the independent variable for at least some of the involved subjects (typically those placed in the experimental group after randomization). The independent variable might be a treatment, a teaching plan, or a medication. The effect of this manipulation is measured to determine the result of the experimental treatment on the dependent variable compared with those who did not receive the treatment.

Box 9-2 provides an illustration of how the three major properties of true experimental design (randomization, control, and manipulation) are used in an intervention study and how the researchers ruled out other potential explanations or bias (threats to internal validity) for the results. This information will help you decide if the study may be helpful in your own clinical setting.

The description in Box 9-2 is also an example of how the researchers used control (along with randomization and manipulation) to minimize bias and its effect on the intervention (Thomas et al., 2012). This control helped rule out the following potential specific internal validity threats (see Chapter 8; not to be confused with instrument threats to validity, described in Chapter 15):

- *Selection:* Representativeness of the sample contributed to the results versus the intervention
- *History:* Events that may have contributed to the results versus the intervention
- *Maturation:* Developmental processes that can occur that potentially could alter the results versus the intervention

However, if any of these threats occurred, the researchers (who implemented random assignment) tested statistically for differences among the groups and found that there were none, reassuring the reader that the randomization process worked.

We have briefly discussed RCTs and how they precisely use control, manipulation, and randomization to test the effectiveness of an intervention. RCTs

- Use an experimental and control group, sometimes referred to as experimental and control arms.
- Have a very specific sampling plan, using clear-cut *inclusion* and *exclusion* criteria (who will be allowed into the study; who will not).
- Administer the intervention in a consistent way, called *intervention fidelity.*
- Typically, carry out statistical comparisons to determine any differences between groups.
- Pay significant attention to the sample size.

It is important that researchers establish a large enough sample size to ensure that there are enough subjects in each study group to statistically detect differences between those who receive the intervention and those who do not. This is called the ability to statistically detect the treatment effect or effect size (see Chapter 12); that is, the impact of the independent variable/intervention on the dependent variable. The mathematical procedure to determine the number for each arm (group) needed to test the study's variables is called a **power analysis** (see Chapter 12). You will usually find power analysis information in the sample section of the research article. For example, you will know there was an appropriate plan for an adequate sample size when a statement like the following is included: "A purposive sample of 249 patients were enrolled. A target sample of 61 per group was selected to achieve a power of at least 80% for detecting group differences in mean change scores" (Sherman et al., 2012). Thus, this information shows you that the researchers sought an adequate sample size. This information is critical to assess because with a small sample size, differences may not be statistically evident, thus creating the potential for a *type II error;* that is, acceptance of the null hypothesis when it is false (see Chapter 16).

Carefully read the intervention and control group section of an article to see exactly what each group received and what the differences between groups were. In Appendix A, Thomas and colleagues (2012) offer the reader a detailed description and illustration of the intervention. The discussion section reports that the patients' in-the-moment priorities may have posed a challenge to adhering to the attitudinal content in the intervention group. That is the kind of inconsistency that should make you wonder if it may have interfered or influenced the findings.

In summary, when reviewing RCTs, carefully assess how well the study incorporates fidelity measures. Fidelity covers several elements of an experimental study (Bellg et al., 2004; Gearing et al., 2011; Keith et al., 2010; Preyde & Burnham, 2011; Santacroce et al., 2004) that must be evaluated and that can enhance a study's internal validity. These elements are as follows:

1. Framework of the study should be considered (e.g., Did the study have a well-defined intervention and procedures? Were the study participant characteristics and environment well described?).
2. **Intervention fidelity** involves the process of enhancing the study's internal validity by ensuring that the intervention is delivered systematically to all subjects in the intervention group. To enhance intervention fidelity, researchers develop a system for evaluating how consistently the intervention was carried out by those delivering the intervention. This system includes a procedure manual that provides for well-defined program *objectives*, including a definition of the treatment *dose; consistent* training of the interventionists and all research staff; *standardized* data collection procedures and/or supervision consisting of *frequent review* of the intervention by observing, videotaping, or audiotaping the sessions; troubleshooting problems; cultural considerations for the intervention; *ongoing training* and supervision of interventionists; and corrective feedback measures (see Chapter 8).
3. Consideration of *internal* and *external validity* threats.
4. Ensuring the *reliability and validity* of instruments.

## Types of Experimental Designs

There are many different experimental designs (Campbell & Stanley, 1966). Each is based on the classic design called the **true experiment** or RCT (Figure 9-1A). The classic RCT is conducted as follows:

1. The researcher recruits a sample from the population.
2. Baseline preintervention demographics, personal characteristics, and measurement of the intended study concepts or dependent variables (sometimes referred to as

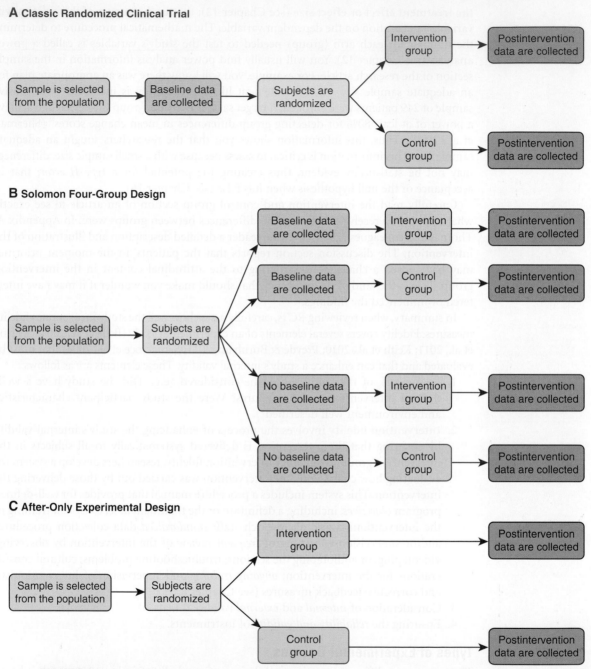

**FIGURE 9-1** Experimental Designs. **A,** Classic randomized clinical trial. **B,** Solomon four-group design. **C,** After-only experimental design.

empirical indicators because they are the outcomes the researcher wishes to assess for change) are collected from the entire sample.

3. Subjects are then randomized to either the intervention or the control group.
4. After each group receives the experimental intervention *or* comparison/control intervention (usual care or standard treatment, education, or placebo), both groups complete postintervention measures to see if any changes have occurred in the dependent variables.

Thus all true experimental designs have subjects randomly assigned to groups, have an experimental treatment introduced to some of the subjects, have a comparison/control group, and have the differential effects of the treatment observed.

### EVIDENCE-BASED PRACTICE TIP

The term *randomized controlled trial (RCT)* is often used to refer to a true experimental design in health care research and is frequently used in nursing research as the gold standard design because it minimizes bias or threats to study validity. Because of ethical issues, rarely is "no treatment" acceptable. Typically either "standard treatment" or another version or dose of "something" is provided to the control group. Only when there is no standard or comparable treatment available is a no-treatment control group appropriate.

The degree of difference between the groups at the end of the study indicates the confidence the researcher has in a causal link (i.e., the intervention caused the difference) between the independent and dependent variables. Because random assignment and control minimizes the effects of many threats to internal study validity or bias (see Chapter 8), it is a strong design for testing cause-and-effect relationships. However, the design is not perfect. Some study threats to internal validity cannot be controlled in true experimental studies:

- **Mortality**: People tend to drop out of studies, especially those that require participation over an extended period of time. When reading experimental studies, examine the sample and the results carefully to see if excessive dropouts or deaths occurred or one group had more dropouts than the other, which can affect the study findings.
- **Testing**: This can be a problem, especially if the same measurement is given twice. Subjects tend to score better the second time just by remembering the test items. Researchers can avoid this problem in one of two ways: They might use different or equivalent forms of the same test for the two measurements (see Chapter 15), or they might use a more complex experimental design called the Solomon four-group design.

*Solomon Four-Group Design.* The **Solomon four-group design**, shown in Figure 9-1B, has two groups that are identical to those used in the classic experimental design, plus two additional groups: an experimental after-group and a control after-group. As the diagram shows, subjects are randomly assigned to one of four groups before baseline data are collected (compared to after baseline data collection as in the classic RCT). This design results in two groups that receive only a posttest (rather than pretest and posttest), which provides an opportunity to rule out result distortions that may have occurred (testing is a threat to internal validity) owing to exposure to the pretest. Common sense tells us that this design would require a larger sample size, which also means this type of study would be more costly. Although this design helps evaluate the effects of testing, the threat of mortality (dropout) remains a problem, as with the classic experimental design.

For example, Rubel and colleagues (2010) used the Solomon four-group design to test the effects of exposure to a prostate cancer screening decision aid versus standard education in men age 50-70 years. They hypothesized that those who received the pretest would have higher posttest knowledge, decreased conflict, and decreased decisional anxiety:

- The subjects were randomly assigned to one of four groups:
    1. pretest, decision aid, immediate posttest
    2. pretest, no decision aid, immediate posttest
    3. no prettest, decision aid, posttest
    4. no pretest, no decision aid, posttest only
- The study found no pretest sensitization, that knowledge increased significantly for those exposed to the decision aid, and that knowledge had some effect on conflict and anxiety.

*After-Only Design.* A less frequently used experimental design is the **after-only design** (Figure 9-1C). This design, which is sometimes called the posttest-only control group design, is composed of two randomly assigned groups, but unlike the true experimental design, neither group is pretested or measured. Again, the independent variable is introduced to the experimental group and not to the control group. The process of randomly assigning the subjects to groups is assumed to be sufficient to ensure lack of bias so that the researcher can still determine whether the intervention created significant differences between the two groups. This design is particularly useful when testing effects that are expected to be a major problem, or when outcomes cannot be measured beforehand (e.g., postoperative pain management).

Thus, when critiquing experimental research to help inform your evidence-based decisions, consider what design type was used; how the groups were formed (i.e., if the researchers used randomization); whether the groups were equivalent at baseline; if they were not equivalent, what the possible threats to internal validity were; what kind of manipulation (i.e., intervention) was administered to the experimental group; and what the control group received.

---

### HELPFUL HINT

Look for evidence of preestablished inclusion and exclusion criteria for the study participants.

---

## Strengths and Weaknesses of the Experimental Design

Experimental designs are the most powerful for testing cause-and-effect relationships due to the control, manipulation, and randomization components. Therefore, the design offers a better chance of measuring if the intervention caused the change or difference in the two groups. For example, Thomas and colleagues (2012) tested several types of psychoeducational interventions for cancer patients and had mixed results. If you were working in an oncology clinic and wanted to start a similar intervention, you could use the strengths and limitations of their evidence as a starting point for putting research findings into clinical practice.

Still, experimental designs have weaknesses as well. They are complicated to design and can be costly to implement. For example, there may not be an adequate number of potential study participants in the accessible population. Another problem with experimental designs is that they may be difficult or impractical to carry out in a clinical setting. An example might be trying to randomly assign patients from one hospital unit to different groups when nurses might talk to each other about the different treatments. Experimental procedures also may be disruptive to the setting's usual routine. If several nurses are involved in administering the experimental program, it may be impossible to ensure that the program is administered in the same way to each subject. Another problem is that many important variables that are related to patient care outcomes are not amenable to manipulation for ethical reasons. For example, cigarette smoking is known to be related to lung cancer, but you could not randomly assign people to smoking or nonsmoking groups. Health status varies with age and socioeconomic status. No matter how careful a researcher is, no one can assign subjects randomly by age or by a certain income level. Because of these problems in carrying out true experiments, researchers frequently turn to another type of research design to evaluate cause-and-effect relationships. Such designs, which look like experiments but lack some of the control of the true experimental design, are called quasi-experimental designs.

## QUASI-EXPERIMENTAL DESIGNS

Quasi-experimental designs also test cause-and-effect relationships. However, in quasi-experimental designs, random assignment or the presence of a control group lacking the characteristics of a true experiment (randomization, control, and manipulation) may not be possible because of the nature of the independent variable or the available subjects.

Without all the characteristics associated with a true experiment, internal validity may be compromised. Therefore, the basic problem with the quasi-experimental approach is a weakened confidence in making causal assertions that the results occurred because of the intervention. Instead, the findings may be a result of other extraneous variables. As a result, quasi-experimental studies provide Level III evidence (versus Level II, as in experimental studies). For example, a pilot study by Bradley (2012) used a quasi-experimental design to examine characteristics of a single sample of nurse practitioners (NPs) investigating aspects of a skin cancer screening tool in a single college health center setting. To assess cognitive ability of the NPs related to the cancer screening and how NPs' attitudes toward participation in skin cancer screening and documentation principles changed based on an educational intervention that they received, pre- and post-tests were conducted, but neither random assignment nor a control group was included as a design feature.

> **HELPFUL HINT**
>
> Remember that researchers often make trade-offs and sometimes use a quasi-experimental design instead of an experimental design because it may be impossible to randomly assign subjects to groups. Not using the "purest" design does not decrease the value of the study even though it may decrease the strength of the findings.

### Types of Quasi-Experimental Designs

There are many different quasi-experimental designs, but we will limit the discussion to only those most commonly used in nursing research. Refer back to the true experimental design shown in Figure 9-1A, and compare it with the nonequivalent control group

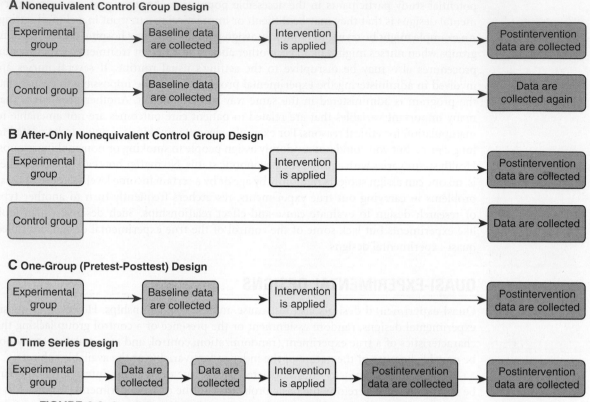

**FIGURE 9-2** Quasi-Experimental Designs. **A,** Nonequivalent control group design. **B,** After-only nonequivalent control group design. **C,** One-group (pretest-posttest) design. **D,** Time series design.

**design** shown in Figure 9-2A. Note that this design looks exactly like the true experiment except that subjects are not randomly assigned to groups. Suppose a researcher is interested in the effects of a new diabetes education program on the physical and psychosocial outcomes of patients newly diagnosed with diabetes. Under certain conditions, the researcher might be able to randomly assign subjects to either the group receiving the new program or the group receiving the usual program, but for any number of reasons, that design might not be possible.

- For example, nurses on the unit where patients are admitted might be so excited about the new program that they cannot help but include the new information for all patients.
- The researcher has two choices: to abandon the study or to conduct a quasi experiment.
- To conduct a quasi experiment, the researcher might use one unit as the intervention group for the new program, find a similar unit that has not been introduced to the new program, and study the newly diagnosed patients with diabetes who are admitted to that unit as a comparison group. The study would then involve a quasi-experimental design.

*Nonequivalent Control Group.* The **nonequivalent control group design** is commonly used in nursing studies conducted in clinical settings. The basic problem with this design is the weakened confidence the researcher can have in assuming that the experimental and comparison groups are similar at the beginning of the study. Threats to internal validity, such as *selection, maturation, testing,* and *mortality,* are possible with this design. However, the design is relatively strong because by gathering pretest data, the researcher can compare the equivalence of the two groups on important antecedent variables before the independent variable is introduced. **Antecedent variables** are variables that occur within the subjects prior to the study, such as in the previous example, where the patients' motivation to learn about their medical condition might be important in determining the effect of the diabetes education program. At the outset of the study, the researcher could include a measure of motivation to learn. Thus differences between the two groups on this variable could be tested, and if significant differences existed, they could be controlled statistically in the analysis. Nonetheless, the strength of the causal assertions that can be made on the basis of such designs depends on the researcher's ability to identify and measure or control possible threats to internal validity.

*After-Only Nonequivalent Control Group.* Sometimes, the outcomes simply cannot be measured before the intervention, as with prenatal interventions that are expected to affect birth outcomes. The study that could be conducted would look like the **after-only nonequivalent control group design** shown in Figure 9-2B. This design is similar to the after-only experimental design, but randomization is not used to assign subjects to groups and makes the assumption that the two groups are equivalent and comparable before the introduction of the independent variable. Thus the soundness of the design and the confidence that we can put in the findings depend on the soundness of this assumption of preintervention comparability. Often it is difficult to support the assertion that the two nonrandomly assigned groups are comparable at the outset of the study because there is no way of assessing its validity.

*One-Group (Pretest-Posttest).* Another quasi-experimental design is a **one-group (pretest-posttest) design** (Figure 9-2C), which is used when only one group is available for study. Data are collected before and after an experimental treatment on one group of subjects. In this design, there is no control group and no randomization, which are important characteristics that enhance internal validity. Therefore it becomes important that the evidence generated by the findings of this type of quasi-experimental design is interpreted with careful consideration of the design limitations.

*Time Series.* Another quasi-experimental approach used by researchers when only one group is available to study over a longer period of time is called a **time series design** (Figure 9-2D). Time series designs are useful for determining trends over time. Data are collected multiple times before the introduction of the treatment to establish a baseline point of reference on outcomes. The experimental treatment is introduced, and data are collected multiple times afterward to determine a change from baseline. The broad range and number of data collection points help rule out alternative explanations, such as history effects. However, a testing threat to internal validity is ever present because of multiple data collection points, and without a control group, the threats of selection and maturation cannot be ruled out (see Chapter 8).

**HELPFUL HINT**

One of the reasons replication is so important in nursing research is that so many problems cannot be subjected to experimental methods. Therefore the consistency of findings across many populations helps support a cause-and-effect relationship even when an experimental study cannot be conducted.

## Strengths and Weaknesses of Quasi-Experimental Designs

Quasi-experimental designs are used frequently because they are practical, less costly, feasible, and generalizable. These designs are more adaptable to the real-world practice setting than the controlled experimental designs. In addition, for some hypotheses, these designs may be the only way to evaluate the effect of the independent variable of interest.

The weaknesses of the quasi-experimental approach involve mainly the inability to make clear cause-and-effect statements. Researchers have other options for ruling out these alternative explanations as well. They may control extraneous variables (alternative events that could explain the findings) a priori (before initiating the intervention) by design or while conducting statistical analyses.

### EVIDENCE-BASED PRACTICE TIP

Experimental designs provide Level II evidence, and quasi-experimental designs provide Level III evidence. Quasi-experimental designs are lower on the evidence hierarchy because of lack of control, which limits the ability to make confident cause-and-effect statements that influence applicability to practice and clinical decision making.

## EVIDENCE-BASED PRACTICE

As the science of nursing expands and the cost of health care rises, nurses must become more cognizant of what constitutes best practice for their patient population. Having a basic understanding of the value of intervention studies that use an experimental or quasi-experimental design is critical for improving clinical outcomes. These study designs provide the strongest evidence for making informed clinical decisions. These designs are those most commonly included in systematic reviews (see Chapter 11).

One cannot assume that because an intervention study has been published it was rigorously done and that the findings apply to your particular practice population. When conducting an evidence-based practice project, the first step after you have identified the clinical question is to collect the strongest, most relevant and current evidence related to your problem. You then need to critically appraise the existing experimental and quasi-experimental literature to evaluate which studies provide the best available evidence. Key points for evaluating the evidence and whether bias has been minimized in experimental and quasi-experimental designs include the following:

- Random group assignment (experimental or intervention and control or comparison)—how subjects are assigned to groups, equivalence of groups at baseline on key demographic variables
- Adequate sample size—calculated sample size and inclusion and exclusion criteria that are relevant to the clinical problem studied
- Recruitment of a homogenous sample
- Intervention fidelity and consistent data collection procedures
- Experimental group is different enough from control group to detect a clinical and statistical difference/effect size (see Chapters 16 and 17)
- Control of antecedent, intervening, or extraneous variables
- Likelihood of changing practice based on one study is low unless it is a large clinical RCT based on prior research work

## CRITIQUING CRITERIA

### *Experimental and Quasi-Experimental Designs*

1. Is the design used appropriate to the research question or hypothesis?
2. Is the design pragmatic for the setting or sample?
3. Is there a detailed description of the intervention?
4. Is there a description of what the intervention group versus control group received, and what the differences are?
5. How is intervention fidelity maintained?
6. Is power analysis used to calculate the appropriate sample size for the study?

#### Experimental Designs

1. What experimental design is used in the study?
2. How are randomization, control, and manipulation applied?
3. Are there any reasons to believe that there are alternative explanations for the findings?
4. Are all threats to internal validity, including mortality, testing, and selection bias addressed in the report?
5. Are the findings generalizable to the larger population of interest?

#### Quasi-Experimental Designs

1. What quasi-experimental design is used in the study, and is it appropriate?
2. What are the most common threats to internal and external validity of the findings of this design?
3. What are the plausible alternative explanations, and have they been addressed?
4. Are the author's explanations of threats to internal and external validity acceptable?
5. What does the author say about the limitations of the study?
6. To what extent are the study findings generalizable?

# APPRAISING THE EVIDENCE
# EXPERIMENTAL AND QUASI-EXPERIMENTAL DESIGNS

As discussed earlier, various designs for research studies differ in the amount of control the researcher has over the antecedent and intervening variables that may affect the results of the study. True experimental designs, which provide Level II evidence, offer the most possibility for control, and nonexperimental designs (Levels IV, V, or VI) offer the least. Quasi-experimental designs, which provide Level III evidence, fall somewhere in between. When conducting an evidence-based practice or quality improvement project, one must always look for studies that provide the highest level of evidence (see Chapter 1). At times for a specific PICO question (see Chapter 2), you will find both Level II and Level III evidence. Research designs must balance the needs for internal validity and external validity to produce useful results. In addition, judicious use of design requires that the chosen design be appropriate to the problem, free of bias, and capable of answering the research question or hypothesis. Therefore using designs of different levels is appropriate.

## HELPFUL HINT

When reviewing the experimental and quasi-experimental literature, do not limit your search only to your patient population. For example, it is possible that if you are working with adult caregivers, related parent caregiver intervention literature may provide you with strategies as well. Many times with some adaptation, interventions used with one sample might be applicable for other populations.

Questions that you should pose when reading studies that test cause-and-effect relationships are listed in the Critiquing Criteria box. All of these questions should help you judge whether a causal relationship exists.

For studies in which either experimental or quasi-experimental designs are used, first try to determine the type of design that was used. Often a statement describing the design of the study appears in the abstract and in the methods section of the article. If such a statement is not present, you should examine the article for evidence of three properties: control, randomization, and manipulation. If all are discussed, the design is probably experimental. On the other hand, if the study involves the administration of an experimental treatment but does not involve the random assignment of subjects to groups, the design is quasi-experimental. Next, try to identify which of the experimental and quasi-experimental designs was used. Determining the answer to these questions gives you a head start, because each design has its inherent validity threats and this step makes it a bit easier to critically evaluate the study. The next question to ask is whether the researcher required a solution to a cause-and-effect problem. If so, the study is suited to these designs. Finally, think about the conduct of the study in the setting. Is it realistic to think that the study could be conducted in a clinical setting without some contamination?

The most important question to ask yourself as you read experimental studies is, "What else could have happened to explain the findings?" Thus it is important that the author provide adequate accounts of how the procedures for randomization, control, and manipulation were carried out. The report should include a description of the procedures for random assignment to such a degree that the reader could determine just how likely it was for any one subject to be assigned to a particular group. The description of the independent variable (intervention) and the control group should also be detailed. The inclusion of this information helps you to decide if it is possible that the treatment given to some subjects in the experimental group might be different from what was given to others in the same group (intervention fidelity). In addition, threats to internal validity, such as testing and mortality, should be addressed, as should threats to external validity. Otherwise, there is the potential for the findings of the study to be in error and less believable to the reader.

This question of potential alternative explanations or threats to internal validity for the findings is even more important when critically evaluating a quasi-experimental study because quasi-experimental designs cannot possibly control many plausible alternative explanations. A well-written report of a quasi-experimental study systematically reviews potential threats to the internal and external validity of the findings. Then your work is to decide if the author's explanations make sense. For either experimental or quasi-experimental studies, you should also check for a reported power analysis that assures you that an appropriate sample size for detecting a treatment effect was planned, a detailed description of the intervention, what both groups received during the trial, and what intervention fidelity strategies were implemented.

## KEY POINTS

- Experimental designs or randomized clinical trials provide the strongest evidence (Level II) for a single study in terms of whether an intervention or treatment affects patient outcomes.
- Two types of design commonly used in nursing research to test hypotheses about cause-and-effect relationships are experimental and quasi-experimental designs. Both

are useful for the development of nursing knowledge because they test the effects of nursing actions and lead to the development of prescriptive theory.

- True experiments are characterized by the ability of the researcher to control extraneous variation, to manipulate the independent variable, and to randomly assign subjects to research groups.
- Experiments conducted either in clinical settings or in the laboratory provide the best evidence in support of a causal relationship because the following three criteria can be met: (1) the independent and dependent variables are related to each other; (2) the independent variable chronologically precedes the dependent variable; and (3) the relationship cannot be explained by the presence of a third variable.
- Researchers frequently turn to quasi-experimental designs to test cause-and-effect relationships because experimental designs often are impractical or unethical.
- Quasi experiments may lack the randomization and/or the comparison group characteristics of true experiments. The usefulness of quasi-experiments for studying causal relationships depends on the ability of the researcher to rule out plausible threats to the validity of the findings, such as history, selection, maturation, and testing effects.
- The level of evidence (Level III) provided by quasi-experimental designs weakens confidence that the findings were the result of the intervention rather than extraneous variables.
- The overall purpose of critiquing such studies is to assess the validity of the findings and to determine whether these findings are worth incorporating into the nurse's personal practice.

## CRITICAL THINKING CHALLENGES

- Describe the ethical issues included in a true experimental research design used by a nurse researcher.
- Describe how a true experimental design could be used in a hospital setting with patients.
- How should a nurse go about critiquing experimental research articles in the research literature so that his or her evidence-based practice is enhanced?
- The nurse researcher is considering using a time series design as a research approach. When would this be an appropriate selection for a research project?
- Identify a clinical quality indicator that is a problem on your unit (e.g., falls, ventilator-acquired pneumonia, catheter-acquired urinary tract infection) and consider how a search for studies using experimental or quasi-experimental designs could provide the foundation for a quality improvement project.

## REFERENCES

Bellg, A. J., Borrelli, B., Resnick, B., et al. (2004). Enhancing treatment fidelity in health behavior change studies: best practices and recommendations from the NIH Behavior Change Consortium. *Health Psychology, 14*, 197–211.

Bradley, H. P. (2012). Implementation of a skin cancer screening tool in a primary care setting: a pilot study. *Journal of the American Academy of Nurse Practitioners, 24*(2), 82–88.

Campbell, D., & Stanley, J. (1966). *Experimental and quasi-experimental designs for research.* Chicago, IL: Rand-McNally.

Gearing, R. E., El-Bassel, N., Ghesquiere, A., et al. (2011). Major ingredients of fidelity: a review and scientific guide to improving quality of intervention research implementation. *Clinical Psychology Review, 31*, 79–88. doi:10.1016/jcpr.2010.09.007.

Keith, R. E., Hopp, F. P., Subramanian, U., et al. (2010). Fidelity of implementation: development and testing of a measure. *Implementation Science, 5,* 991–911. doi: 10.1186/1748-5908-5-99.

Preyde, M., & Burnham, P. V. (2011). Intervention fidelity in psychosocial oncology. *Journal of Evidence-Based Social Work, 8,* 379–396. doi: 10.1080/15433714.2011.54234.

Rubel, S. K., Miller, J. W., Stephens, R. L, et al. (2010). Testing decision aid for prostate cancer screening. *Journal of Health Communications, 15,* 307–321. doi: 10.1080/10810731003686614.

Santacroce, S. J., Marccarelli, L., & Grey, M. (2004). Intervention fidelity. *Nursing Research, 53,* 63–66.

Suresh, K. P. (2011). An overview of randomization techniques: an unbiased assessment of outcome in clinical research. *Journal of Human Reproductive Science, 4,* 8–11.

Sherman, D. W., Haber, J., Hoskins, C. N., et al. (2012). The effects of psychoeducation and telephone counseling on the adjustment of women with early-stage breast cancer. *Applied Nursing Research,* 25, 3–16.

Thomas, M. L., Elliott, J. E., Rao, S. M., et al. (2012). A randomized clinical trial of education or motivational-interviewing–based coaching compared to usual care to improve cancer pain management. *Oncology Nursing, Forum,* 39(1), 39–49.

# evolve WEBSITE

*Go to Evolve at http://evolve.elsevier.com/LoBiondo/ for review questions, critiquing exercises, and additional research articles for practice in reviewing and critiquing.*

# CHAPTER 10

# Nonexperimental Designs

*Geri LoBiondo-Wood and Judith Haber*

## ⊖volve WEBSITE

*Go to Evolve at http://evolve.elsevier.com/LoBiondo/ for review questions, critiquing exercises, and additional research articles for practice in reviewing and critiquing.*

## LEARNING OUTCOMES

*After reading this chapter, you should be able to do the following:*

- Describe the overall purpose of nonexperimental designs.
- Describe the characteristics of survey, relationship, and difference designs.
- Define the differences between survey, relationship, and difference designs. List the advantages and disadvantages of surveys and each type of relationship and difference designs.
- Identify methodological and secondary analysis methods of research.
- Identify the purposes of methodological and secondary analysis methods of research.
- Describe the purposes of a systematic review, meta-analysis, integrative review, and clinical practice guidelines.
- Define the differences between a systematic review, meta-analysis, integrative review, and clinical practice guidelines.

- Discuss relational inferences versus causal inferences as they relate to nonexperimental designs.
- Identify the critical appraisal criteria used to critique nonexperimental research designs.
- Apply the critiquing criteria to the evaluation of nonexperimental research designs as they appear in research reports.
- Apply the critiquing criteria to the evaluation of systematic reviews and clinical practice guidelines.
- Evaluate the strength and quality of evidence by nonexperimental designs.
- Evaluate the strength and quality of evidence provided by systematic reviews, meta-analysis, integrative reviews, and clinical practice guidelines.

Many phenomena relevant to nursing do not lend themselves to an experimental design. For example, nurses studying cancer-related fatigue may be interested in the amount of fatigue, variations in fatigue, and patient fatigue in response to chemotherapy. The investigator would not design an experimental study that would potentially intensify an aspect of a patient's fatigue just to study the fatigue experience. Instead, the researcher would examine the factors that contribute to the variability in a patient's cancer-related fatigue experience using a nonexperimental design. Nonexperimental designs are used in studies in which the researcher wishes to construct a picture of a phenomenon (variable); explore events, people, or situations as they naturally occur; or test relationships and differences among variables. Nonexperimental designs may construct a picture of a phenomenon at one point or over a period of time.

In experimental research the independent variable is actively manipulated; in nonexperimental research it is not. In nonexperimental research the independent variables have naturally occurred, so to speak, and the investigator cannot directly control them by manipulation. In a nonexperimental design the researcher explores relationships or differences among the variables. Even though the researcher does not actively manipulate the variables, the concepts of control and potential sources of bias (see Chapter 8) should be considered as much as possible. Nonexperimental research designs provide Level IV evidence. The strength of evidence provided by nonexperimental designs is not as strong as that for experimental designs because there is a different degree of control within the study; that is, the independent variable is not manipulated, subjects are not randomized, and there is no control group. Yet the information yielded by these types of studies is critical to developing a base of evidence for practice and may represent the best evidence available to answer research or clinical questions.

Researchers are not in agreement on how to classify nonexperimental studies. A continuum of quantitative research design is presented in Figure 10-1. Nonexperimental studies explore the relationships or the differences between variables. This chapter divides nonexperimental designs into survey studies and relationship/difference studies as illus-

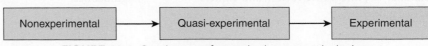

**FIGURE 10-1** Continuum of quantitative research design.

BOX 10-1    **SUMMARY OF NONEXPERIMENTAL RESEARCH DESIGNS**

**I. Survey Studies**
A. Descriptive
B. Exploratory
C. Comparative

**II. Relationship/Difference Studies**
A. Correlational studies
B. Developmental studies
   1. Cross-sectional
   2. Longitudinal, cohort, and prospective
   3. Retrospective, ex post facto, and case control

TABLE 10-1    **EXAMPLES OF STUDIES WITH MORE THAN ONE DESIGN LABEL**

| DESIGN TYPE | STUDY'S PURPOSE |
| --- | --- |
| Descriptive, longitudinal with retrospective, longitudinal with medical records review | To assess patient and provider responses to a computerized symptom assessment system (Carpenter et al., 2008) |
| Descriptive, exploratory, secondary analysis of a randomized controlled trial | To identify the predictors of fatigue 30 days after completing adjuvant chemotherapy for breast cancer and whether differences are observed between a sleep intervention and a healthy eating attention control group in predicting fatigue (Wielgus et al., 2009) |
| Longitudinal, descriptive | This longitudinal, descriptive study was conducted to examine the relationships of maternal-fetal attachment, health practices during pregnancy and neonatal outcomes (Alhusen et al., 2012) |

trated in Box 10-1. These categories are somewhat flexible, and other sources may classify nonexperimental studies in a different way. Some studies fall exclusively within one of these categories, whereas many other studies have characteristics of more than one category (Table 10-1). As you read the research literature you will often find that researchers who are conducting a nonexperimental study use several design classifications for one study. This chapter introduces the various types of nonexperimental designs and discusses their advantages and disadvantages, the use of nonexperimental research, the issues of causality, and the critiquing process as it relates to nonexperimental research. The Critical Thinking Decision Path outlines the path to the choice of a nonexperimental design.

**EVIDENCE-BASED PRACTICE TIP**

When critically appraising nonexperimental studies, you need to be aware of possible sources of bias that can be introduced at any point in the study.

**CRITICAL THINKING DECISION PATH**

*Nonexperimental Design Choice*

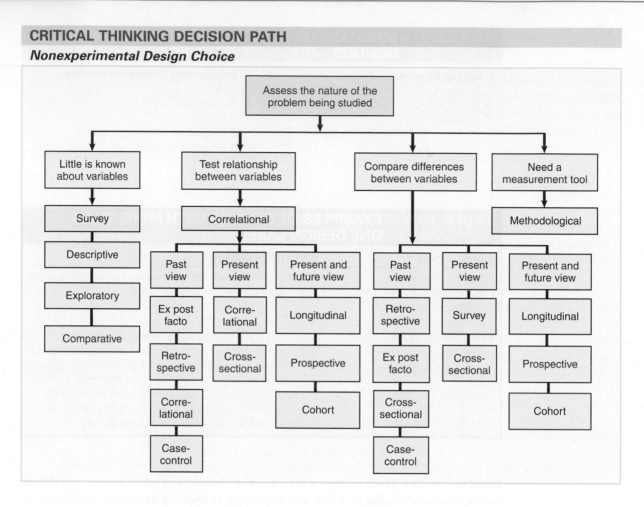

## SURVEY STUDIES

The broadest category of nonexperimental designs is the survey study. **Survey studies** are further classified as *descriptive, exploratory, or comparative. Surveys* collect detailed descriptions of variables and use the data to justify and assess conditions and practices or to make plans for improving health care practices. You will find that the terms *exploratory, descriptive, comparative,* and *survey* are used either alone, interchangeably, or together to describe a study's design (see Table 10-1).

- Investigators use a survey design to search for accurate information about the characteristics of particular subjects, groups, institutions, or situations or about the frequency of a variable's occurrence, particularly when little is known about the variable. Box 10-2 provides examples of survey studies.
- The types of variables in a survey can be classified as opinions, attitudes, or facts.
- Fact variables include attributes of an individual such as gender, income level, political and religious affiliations, ethnicity, occupation, and educational level.
- Surveys provide the basis for further development of programs and interventions.

> **BOX 10-2    SURVEY DESIGN EXAMPLES**
>
> - Williams and colleagues (2012) conducted a survey of 150 family caregivers to adults with cancer visiting an outpatient chemotherapy center. The purpose of the survey was to determine whether barriers to meditation differ by age and gender among a sample of cancer family caregivers who were chosen because they represent a highly stressed segment of the general population who would likely benefit from meditation practice.
> - Moceri and Drevdahl (2012) conducted a survey to investigate emergency nurses' knowledge and attitudes about pain using the Knowledge and Attitudes Survey Regarding Pain.

- Surveys are described as comparative when used to determine differences between variables.
- Survey data can be collected with a questionnaire or an interview (see Chapter 14).
- Surveys have either small or large samples of subjects drawn from defined populations, can be either broad or narrow, and can be made up of people or institutions.
- The data might provide the basis for projecting programmatic needs of groups.
- A survey's scope and depth depend on the nature of the problem.
- Surveys attempt to relate one variable to another or assess differences between variables, but do not determine causation.

The advantages of surveys are that a great deal of information can be obtained from a large population in a fairly economical manner, and that survey research information can be surprisingly accurate. If a sample is representative of the population (see Chapter 12), even a relatively small number of subjects can provide an accurate picture of the population.

Survey studies have several disadvantages. First, the information obtained in a survey tends to be superficial. The breadth rather than the depth of the information is emphasized. Second, conducting a survey requires a great deal of expertise in various research areas. The survey investigator must know sampling techniques, questionnaire construction, interviewing, and data analysis to produce a reliable and valid study.

> **EVIDENCE-BASED PRACTICE TIP**
>
> Evidence gained from a survey may be coupled with clinical expertise and applied to a similar population to develop an educational program to enhance knowledge and skills in a particular clinical area (e.g., a survey designed to measure the nursing staff's knowledge and attitudes about evidence-based practice where the data are used to develop an evidence-based practice staff development course).

> **HELPFUL HINT**
>
> You should recognize that a well-constructed survey can provide a wealth of data about a particular phenomenon of interest, even though causation is not being examined.

## RELATIONSHIP AND DIFFERENCE STUDIES

Investigators also try to trace the relationships or differences between variables that can provide a deeper insight into a phenomenon. These studies can be classified as relationship or difference studies. The following types of relationship/difference studies are discussed: correlational studies and developmental studies.

## Correlational Studies

In a **correlational study** the *relationship* between two or more variables is examined. The researcher is:

- Not testing whether one variable causes another variable.
- Testing whether the variables co-vary; that is, as one variable changes, does a related change occur in another variable.
- Interested in quantifying the strength of the relationship between variables, or in testing a hypothesis or research question about a specific relationship.

The direction of the relationship is important (see Chapter 16 for an explanation of the correlation coefficient). For example, in their correlational study, Pinar and colleagues (2012) assessed the relationship between social support and anxiety levels, depression, and quality of life in Turkish women with gynecologic cancer. This study tested multiple variables to assess the relationship and differences among the sample. The researchers concluded that having higher levels of social support were significantly related to lower levels of depression and anxiety, and higher levels of quality of life. Thus the variables were related to (not causal of) outcomes. Each step of this study was consistent with the aims of exploring the relationship among variables.

When reviewing a correlational study, remember what relationship the researcher tested and notice whether the researcher implied a relationship that is consistent with the theoretical framework and hypotheses being tested. Correlational studies offer the following advantages:

- An increased flexibility when investigating complex relationships among variables.
- An efficient and effective method of collecting a large amount of data about a problem.
- A potential for evidence-based application in clinical settings.
- A potential foundation for future experimental research studies.
- A framework for exploring the relationship between variables that cannot be inherently manipulated.
- A correlational study has a quality of realism and is appealing because it can suggest the potential for practical solutions to clinical problems.

The following are disadvantages of correlational studies:

- The researcher is unable to manipulate the variables of interest.
- The researcher does not use randomization in the sampling procedures as the groups are preexisting and therefore generalizability is decreased.
- The researcher is unable to determine a causal relationship between the variables because of the lack of manipulation, control, and randomization.
- The strength and quality of evidence is limited by the associative nature of the relationship between the variables.
- A misuse of a correlational design would be if the researcher concluded that a causal relationship exists between the variables.

Correlational studies may be further labeled as *descriptive correlational* or *predictive correlational*. Given the level of evidence provided by these studies, the ability to generalize the findings has some limitations, but often authors conclude the article with some very thoughtful recommendations for future studies in the specific area. The inability to draw causal statements should not lead you to conclude that a nonexperimental correlational study uses a weak design. In terms of evidence for practice, the researchers, based on the literature review and their findings, frame the utility of the results in light of previous research, and therefore help to establish the "best available" evidence that, combined with clinical expertise, informs clinical decisions regarding the study's applicability to a specific patient population. A correlational design is a very useful design for clinical research studies because many of the phenomena of clinical interest are beyond the researcher's ability to manipulate, control, and randomize.

---

### EVIDENCE-BASED PRACTICE TIP

Establishment of a strong relationship in predictive correlational studies often lends support for attempting to influence the independent variable in a future intervention study.

---

## Developmental Studies

There are also classifications of nonexperimental designs that use a time perspective. Investigators who use **developmental studies** are concerned not only with the existing status and the relationship and differences among phenomena at one point in time, but also with changes that result from elapsed time. The following three types of developmental study designs are discussed: cross-sectional, longitudinal, cohort or prospective and retrospective (also labeled as ex post facto or case control). Remember that in the literature, however, studies may be designated by more than one design name. This practice is accepted because many studies have elements of several designs. Table 10-1 provides examples of studies classified with more than one design label.

---

### EVIDENCE-BASED PRACTICE TIP

Replication of significant findings in nonexperimental studies with similar and/or different populations increases your confidence in the conclusions offered by the researcher and the strength of evidence generated by consistent findings from more than one study.

---

## Cross-Sectional Studies

A **cross-sectional study** examines data at one point in time; that is, data collected on only one occasion with the same subjects rather than with the same subjects at several time points. For example, in a study of post-traumatic stress symptoms Melvin and colleagues (2012; see Appendix D) hypothesized that couple functioning, as perceived by each member of the couple, would be negatively associated with post-traumatic stress symptoms (PTSS). This study tested multiple variables (age, gender, military ranks, and marital stress) to assess the relationship and differences among the sample. The researchers concluded that having higher levels of PTSS were associated with lower couple functioning and resilience, thus the variables were related to (not causal of) outcomes. Each step of this study was consistent with the aims of exploring the relationship and differences among variables in a cross-sectional design.

In this study the sample subjects participated on one occasion; that is, data were collected on only one occasion from each subject and represented a cross section of military couples rather than the researchers following a group of military couples over time. The purpose of this study was not to test causality, but to explore the potential relationships between and among variables that can be related to PTSS. Cross-sectional studies can explore relationships and correlations, or differences and comparisons, or both.

## Longitudinal/Prospective/Cohort Studies

Like cross-sectional studies, longitudinal, prospective, or cohort studies explore differences and relationships among variables. However, in contrast to the cross-sectional design, **longitudinal/prospective/cohort studies** collect data from the same group at different points in time. Longitudinal/prospective/or cohort studies are also referred to as **repeated measures studies**. These terms are interchangeable. An example of a longitudinal study is found in Alhusen and colleagues (2012; Appendix B). In this study the research team examined the relationships among maternal-fetal attachment, health practices during pregnancy, and adverse neonatal outcomes in a sample of low-income women.

Cross-sectional and longitudinal designs have advantages and disadvantages. When assessing the appropriateness of a cross-sectional study versus a longitudinal study, first assess the nature of the research question: What is the researcher's goal in light of the theoretical framework and the strength of evidence that will be provided by the findings? Longitudinal research allows clinicians to assess the incidence of a problem over time and potential reasons for changes in the variables of the study. However, the disadvantages inherent in a longitudinal design also must be considered. Data collection may be of long duration; therefore, costs can be high due to the time it takes for the subjects to progress to each data collection point. Internal validity threats, such as testing and mortality, are also ever-present and unavoidable in a longitudinal study. Subject loss to follow-up and attrition, whether due to dropout or death, may lead to unintended sample bias affecting both the internal validity and external validity of the study.

These realities make a longitudinal design costly in terms of time, effort, and money. There is also a chance of confounding variables that could affect the interpretation of the results. Subjects in such a study may respond in a socially desirable way that they believe is congruent with the investigator's expectations (see Hawthorne effect in Chapter 8). However, despite the pragmatic constraints imposed by a longitudinal study, the researcher should proceed with this design if the theoretical framework supports a longitudinal developmental perspective.

Advantages of a longitudinal study are as follows:
- Each subject is followed separately and thereby serves as his or her own control.
- Increased depth of responses can be obtained and early trends in the data can be analyzed.
- The researcher can assess changes in the variables of interest over time, and both relationships and differences can be explored between variables.
- Additional advantages and disadvantages of cross-sectional are as follows: Cross-sectional studies, when compared to longitudinal/prospective/cohort studies are less time-consuming, less expensive, and thus more manageable.
- Large amounts of data can be collected at one point, making the results more readily available.
- The confounding variable of maturation, resulting from the elapsed time, is not present.
- The investigator's ability to establish an in-depth developmental assessment of the interrelationships of the variables being studied is lessened.

Thus the researcher is unable to determine whether the change that occurred is related to the change that was predicted because the same subjects were not followed over a period of time. In other words, the subjects are unable to serve as their own controls (see Chapter 8). In summary, longitudinal studies begin in the present and end in the future, and cross-sectional studies look at a broader perspective of a cross section of the population at a specific point in time.

| TABLE 10-2 | **PARADIGM FOR THE EX POST FACTO DESIGN** | |
|---|---|---|
| **GROUPS (NOT RANDOMLY ASSIGNED)** | **INDEPENDENT VARIABLE (NOT MANIPULATED BY INVESTIGATOR)** | **DEPENDENT VARIABLE** |
| Exposed group: cigarette smokers | $X$ Cigarette smoking | $Y_e$ Lung cancer |
| Control group: nonsmokers | | $Y_c$ No lung cancer |

### Retrospective/Ex Post Facto/Case Control Studies

A retrospective study is essentially the same as an ex post facto study and a case control study. In either case, the dependent variable already has been affected by the independent variable, and the investigator attempts to link present events to events that occurred in the past. When researchers wish to explain causality or the factors that determine the occurrence of events or conditions, they prefer to use an experimental design. However, they cannot always manipulate the independent variable, X, or use random assignments. When experimental designs that test the effect of an intervention or condition cannot be employed, ex post facto/case control studies may be used. Ex post facto literally means "from after the fact." Ex post facto, retrospective, or case control studies also are known as *causal-comparative* studies or *comparative* studies. As we discuss this design further, you will see that many elements of this category are similar to quasi-experimental designs because they explore differences between variables (Campbell & Stanley, 1963).

In retrospective/ex post facto/case control studies, a researcher hypothesizes, for instance:

- That $X$ (cigarette smoking) is related to and a determinant of $Y$ (lung cancer).
- But $X$, the presumed cause, is not manipulated and subjects are not randomly assigned to groups.
- Rather, a group of subjects who have experienced $X$ (cigarette smoking) in a normal situation is located and a control group of subjects who have not experienced $X$ is chosen.
- The behavior, performance, or condition (lung tissue) of the two groups is compared to determine whether the exposure to $X$ had the effect predicted by the hypothesis.

Table 10-2 illustrates this example. Examination of Table 10-2 reveals that although cigarette smoking appears to be a determinant of lung cancer, the researcher is still not able to conclude that a causal relationship exists between the variables because the independent variable has not been manipulated and subjects were not randomly assigned to groups.

Abbass and colleagues (2012) conducted a retrospective study to explore the impact of electronic health records (EHR) on nurses' productivity, and to examine whether the impact is moderated through a case-mix index or adjusted patient days. Two sources of data were linked and analyzed for 2007 and 2008: the American Hospital Association

### EVIDENCE-BASED PRACTICE TIP

The quality of evidence provided by a longitudinal, prospective, or cohort study is stronger than that from other nonexperimental designs because the researcher can determine the incidence of a problem and its possible causes.

survey and the Center for Medicare and Medicaid Services data. The study findings do not suggest significant financial savings or superior productivity related to the use of EHRs.

The advantages of the retrospective/ex post facto/case control design are similar to those of the correlational design. The additional benefit is that it offers a higher level of control than a correlational study, thereby increasing the confidence the research consumer would have in the evidence provided by the findings. For example, in the cigarette smoking study, a group of nonsmokers' lung tissue samples are compared with samples of smokers' lung tissue. This comparison enables the researcher to establish the existence of a differential effect of cigarette smoking on lung tissue. However, the researcher remains unable to draw a causal linkage between the two variables, and this inability is the major disadvantage of the retrospective/ex post facto/case control design.

Another disadvantage of retrospective research is the problem of an alternative hypothesis being the reason for the documented relationship. If the researcher obtains data from two existing groups of subjects, such as one that has been exposed to $X$ and one that has not, and the data support the hypothesis that $X$ is related to $Y$, the researcher cannot be sure whether $X$ or some extraneous variable is the real cause of the occurrence of $Y$. As such, the impact or effect of the relationship cannot be estimated accurately. Finding naturally occurring groups of subjects who are similar in all respects except for their exposure to the variable of interest is very difficult. There is always the possibility that the groups differ in some other way, such as exposure to other lung irritants, such as asbestos, that can affect the findings of the study and produce spurious or unreliable results. Consequently, you need to cautiously evaluate the conclusions drawn by the investigator.

### HELPFUL HINT

When reading research reports, you will note that at times researchers classify a study's design with more than one design type label. This is correct because research studies often reflect aspects of more than one design label.

The threats to internal validity or bias that may arise in a **prospective study** are related to the internal validity threats of mortality, instrumentation, and testing. However, longitudinal/prospective/cohort studies are considered to be stronger than retrospective studies because of the degree of control that can be imposed on extraneous variables that might confound the data and lead to bias.

### HELPFUL HINT

Remember that nonexperimental designs can test relationships, differences, comparisons, or predictions, depending on the purpose of the study.

## PREDICTION AND CAUSALITY IN NONEXPERIMENTAL RESEARCH

A concern of researchers and research consumers are the issues of prediction and causality. Researchers are interested in explaining cause-and-effect relationships; that is, estimating the effect of one phenomenon on another without bias. Historically, researchers have said that only experimental research can support the concept of causality. For example, nurses are interested in discovering what causes anxiety in many settings. If we can uncover the causes, we could develop interventions that would prevent or decrease the anxiety. Causality makes it necessary to order events chronologically; that is, if we find in a randomly assigned experiment that event 1 (stress) occurs before event 2 (anxiety) and that those in the stressed group were anxious whereas those in the unstressed group were not, we can say that the hypothesis of stress causing anxiety is supported by these empirical observations. If these results were found in a nonexperimental study where some subjects underwent the stress of surgery and were anxious and others did not have surgery and were not anxious, we would say that there is an association or relationship between stress (surgery) and anxiety. But on the basis of the results of a nonexperimental study, we could not say that the stress of surgery caused the anxiety.

Many variables (e.g., anxiety) that nurse researchers wish to study cannot be manipulated, nor would it be wise or ethical to try to manipulate them. Yet there is a need to have studies that can assert a predictive or causal sequence. In light of this need, many nurse researchers are using several analytical techniques that can explain the relationships among variables to establish predictive or causal links. These analytical techniques are called *causal modeling, model testing,* and *associated causal analysis techniques* (Kaplan, 2008; Kline, 2005). The reader of research also will find the terms *path analysis, LISREL, analysis of covariance structures, structural equation modeling (SEM),* and *hierarchical linear modeling (HLM)* to describe the statistical techniques (see Chapter 16) used in these studies. These terms do not designate the design of a study, but are statistical tests that are used in many nonexperimental designs to predict how precisely a dependent variable can be predicted based on an independent variable. A national internet survey was conducted by Im and colleagues (2012) to explore midlife women's (n = 542) attitudes toward physical activity, and to determine the relationship between their attitudes and actual participation in physical activity considering other influencing factors, such as ethnicity. Path Analysis was used to establish a model of how the variables predicted, or were related to, each other. Direct paths from attitude scores ($p < .01$), self-efficacy scores ($p < .01$), and barrier scores to physical activity ($p < .05$) were statistically significant in all ethnic groups. However, the path from social influence to physical activity were not significant. This sophisticated study design aids nursing conceptualization of ethnic differences in midlife women's attitudes toward physical activity.

Sometimes researchers want to make a forecast or prediction about how patients will respond to an intervention or a disease process, or how successful individuals will be in a particular setting or field of specialty. In this case, a model may be tested to assess which physical activity scores were not significant.

Many nursing studies test models. The statistics used in model-testing studies are advanced, but you should be able to read the article, understand the purpose of the study, and determine if the model generated was logical and developed with a solid basis from the literature and past research. This section cites several studies that conducted sound tests of theoretical models. A full description of the techniques and principles of causal modeling is beyond the scope of this text; however, if you want to read about these advanced techniques, a book such as that by Kaplan (2008) is appropriate to consult.

**HELPFUL HINT**

Nonexperimental clinical research studies have progressed to the point where prediction models are often used to explore or test relationships between independent and dependent variables.

## ADDITIONAL TYPES OF QUANTITATIVE METHODS

Other types of quantitative studies complement the science of research. The additional research methods provide a means of viewing and interpreting phenomena that give further breadth and knowledge to nursing science and practice. The additional types include methodological research and secondary analysis.

### Methodological Research

Methodological research is the development and evaluation of data collection instruments, scales, or techniques. As you will find in Chapters 14 and 15, methodology greatly influences research and the evidence produced.

The most significant and critically important aspect of methodological research addressed in measurement development is called **psychometrics**. Psychometrics focuses on the theory and development of measurement instruments (such as questionnaires) or measurement techniques (such as observational techniques) through the research process. Nurse researchers have used the principles of psychometrics to develop and test measurement instruments that focus on nursing phenomena. Many of the phenomena of interest to practice and research are intangible, such as interpersonal conflict, resilience, quality of life, coping, and symptom management. The intangible nature of various phenomena—yet the recognition of the need to measure them—places methodological research in an important position. Methodological research differs from other designs of research in two ways. First, it does not include all of the research process steps as discussed in Chapter 1. Second, to implement its techniques the researcher must have a sound knowledge of psychometrics or must consult with a researcher knowledgeable in psychometric techniques. The methodological researcher is not interested in the relationship of the independent variable and dependent variable or in the effect of an independent variable on a dependent variable. The methodological researcher is interested in identifying an intangible construct (concept) and making it tangible with a paper-and-pencil instrument or observation protocol.

A methodological study basically includes the following steps:
- Defining the concept or behavior to be measured
- Formulating the instrument's items
- Developing instructions for users and respondents
- Testing the instrument's reliability and validity

These steps require a sound, specific, and exhaustive literature review to identify the theories underlying the concept. The literature review provides the basis of item formulation. Once the items have been developed, the researcher assesses the tool's reliability and validity (see Chapter 15). As an example of methodological research, Bova and colleagues (2012) identified the concept of trust between patients and health care providers. They defined this concept as collaborative trust "level that develops between patient and health care provider in a partnership where goals are shared and there is a mutual respect for each other's contribution to the process" (Bova et al., 2012; p. 482). The researchers defined the concept operationally and conceptually and followed through by testing the Health Care Relationship Trust (HCR) Scale for reliability and validity (see Chapter 15). Common considerations that researchers incorporate into methodological research are outlined in Table 10-3. Many more examples of methodological research can be found in nursing research literature. Psychometric or methodological studies are found primarily in journals that report research. The *Journal of Nursing Measurement* is devoted to the publication of information on instruments and approaches for measurement of variables. The specific procedures of methodological research are beyond the scope of this book, but you are urged to closely review the instruments used in studies.

| TABLE 10-3 | COMMON CONSIDERATIONS IN THE DEVELOPMENT OF MEASUREMENT TOOLS |
|---|---|
| **CONSIDERATION** | **EXAMPLE** |
| A well-constructed scale, test, or interview schedule should consist of an objective, standardized measure of a behavior that has been clearly defined. Observations should be made on a small but carefully chosen sampling of the behavior of interest, thus permitting the reader to feel confident that the samples are representative. | In the report of the Health Care Relationship (HCR) Trust Scale, the relationship of trust to improved patient outcomes as demonstrated by several trust scales developed by other research teams is discussed. The strengths and weaknesses of those scales were highlighted, thus providing the rationale for the development of the HCR first piloted by Bova and colleagues (2006) as an instrument that studies collaborative trust between patients and health care providers in primary care settings. The scale also was based on a thorough review of the theoretical framework of collaborative trust and other research literature (Bova et al., 2012). |
| The measure should be standardized, that is, it should be a set of uniform items and response possibilities, uniformly administered and scored. | In the Bova and colleagues (2012) study, the HCR has evolved to a 13-item scale with items measuring diabetes trust in the patient health care provider relationship. The HCR is scored from 0-4; 3 items are reverse scored with higher scores indicating greater trust levels. The items are completed by the patient, or they can be read to the patient. The total score is obtained by summation of the ratings for each response. |
| The items of the instrument should be unambiguous; clear-cut, concise, exact statements with only one idea per item. | A pilot study was conducted to evaluate the HCR's items and the study administration procedures. The pilot data indicated that only one item needed to be reworded and no items needed to be discarded. They based the item revision on the fact that 2 participants left an item blank and 1 participant indicated that he did not understand the question. |
| The type of items used in any instrument should be restricted to a limited number of variations. Subjects who are expected to shift from one kind of item to another may fail to provide a true response as a result of the distraction of making such a change. | Mixing true-or-false items with questions that require a yes-or-no response and items that provide a response format of five possible answers is conducive to a high level of measurement error. The HCR contained only a Likert scale format ranging from 0-4. |

*Continued*

| CONSIDERATION | EXAMPLE |
|---|---|

**TABLE 10-3   COMMON CONSIDERATIONS IN THE DEVELOPMENT OF MEASUREMENT TOOLS—cont'd**

| CONSIDERATION | EXAMPLE |
|---|---|
| Items should not provide irrelevant clues. Unless carefully constructed, an item may furnish an indication of the expected response or answer. Furthermore, the correct answer or expected response to one item should not be given by another item. | An item that provides a clue to the expected answer may contain value words that convey cultural expectations, such as the following: "A good wife enjoys caring for her home and family." |
| Instruments should not be made difficult by requiring unnecessarily complex or exact operations. Furthermore, the difficulty of an instrument should be appropriate to the level of the subjects being assessed. Limiting each item to one concept or idea helps accomplish this objective. | A test constructed to evaluate learning in an introductory course in research methods may contain an item that is inappropriate for the designated group, such as the following: "A nonlinear transformation of data to linear data is a useful procedure before testing a hypothesis of curvilinearity." |
| The diagnostic, predictive, or measurement value of an instrument depends on the degree to which it serves as an indicator of a relatively broad and significant behavior area, known as the universe of content for the behavior. As already emphasized, a behavior must be clearly defined before it can be measured. The extent to which test items appear to accomplish this objective is an indication of the content and/or construct validity of the instrument. | The HCR development included establishment of acceptable content validity. The HCR items were submitted to a panel of experts in trust; the Content Validity Index = .88, which means that the items are deemed to reflect the universe of content related to collaborative trust. Construct validity was established using factor analysis which confirmed a uni-dimensional factor structure for 13 of the 15 items. |
| The instrument also should adequately cover the defined behavior. The primary consideration is whether the number and nature of items in the sample are adequate. If there are too few items, the accuracy or reliability of the measure must be questioned. | Very few people would be satisfied with an assessment of such traits as trust if the scales were limited to three items. Bova and colleagues (2012) discuss that the HCR was originally 15 items, but based on validity testing, theoretical considerations, and practical considerations, 2 items were deleted. This resulted in the current 13-item HCR scale. |
| The measure must prove its worth empirically through tests of reliability and validity. | A researcher should demonstrate that a scale is accurate and measures what it purports to measure (see Chapter 15). Bova and colleagues (2012) provide the data on the reliability and validity testing of the HCR scale (pp. 402-403). |

## Secondary Analysis

Secondary analysis is also not a design, but rather a research method in which the researcher takes previously collected and analyzed data from *one* study and reanalyzes the data or a subset of the data for a *secondary* purpose. The original study may be either an experimental or a nonexperimental design. For example, Fantasia and colleagues (2012) conducted a secondary analysis of data from a larger behavioral health intervention trial that targeted drinking behaviors among adolescents (Bernstein et al., 2010). Data from a total of 2560 male and female urban adolescents between the ages of 14 and 21 were analyzed for personal, interpersonal, and community exposure to violence and risky sexual behavior. Findings of the secondary analysis demonstrated that violence has an impact on sexual risk. For females, carrying a weapon ($p < .020$) and feeling safe in intimate relationships ($p < .029$) were individual correlates for risky sexual behavior, while for males, race/ethnicity ($p < .019$) and being in a physical fight ($p < .001$) were significant correlates of risky sexual behavior. The data from this study allowed further in-depth exploration of gender differences in risky sexual behavior among urban adolescents exposed to violence. The data cannot be used to infer causality but to provide information for identifying adolescents in urban settings at high risk for risky sexual behavior and the potential negative reproductive health outcomes.

### HELPFUL HINT

As you read the literature, you will find labels such as *outcomes research, needs assessments, evaluation research*, and *quality assurance*. These studies are not designs per se. These studies use either experimental or nonexperimental designs. Studies with these labels are designed to test the effectiveness of health care techniques, programs, or interventions. When reading such a research study, the reader should assess which design was used and if the principles of the design, sampling strategy, and analysis are consistent with the study's purpose.

## APPRAISING THE EVIDENCE
## NONEXPERIMENTAL DESIGNS

Criteria for appraising nonexperimental designs are presented in the Critiquing Criteria box. When appraising nonexperimental research designs, you should keep in mind that such designs offer the researcher a lower level of control and an increased risk of bias. As such, the level of evidence provided by nonexperimental designs is not as strong as evidence generated by experimental designs in which manipulation, randomization, and control are used; however, there are other important clinical research questions that need to be answered beyond the testing of interventions and experimental or quasi-experimental designs.

The first step in critiquing nonexperimental designs is to determine which type of design was used in the study. Often a statement describing the design of the study appears in the abstract and in the methods section of the report. If such a statement is not present, you should closely examine the paper for evidence of which type of design was employed. You should be able to discern that either a survey or a relationship design was used, as well as the specific subtype. For example, you would expect an investigation of self-concept development in children from birth to 5 years of age to be a relationship study using a longitudinal design. If a longitudinal study was used, you should assess for possible threats to internal validity or bias, such as mortality, testing, and instrumentation. Potential threats to internal or external validity should be recognized by the researchers at the end of the study and, in particular, the limitations section.

Next, evaluate the theoretical framework and underpinnings of the study to determine if a nonexperimental design was the most appropriate approach to the research question or hypothesis. For example, many of the studies on pain (e.g., intensity, severity, perception) discussed throughout this text are suggestive of a relationship between pain and any of the independent variables (diagnosis, coping style, ethnicity) under consideration where the independent variable cannot be manipulated. As such, these studies suggest a nonexperimental correlational, longitudinal/prospective/cohort, a retrospective/ex post facto/case control, or a cross-sectional design. Investigators will use one of these designs to examine the relationship between the variables in naturally occurring groups. Sometimes you may think that it would have been more appropriate if the investigators had used an experimental or a quasi-experimental design. However, you must recognize that pragmatic or ethical considerations also may have guided the researchers in their choice of design (see Chapters 8 through 18).

Finally, the factor or factors that actually influence changes in the dependent variable can be ambiguous in nonexperimental designs. As with all complex phenomena, multiple factors can contribute to variability in the subjects' responses. When an experimental design is not used for controlling some of these extraneous variables that can influence results, the researcher must strive to provide as much control of them as possible within the context of a nonexperimental design, to decrease bias. For example, when it has not been possible to randomly assign subjects to treatment groups as an approach to controlling an independent variable, the researchers will most often use strict inclusion and exclusion criteria and calculate an adequate sample size using power analysis that will support a valid testing of how correlated (or predictive) the independent variable is to the dependent variable (see Chapter 12). Threats to internal and external validity or potential sources of bias represent a major influence when interpreting the findings of a nonexperimental study because they impose limitations to the generalizability of the results and applicability to practice. It is also important to remember that prediction of patient clinical outcomes is of critical value for clinical researchers. Nonexperimental designs can be used to make predictions if the study is designed with an adequate sample size (see Chapter 12), collects data consistently, and uses reliable and valid instruments (see Chapter 15).

If you are appraising methodological research, you need to apply the principles of reliability and validity (see Chapter 15). A secondary analysis needs to be reviewed from several perspectives. First, you need to understand if the researcher followed sound scientific logic in the secondary analysis completed. Second, you need to review the original study that the data were extracted from to assess the reliability and validity of the original study. Even though the format and methods vary, it is important to remember that all research has a central goal: to answer questions scientifically and provide the strongest, most consistent evidence possible, while controlling for potential bias.

## KEY POINTS

- Nonexperimental research designs are used in studies that construct a picture or make an account of events as they naturally occur. The major difference between nonexperimental and experimental research is that in nonexperimental designs the independent variable is not actively manipulated by the investigator.
- Nonexperimental designs can be classified as either survey studies or relationship/difference studies.
- Survey studies and relationship/difference studies are both descriptive and exploratory in nature.
- Survey research collects detailed descriptions of existing phenomena and uses the data either to justify current conditions and practices or to make more intelligent plans for improving them.
- Relationship studies endeavor to explore the relationships between variables that provide deeper insight into the phenomena of interest.
- Correlational studies examine relationships.
- Developmental studies are further broken down into categories of cross-sectional studies, longitudinal/prospective/cohort studies, retrospective/ex post facto studies, and case control studies.
- Methodological research and secondary analysis are examples of other means of adding to the body of nursing research. Both the researcher and the reader must consider the advantages and disadvantages of each design.
- Nonexperimental research designs do not enable the investigator to establish cause-and-effect relationships between the variables. Consumers must be wary of nonexperimental studies that make causal claims about the findings unless a causal modeling technique is used.
- Nonexperimental designs also offer the researcher the least amount of control. Threats to validity impose limitations on the generalizability of the results and as such should be fully assessed by the critical reader.
- The critiquing process is directed toward evaluating the appropriateness of the selected nonexperimental design in relation to factors, such as the research problem, theoretical framework, hypothesis, methodology, and data analysis and interpretation.
- Though nonexperimental designs do not provide the highest level of evidence (Level I), they do provide a wealth of data that become useful pieces for formulating both Level I and Level II studies that are aimed at developing and testing nursing interventions.

## CRITICAL THINKING CHALLENGES

- The mid-term assignment for your research course is to critique an assigned study on the relationship of perception of pain severity and quality of life in advanced cancer patients. Your first job is to decide what kind of design was used and whether it was appropriate for the overall purpose of the study. You think it is a cross-sectional design, but other students think it is a quasi-experimental design because it has several specific hypotheses. How would you support your argument that you are correct?

- You are completing your senior practicum on a surgical unit, and for preconference your student group has just completed a search for studies related to the effectiveness of hand washing in decreasing the incidence of nosocomial infections, but the studies all use an ex post facto/case control design. You want to approach the nurse manager on the unit to present the evidence you have collected and critically appraised, but you are concerned about the strength of the evidence because the studies all use a nonexperimental design. How would you justify that this is the "best available evidence"?

- You are a member of a journal club at your hospital. Your group is interested in the effectiveness of smoking cessation interventions provided by nurses. An electronic search indicates that 12 individual research studies and one meta-analysis meet your inclusion criteria. Would your group begin with critically appraising the 12 individual studies or the one meta-analysis? Provide rationale for your choice, including consideration of the strength and quality of evidence provided by individual studies versus a meta-analysis.

- A patient in a primary care practice who had a history of a "heart murmur" called his nurse practitioner for a prescription for an antibiotic before having a periodontal (gum) procedure. When she responded that according to the new American Heart Association (AHA) clinical practice guideline, antibiotic prophylaxis is no longer considered appropriate for his heart murmur, the patient got upset, stating, "But I always take antibiotics! I want you to tell me why I should believe this guideline. How do I know my heart will not be damaged by listening to you?" What is the purpose of a clinical practice guideline and how would you as an NP respond to this patient?

## REFERENCES

Abbass, J., Helton, J., Mhaure, S., & Sansgiry, S. S. (2012). Impact of electronic health records on nurses' productivity. *Computers Informatics Nursing, 30*(5), 237–241.

Alhusen, J. L, Gross, D., Hayat, M. J., et al. (2012). The influence of maternal-fetal attachment and health practices on neonatal outcomes in low-income, urban women. *Research in Nursing & Health, 35*(2), 112–120.

Bernstein, J., Heeren, T., Edward, E., et al. (2010). A brief motivational interview in a pediatric emergency department, plus 10-day telephone follow-up, increases attempts to quit drinking among youth and young adults who screen positive for problematic drinking. *Academic Emergency Medicine, 17*, 890–902.

Bova, C., Fennie, K. P., Watrous, E., et al. (2006). The health care relationship (HCR) trust scale: development and psychometric evaluation. *Nursing in Research & Health, 29*, 477–488.

Bova, C., Route, P. S., Fennie, K., et al. (2012). Measuring patient-provider trust in a primary care population: refinement of the health care relationship trust scale. *Research in Nursing & Health, 35*, 397–408.

Campbell, D. T., & Stanley, J.C. (1963). *Experimental and quasi-experimental designs for research.* Chicago, IL: Rand-McNally.

Carpenter, J. S., Rawl, S., Porter, J., et al. (2008). Oncology outpatient and provider responses to a computerized symptom assessment system. *Oncology Nursing Forum, 35*(4), 661–670.

Fantasia, H. C. (2012). Gender differences in risky sexual behavior among urban adolescents exposed to violence. *Journal of the American Academy of Nurse Practitioners, 24*(7), 436–442.

Im, E., Chang, S. J., Ko, Y., et al. (2012). A national internet survey on midlife women's attitudes toward physical activity. *Nursing Research, 61*(5), 342–352.

Kaplan, D. W. (2008). *Structure equation modeling: foundations and extensions.* Thousand Oaks, CA: Sage.

Kline, R. (2005). *Principles and practices of structural equation modeling* (2nd ed.). New York, NY: Guilford Press.

Melvin, K. C., Gross, D., Hayat, M. J., et al. (2012). Couple functioning and post-traumatic stress symptoms in U.S. army couples: the role of resilience. *Research in Nursing & Health, 35*(2), 164–177.

Moceri, J. T., & Drevdahl, D. J. (2012). Nurses' knowledge and attitudes toward pain in the emergency department. *Journal of Emergency Nurses Online, 38*, 1–7. doi: 10.1016/jen2012.04.014.

Pinar, G., Okdem, S., Buyukgonenc, L., & Ayhan, A. (2012). The relationship between social support and the level of anxiety, depression, and quality of life of Turkish women with gynecologic cancer. *Cancer Nursing, 35*(2), 229–235.

Wielgus, K. K., Berger, A. M., & Hertoz, M. (2009). Predictors of fatigue 30 days after completing anthracycline plus taxane adjuvant chemotherapy for breast cancer. *Oncology Nursing Forum, 36*(1), 38–48.

Williams, A., Van Ness, P., Dixon, J., & McCorkle, R. (2012). Barriers to meditation by gender and age among cancer family caregivers. *Nursing Research, 61*(1), 22–27.

# ⊖volve WEBSITE

*Go to Evolve at http://evolve.elsevier.com/LoBiondo/ for review questions, critiquing exercises, and additional research articles for practice in reviewing and critiquing.*

# CHAPTER 11

# Systematic Reviews and Clinical Practice Guidelines

*Geri LoBiondo-Wood*

## ⊖volve WEBSITE

*Go to Evolve at http://evolve.elsevier.com/LoBiondo/ for review questions, critiquing exercises, and additional research articles for practice in reviewing and critiquing.*

## LEARNING OUTCOMES

*After reading this chapter, you should be able to do the following:*

- Describe the types of research reviews.
- Describe the components of a systematic review.
- Differentiate between a systematic review, meta-analysis, and integrative review.
- Describe the purpose of clinical guidelines.

- Differentiate between an expert and an evidence-based clinical guideline.
- Critically appraise systematic reviews and clinical practice guidelines.

## KEY TERMS

| | | | |
|---|---|---|---|
| AGREE II | effect size | expert-based practice | integrative review |
| CASP tools | evidence-based practice | guidelines | meta-analysis |
| clinical practice | guidelines | forest plot | systematic review |
| guidelines | | | |

The breadth and depth of clinical research has grown. As the number of research studies focused on similar content conducted by multiple researchers has grown, it has become important to have a means of organizing and assessing the quality, quantity, and consistency among the findings of a group of like studies. The previous chapters have introduced the types of qualitative and quantitative designs and how to critique these studies for quality and applicability to practice. The purpose of this chapter is to acquaint you with systematic reviews and clinical guidelines that assess multiple studies focused on the same clinical

---

**BOX 11-1    SYSTEMATIC REVIEW COMPONENTS WITH OR WITHOUT META-ANALYSIS**

**Introduction**
Review rationale and a clear clinical question (PICO)

**Methods**
Information sources, databases used, and search strategy identified: how studies were selected and data extracted as well as the variables extracted and defined
Description of methods used to assess risk of bias, summary measures identified (e.g., risk, ratio); identification of how data is combined, if studies are graded what quality appraisal system was used (see Chapters 1, 17, and 18)

**Results**
Number of studies screened and characteristics, risk of bias within studies, if a meta-analysis there will be a synthesis of results including confidence intervals, risk of bias for each study, and all outcomes considered

**Discussion**
Summary of findings including the strength, quality, quantity and consistency of the evidence for each outcome
Any limitations of the studies, conclusions and recommendations of findings for practice

**Funding**
Sources of funding for the systematic review

---

question, and how these reviews and guidelines can support evidence-based practice. Terminology used to define systematic reviews and clinical guidelines has changed as this area of research and literature assessment has grown. The definitions used in this textbook are consistent with the definitions from the Cochrane Collaboration and the PRISMA Group (Higgins & Green, 2011; Moher et al, 2009). Systematic reviews and clinical guidelines are critical and meaningful for the development of quality improvement practices.

## SYSTEMATIC REVIEW TYPES

As defined in Chapter 1, a **systematic review** is a summation and assessment of research studies found in the literature based on a clearly focused question that uses systematic and explicit methods to identify, select, critically appraise, and analyze relevant data from the selected studies to summarize the findings in a focused area (Liberati et al., 2009; Moher et al., 2009). Statistical methods may or may not be used to analyze the studies reviewed. Multiple terms and methods are used to systematically review the literature, depending on the review's purpose. See Box 11-1 for the components of a systematic review. At times, some of these terms are used interchangeably. The terms *systematic review* and *meta-analysis* are often used interchangeably or together. The only review type that can be labeled a meta-analysis is one that reviewed studies using statistical methods. An important concept to remember when reading a systematic review is how well the studies reviewed minimized bias or maintained the concept of control (see Chapters 8 and 9).

You will also find reviews of an area of research or theory synthesis termed **integrative reviews.** *Integrative reviews* critically appraise the literature in an area but without a statistical analysis and are the broadest category of review (Whittemore, 2005; Whittemore & Knafl, 2005). Systematic and integrative reviews are not designs per se, but methods for

## CRITICAL THINKING DECISION PATH
### Completing a Systematic Review

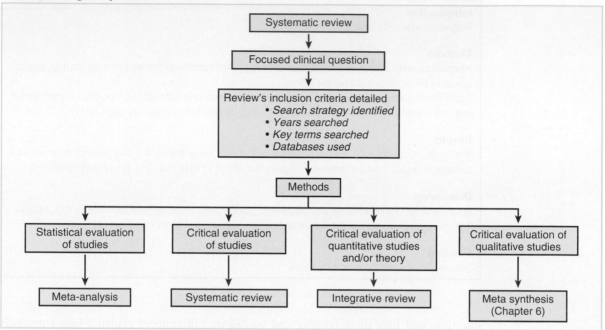

searching, and integrating the literature related to a specific clinical issue. These methods take the results of many studies in a specific area; assesses the studies critically for reliability and validity (quality, quantity, and consistency) (see Chapters 1, 7, 17, and 18); and synthesize findings to inform practice. Meta-analysis provides Level I evidence; the highest level of evidence as it statistically analyzes and integrates the results of many studies. Systematic reviews and meta-analyses also grade the level of design or evidence of the studies reviewed (see Chapters 1 and 17). Of all the review types, a meta-analysis provides the strongest summary support because it summarizes studies using data analysis. The Critical Thinking Decision Path outlines the path for completing a systematic review.

## SYSTEMATIC REVIEW

A systematic review is a summary of the quantitative research literature that used similar designs based on a focused clinical question. The goal is to bring together all of the studies concerning a focused clinical question and, using rigorous inclusion and exclusion criteria, assess the strength and quality of the evidence provided by the chosen studies in relation to:

- Sampling issues
- Internal validity (bias) threats
- External validity
- Data analysis

The purpose is to report, in a consolidated fashion, the most current and valid research on intervention effectiveness and clinical knowledge, which will ultimately inform evidence-based decision making about the applicability of findings to clinical practice.

Once the studies in a systematic review are gathered from a comprehensive literature search (see Chapter 3), they are assessed for quality and synthesized according to quality or focus; then practice recommendations are made and presented in an article. More than one person independently evaluates the studies to be included or excluded in the review. Generally, the articles critically appraised are discussed in the article and presented in a table format within the article, which helps you to easily identify the specific studies gathered for the review and their quality. The most important principle to assess when reading a systematic review is how the author(s) of the review identified the studies to evaluate and how they systematically reviewed and appraised the literature that leads to the reviewers' conclusions.

The components of a systematic review are the same as a meta-analysis (see Box 11-1) except for the analysis of the studies. An example of a systematic review was completed by Fowles and colleagues (2012) on the effectiveness of maternal health promoting interventions. In this review, the authors

- Synthesized the literature from studies on the effectiveness of interventions promoting maternal health in the first year after childbirth.
- Included a clear clinical question; all of the sections of a systematic review were presented, except there was no statistical meta-analysis (combination of studies data) of the studies as a whole because the interventions and outcomes varied across the studies reviewed.

Each study in this review was considered *individually, not collectively,* for its sample size, effect size, and its contribution to knowledge in the area based on a set of criteria.

Although systematic reviews are highly useful, they also have to be reviewed for potential bias. Thus the studies in a review need to be carefully critiqued for scientific rigor in each step of the research process.

## META-ANALYSIS

A **meta-analysis** is a systematic summary using *statistical techniques* to assess and combine studies of the same design to obtain a precise estimate of *effect* (impact of an intervention on the dependent variable/outcomes or association between variables). The terms meta-analysis and systematic review are often used interchangeably. The main difference is *only* a meta-analysis includes a statistical assessment of the studies reviewed. A meta-analysis statistically analyzes the data from each of the studies, treating all the studies reviewed as one large data set in order to obtain a precise estimate of the effect (impact) of the results (outcomes) of the studies in the review.

Meta-analysis uses a rigorous process of summary and determining the impact of a number of studies rather than the impact derived from a single study alone (see Chapter 10). After the clinical question is identified and the search of the review of published and unpublished literature is completed, a meta-analysis is conducted in two phases:

Phase I: The data are extracted (i.e., outcome data, sample sizes, and measures of variability from the identified studies).

Phase II: The decision is made as to whether it is appropriate to calculate what is known as a pooled average result (effect) of the studies reviewed.

Effect sizes are calculated using the difference in the average scores between the intervention and control groups from each study (Cochrane Handbook of Systematic Reviews for Interventions, 2011). Each study is considered a unit of analysis. A meta-analysis takes the effect size (see Chapter 12) from each of the studies reviewed to obtain an estimate of the population (or the whole) to create a single effect size of all the studies. Thus the effect size is an estimate of how large of a difference there is between intervention and control groups in the *summarized* studies. For example, the meta-analysis in Appendix E studied the question "Does counseling follow-up of women who had a miscarriage improve psychological well-being?" (Murphy et al., 2012). The studies that assessed this question were reviewed and each weighted for its impact or effect on improving psychological well-being. This estimate helps health care providers decide which intervention, if any, was more useful for improving well-being after a miscarriage. Detailed components of a systematic review with or without meta-analysis (Moher et al., 2009) are listed in Box 11-1.

In addition to calculating effect sizes, meta-analyses use multiple statistical methods to present and depict the data from studies reviewed (see Chapters 19 and 20). One of these methods is a forest plot, sometimes called a blobbogram. A forest plot graphically depicts the results of analyzing a number of studies. Figure 11-1 is an example of a forest plot from Murphy and colleagues (Cochrane Review, 2012; see Appendix E). This review identified whether follow-up by health care professionals or lay organizations at any time affects the psychological well-being of women following miscarriage.

## EVIDENCE-BASED PRACTICE TIP

Evidence-based practice methods such as meta-analysis increase your ability to manage the ever-increasing volume of information produced to develop the best evidence-based practices.

Figure 11-1 displays three studies that compared one counseling session versus no counseling sessions at 4 months after miscarriage using different psychological measures of well-being. Each study analyzed is listed. To the right of the listed study is a horizontal line that identifies the effect size estimate for each study. The box on the vertical line represents the effect size of each study and the diamond is the effect or significance of the combined studies. The boxes to the left of the 0 line mean that counseling was favored or produced a significant effect. The box to the right of the line indicates studies in which counseling was not favored or significant. The diamond is a more precise estimate of the interventions as it combines the data from the studies. The exemplar provided is basic as meta-analysis is a sophisticated methodology. For a fuller understanding, several references are provided (Borenstein et al., 2009; Higgins & Green, 2011); also see Chapters 19 and 20.

A well done meta-analysis assesses for bias in studies and provides clinicians a means of deciding the merit of a body of clinical research. Besides the repository of meta-analyses found in The Cochrane Library published by The Cochrane Collaboration (see Appendix E), meta-analyses can be found published in journals. For example, Cullen and colleagues (2011) conducted a meta-analysis with studies that assessed the feasibility and safety of prehospital hypothermia via data extraction from randomized controlled studies. The article presents

| Study or Subgroup | One Counselling Session | | | No Counselling | | Std. Mean Difference | | Std. Mean Difference |
|---|---|---|---|---|---|---|---|---|
| | N | Mean (SD) | | N | Mean (SD) | IV, Fixed, 95% CI | Weight | IV, Fixed, 95% CI |
| **1 Anxiety** | | | | | | | | |
| Lee 1996 | 21 | 7.4 (5.9) | | 18 | 8.1 (6.2) | | 37.3% | −0.11 [ −0.74, 0.52 ] |
| Nikcevic 2007 | 33 | 5.6 (4.5) | | 33 | 7 (4.4) | | 62.7% | −0.31 [ −0.80, 0.17 ] |
| **Subtotal (95% CI)** | **54** | | | **51** | | | **100.0%** | **−0.24 [ −0.62, 0.15 ]** |
| Heterogeneity: Chi² = 0.24, df = 1 (P = 0.63); I² = 0.0% | | | | | | | | |
| Test for overall effect: Z = 1.21 (P = 0.23) | | | | | | | | |
| **2 Depression** | | | | | | | | |
| Lee 1996 | 21 | 3.2 (4.2) | | 18 | 4.8 (7) | | 36.9% | −0.28 [ −0.91, 0.36 ] |
| Nikcevic 2007 | 33 | 2.8 (4.1) | | 33 | 3.7 (3.7) | | 63.1% | −0.23 [ −0.71, 0.26 ] |
| **Subtotal (95% CI)** | **54** | | | **51** | | | **100.0%** | **−0.25 [ −0.63, 0.14 ]** |
| Heterogeneity: Chi² = 0.01, df = 1 (P = 0.90); I² = 0.0% | | | | | | | | |
| Test for overall effect: Z = 1.21 (P = 0.21) | | | | | | | | |
| **3 Grief** | | | | | | | | |
| Adolfsson 2006 | 43 | 31 (19.2) | | 45 | 32.7 (20) | | 57.2% | −0.09 [ −0.50, 0.33 ] |
| Nikcevic 2007 | 33 | 39.9 (12.4) | | 33 | 42 (13.4) | | 42.8% | −0.16 [ −0.64, 0.32 ] |
| **Subtotal (95% CI)** | **76** | | | **78** | | | **100.0%** | **−0.12 [ −0.43, 0.20 ]** |
| Heterogeneity: Chi² = 0.05, df = 1 (P = 0.82); I² = 0.0% | | | | | | | | |
| Test for overall effect: Z = 0.73 (P = 0.46) | | | | | | | | |
| **4 Avoidance** | | | | | | | | |
| Lee 1996 | 21 | 13.5 (12) | | 18 | 11.4 (11.3) | | 100.0% | 0.18 [ −0.45, 0.81 ] |
| **Subtotal (95% CI)** | **21** | | | **18** | | | **100.0%** | **0.18 [ −0.45, 0.81 ]** |
| Heterogeneity: not applicable | | | | | | | | |
| Test for overall effect: Z = 0.55 (P = 0.58) | | | | | | | | |
| **5 Intrusion** | | | | | | | | |
| Lee 1996 | 21 | 13.2 (11.3) | | 18 | 18.1 (11.5) | | 100.0% | −0.42 [ −1.06, 0.22 ] |
| **Subtotal (95% CI)** | **21** | | | **18** | | | **100.0%** | **−0.42 [ −1.06, 0.22 ]** |
| Heterogeneity: not applicable | | | | | | | | |
| Test for overall effect: Z = 1.30 (P = 0.20) | | | | | | | | |
| **6 Difficulty in Coping** | | | | | | | | |
| Adolfsson 2006 | 43 | 21.7 (13.2) | | 45 | 22.9 (15.8) | | 100.0% | −0.08 [ −0.50, 0.34 ] |
| **Subtotal (95% CI)** | **43** | | | **45** | | | **100.0%** | **−0.08 [ −0.50, 0.34 ]** |
| Heterogeneity: not applicable | | | | | | | | |
| Test for overall effect: Z = 0.38 (P = 0.70) | | | | | | | | |
| **7 Despair** | | | | | | | | |
| Adolfsson 2006 | 43 | 20.7 (13.5) | | 45 | 20.6 (13.8) | | 100.0% | 0.01 [ −0.41, 0.43 ] |
| **Subtotal (95% CI)** | **43** | | | **45** | | | **100.0%** | **0.01 [ −0.41, 0.43 ]** |
| Heterogeneity: not applicable | | | | | | | | |
| Test for overall effect: Z = 0.03 (P = 0.97) | | | | | | | | |
| **8 Self Blame** | | | | | | | | |
| Nikcevic 2007 | 33 | 5.7 (3.6) | | 33 | 5.6 (3.2) | | 100.0% | 0.03 [ −0.45, 0.51 ] |
| **Subtotal (95% CI)** | **33** | | | **33** | | | **100.0%** | **0.03 [ −0.45, 0.51 ]** |
| Heterogeneity: not applicable | | | | | | | | |
| Test for overall effect: Z = 0.12 (P = 0.91) | | | | | | | | |
| **9 Worry** | | | | | | | | |
| Nikcevic 2007 | 33 | 11.9 (3.3) | | 33 | 13.5 (4.1) | | 100.0% | −0.42 [ −0.91, 0.06 ] |
| **Subtotal (95% CI)** | **33** | | | **33** | | | **100.0%** | **−0.42 [ −0.91, 0.06 ]** |
| Heterogeneity: not applicable | | | | | | | | |
| Test for overall effect: Z = 1.71 (P = 0.088) | | | | | | | | |
| Test for subgroup differences: Chi² = 4.59, df = 8 (P = 0.80); I² = 0.0% | | | | | | | | |

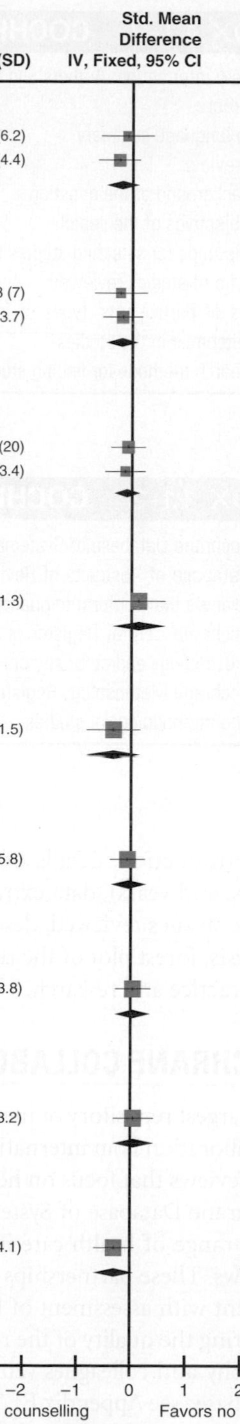

−2    −1    0    1    2

Favors counselling          Favors no counselling

**FIGURE 11-1** An example of a forest plot.

---

**BOX 11-2    COCHRANE REVIEW SECTIONS**

Review information: Authors and contact person
Abstract
Plain language summary
The review:
   Background of the question
   Objectives of the search
   Methods for selecting studies for review
   Type of studies reviewed
Types of participants, types of intervention, types of
   outcomes in the studies
   Search methods for finding studies

Data collection
Analysis of the located studies, including effect sizes
Results including description of studies, risk of bias,
   intervention effects
Discussion
Implications for research and practice
References and tables to display the data
   Supplementary information (e.g., appendices, data
   analysis

---

**BOX 11-3    COCHRANE LIBRARY DATABASES**

- Cochrane Database of Systematic Reviews: Full-text Cochrane reviews
- Database of Abstracts of Review of Effects (DARE): Critical assessments and abstracts of other systematic reviews that conform to quality criteria
- Cochrane Central Register of Controlled Trials (CENTRAL): Information of studies published in conference proceedings and other sources not available in other databases
- Cochrane Methodology Register (CMR): Bibliographic information on articles and books on reviewing research and methodological studies

---

an introduction, details of the methods used to search the literature (databases, search terms, and years), data extraction, and analysis. The article also includes an evidence table of the studies reviewed, description of how the data were summarized, results of the meta-analysis, forest plot of the reviewed studies (see Chapter 19), conclusions, and implications for practice and research.

## COCHRANE COLLABORATION

The largest repository of meta-analyses is the Cochrane Collaboration/Review. The Cochrane Collaboration is an international organization that prepares and maintains a body of systematic reviews that focus on health care interventions (Box 11-2). The reviews are found in the Cochrane Database of Systematic Reviews. The Cochrane Collaboration collaborates with a wide range of health care individuals with different skills and backgrounds for developing reviews. These partnerships assist with developing reviews that minimize bias while keeping current with assessment of health care interventions, promoting access to the database, and ensuring the quality of the reviews (Cochrane Handbook for Systematic Reviews, 2011). The Murphy and colleagues (2012) meta-analysis can be found in the Cochrane Collaboration Database (see Appendix E). The steps of a Cochrane Report mirror those of a standard meta-analysis except for the plain language summary. This useful feature is a straightforward summary of the meta-analysis. The Cochrane Library also publishes several other useful databases (Box 11-3).

> **BOX 11-4   INTEGRATIVE REVIEW EXAMPLES**
>
> - Cahill and colleagues (2012) published an integrative review of brain tumor symptoms as an antecedent to uncertainty. This review included a purpose, description of the methods used (databases searched, years included), key terms used, and parameters of the search. These components allow others to evaluate and replicate the search. Twenty-one nonexperimental design studies that assessed brain tumor symptoms and uncertainty were found and reviewed in the text and via a table format.
> - Kestler & LoBiondo-Wood (2012) published an integrative review of symptom experience in children and adolescents with cancer. The review was a follow-up of a 2003 review published by Docherty (2003) and was completed to assess the progress that has been made since the 2003 research publication on the symptoms of pediatric oncology patients. The review included a description of the search strategy used including databases, years searched, terms used, and the results of the search. Literature on each symptom was described, and a table of the 52 studies reviewed was included.

## INTEGRATIVE REVIEW

You will also find critical reviews of an area of research without a statistical analysis or a theory synthesis termed **integrative reviews.** An integrative review is the broadest category of review (Whittemore, 2005; Whittemore & Knafl, 2005). It can include theoretical literature, research literature, or both. An integrative review may include methodology studies, a theory review, or the results of differing research studies with wide-ranging clinical implications (Whittemore, 2005). An integrative review can include quantitative or qualitative research, or both. Statistics are not used to summarize and generate conclusions about the studies. Several examples of an integrative review are found in Box 11-4. Recommendations for future research are suggested in each review.

## TOOLS FOR EVALUATING INDIVIDUAL STUDIES

As the importance of practicing from a base of evidence has grown, so has the need to have tools or instruments available that can assist practitioners in evaluating studies of various types. When evaluating studies for clinical evidence, it is first important to assess if the study is valid. At the end of each chapter of this text are critiquing questions that will aid you in assessing if studies are valid and if the results are applicable to your practice. In addition to these questions, there are standardized appraisal tools that can assist with appraising the evidence. The international collaboration Critical Appraisal Skills Programme (CASP), whose focus is on teaching critical appraisal, developed tools known as Critical Appraisal Skills Programme Checklists that provide an evidence-based approach for assessing the quality, quantity, and consistency of specific study designs (CASP, 2012). These instruments are part of an international network that provides consumers with specific questions to help assess study quality. Each checklist has a number of general questions as well as design-specific questions. The tools center on assessing a study's methodology, validity, and reliability. The questions focus on the following:

1. Are the study's results valid? Understanding the steps of *research methodology,* especially threats to internal validity as described in the previous and subsequent chapters, will assist in this process (see Chapters 8 through 16).
2. What are the results? This means can you rely on the results (analysis) or the study's findings (see Chapters 16 and 17).

3. Are the findings applicable to your practice? Chapters 19 and 20 are aimed at helping you with this decision.

Each CASP guideline is divided into one of the above three areas in a study. There are eight critical appraisal checklists. The checklist with instructions can be found at www.casp-uk-net. The design specific **CASP tools** with checklists are available online and include:

- Systematic reviews
- Randomized controlled studies
- Cohort studies
- Diagnostic studies
- Case-control studies
- Economic evaluations
- Qualitative studies
- Clinical prediction rule

## CLINICAL PRACTICE GUIDELINES

**Clinical practice guidelines** are systematically developed statements or recommendations that link research and practice and serve as a guide for practitioners. Guidelines have been developed to assist in bridging practice and research. Guidelines are developed by professional organizations, government agencies, institutions, or convened expert panels. Guidelines provide clinicians with an algorithm for clinical management, or decision making for specific diseases (e.g., colon cancer) or treatments (e.g., pain management). Not all guidelines are well developed and, like research, must be assessed before implementation (see Chapter 9). Guidelines should present scope and purpose of the practice, detail who the development group included, demonstrate scientific rigor, be clear in its presentation, demonstrate clinical applicability, and demonstrate editorial independence. An example is the National Comprehensive Cancer Network, which is an interdisciplinary consortium of 21 cancer centers across the world. Interdisciplinary groups develop practice guidelines for practitioners and education guidelines for patients. These guidelines are accessible at www.nccn.org.

The research findings in a clinical practice guideline need to be evaluated for quality, quantity, and consistency. Practice guidelines can be either expert-based or evidence-based. **Evidence-based practice guidelines** are those developed using a scientific process. This process includes first assembling a multidisciplinary group of experts in a specific field. This group is charged with completing a rigorous search of the literature and completing an evidence table that summarizes the quality and strength of the evidence on which the practice guideline is derived (see Chapters 19 and 20). For various reasons, not all areas of clinical practice have a sufficient research base; therefore, **expert-based practice guidelines** are developed. Expert-based guidelines depend on having a group of nationally known experts in the field who meet and solely use opinions of experts along with whatever research evidence is developed to date. If limited research is available for such a guideline, a rationale should be presented for the practice recommendations.

Many national organizations develop clinical practice guidelines. It is important to know which one to apply to your patient population. For example, there are numerous evidence-based practice guidelines developed for the management of pain. These guidelines are available from organizations such as the Oncology Nurses Society, American Academy of Pediatrics, National Comprehensive Cancer Network, National Cancer Institute, American College of Physicians, and American Academy of Pain Medicine. You, as a consumer of evidence, need to be able to evaluate each of the guidelines and decide which is the most appropriate for your patient population.

The Agency for Healthcare Research and Quality supports the National Guideline Clearinghouse (NGC). The NGC's mission is to provide health care professionals from all disciplines with objective, detailed information on clinical practice guidelines that are disseminated, implemented, and issued. The NGC encourages groups to develop guidelines for implementation via their site; it is a very useful site to find well-developed clinical guidelines on a wide range of health- and illness-related topics. Specific guidelines can be found on the AHRQ Effective Health Care Program website.

## EVALUATING CLINICAL PRACTICE GUIDELINES

As the number of evidence-based practice guidelines proliferate, it becomes increasingly important that you critique these guidelines with regard to the methods used for guideline formulation and consider how they might be used in practice. Critical areas that should be assessed when critiquing evidence-based practice guidelines include the following:

- Date of publication or release and authors
- Endorsement of the guideline
- Clear purpose of what the guideline covers and patient groups for which it was designed
- Types of evidence (research, nonresearch) used in guideline formulation
- Types of research included in formulating the guideline (e.g., "We considered only randomized and other prospective controlled trials in determining efficacy of therapeutic interventions.")
- Description of the methods used in grading the evidence
- Search terms and retrieval methods used to acquire evidence used in the guideline
- Well-referenced statements regarding practice
- Comprehensive reference list
- Review of the guideline by experts
- Whether the guideline has been used or tested in practice, and if so, with what types of patients and what types of settings

Evidence-based practice guidelines that are formulated using rigorous methods provide a useful starting point for nurses to understand the evidence base of practice. However, more research may be available since the publication of the guideline, and refinements may be needed. Although information in well-developed, national, evidence-based practice guidelines are a helpful reference, it is usually necessary to localize the guideline using institution-specific evidence-based policies, procedures, or standards before application within a specific setting.

There are several tools for appraising the quality of clinical practice guidelines. The **Appraisal of Guidelines Research and Evaluation II (AGREE II)** instrument is one of the most widely used to evaluate the applicability of a guideline to practice (Brouwers et al., AGREE Collaboration, 2010). The AGREE II was developed to assist in evaluating guideline quality, provide a methodological strategy for guideline development, and inform practitioners about what information should be reported in guidelines and how it should be reported. The AGREE II is available online and replaces the original AGREE tool. The instrument focuses on six domains with a total of 23 questions rated on a 7-point scale and two final assessment items that require the appraiser to make overall judgments of the guideline based on how the 23 items were rated. Along with the instrument itself, the

---

**CRITIQUING CRITERIA**

***Systematic Reviews***

1. Does the PICO question used as the basis of the review match the studies included in the review?
2. Are the review methods clearly stated and comprehensive?
3. Are the dates of the review's inclusion clear and relevant to the area reviewed?
4. Are the inclusion and exclusion criteria for studies in the review clear and comprehensive?
5. What criteria were used to assess each of the studies in the review for quality and scientific merit?
6. If studies were analyzed individually, were the data clear?
7. Were the methods of study combination clear and appropriate?
8. If the studies were reviewed collectively, how large was the effect?
9. Are the clinical conclusions drawn from the studies relevant and supported by the review?

---

AGREE Enterprise website offers guidance on tool usage and development. The AGREE II has been tested for reliability and validity. The guideline assesses the following components of a practice guideline:

1. Scope and purpose of the guideline
2. Stakeholder involvement
3. Rigor of the guideline development
4. Clarity and presentation of the guideline
5. Applicability of the guideline to practice
6. Demonstrated editorial independence of the developers

Clinical practice guidelines, although they are systematically developed and make explicit recommendations for practice, may be formatted differently. Practice guidelines should reflect the components listed. Guidelines can be located on an organization's website, at the AHRQ, on the National Guideline Clearinghouse website (www.AHRQ.gov), or on MEDLINE (see Chapters 3 and 20). Well-developed guidelines are constructed using the principles of a systematic review.

# APPRAISING THE EVIDENCE
## SYSTEMATIC REVIEWS AND CLINICAL GUIDELINES

For each of the review methods described—systematic, meta-analysis, integrative and clinical guidelines—think about each method as one that progressively sifts and sorts research studies and the data until the highest quality of evidence is used to arrive at the conclusions. First the researcher combines the results of all the studies that focus on a specific question. The studies considered of lowest quality are then excluded and the data are re-analyzed. This process is repeated sequentially, excluding studies until only the studies of highest quality available are included in the analysis. An alteration in the overall results as an outcome of this sorting and separating process suggests how sensitive the conclusions are to the quality of studies included (Whittemore, 2005). No matter which type of review is completed, it is important to understand that the research studies reviewed still must be examined through your evidence-based practice lens. This means that evidence that you have derived through your critical appraisal and synthesis or derived through other researchers' review must be integrated with an individual clinician's expertise and patients' wishes.

You should note that a researcher who uses any of the systematic review methods of combining evidence does not conduct the original studies or analysis of data in the area, but rather takes the data from already published studies and synthesizes the information by following a set of controlled and systematic steps. Systematic methods for combining evidence are used to synthesize both nonexperimental and experimental research studies.

Finally, evidence-based practice requires that you determine—based on the strength and quality of the evidence provided by the systematic review coupled with your clinical expertise and patient values—whether or not you would consider a change in practice. For example, the meta-analysis by Murphy and colleagues (2012) in Appendix E details the important findings from the literature, some that could be used in nursing practice and some that need further research.

Systematic reviews that use multiple randomized controlled trials (RCTs) to combine study results offer stronger evidence (Level I) in estimating the magnitude of an effect for an intervention (see Chapter 2, Table 2-3). The strength of evidence provided by systematic reviews is a key component for developing a practice based on evidence. The qualitative counterpart to systematic reviews is *meta-synthesis*, which uses qualitative principles to assess qualitative research and is described in Chapter 5.

# REFERENCES

Borenstein, M., Hedges, L. V., Higgins, J. P. T., & Rothstein, H. R. (2009). *Introduction to meta-analysis.* United Kingdom: Wiley.

Brouwers, M., Kho, M. E., Browman, G. P., et al. for the AGREE Next Steps Consortium. (2010). AGREE II: advancing guideline development, reporting and evaluation in healthcare. Canadian Medical Association Journal, *182*, E839–E842. doi:10.1503/090449.

Cahill, J., LoBiondo-Wood, G., Bergstrom, N., & Armstrong, T. (2012). Brain tumor symptoms as antecedents to uncertainty: an integrative review. *Journal of Nursing Scholarship, 44*(2), 145–155. doi10.1111/j.1547-5069.2012.01445.x.

Critical Appraisal Skill Programme (CASP). (2012). *Critical appraisal skills programme: making sense of evidence.* Available at www.casp-uk.net.

Cullen, D., Augenstine, D., Kaper, L. L., et al. (2011). Therapeutic hypothermia initiated in the pre-hospital setting. *Advanced Emergency Nursing Journal, 33*(4), 314–321. doi: 10.1097/TME. ob013e3182343ch6.

Docherty, S. L. (2003). Symptom experiences of children and adolescents with cancer. *Annual Review Nursing Research, 21*(2), 123–149.

Fowles, E. R., Cheng, H. R., & Mills, S. (2012). Postpartum health promotion interventions: a systematic review. *Nursing Research, 61*(4), 269–282. doi: 10.109/NNR.0b013e3182556d29.

Higgins, J. P. T., & Green, S. (2011). *Cochrane handbook for systematic reviews of interventions version 5.1.0.* Available at http://www.cochrane-handbook.org.

Kestler, S. A., & LoBiondo-Wood, G. (2012). Review of symptom experiences in children and adolescents with cancer. *Cancer Nursing, 35*(2), E31–E49. doi:10.1097/NCC.0b013e3182207a2a.

Liberati, A., Altman, D. G., Tetzlaff, J., et al. (2009). The PRISMA statement for reporting systematic reviews and meta-analyses of studies that evaluate health care interventions: explanation and elaboration. *Annuals of Internal Medicine, 151*(4), w65–w94.

Moher, D., Liberati, A., Tetzlaff, J., & Altman, D. G. (2009). Preferred reporting items for systematic reviews and meta-analyses: the PRISMA statement. *PLOS Medicine*, Oct; *62*(10), 1006–1012, doi:10.1016/j.jclinepi.2009.06.005.

Murphy, F. A., Lipp, A., & Powles, D. L. (2012). Follow-up for improving psychological well-being for women after a miscarriage (review). *Cochrane Database System Review, 3*, 1–39.

Whittemore, R. (2005). Combining evidence in nursing research: methods and implications. *Nursing Research, 54*(1), 56–62.

Whittemore, R., & Knafl, K. (2005). The integrative review: updated methodology. *Journal of Advanced Nursing, 52*(5), 546–553.

# ⊝volve WEBSITE

*Go to Evolve at http://evolve.elsevier.com/LoBiondo/ for review questions, critiquing exercises, and additional research articles for practice in reviewing and critiquing.*

# CHAPTER 12

# Sampling

*Judith Haber*

e**volve** WEBSITE

*Go to Evolve at http://evolve.elsevier.com/LoBiondo/ for review questions, critiquing exercises, and additional research articles for practice in reviewing and critiquing.*

## LEARNING OUTCOMES

*After reading this chapter, you should be able to do the following:*

- Identify the purpose of sampling.
- Define *population, sample,* and *sampling.*
- Compare a population and a sample.
- Discuss the importance of inclusion and exclusion criteria.
- Define *nonprobability* and *probability sampling.*
- Identify the types of nonprobability and probability sampling strategies.
- Compare the advantages and disadvantages of nonprobability and probability sampling strategies.
- Discuss the contribution of nonprobability and probability sampling strategies to strength of evidence provided by study findings.
- Discuss the factors that influence determination of sample size.
- Discuss potential threats to internal and external validity as sources of sampling bias.
- Use the critiquing criteria to evaluate the "Sample" section of a research report.

## KEY TERMS

| | | | |
|---|---|---|---|
| accessible population | matching | population | sampling frame |
| convenience sampling | multistage (cluster) | probability sampling | sampling unit |
| data saturation | sampling | purposive sampling | simple random |
| delimitations | network (snowball | quota sampling | sampling |
| element | effect) sampling | random selection | snowballing |
| eligibility criteria | nonprobability | representative sample | stratified random |
| exclusion criteria | sampling | sample | sampling |
| inclusion | pilot study | sampling | target population |

The sampling section of a study is usually found in the "Methods" section of a research article. It is important for you to understand the sampling process and the ingredients that contribute to a researcher using the most appropriate sampling strategy for the type of research being conducted. Equally important, is knowing how to critically appraise the sampling section of a study to identify how the strengths and weaknesses of the sampling process contributed to the overall strength and quality of evidence provided by the findings of a study.

When you are critically appraising the sampling section of a study, the threats to internal and external validity as sources of bias need to be considered (see Chapter 8). Your evaluation of the sampling section of a study is very important in your overall critical appraisal of a study's findings and their applicability to practice.

**Sampling** is the process of selecting representative units of a population in a study. Although sampling is a complex process, it is a familiar one. In our daily lives, we gather knowledge, make decisions, and formulate predictions based on sampling procedures. For example, nursing students may make generalizations about the overall quality of nursing professors as a result of their exposure to a sample of nursing professors during their undergraduate programs. Patients may make generalizations about a hospital's food or quality of nursing care during a 3-day hospital stay. You can see how exposure to a limited portion of these experiences forms the basis of our conclusions, and how much of our knowledge and decisions are based on our experience with samples.

Researchers also derive knowledge from samples. Many problems in research cannot be solved without employing rigorous sampling procedures. For example, when testing the effectiveness of a medication for patients with asthma, the drug is administered to a sample of the population for whom the drug is potentially appropriate. The researcher must come to some conclusions without giving the drug to every patient with asthma or laboratory animal. But because human lives are at stake, the researcher cannot afford to arrive casually at conclusions that are based on the first dozen patients available for study.

The impact of arriving at conclusions that are not accurate or making generalizations from a small nonrepresentative sample is much more severe in research than in everyday life. Essentially, researchers sample representative segments of the population because it is rarely feasible or necessary to sample the entire population of interest to obtain relevant information.

This chapter will familiarize you with the basic concepts of sampling as they primarily pertain to the principles of quantitative research design, nonprobability and probability sampling, sample size, and the related appraisal process. Sampling issues that relate to qualitative research designs are discussed in Chapters 5, 6, and 7.

## SAMPLING CONCEPTS

### Population

A **population** is a well-defined set that has specified properties. A population can be composed of people, animals, objects, or events. Examples of clinical populations might be all of the female patients older than 65 years admitted to a certain hospital for congestive heart failure (CHF) during the year 2013, all of the children with asthma in the state of New York, or all of the men and women with a diagnosis of clinical depression in the United States. These examples illustrate that a population may be broadly defined and potentially involve millions of people or narrowly specified to include only several hundred people.

The population criteria establish the **target population**; that is, the entire set of cases about which the researcher would like to make generalizations. A target population might include all undergraduate nursing students enrolled in accelerated baccalaureate programs in the United States. Because of time, money, and personnel, however, it is often not feasible to pursue a study using a target population.

An **accessible population,** one that meets the target population criteria and that is available, is used instead. For example, an accessible population might include all full-time accelerated baccalaureate students attending school in Ohio. Pragmatic factors must also be considered when identifying a potential population of interest.

It is important to know that a population is not restricted to humans. It may consist of hospital records; blood, urine, or other specimens taken from patients at a clinic; historical documents; or laboratory animals. For example, a population might consist of all the $HgbA_{1C}$ blood test specimens collected from patients in the Upper City Hospital diabetes clinic or all of the patient charts on file who had been screened during pregnancy for HIV infection. It is apparent that a population can be defined in a variety of ways. The important point to remember is that the basic unit of the population must be clearly defined because the generalizability of the findings will be a function of the population criteria.

## Inclusion and Exclusion Criteria

When reading a research report, you should consider whether the researcher has identified the population characteristics that form the basis for the inclusion (eligibility) or exclusion (delimitations) criteria used to select the sample—whether people, objects, or events. The terms **inclusion** or **eligibility criteria** and **exclusion criteria** or **delimitations** are applied to define attributes that restrict the population to a homogenous group of subjects. The population characteristics that provide the basis for inclusion (eligibility) criteria should be evident in the sample; that is, the characteristics of the population and the sample should be congruent. Examples of inclusion or eligibility criteria and exclusion criteria or delimitations include the following: gender, age, marital status, socioeconomic status, religion, ethnicity, level of education, age of children, health status, and diagnosis. The degree of congruence between the criteria and the population is evaluated to assess the representativeness of the sample.

Think about the concept of inclusion or eligibility criteria applied to a study where the subjects are patients. For example, participants in a study investigating the effectiveness of a motivational-interviewing–based coaching intervention compared to usual care to improve cancer pain management (Thomas et al., 2012; see Appendix A) had to meet the following inclusion (eligibility) criteria:

1. Age: at least 21 years
2. Pain Intensity Status: pain intensity score of 2 or higher on a scale of 0-10
3. Health status: life expectancy longer than 6 months
4. Available resources: access to a telephone
5. Language: read and understand the English language

Remember that inclusion and exclusion criteria are established to control for extraneous variability or bias that would limit the strength of evidence contributed by the sampling plan in relation to the study's design. Each inclusion or exclusion criterion should have a rationale, presumably related to a potential contaminating effect on the dependent variable. For example, subjects were excluded from this study if they had:

- A concurrent cognitive or psychiatric condition or substance abuse problem that would prevent adherence to the protocol

- Severe pain unrelated to their cancer
- A housing setting where the patient could not self-administer pain medication (e.g., skilled nursing facility)

The careful establishment of sample inclusion or exclusion criteria will increase the study's precision and strength of evidence, thereby contributing to the accuracy and generalizability of the findings (see Chapter 8).

---

**HELPFUL HINT**

Often, researchers do not clearly identify the population under study, or the population is not clarified until the "Discussion" section when the effort is made to discuss the group (population) to which the study findings can be generalized.

---

## Samples and Sampling

Sampling is a process of selecting a portion or subset of the designated population to represent the entire population. A **sample** is a set of elements that make up the population; an **element** is the most basic unit about which information is collected. The most common element in nursing research is individuals, but other elements (e.g., places, objects) can form the basis of a sample or population. For example, a researcher was planning a study that compared the effectiveness of different nursing interventions on reducing falls in the elderly in long-term care facilities (LTCs). Four LTCs, each using a different falls prevention treatment protocol, were identified as the sampling units rather than the nurses themselves or the treatment alone.

The purpose of sampling is to increase a study's efficiency. As a new evaluator of research you must realize that it would not be feasible to examine every element in the population. When sampling is done properly, the researcher can draw inferences and make generalizations about the population without examining each element in the population. Sampling procedures that formulate specific criteria for selection ensure that the characteristics of the phenomena of interest will be, or are likely to be, present in all of the units being studied. The researcher's efforts to ensure that the sample is representative of the target population strengthens the evidence generated by the sample composition, which puts the researcher in a stronger position to draw conclusions that are generalizable to the population and applicable to practice (see Chapter 8).

After having reviewed a number of research studies, you will recognize that samples and sampling procedures vary in terms of merit. The foremost criterion in appraising a sample is its representativeness. A **representative sample** is one whose key characteristics closely approximate those of the population. If 70% of the population in a study of child-rearing

---

**EVIDENCE-BASED PRACTICE TIP**

Consider whether the choice of participants was biased, thereby influencing the strength of evidence provided by the outcomes of the study.

| | | | |
|---|---|---|---|
| TABLE 12-1 | **SUMMARY OF SAMPLING STRATEGIES** | | |

| SAMPLING STRATEGY | EASE OF DRAWING SAMPLE | RISK OF BIAS | REPRESENTATIVENESS OF SAMPLE |
|---|---|---|---|
| **NONPROBABILITY** | | | |
| Convenience | Easy | Greater than any other sampling strategy | Because samples tend to be self-selecting, representativeness is questionable |
| Quota | Relatively easy | Contains unknown source of bias that affects external validity | Builds in some representativeness by using knowledge about population of interest |
| Purposive | Relatively easy | Bias increases with greater heterogeneity of population; conscious bias is also a danger | Very limited ability to generalize because sample is handpicked |
| **PROBABILITY** | | | |
| Simple random | Time consuming | Low | Maximized; probability of nonrepresentativeness decreases with increased sample size |
| Stratified random | Time consuming | Low | Enhanced |
| Cluster | Less or more time consuming depending on the strata | Subject to more sampling errors than simple or stratified | Less representative than simple or stratified |

practices consisted of women and 40% were full-time employees, a representative sample should reflect these characteristics in the same proportions.

## TYPES OF SAMPLES

Sampling strategies are generally grouped into two categories: nonprobability sampling and probability sampling. In **nonprobability sampling**, elements are chosen by nonrandom methods. The drawback of this strategy is that there is no way of estimating each element's probability of being included in a particular sample. Essentially, there is no way of ensuring that every element has a chance for inclusion in the nonprobability sample.

Probability sampling uses some form of random selection when the sample is chosen. This type of sample enables the researcher to estimate the probability that each element of the population will be included in the sample. Probability sampling is the more rigorous type of sampling strategy and is more likely to result in a representative sample. The remainder of this section is devoted to a discussion of different types of nonprobability and probability sampling strategies. A summary of sampling strategies appears in Table 12-1. You may wish to refer to this table as the various nonprobability and probability strategies are discussed in the following sections.

| |
|---|
| **EVIDENCE-BASED PRACTICE TIP** |
| Determining whether the sample is representative of the population being studied will influence your interpretation of the evidence provided by the findings and decision making about their relevance to the patient population and practice setting. |

## Nonprobability Sampling

Because of lack of randomization, the findings of studies using nonprobability sampling are less generalizable than those using a probability sampling strategy, and they tend to produce fewer representative samples. Such samples are easier for the researcher to obtain, however, and many samples—not only in nursing research, but also in other disciplines—are nonprobability samples. When a nonprobability sample is carefully chosen to reflect the target population through the careful use of inclusion and exclusion criteria and adequate sample size, you can have more confidence in the sample's representativeness and the external validity of the findings. The three major types of nonprobability sampling are convenience, quota, and purposive sampling strategies.

## Convenience Sampling

Convenience sampling is the use of the most readily accessible persons or objects as subjects. The subjects may include volunteers, the first 100 patients admitted to hospital X with a particular diagnosis, all of the people enrolled in program Y during the month of September, or all of the students enrolled in course Z at a particular university during 2014. The subjects are convenient and accessible to the researcher and are thus called a *convenience sample.* For example, a researcher studying the relationship among maternal-fetal attachment (MFA), health practices during pregnancy, and neonatal outcomes in a sample of low-income predominantly African-American women and their neonates recruited a convenience sample of 167 women from three urban obstetrical clinics in the Mid Atlantic region who met the eligibility criteria and volunteered to participate in the study (Alhusen et al., 2012; see Appendix B).

The advantage of a convenience sample is that generally it is easier for the researcher to obtain subjects. The researcher may have to be concerned only with obtaining a sufficient number of subjects who meet the same criteria. A convenience sample may be the most appropriate sampling strategy to use even though it is not the strongest approach. The major disadvantage of a convenience sample is that the risk of bias is greater than in any other type of sample (see Table 12-1). The fact that convenience samples use voluntary participation increases the probability of researchers recruiting those people who feel strongly about the issue being studied, which may favor certain outcomes (Sousa et al., 2004). In this case, you can ask yourself the following as you think about the strength and quality of evidence contributed by the sampling component of a study:

- What motivated some people to participate and others not to participate (self-selection)?
- What kind of data would have been obtained if nonparticipants had also responded?
- How representative are the people who did participate in relation to the population?
- What kind of confidence can you have in the evidence provided by the findings?

Researchers may recruit subjects when they stop people on a street corner to ask their opinion on some issue, place advertisements in the newspaper, or place signs in local

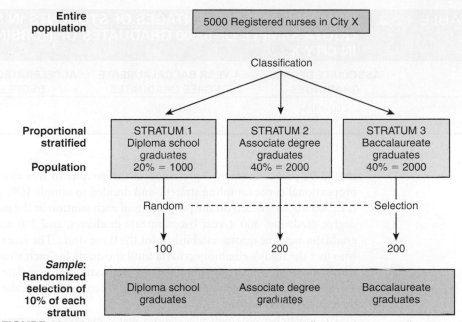

FIGURE 12-1 Subject selection using a proportional stratified random sampling strategy.

churches, community centers, or supermarkets indicating that volunteers are needed for a particular study. To assess the degree to which a convenience sample approximates a random sample, the researcher checks for the representativeness of the convenience sample by comparing the sample to population percentages and, in that way, assesses the extent to which bias is or is not evident (Sousa et al., 2004).

Because acquiring research subjects is a problem that confronts many nurse researchers, innovative recruitment strategies may be used. A unique method of accessing and recruiting subjects is the use of online computer networks (e.g., disease-specific chat rooms, blogs, and bulletin boards). In the evidence hierarchy in Figure 1-1, nonprobability sampling is most commonly associated with quantitative nonexperimental or qualitative studies that contribute Level IV through Level VI evidence.

When you appraise a study you should recognize that the convenience sample strategy, although the most common, is the weakest sampling strategy with regard to strength of evidence and generalizability. When a convenience sample is used, caution should be exercised in interpreting the data. When critiquing a study that has employed this sampling strategy, the reviewer should be justifiably skeptical about the external validity and applicability of the findings (see Chapter 8).

## Quota Sampling

**Quota sampling** refers to a form of nonprobability sampling in which knowledge about the population of interest is used to build some representativeness into the sample (see Table 12-1). A quota sample identifies the strata of the population and proportionally represents the strata in the sample. For example, the data in Table 12-2 reveal that 40% of the 5000 nurses in city X are associate degree graduates, 30% are 4-year baccalaureate degree graduates, and 30% are accelerated baccalaureate graduates. Each stratum of the population

| TABLE 12-2 | NUMBERS AND PERCENTAGES OF STUDENTS IN STRATA OF A QUOTA SAMPLE OF 5,000 GRADUATES OF NURSING PROGRAMS IN CITY X | | |
|---|---|---|---|
| | ASSOCIATE DEGREE GRADUATES | 4-YEAR BACCALAUREATE DEGREE GRADUATES | ACCELERATED BACCALAUREATE DEGREE GRADUATES |
| Population | 2,000 (40%) | 1,500 (30%) | 1,500 (30%) |
| Strata | 200 | 150 | 150 |

should be proportionately represented in the sample. In this case, the researcher used a proportional quota sampling strategy and decided to sample 10% of a population of 5000 (i.e., 500 nurses). Based on the proportion of each stratum in the population, 400 associate degree graduates, 300 4-year baccalaureate graduates, and 300 accelerated baccalaureate graduates were the quotas established for the three strata. The researcher recruited subjects who met the study's eligibility criteria until the quota for each stratum was filled. In other words, once the researcher obtained the necessary 400 associate degree graduates, 300 4-year baccalaureate degree graduates, and 300 accelerated baccalaureate degree graduates, the sample was complete.

The researcher systematically ensures that proportional segments of the population are included in the sample. The quota sample is not randomly selected (i.e., once the proportional strata have been identified, the researcher recruits and enrolls subjects until the quota for each stratum has been filled) but does increase the sample's representativeness. This sampling strategy addresses the problem of overrepresentation or underrepresentation of certain segments of a population in a sample.

The characteristics chosen to form the strata are selected according to a researcher's knowledge of the population and the literature review. The criterion for selection should be a variable that reflects important differences in the dependent variables under investigation. Age, gender, religion, ethnicity, medical diagnosis, socioeconomic status, level of completed education, and occupational rank are among the variables that are likely to be important stratifying variables in nursing research studies. For example, Im and colleagues (2012) conducted a national Internet survey on midlife women's attitudes toward physical activity and stratified a quota sample of 542 subjects by ethnicity and socioeconomic status (SES). When the ethnicity or SES of the stratum did not need more participants, the participants received an electronic message saying, "Thank you, but the group you belong to is already filled."

As you critically appraise a study, your aim is to determine whether the sample strata appropriately reflect the population under consideration and whether the stratifying variables are homogeneous enough to ensure a meaningful comparison of differences among strata. Establishment of strict inclusion and exclusion criteria and using power analysis to determine appropriate sample size increase the rigor of a quota sampling strategy by creating homogeneous subject categories that facilitate making meaningful comparisons across strata.

### Purposive Sampling

Purposive sampling is a common strategy. The researcher selects subjects who are considered to be typical of the population. When a researcher is considering the sampling strategy

---

**BOX 12-1**   **CRITERIA FOR USE OF A PURPOSIVE SAMPLING STRATEGY**

- Effective pretesting of newly developed instruments with a purposive sample of divergent types of people
- Validation of a scale or test with a known-group technique
- Collection of exploratory data in relation to an unusual or highly specific population, particularly when the total target population remains an unknown to the researcher
- Collection of descriptive data (e.g., as in qualitative studies) that seek to describe the lived experience of a particular phenomenon (e.g., postpartum depression, caring, hope, surviving childhood sexual abuse)
- Focus of the study population relates to a specific diagnosis (e.g., type 1 diabetes, ovarian cancer) or condition (e.g., legal blindness, terminal illness) or demographic characteristic (e.g., same-sex twin pairs)

---

for a randomized clinical trial focusing on a specific diagnosis or patient population, the sampling strategy is often purposive in nature. For example, Sherman and colleagues (2012) explored the differential effect of a phase-specific psychoeducation and telephone counseling intervention on the emotional, social, and physical adjustment of women with breast cancer. A purposive sample in which 249 patients with early stage breast cancer were randomly assigned to one of four groups: one control group and three intervention groups.

Purposive sampling is also commonly used in qualitative research studies. For example, the purpose of the qualitative study by Seiler and Moss (2012; see Appendix C) was to gain insight into the unique experiences of nurse practitioners (NPs) who provide health care to homeless people. A purposive sample of nine NPs practicing at least 6 months were recruited through NP managed clinics in the Midwest that provided health care for the homeless. The NP subjects were chosen because they were typical (homogeneous) of the population under study, which enhances the representativeness of this sampling strategy used to describe a specific, and sometimes underrepresented, population.

A purposive sample is used also when a highly unusual group is being studied, such as a population with a rare genetic disease (e.g., Huntington's chorea). In this case, the researcher would describe the sample characteristics precisely to ensure that the reader will have an accurate picture of the subjects in the sample.

Today, computer networks (e.g., online services) can be of great value in helping researchers access and recruit subjects for purposive samples. Online support group bulletin boards that facilitate recruitment of subjects for purposive samples exist for people with cancer, rheumatoid arthritis, systemic lupus erythematosus, human immunodeficiency virus/acquired immunodeficiency syndrome (HIV/AIDS), bipolar disorder, Lyme disease, and many others.

The researcher who uses a purposive sample assumes that errors of judgment in overrepresenting or underrepresenting elements of the population in the sample will tend to balance out. There is no objective method, however, for determining the validity of this assumption. You should be aware that the more heterogeneous the population, the greater the chance of bias being introduced in the selection of a purposive sample. As indicated in Table 12-1, conscious bias in the selection of subjects remains a constant danger. Therefore the findings from a study using a purposive sample should be regarded with caution. As with any nonprobability sample, the ability to generalize from the evidence provided by the findings is very limited. Box 12-1 lists examples of when a purposive sample may be appropriate.

---

**HELPFUL HINT**

When purposive sampling is used as the first step in recruiting a sample for a randomized clinical trial, as illustrated in Figure 12-1, it is often followed by random assignment of subjects to an intervention or control group, which increases the generalizability of the findings.

---

## Probability Sampling

The primary characteristic of **probability sampling** is the random selection of elements from the population. **Random selection** occurs when each element of the population has an equal and independent chance of being included in the sample. In an evidence hierarchy, probability sampling, which is most closely associated with experimental and quasi-experimental designs, represents the strongest sampling type. The research consumer has greater confidence that the sample is representative rather than biased and more closely reflects the characteristics of the population of interest. Three commonly used probability sampling strategies are: simple random, stratified random, and cluster.

Random selection of sample subjects should not be confused with random assignment of subjects. The latter, as discussed in Chapter 8, refers to the assignment of subjects to either an experimental or a control group on a purely random basis.

## Simple Random Sampling

**Simple random sampling** is a carefully controlled process. The researcher defines the population (a set), lists all of the units of the population (a **sampling frame**), and selects a sample of units (a subset) from which the sample will be chosen. For example, if American hospitals specializing in the treatment of cancer were the sampling unit, a list of all such hospitals would be the sampling frame. If certified critical care nurses (CCRNs) constituted the accessible population, a list of those nurses would be the sampling frame.

Once a list of the population elements has been developed, the best method of selecting a random sample is to use a computer program that generates the order in which the random selection of subjects is to be carried out.

The advantages of simple random sampling are as follows:

- Sample selection is not subject to the conscious biases of the researcher.
- Representativeness of the sample in relation to the population characteristics is maximized.
- Differences in the characteristics of the sample and the population are purely a function of chance.
- Probability of choosing a nonrepresentative sample decreases as the size of the sample increases.

Simple random sampling was used in a study examining whether rural and urban nurse practitioner attitudes and treatment practices for childhood overweight and obesity differ (Hessler & Siegrist, 2012). Of interest to the researchers were differences in the following:

- Rural and urban NP attitudes toward overweight and obese pediatric patients
- Strategies used to assess and treat overweight and obese pediatric patients
- Resources available to NPs for treatment and referral of overweight and obese pediatric patients

The membership services of the American Academy of Nurse Practitioners (AANP) mailing list provided the participants for the study. A random sample of 7000 family and pediatric nurse practitioners were drawn from the AANP membership list of 25,000 that represented NPs in all 50 states. Inspection of the final random sample indicated that NPs from all 50 states were represented in the sample.

When appraising the sample of a study, you must remember that despite the use of a carefully controlled sampling procedure that minimizes error, there is no guarantee that the sample will be representative. Factors such as sample heterogeneity and subject dropout may jeopardize the representativeness of the sample despite the most stringent random sampling procedure.

The major disadvantage of simple random sampling is that it can be a time-consuming and inefficient method of obtaining a random sample; for example, consider the task of listing all of the baccalaureate nursing students in the United States. With random sampling, it may also be impossible to obtain an accurate or complete listing of every element in the population; for example, imagine trying to obtain a list of all completed suicides in New York City for the year 2012. It often is the case that although suicide may have been the cause of death, another cause (e.g., cardiac failure) appears on the death certificate. It would be difficult to estimate how many elements of the target population would be eliminated from consideration. The issue of bias would definitely enter the picture despite the researcher's best efforts. In the final analysis, you, as the evaluator of a research article, must be cautious about generalizing from reported findings, even when random sampling is the stated strategy, if the target population has been difficult or impossible to list completely.

## EVIDENCE-BASED PRACTICE TIP

When thinking about applying study findings to your clinical practice, consider whether the participants making up the sample are similar to your own patients.

### Stratified Random Sampling

Stratified random sampling requires that the population be divided into strata or subgroups as illustrated in Figure 12-1 on p. 237. The subgroups or subsets that the population is divided into are homogeneous. An appropriate number of elements from each subset are randomly selected on the basis of their proportion in the population. The goal of this strategy is to achieve a greater degree of representativeness. Stratified random sampling is similar to the proportional stratified quota sampling strategy discussed earlier in the chapter. The major difference is that stratified random sampling uses a random selection procedure for obtaining sample subjects.

The population is stratified according to any number of attributes, such as age, gender, ethnicity, religion, socioeconomic status, or level of education completed. The variables selected to form the strata should be adaptable to homogeneous subsets with regard to the attributes being studied. For example, the prevalence of mental health issues appears to be increasing in the college student population. Stress that leads to depression may be mediated if people believe that they have the resources to manage it. A study by Sawatzky and colleagues (2012) examined the extent to which the relationship between adverse stress and depression is mediated by university students' perceived ability to manage their stress. The data were obtained via one Canadian university's spring 2006 (n = 2147) and 2008 (n = 2292) National College Health Assessment (NCHA) surveys. Students were randomly selected and then stratified according to undergraduate, graduate, or international, and by campus location.

As illustrated in Table 12-1, several advantages to a stratified sampling strategy are the following: (1) the representativeness of the sample is enhanced; (2) the researcher has a valid basis for making comparisons among subsets if information on the critical variables has been available; and (3) the researcher is able to oversample a disproportionately small stratum to adjust for their underrepresentation, statistically weigh the data accordingly, and continue to make legitimate comparisons.

The obstacles encountered by a researcher using this strategy include the following: (1) the difficulty of obtaining a population list containing complete critical variable information; (2) the time-consuming effort of obtaining multiple enumerated lists; (3) the challenge of enrolling proportional strata; and (4) the time and money involved in carrying out a large-scale study using a stratified sampling strategy.

## Multistage Sampling (Cluster Sampling)

Multistage (cluster) sampling involves a successive random sampling of units (clusters) that progress from large to small and meet sample eligibility criteria. The first-stage sampling unit consists of large units or clusters. The second-stage sampling unit consists of smaller units or clusters. Third-stage sampling units are even smaller. For example, if a sample of critical care nurses is desired, the first sampling unit would be a random sample of hospitals, obtained from an American Hospital Association list, that meet the eligibility criteria (e.g., size, type). The second-stage sampling unit would consist of a list of critical care nurses practicing at each hospital selected in the first stage (i.e., the list obtained from the vice president for nursing at each hospital). The criteria for inclusion in the list of critical care nurses would be as follows:

1. Certified as a CCRN with at least 3 years' experience as a critical care nurse
2. At least 75% of the CCRN's time spent in providing direct patient care in a critical care unit
3. Full-time employment at the hospital

The second-stage sampling unit would obtain a random selection of ten CCRNs from each hospital who met the previously mentioned eligibility criteria.

When multistage sampling is used in relation to large national surveys, states are used as the first-stage sampling unit, followed by successively smaller units such as counties, cities, districts, and blocks as the second-stage sampling unit, and finally households as the third-stage sampling unit.

Sampling units or clusters can be selected by simple random or stratified random sampling methods. For example, a study by Zhu and colleagues (2012) investigated whether nurse staffing levels make a difference on patient outcomes in Chinese hospitals. The study was conducted in 181 hospitals from nine provinces, municipalities, and autonomous regions (PMAs) across eight economic zones in mainland China using a four-stage sampling strategy to ensure geographic representation of the sample. First, hospitals were stratified by hospital level and location. Twenty general hospitals with equal numbers of Levels 2 and 3 hospitals were drawn from each of the nine PMAs. Second, at least four units, including intensive care units (ICUs) were drawn by systematic sampling according to a unit list. Third, three to eight units from each participating hospital participated, with a final participation of 780 units. Fourth, patients who stayed at least three nights on a unit, who were conscious and able to communicate, were drawn by systematic sampling based on their bed code.

The main advantage of cluster sampling, as illustrated in Table 12-1, is that it can be more economical in terms of time and money than other types of probability sampling. There are two major disadvantages: (1) more sampling errors tend to occur than with simple random or stratified random sampling, and (2) the appropriate handling of the statistical data from cluster samples is very complex. When you are critically appraising a study, you will need to consider whether the use of cluster sampling is justified in light of the research design, as well as other pragmatic matters, such as economy.

### EVIDENCE-BASED PRACTICE TIP

The sampling strategy, whether probability or nonprobability, must be appropriate to the design and evaluated in relation to the level of evidence provided by the design.

## Special Sampling Strategies

Several special sampling strategies are used in nonprobability sampling. Matching is a strategy used to construct an equivalent comparison sample group by filling it with subjects who are similar to each subject in another sample group in relation to preestablished variables such as age, gender, level of education, medical diagnosis, or socioeconomic status. Theoretically, any variable other than the independent variable that could affect the dependent variable should be matched. In reality, the more variables matched, the more difficult it is to obtain an adequate sample size. For example, in a study examining the effect of an ankle strengthening and walking exercise program on improving fall-related outcomes in the elderly, Graziotti and colleagues (2012) examined retention strategies to maximize retention in longitudinal studies involving high-risk families. The researchers conducted a follow-up study of 1388 children, half of whom were initially identified as cocaine or opiate exposed (n = 658) who were then matched to a non-cocaine or non-opiate exposed control (n = 730), based on gestational age, race, and gender.

Networking sampling, sometimes referred to as snowballing, is used for locating samples that are difficult or impossible to locate in other ways. This strategy takes advantage of social networks and the fact that friends tend to have characteristics in common. When a few subjects with the necessary eligibility criteria are found, the researcher asks for their assistance in getting in touch with others with similar criteria. For example, Othman and colleagues (2012) used networking and snowballing to recruit women from the community to expand recruitment beyond those seeking care for a study identifying factors that influence Jordanian women's intention to engage in mammography screening. Today, online computer networks, as described in the section on purposive sampling and in this last example, can be used to assist researchers in acquiring otherwise difficult to locate subjects, thereby taking advantage of the networking or snowball effect.

**CRITICAL THINKING DECISION PATH**

*Assessing the Relationship Between the Type of Sampling Strategy and the Appropriate Generalizability*

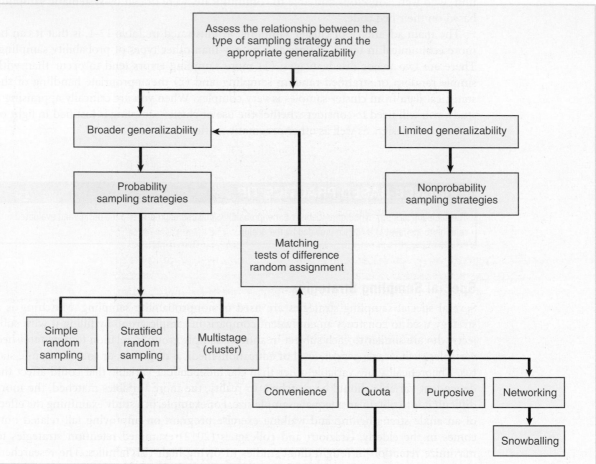

The Critical Thinking Decision Path illustrates the relationship between the type of sampling strategy and the appropriate generalizability.

# SAMPLE SIZE

There is no single rule that can be applied to the determination of a sample's size. When arriving at an estimate of sample size, many factors, such as the following, must be considered:

- Type of design used
- Type of sampling procedure used
- Type of formula used for estimating optimum sample size
- Degree of precision required
- Heterogeneity of the attributes under investigation

- Relative frequency that the phenomenon of interest occurs in the population (i.e., a common versus a rare health problem)
- Projected cost of using a particular sampling strategy

The sample size should be determined before a study is conducted. A general rule is always to use the largest sample possible. The larger the sample, the more representative of the population it is likely to be; smaller samples produce less accurate results.

One exception to this principle occurs when using qualitative designs. In this case, sample size is not predetermined. Sample sizes in qualitative research tend to be small because of the large volume of verbal data that must be analyzed and because this type of design tends to emphasize intensive and prolonged contact with subjects (Speziale & Carpenter, 2011). Subjects are added to the sample until **data saturation** is reached (i.e., new data no longer emerge during the data-collection process). Fittingness of the data is a more important concern than representativeness of subjects (see Chapters 5, 6, and 7).

Another exception is in the case of a **pilot study,** which is defined as a small sample study conducted as a prelude to a larger-scale study that is often called the "parent study." The pilot study is typically a smaller scale of the parent study with similar methods and procedures that yield preliminary data to determine the feasibility of conducting a larger-scale study and establish that sufficient scientific evidence exists to justify subsequent, more extensive research.

The principle of "larger is better" holds true for both probability and nonprobability samples. Results based on small samples (under 10) tend to be unstable—the values fluctuate from one sample to the next and it is difficult to apply statistics meaningfully. Small samples tend to increase the probability of obtaining a markedly nonrepresentative sample. As the sample size increases, the mean more closely approximates the population values, thus introducing fewer sampling errors.

A hypothetical example of this concept is illustrated by a study in which the average monthly sleeping pill consumption is being investigated for patients on a rehabilitation unit after a total knee replacement. The data in Table 12-3 indicate that the population consists of 20 patients whose average consumption of sleeping pills is 15.15 per month. Two simple random samples with sample sizes of 2, 4, 6, and 10 have been drawn from the population of 20 patients. Each sample average in the right-hand column represents an estimate of the population average, which is known to be 15.15. In most cases, the population

| TABLE 12-3 | COMPARISON OF POPULATION AND SAMPLE VALUES AND AVERAGES IN STUDY OF SLEEPING PILL CONSUMPTION | | |
| --- | --- | --- | --- |
| **NUMBER IN GROUP** | **GROUP** | **NUMBER OF SLEEPING PILLS CONSUMED (VALUES EXPRESSED MONTHLY)** | **AVERAGE** |
| 20 | Population | 1, 3, 4, 5, 6, 7, 9, 11, 13, 15, 16, 17, 19, 21, 22, 23, 25, 27, 29, 30 | 15.15 |
| 2 | Sample 1A | 6, 9 | 7.5 |
| 2 | Sample 1B | 21, 25 | 23.0 |
| 4 | Sample 2A | 1, 7, 15, 25 | 12.0 |
| 4 | Sample 2B | 5, 13, 23, 29 | 17.5 |
| 6 | Sample 3A | 3, 4, 11, 15, 21, 25 | 13.3 |
| 6 | Sample 3B | 5, 7, 11, 19, 27, 30 | 16.5 |
| 10 | Sample 4A | 3, 4, 7, 9, 11, 13, 17, 21, 23, 30 | 13.8 |
| 10 | Sample 4B | 1, 4, 6, 11, 15, 17, 19, 23, 25, 27 | 14.8 |

value is unknown to the researchers, but because the population is so small, it could be calculated. As we examine the data in Table 12-3, we note that with a sample size of 2, the estimate might have been wrong by as many as 8 sleeping pills in sample 1B. As the sample size increases, the averages get closer to the population value, and the differences in the estimates between samples A and B also get smaller. Large samples permit the principles of randomization to work effectively (i.e., to counterbalance atypical values in the long run).

It is possible to estimate the sample size needed with the use of a statistical procedure known as power analysis (Cohen, 1988). Power analysis is an advanced statistical technique that is commonly used by researchers and is a requirement for external funding. When it is not used, research consumers will have less confidence provided by the findings because the study may be based on a sample that is too small. A researcher may commit a type II error of accepting a null hypothesis when it should have been rejected if the sample is too small (see Chapter 16). No matter how high a research design is located on the evidence hierarchy (e.g., Level II—experimental design consisting of a randomized clinical trial), the findings of a study and their generalizability are weakened when power analysis is not calculated to ensure an adequate sample size to determine the effect of the intervention.

It is beyond the scope of this chapter to describe this complex procedure in great detail, but a simple example will illustrate its use. Im and colleagues (2012) wanted to determine ethnic differences in midlife women's attitudes toward physical activity among four ethnic groups in the United States. 542 middle-aged women (127 Hispanics, 157 whites, 135 African Americans, and 123 Asians) were recruited through Internet and community settings.

How would a research team such as Im and colleagues know the appropriate number of patients that should be used in the study? When using power analysis, the researcher must estimate how large of a difference will be observed between the four ethnic groups (i.e., to test differences in attitudes toward exercise, stratified by ethnicity and socioeconomic status). If a moderate difference is expected, a conventional effect size of .20 is assumed. With a significance level of .05, a total of 105 participants would be needed for each ethnic group to detect a statistically significant difference between the groups with a power of .80. The total sample in this study ($n = 542$) exceeded the minimum number of 105 per ethnic group.

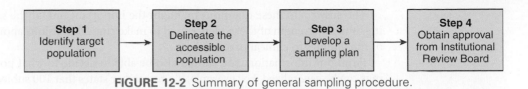

**FIGURE 12-2** Summary of general sampling procedure.

When calculating sample size using power analysis, the total sample size needs to consider that attrition, or dropouts, will occur and build in approximately 15% extra subjects to make sure that the ability to detect differences between groups or the effect of an intervention remains intact. When expected differences are large, it does not take a very large sample to ensure that differences will be revealed through statistical analysis.

When critically appraising a study, you should evaluate the sample size in terms of the following: (1) how representative the sample is relative to the target population; and (2) to whom the researcher wishes to generalize the study's results. The goal is to have a sample as representative as possible with as little sampling error as possible. Unless representativeness is ensured, all the data in the world become inconsequential. When an appropriate sample size, including power analysis for calculation of sample size, and sampling strategy have been used, you can feel more confident that the sample is representative of the accessible population rather than biased (Figure 12-2) and the potential for generalizability of findings is greater (Chapter 8).

# APPRAISING THE EVIDENCE
## SAMPLING

The criteria for critical appraisal of a study's sample are presented in the Critiquing Criteria box. As you evaluate the sample section of a study, you must raise two questions:

1. If this study were to be replicated, would there be enough information presented about the nature of the population, the sample, the sampling strategy, and sample size of another investigator to carry out the study?
2. What are the sampling threats to internal and external validity that are sources of bias?

The answers to these questions highlight the important link of the sample to the findings and the strength of the evidence used to make clinical decisions about the applicability of the findings to clinical practice.

From this information, you should also be able to decide to what population the findings can be generalized. For example, if a researcher states that 100 subjects were randomly drawn from a population of women 14 years and older, diagnosed with cervical intraepithelial neoplasia II or III who were willing to postpone standard ablative therapy and receive topical retinoic acid treatment at affiliated clinics within hospital X during the year 2013, you can specifically evaluate the population's parameters. Demographic characteristics of the sample (e.g., age, diagnosis, ethnicity, religion, level of education, socioeconomic status [SES], marital status) should be presented in either a tabled or a narrative summary because they provide further explication about the nature of the sample and enable you to appraise the sampling procedure more accurately.

For example, in their study titled Couple Functioning and Post-Traumatic Stress Symptoms in U.S. Army Couples, Melvin and colleagues (2012; see Appendix D) present detailed data summarizing demographic variables of importance in Table 1. Analysis of findings related to demographic variables indicates that there were no statistically significant differences between responding and non-responding individuals.

The information that the responding and non-responding groups were equivalent on demographic, clinical, or adherence variables is important because it means that bias related to attrition is minimized and that resilience is more likely to be an accurate predictor of couple functioning even when the individual post-traumatic stress levels were high. This example illustrates how a detailed description of the sample both provides you with a frame of reference for the study population and sample and highlights questions about replicability and bias that need to be raised.

In Chapter 8, we talked about how selection effect as a threat to internal validity could occur in studies where a convenience, quota, or purposive sampling strategy was used. In these studies individuals themselves decide whether or not to participate. Subject mortality or attrition is another threat to internal validity related to sampling (see Chapter 8). Mortality is the loss of subjects from the study, usually from the first data-collection point to the second. If the subjects who remain in the study are different from those who drop out, the results can be affected. When more of the subjects in one group drop out than the other group, the results can also be influenced. It is common for journals to require authors reporting research results to include a flow chart that diagrams the screening, recruitment, enrollment, random assignment, and attrition process and results. For example, see Figure 1 in the study by Thomas and colleagues (2012; Appendix A), which studied the effect of a motivational-interviewing–based coaching intervention compared with usual care in decreasing attitudinal barriers to cancer pain management and improving functional status and quality of life for people with cancer.

Threats to external validity related to sampling are concerned with generalizability of the results to other populations. Generalizability depends on who actually participates in a study. Not everyone who is approached meets the inclusion criteria, agrees to enroll, or completes the study. Bias in sample representativeness and generalizability of findings are important sampling issues that have generated national concern because the presence of these factors decreases confidence in the evidence provided by the findings and limits applicability. Historically, many of the landmark adult health studies (e.g., the Framingham

## CRITIQUING CRITERIA

### Sampling

1. Have the sample characteristics been completely described?
2. Can the parameters of the study population be inferred from the description of the sample?
3. To what extent is the sample representative of the population as defined?
4. Are the eligibility/inclusion criteria for the sample clearly identified?
5. Have sample exclusion criteria/delimitations for the sample been established?
6. Would it be possible to replicate the study population?
7. How was the sample selected? Is the method of sample selection appropriate?
8. What kind of bias, if any, is introduced by this sampling method?
9. Is the sample size appropriate? How is it substantiated?
10. Are there indications that rights of subjects have been ensured?
11. Does the researcher identify limitations in generalizability of the findings from the sample to the population? Are they appropriate?
12. Is the sampling strategy appropriate for the design of the study and level of evidence provided by the design?
13. Does the researcher indicate how replication of the study with other samples would provide increased support for the findings?

heart study, the Baltimore longitudinal study on aging) excluded women as subjects. Despite the all-male samples, the findings of these studies were generalized from males to all adults, in spite of the lack of female representation in the samples. Similarly, the use of largely European-American subjects in clinical trials limits the identification of variant responses to interventions or drugs in ethnic or racially distinct groups (Ward, 2003). Findings based on European-American data cannot be generalized to African Americans, Asians, Hispanics, or any other cultural group.

Probability sampling is clearly the ideal sampling procedure for ensuring the representativeness of a study population. Use of random selection procedures (e.g., simple random, stratified, cluster, or systematic sampling strategies) minimizes the occurrence of conscious and unconscious biases, which affect the researcher's ability to generalize about the findings from the sample to the population. You should be able to identify the type of probability strategy used and determine whether the researcher adhered to the criteria for a particular sampling plan.

When a purposive sample is used in experimental and quasi-experimental studies, you should determine whether or how the subjects were randomly assigned to groups. If criteria for random assignment have not been followed, you have a valid basis for being cautious about the strength of evidence provided by the proposed conclusions of the study.

Although random selection is the ideal in establishing the representativeness of a study population, more often realistic barriers (e.g., institutional policy, inaccessibility of subjects, lack of time or money, and current state of knowledge in the field) necessitate the use of nonprobability sampling strategies. Many important research questions that are of interest to nursing do not lend themselves to levels of evidence provided by experimental designs and probability sampling. This is particularly true with qualitative research designs.

A well-designed, carefully controlled study using a nonprobability sampling strategy can yield accurate and meaningful evidence that makes a significant contribution to nursing's scientific body of knowledge.

As the evaluator, you must ask a philosophical question: "If it is not possible or appropriate to conduct an experimental or quasi-experimental investigation that uses probability sampling, should the study be abandoned?" The answer usually suggests that it is better to carry out the study and be fully aware of the limitations of the methodology and evidence provided than to lose the knowledge that can be gained. The researcher is always able to move on to subsequent studies that reflect a stronger and more consistent level of evidence either by replicating the study or by using more stringent design and sampling strategies to refine the knowledge derived from a nonexperimental study.

The greatest difficulty in nonprobability sampling stems from the fact that not every element in the population has an equal chance of being represented in the sample. Therefore it is likely that some segment of the population will be systematically underrepresented. If the population is homogeneous on critical characteristics, such as age, gender, socioeconomic status, and diagnosis, systematic bias will not be very important. Few of the attributes that researchers are interested in, however, are sufficiently homogeneous to make sampling bias an irrelevant consideration.

Basically you will decide whether the sample size for a quantitative study is appropriate and its size is justifiable. You want to make sure that the researcher indicated how the sample size was determined. The method of arriving at the sample size and the rationale should be briefly mentioned. In the study titled Couple Functioning and Post-Traumatic Stress Symptoms in U.S. Army Couples (Melvin et al., 2012; Appendix D), the power analysis indicated that based on a power of .80, a sample of 45 couples was adequate to detect a medium effect size of .70 that differentiated between distressed and non-distressed couples using couple functioning scores.

When appraising qualitative research designs, you also apply criteria related to sampling strategies that are relevant for a particular type of qualitative study. In general, sampling strategies for qualitative studies are purposive because the study of specific phenomena in their natural setting is emphasized; any subject belonging to a specified group is considered to represent that group. For example, in the qualitative study titled The Experiences of Nurse Practitioners Providing Health Care to the Homeless (Seiler & Moss, 2012; Appendix C), the specified group was nurse practitioners directly involved in providing health care to the homeless. Keep in mind that qualitative studies will not discuss predetermining sample size or mehod of arriving at sample size. Rather, sample size will tend to be small and a function of data saturation. In the study by Seiler and Moss the sample consisted of nine nurse practitioners in community clinic sites.

Finally, evidence that the rights of human subjects have been protected should appear in the "Sample" section of the research report and probably consists of no more than one sentence. Remember to evaluate whether permission was obtained from an institutional review board that reviewed the study relative to the maintenance of ethical research standards (see Chapter 13). For example, the review board examines the research proposal to determine whether the introduction of an experimental procedure may be potentially harmful and therefore undesirable. You also examine the report for evidence of the subjects' informed consent, as well as protection of their confidentiality or anonymity. It is highly unusual for research studies not to demonstrate evidence of having met these criteria. Nevertheless, you will want to be certain that ethical standards that protect sample subjects have been maintained.

## ■ KEY POINTS

- Sampling is a process that selects representative units of a population for study. Researchers sample representative segments of the population because it is rarely feasible or necessary to sample entire populations of interest to obtain accurate and meaningful information.
- Researchers establish eligibility criteria; these are descriptors of the population and provide the basis for selection of a sample. Eligibility criteria, which are also referred to as delimitations, include the following: age, gender, socioeconomic status, level of education, religion, and ethnicity.
- The researcher must identify the target population (i.e., the entire set of cases about which the researcher would like to make generalizations). Because of the pragmatic constraints, however, the researcher usually uses an accessible population (i.e., one that meets the population criteria and is available).
- A sample is a set of elements that makes up the population.
- A sampling unit is the element or set of elements used for selecting the sample. The foremost criterion in appraising a sample is the representativeness or congruence of characteristics with the population.
- Sampling strategies consist of nonprobability and probability sampling.
- In nonprobability sampling, the elements are chosen by nonrandom methods. Types of nonprobability sampling include convenience, quota, and purposive sampling.
- Probability sampling is characterized by the random selection of elements from the population. In random selection, each element in the population has an equal and independent chance of being included in the sample. Types of probability sampling include simple random, stratified random, and multistage sampling.
- Sample size is a function of the type of sampling procedure being used, the degree of precision required, the type of sample estimation formula being used, the heterogeneity of the study attributes, the relative frequency of occurrence of the phenomena under consideration, and cost.
- Criteria for drawing a sample vary according to the sampling strategy. Systematic organization of the sampling procedure minimizes bias. The target population is identified, the accessible portion of the target population is delineated, permission to conduct the research study is obtained, and a sampling plan is formulated.
- When critically appraising a research report, the sampling plan needs to be evaluated for its appropriateness in relation to the particular research design and level of evidence generated by the design.
- Completeness of the sampling plan is examined in light of potential replicability of the study. The critiquer appraises whether the sampling strategy is the strongest plan for the particular study under consideration.
- An appropriate systematic sampling plan will maximize the efficiency of a research study. It will increase the strength, accuracy, and meaningfulness of the evidence provided by the findings and enhance the generalizability of the findings from the sample to the population.

## CRITICAL THINKING CHALLENGES

- How do inclusion and exclusion criteria contribute to increasing the strength of evidence provided by the sampling strategy of a research study?
- Why is it important for a researcher to use power analysis to calculate sample size? How does adequate sample size affect subject mortality, representativeness of the sample, the researcher's ability to detect a treatment effect, and your ability to generalize from the study findings to your patient population?
- How does a flowchart such as the one in Figure 1 of the Thomas article in Appendix A contribute to the strength and quality of evidence provided by the findings of research study and their potential for applicability to practice?
- Evaluate the overall strengths and weaknesses of the sampling section of the Thomas research report in Appendix A. What are the sources of bias, if any, that present threats to internal or external validity? How does the sampling strategy contribute to the strength and quality of evidence provided by the findings and their applicability to clinical practice?
- Your research classmate argues that a random sample is always better, even if it is small and represents only one site. Another student counters that a very large convenience sample representing multiple sites can be very significant. Which classmate would you defend and why? How would each scenario affect the strength and quality of evidence provided by the findings?

## REFERENCES

Alhusen, J. L., Gross, D., Hayat, M. J., et al. (2012). The influence of maternal-fetal attachment and health practices on neonatal outcomes in low-income, urban women. *Research in Nursing & Health, 35*, 112–120.

Cohen, J. (1988). *Statistical power analysis for the behavioral sciences* (2nd ed.). New York, NY: Academic Press.

Graziotti, A. L., Hammond, J., Messinger, D. S., et al. (2012). Maintaining participation and momentum in longitudinal research involving high-risk families. *Journal of Nursing Scholarship, 44*(2), 120–126.

Hessler, K., & Siegrist, M. (2012). Nurse practitioner attitudes and treatment practices for childhood overweight: how do rural and urban practitioners differ? *Journal of the American Academy of Nurse Practitioners, 24*(2), 97–106.

Im, E., Chang, S. J., Ko, Y., et al. (2012). A national internet survey on midlife women's attitudes toward physical activity. *Nursing Research, 61*(5), 342–352.

Melvin, K. C., Gross, D., Hayat, X., et al. (2012). Couple functioning and post-traumatic stress symptoms in US Army couples: the role of resilience. *Research in Nursing & Health, 35*, 164–177.

Othman, A. K., Kiviniemi, M. T., Wu, Y. B., & Lally, R. M. (2012). Influence of demographic factors, knowledge, and beliefs on Jordanian women's intention to undergo mammography screening. *Journal of Nursing Scholarship, 44*(1), 19–26.

Seiler, A. J., & Moss, V. A. (2012). The experiences of nurse practitioners providing health care to the homeless. *Journal of the American Academy of Nurse Practitioners, 24*(5), 303–312.

Sherman, D. W., Haber, J., Hoskins, C. N., et al. (2012). The effects of psychoeducation and telephone counseling on the adjustment of women with early stage breast cancer. *Applied Nursing Research, 25*, 13–16.

Sousa, V. D., Zauszniewski, J. A., & Musil, C. M. (2004). How to determine whether a convenience sample represents the population. *Applied Nursing Research, 17*(2), 130–133.

Speziale, S., & Carpenter, D. R. (2011). *Qualitative research in nursing* (4th ed.). Philadelphia, PA: Lippincott.

Swatzky RG, Ratner PA, Richardson CG, Washburn C, Sudament W, Mirwaldt P (2012). Stress and depression in students: The mediating role of stress management self-efficacy. *Nursing Research*, 61(1), 13–21.

Thomas, M. L., Elliott, J. E., Rao, S. M., et al. (2012). A randomized clinical trial of education or motivational-interviewing–based coaching compared to usual care to improve cancer pain management. *Oncology Nursing Forum*, 39(1), 39–49.

Ward, L. S. (2003). Race as a variable in cross-cultural research. *Nursing Outlook*, 51(3), 120–125.

Zhu, X., You, L., Zheng, J., et al. (2012). Nurse staffing levels make a difference on patient outcomes: a multisite study in Chinese hospitals. *Journal of Nursing Scholarship*, 44(3), 266–273.

# evolve WEBSITE

*Go to Evolve at http://evolve.elsevier.com/LoBiondo/ for review questions, critquing exercises, and additional research articles for practice in reviewing and critiquing.*

# CHAPTER
# 13

# Legal and Ethical Issues

*Judith Haber and Geri LoBiondo-Wood*

"In the 'court of imagination,' where Americans often play out their racial politics, a ceremony, starring a southern white President of the United States offering an apology and asking for forgiveness from a 94-year-old African-American man, seemed like a fitting close worthy in its tableaux quality of a William Faulkner or Toni Morrison novel. The reason for this drama was the federal government's May 16th formal ceremony of repentance tendered to the aging and ailing survivors of the infamous Tuskegee Syphilis Study. The study is a morality play for many among the African-American public and the scientific research community, serving as our most horrific example of a racist 'scandalous story,' when government doctors played God and science went mad. At the formal White House gathering, when President William J. Clinton apologized on behalf of the American government to the eight remaining survivors of the study, their families, and heirs, seemingly a sordid chapter in American research history was closed 25 years after the study itself was forced to end. As the room filled with members of the Black Congressional Caucus, cabinet members, civil rights leaders, members of the Legacy Committee, the Centers for Disease Control (CDC), and five of the survivors, the sense of a dramatic restitution was upon us."

*Reverby (2000)*

## ⊖volve WEBSITE

*Go to Evolve at http://evolve.elsevier.com/LoBiondo/ for review questions, critiquing exercises, and additional research articles for practice in reviewing and critiquing.*

## LEARNING OUTCOMES

*After reading this chapter, you should be able to do the following:*

- Describe the historical background that led to the development of ethical guidelines for the use of human subjects in research.
- Identify the essential elements of an informed consent form.
- Evaluate the adequacy of an informed consent form.
- Describe the institutional review board's role in the research review process.
- Identify populations of subjects who require special legal and ethical research considerations.

- Appreciate the nurse researcher's obligations to conduct and report research in an ethical manner.

- Describe the nurse's role as patient advocate in research situations.
- Critique the ethical aspects of a research study.

## KEY TERMS

| | | |
|---|---|---|
| anonymity | consent | justice |
| assent | ethics | respect for persons |
| beneficence | informed consent | risk/benefit ratio |
| confidentiality | institutional review boards | |

Nurses are in an ideal position to promote patients' awareness of the role played by research in the advancement of science and improvement in patient care. Embedded in our professional Code of Ethics (American Nurses Association [ANA], 2001) is the charge to protect patients from harm. Code of ethics not only state the rules and regulations regarding the involvement of human research subjects to ensure that research is conducted legally and ethically, but also address appropriate conduct of researchers governed by those rules. Researchers themselves and caregivers providing care to patients, who also happen to be research subjects, must be fully committed to the tenets of informed consent and patients' rights. The principle "the ends justify the means" must never be tolerated. Researchers and caregivers of research subjects must take every precaution to protect those being studied from physical or mental harm or discomfort. It is not always clear what constitutes harm or discomfort.

The focus of this chapter is the legal and ethical considerations that must be addressed before, during, and after the conduct of research. Informed consent, institutional review boards, and research involving vulnerable populations—elderly people, pregnant women, children, prisoners, persons with acquired immunodeficiency syndrome (AIDS)—are discussed. The nurse's role as patient advocate, whether functioning as researcher, caregiver, or research consumer, is addressed. This focus is consistent with the definition of ethics; that is, the theory or discipline dealing with principles of moral values and moral conduct.

## ETHICAL AND LEGAL CONSIDERATIONS IN RESEARCH: A HISTORICAL PERSPECTIVE

### Past Ethical Dilemmas in Research

Ethical and legal considerations with regard to research first received attention after World War II. When the reigning U.S. Secretary of State and Secretary of War learned that the trials for war criminals would focus on justifying the atrocities committed by Nazi physicians as "medical research," the American Medical Association was asked to appoint a group to develop a code of ethics for research that would serve as a standard for judging the medical atrocities committed by physicians on concentration camp prisoners.

The Nuremberg Code and its definitions of the terms *voluntary, legal capacity, sufficient understanding,* and *enlightened decision* have been the subject of numerous court cases and presidential commissions involved in setting ethical standards in research (Amdur & Bankert, 2011). The code that was developed requires informed consent in all cases but makes no provisions for any special treatment of children, the elderly, or the mentally

## BOX 13-1 BASIC ETHICAL PRINCIPLES RELEVANT TO THE CONDUCT OF RESEARCH

**Respect for Persons**
People have the right to self-determination and to treatment as autonomous agents. Thus they have the freedom to participate or not participate in research. Persons with diminished autonomy are entitled to protection.

**Beneficence**
Beneficence is an obligation to do no harm and maximize possible benefits. Persons are treated in an ethical manner, their decisions are respected, they are protected from harm, and efforts are made to secure their well-being.

**Justice**
Human subjects should be treated fairly. An injustice occurs when a benefit to which a person is entitled is denied without good reason or when a burden is imposed unduly.

incompetent. Several other international standards have followed, the most notable of which was the Declaration of Helsinki, which was adopted in 1964 by the World Medical Assembly and later revised in 1975.

In the United States, federal guidelines for the ethical conduct of research involving human subjects were not developed until the 1970s. Despite the supposed safeguards provided by the federal guidelines, some of the most atrocious, and hence memorable, examples of unethical research studies took place in the United States as recently as the 1990s. These examples are highlighted in Table 13-1. They are sad reminders of our own tarnished research heritage and illustrate the human consequences of not adhering to ethical research standards.

The conduct of harmful, illegal research made additional controls necessary. In 1973 the U.S. Department of Health, Education, and Welfare published the first set of proposed regulations on the protection of human subjects. The most important provision was a regulation mandating that an institutional review board functioning in accordance with specifications of the department must review and approve all studies. The National Research Act, passed in 1974 (Public Law 93-348), created the National Commission for the Protection of Human Subjects of Biomedical and Behavioral Research. A major charge of the Commission was to identify the basic principles that should underlie the conduct of biomedical and behavioral research involving human subjects and to develop guidelines to ensure that research is conducted in accordance with those principles (Amdur & Bankert, 2011). Three ethical principles were identified as relevant to the conduct of research involving human subjects: the principles of respect for persons, beneficence, and justice. They are defined in Box 13-1. Included in a report issued in 1979, called the Belmont Report, these principles provided the basis for regulations affecting research sponsored by the federal government. The Belmont Report also served as a model for many of the ethical codes developed by scientific disciplines (National Commission, 1978).

In 1980, the U.S. Department of Health and Human Services (DHHS) developed a set of regulations in response to the Commission's recommendations. These regulations were published in 1981 and have been revised several times (DHHS, 2009). They include
- General requirements for informed consent
- Documentation of informed consent
- IRB review of research proposals
- Exempt and expedited review procedures for certain kinds of research
- Criteria for IRB approval of research

| RESEARCH STUDY | YEAR(S) | FOCUS OF STUDY | ETHICAL PRINCIPLE VIOLATED |
|---|---|---|---|
| Hyman vs. Jewish Chronic Disease Hospital case | 1965 | Doctors injected cancer-ridden aged and senile patients with their own cancer cells to study the rejection response. | Informed consent was not obtained. There was no indication that the study was reviewed and approved by an ethics committee. The two physicians claimed they did not wish to evoke emotional reactions or refusals to participate by informing the subjects of the nature of the study (Hershey & Miller, 1976). |
| Ivory Coast, Africa, AIDS/AZT case | 1994 | In clinical trials supported by the U.S. government and conducted in the Ivory Coast, Dominican Republic, and Thailand, some pregnant women infected with the human immunodeficiency virus (HIV) were given placebo pills rather than AZT, a drug known to prevent mothers from passing the virus to their babies. Babies were in danger of contracting HIV unnecessarily. | Subjects who consented to participate and who were randomized to the control group were denied access to a medication regimen with a known benefit. This violates the subjects' right to fair treatment and protection (French, 1997; Wheeler, 1997). |
| Midgeville, Georgia, case | 1969 | Investigational drugs were used on mentally disabled children without first obtaining the opinion of a psychiatrist. | There was no review of the study protocol or institutional approval of the program before implementation (Levine, 1986). |
| Tuskegee, Alabama, Syphilis Study | 1932-1973 | For 40 years the U.S. Public Health Service conducted a study using two groups of poor black male sharecroppers. One group consisted of those who had untreated syphilis; the other group was judged to be free of the disease. Treatment was withheld from the group having syphilis even after penicillin became generally available and accepted as effective treatment in the 1950s. Steps were taken to prevent the subjects from obtaining it. The researcher wanted to study the untreated disease. | Many of the subjects who consented to participate in the study were not informed about the purpose and procedures of the research. Others were unaware that they were subjects. The degree of risk outweighed the potential benefit. Withholding of known effective treatment violates the subjects' right to fair treatment and protection from harm (Levine, 1986). |
| San Antonio Contraceptive Study | 1969 | In a study examining the side effects of oral contraceptives, 76 impoverished Mexican-American women were randomly assigned to an experimental group receiving birth control pills or a control group receiving placebos. Subjects were not informed about the placebo and pregnancy risk; 11 subjects became pregnant, 10 of whom were in the placebo control group. | Informed consent principles were violated; full disclosure of potential risk, harm, results, or side effects was not evident in the informed consent document. The potential risk outweighed the benefits of the study. The subjects' right to fair treatment and protection from harm was violated (Levine, 1986). |

*Continued*

| TABLE 13-1 | | HIGHLIGHTS OF UNETHICAL RESEARCH STUDIES CONDUCTED IN THE UNITED STATES—cont'd | |
|---|---|---|---|
| **RESEARCH STUDY** | **YEAR(S)** | **FOCUS OF STUDY** | **ETHICAL PRINCIPLE VIOLATED** |
| Willowbrook Hospital study | 1972 | Mentally incompetent children ($n = 350$) were not admitted to Willowbrook Hospital, a residential treatment facility, unless parents consented to their children being subjects in a study examining the natural history of infectious hepatitis and the effect of gamma globulin. The children were deliberately infected with the hepatitis virus under various conditions; some received gamma globulin, others did not. | Principle of voluntary consent was violated. Parents were coerced to consent to their children's participation as research subjects. Subjects or their guardians have a right to self-determination; that is, they should be free of constraint, coercion, or undue influence of any kind. Many subjects feel pressured to participate in studies if they are in powerless, dependent positions (Rothman, 1982). |
| UCLA Schizophrenia Medication Study | 1983 | In a study examining the effects of withdrawing psychotropic medications of 50 patients under treatment for schizophrenia, 23 subjects suffered severe relapses after their medication was stopped. The goal of the study was to determine if some schizophrenics might do better without medications that had deleterious side effects. | Although subjects signed informed consent documents, they were not informed about how severe their relapses might be, or that they could suffer worsening symptoms with each recurrence. Principles of informed consent were violated; full disclosure of potential risk, harm, results, or side effects was not evident in informed consent document. Potential risks outweighed the benefits of the study. The subjects' right to fair treatment and protection from harm was violated (Hilts, 1995). |

## Protection of Human Rights

*Human rights* are the claims and demands that have been justified in the eyes of an individual or by a group of individuals. The term refers to the rights outlined in the ANA (2001) guidelines:

1. Right to self-determination
2. Right to privacy and dignity
3. Right to anonymity and confidentiality
4. Right to fair treatment
5. Right to protection from discomfort and harm

These rights apply to all involved in research, including research team members who may be involved in data collection, practicing nurses involved in the research setting, and subjects participating in the study. As you read a research article, you must realize that any issues highlighted in Table 13-2 should have been addressed and resolved before a research study is approved for implementation.

## Procedures for Protecting Basic Human Rights
### Informed Consent

Elements of informed consent illustrated by the ethical principles of respect and by its related right to self-determination are outlined in Box 13-2 and Table 13-2. It is important to understand the elements of informed consent so that you are a knowledgeable participant in obtaining informed consents from patients and/or in

## TABLE 13-2    PROTECTION OF HUMAN RIGHTS

| DEFINITION | VIOLATION OF BASIC HUMAN RIGHT | EXAMPLE |
|---|---|---|
| **RIGHT TO SELF-DETERMINATION** | | |
| Based on the principle of respect for persons, people should be treated as autonomous agents who have the freedom to choose without external controls. An autonomous agent is one who is informed about a proposed study and allowed to choose to participate or not to participate; subjects have the right to withdraw from a study without penalty. Subjects with diminished autonomy are entitled to protection. They are more vulnerable because of age, legal or mental incompetence, terminal illness, or confinement to an institution. Justification for use of vulnerable subjects must be provided. | A subject's right to self-determination is violated through use of coercion, covert data collection, and deception. <br>• Coercion occurs when an overt threat of harm or excessive reward is presented to ensure compliance. <br>• Covert data collection occurs when people become research subjects and are exposed to research treatments without their knowledge. <br>• Deception occurs when subjects are actually misinformed about the purpose of the research. <br>• Potential for violation of the right to self-determination is greater for subjects with diminished autonomy; they have decreased ability to give informed consent and are vulnerable. | Subjects may feel that their care will be adversely affected if they refuse to participate in research. The Jewish Chronic Disease Hospital Study (see Table 13-1) is an example in which patients and their doctors did not know that cancer cells were being injected. In the Milgrim (1963) study, subjects were deceived when asked to administer electric shocks to another person; the person was really an actor who pretended to feel the shocks. Subjects administering the shocks were very stressed by participating in this study, although they were not administering shocks at all. The Willowbrook Study (see Table 13-1) is an example of how coercion was used to obtain parental consent of vulnerable mentally retarded children who would not be admitted to the institution unless the children participated in a study in which they were deliberately injected with the hepatitis virus. |
| **RIGHT TO PRIVACY AND DIGNITY** | | |
| Based on the principle of respect, privacy is the freedom of a person to determine the time, extent, and circumstances under which private information is shared or withheld from others. | The Privacy Act of 1974 was instituted to protect subjects from such violations. These occur most frequently during data collection when invasive questions are asked that might result in loss of job, friendships, or dignity; or might create embarrassment and mental distress. It also may occur when subjects are unaware that information is being shared with others. | Subjects may be asked personal questions such as the following: "Were you sexually abused as a child?" "Do you use drugs?" "What are your sexual preferences?" When questions are asked using hidden microphones or hidden tape recorders, the subjects' privacy is invaded because they have no knowledge that the data are being shared with others. Subjects also have a right to control access of others to their records. |
| **RIGHT TO ANONYMITY AND CONFIDENTIALITY** | | |
| Based on the principle of respect, **anonymity** exists when a subject's identity cannot be linked, even by the researcher, with their individual responses. | Anonymity is violated when the subjects' responses can be linked with their identity. | Subjects are given a code number instead of using names for identification purposes. Subjects' names are never used when reporting findings. |
| **Confidentiality** means that individual identities of subjects will not be linked to the information they provide and will not be publicly divulged. | Confidentiality is breached when a researcher, either by accident or by direct action, allows an unauthorized person to gain access to study data that contains subjects' identity information or responses that create a potentially harmful situation for subjects. | Breaches of confidentiality with regard to sexual preference, income, drug use, prejudice, or personality variables can be harmful to subjects. Data are analyzed as group data so individuals cannot be identified by their responses. |

*Continued*

## TABLE 13-2    PROTECTION OF HUMAN RIGHTS—cont'd

| DEFINITION | VIOLATION OF BASIC HUMAN RIGHT | EXAMPLE |
|---|---|---|
| **RIGHT TO FAIR TREATMENT** | | |
| Based on the principle of justice, people should be treated fairly and receive what they are due or owed. Fair treatment is equitable subject selection and treatment during a study including: selection of subjects for reasons directly related to the problem studied vs. convenience, compromised position, or vulnerability. Also included is fair treatment of subjects during a study, including fair distribution of risks and benefits regardless of age, race, or socioeconomic status. | Injustices with regard to subject selection have occurred as a result of social, cultural, racial, and gender biases in society. Historically, research subjects often have been obtained from groups of people who were regarded as having less "social value," such as the poor, prisoners, slaves, the mentally incompetent, and the dying. Often subjects were treated carelessly, without consideration of physical or psychological harm. | The Tuskegee Syphilis Study (1973), the Jewish Chronic Disease Study (1965), the San Antonio Contraceptive Study (1969), and the Willowbrook Study (1972) (see Table 13-1) all provide examples related to unfair subject selection. Investigators should not be late for data collection appointments, should terminate data collection on time, should not change agreed-on procedures or activities without consent, and should provide agreed-on benefits such as a copy of the study findings or a participation fee. |
| **RIGHT TO PROTECTION FROM DISCOMFORT AND HARM** | | |
| Based on the principle of beneficence, people must take an active role in promoting good and preventing harm in the world around them, as well as in research studies. Discomfort and harm can be physical, psychological, social, or economic in nature. There are five categories of studies based on levels of harm and discomfort: <br>1. No anticipated effects <br>2. Temporary discomfort <br>3. Unusual level of temporary discomfort <br>4. Risk of permanent damage <br>5. Certainty of permanent damage | Subjects' right to be protected is violated when researchers know in advance that harm, death, or disabling injury will occur and thus the benefits do not outweigh the risk. | Temporary physical discomfort involving minimal risk includes fatigue or headache; emotional discomfort including travel expenses incurred to and from the data collection site. Studies examining sensitive issues, such as rape, incest, or spouse abuse, might cause unusual levels of temporary discomfort by opening up current and/or past traumatic experiences. In these situations, researchers assess distress levels and provide debriefing sessions during which the subject may express feelings and ask questions. The researcher makes referrals for professional intervention. Studies having the potential to cause permanent damage are more likely to be medical rather than nursing in nature. A recent clinical trial of a new drug, a recombinant activated protein C (rAPC) (Zovan) for treatment of sepsis, was halted when interim findings from the Phase III clinical trials revealed a reduced mortality rate for the treatment group vs. the placebo group. Evaluation of the data led to termination of the trial to make available a known beneficial treatment to all patients. In some research, such as the Tuskegee Syphilis Study or the Nazi medical experiments, subjects experienced permanent damage or death. |

> ## BOX 13-2  ELEMENTS OF INFORMED CONSENT
>
> 1. Title of Protocol
> 2. Invitation to Participate
> 3. Basis for Subject Selection
> 4. Overall Purpose of Study
> 5. Explanation of Procedures
> 6. Description of Risks and Discomforts
> 7. Potential Benefits
> 8. Alternatives to Participation
> 9. Financial Obligations
> 10. Assurance of Confidentiality
> 11. In Case of Injury Compensation
> 12. HIPAA Disclosure
> 13. Subject Withdrawal
> 14. Offer to Answer Questions
> 15. Concluding Consent Statement
> 16. Identification of Investigators

From Code of Federal Regulations: Protection of human subjects, 45 CFR 46, *OPRR Reports,* 2009.

critiquing this process as it is presented in research articles. It is critical to note that informed consent is not just giving a potential subject a consent form, but is a *process* that must be completed with each subject. Informed consent is documented by a consent form that is given to prospective subjects and must contain standard elements.

Informed consent is a legal principle that means that potential subjects understand the implications of participating in research and they knowingly agree to participate (Amdur & Bankert, 2011). The Code of Federal Regulations Title 45 Department of Health and Human Services (DHHS, 2009; Food and Drug Administration, 2012a) defines the meaning of informed consent as follows:

> *The knowing consent of an individual or his/her legally authorized representative, under circumstances that provide the prospective subject or representative sufficient opportunity to consider whether or not to participate without undue inducement or any element of force, fraud, deceit, duress, or other forms of constraint or coercion.*

No investigator may involve a person as a research subject before obtaining the legally effective informed consent of a subject or legally authorized representative. The study must be explained to all potential subjects, including the study's purpose; procedures; risks, discomforts and benefits; and expected duration of participation (i.e., when the study's procedures will be implemented, how many times, and in what setting). Potential subjects must also be informed about any appropriate alternative procedures or treatments, if any, that might be advantageous to the subject. For example, in the Tuskegee Syphilis Study, the researchers should have disclosed that penicillin was an effective treatment for syphilis. Any compensation for subjects' participation must be delineated when there is more than minimal risk through disclosure about medical treatments and/or compensation that is available if injury occurs.

Prospective subjects must have time to decide whether to participate in a study. The researcher must not coerce the subject into participating, nor may researchers collect data on subjects who have explicitly refused to participate in a study. An ethical violation of this

> ## HELPFUL HINT
>
> Recognize that the right to personal privacy may be more difficult to protect when carrying out qualitative studies because of the small sample size and because the subjects' verbatim quotes are often used in the results/findings section of the research report to highlight the findings.

principle is illustrated by the halting of eight experiments by the U.S. Food and Drug Administration (FDA) at the University of Pennsylvania's Institute for Human Gene Therapy 4 months after the death of an 18-year-old man, Jesse Gelsinger, who received experimental treatment as part of the Institute's research. The Institute could not document that all patients had been informed of the risks and benefits of the procedures. Furthermore, some patients who received the therapy should have been considered ineligible because their illnesses were more severe than allowed by the clinical protocols. Mr. Gelsinger had a non–life-threatening genetic disorder that permits toxic amounts of ammonia to build up in the liver. Nevertheless, he volunteered for an experimental treatment in which normal genes were implanted directly into his liver and he subsequently died of multiple organ failure. The Institute failed to report to the FDA that two patients in the same trial as Mr. Gelsinger had suffered severe side effects, including inflammation of the liver as a result of the treatment. This should have triggered a halt to the trial (Brainard & Miller, 2000). Of course, subjects may discontinue participation or withdraw from a study at any time without penalty or loss of benefits.

---

### HELPFUL HINT

Remember that research reports rarely provide readers with detailed information regarding the degree to which the researcher adhered to ethical principles, such as informed consent, because of space limitations in journals that make it impossible to describe all aspects of a study. Failure to mention procedures to safeguard subjects' rights does not necessarily mean that such precautions were not taken.

---

The language of the consent form must be understandable. The reading level should be no higher than eighth grade for adults, and lay language and the avoidance of technical terms should be used (DHHS, 2009). According to the Code of Federal Regulations, subjects should not be asked to waive their rights or release the investigator from liability for negligence. The elements for an informed consent form are listed in Box 13-2.

Investigators obtain **consent** through personal discussion with potential subjects. This process allows the person to obtain immediate answers to questions. However, consent forms, which are written in narrative or outline form, highlight elements that both inform and remind subjects of the nature of the study and their participation (Amdur & Bankert, 2011).

Assurance of anonymity and confidentiality (defined in Table 13-2) is conveyed in writing and describes how confidentiality of the subjects' records will be maintained. The right to privacy is also protected through protection of individually identifiable health information (IIHI). The DHHS developed the following guidelines to help researchers, health care organizations, health care providers, and academic institutions determine when they can use and disclose IIHI:

- IIHI has to be "de-identified" under the HIPAA Privacy Rule.
- Data are part of a limited data set, and a data use agreement with the researcher is in place.
- The individual who is a potential subject provides authorization for the researcher to use and disclose protected health information (PHI).
- A waiver or alteration of the authorization requirement is obtained from the IRB.

- The consent form must be signed and dated by the subject. The presence of witnesses is not always necessary but does constitute evidence that the subject actually signed the form. If the subject is a minor or is physically or mentally incapable of signing the consent, the legal guardian or representative must sign. The investigator also signs the form to indicate commitment to the agreement.

A copy of the signed informed consent is given to the subject. The researcher maintains the original for their records. Some research, such as a retrospective chart audit, may not require informed consent—only institutional approval. In some cases when minimal risk is involved, the investigator may have to provide the subject only with an information sheet and verbal explanation. In other cases, such as a volunteer convenience sample, completion and return of research instruments provide evidence of consent. The IRB will help advise on exceptions to these guidelines, and there are cases in which the IRB might grant waivers or amend its guidelines in other ways. The IRB makes the final determination regarding the most appropriate documentation format. You should note whether and what kind of evidence of informed consent has been provided in a research article.

---

## HELPFUL HINT

Note that researchers often do not obtain written, informed consent when the major means of data collection is through self-administered questionnaires. The researcher usually assumes implied consent in such cases; that is, the return of the completed questionnaire reflects the respondent's voluntary consent to participate.

---

### Institutional Review Board

**Institutional Review Boards** (IRBs) are boards that review studies to assess that ethical standards are met in relation to the protection of the rights of human subjects. The National Research Act (1974) requires that agencies such as universities, hospitals, and other health care organizations (e.g., managed care companies) applying for a grant or contract for any project or program that involves the conduct of biomedical or behavioral research involving human subjects must submit with their application assurances that they have established an IRB, sometimes called a human subjects' committee, that reviews the research projects and protects the rights of the human subjects (FDA, 2012b). At agencies where no federal grants or contracts are awarded, there is usually a review mechanism similar to an IRB process, such as a research advisory committee. The National Research Act requires that the IRB have at least five members of various research backgrounds to promote complete and adequate project review. The members must be qualified by virtue of their expertise and experience and reflect professional, gender, racial, and cultural diversity. Membership must include one member whose concerns are primarily nonscientific (lawyer, clergy, ethicist) and at least one member from outside the agency. Members of IRBs have mandatory training in scientific integrity and prevention of scientific misconduct, as do the principal investigator of a research study and his or her research team members. In an effort to protect research subjects, the HIPAA Privacy Rule has made IRB requirements much more stringent for researchers to meet (Code of Federal Regulations, Part 46, 2009).

The IRB is responsible for protecting subjects from undue risk and loss of personal rights and dignity. The **risk/benefit ratio**, the extent to which a study's benefits are maximized and the risks are minimized such that the subjects are protected from harm

---

### BOX 13-3    CODE OF FEDERAL REGULATIONS FOR IRB APPROVAL OF RESEARCH STUDIES

To approve research, the IRB must determine that the following Code of Federal Regulations has been satisfied:
1. Risks to subjects are minimized.
2. Risks to subjects are reasonable in relation to anticipated benefits.
3. Selection of the subjects is equitable.
4. Informed consent must be and will be sought from each prospective subject or the subject's legally authorized representative.
5. Informed consent form must be properly documented.
6. Where appropriate, the research plan makes adequate provision for monitoring the data collected to ensure subject safety.
7. There are adequate provisions to protect the privacy of subjects and the confidentiality of data.
8. Where some or all of the subjects are likely to be vulnerable to coercion or undue influence additional safeguards are included.

---

during the study, is always a major consideration. For a research proposal to be eligible for consideration by an IRB, it must already have been approved by a departmental review group such as a nursing research committee that attests to the proposal's scientific merit and congruence with institutional policies, procedures, and mission. The IRB reviews the study's protocol to ensure that it meets the requirements of ethical research that appear in Box 13-3.

IRBs provide guidelines that include steps to be taken to receive IRB approval. For example, guidelines for writing a standard consent form or criteria for qualifying for an expedited rather than a full IRB review may be made available. The IRB has the authority to approve research, require modifications, or disapprove a research study. A researcher must receive IRB approval before beginning to conduct research. IRBs have the authority to audit, suspend, or terminate approval of research that is not conducted in accordance with IRB requirements or that has been associated with unexpected serious harm to subjects.

IRBs also have mechanisms for reviewing research in an expedited manner when the risk to research subjects is minimal (Code of Federal Regulations, 2009). An expedited review usually shortens the length of the review process. Keep in mind that although a researcher may determine that a project involves minimal risk, the IRB makes the final determination, and the research may not be undertaken until approved. A full list of research categories eligible for expedited review is available from any IRB office. Examples include the following:

- Prospective collection of specimens by noninvasive procedure (e.g., buccal swab, deciduous teeth, hair/nail clippings)
- Research conducted in established educational settings in which subjects are de-identified
- Research involving materials collected for clinical purposes
- Research on taste, food quality, and consumer acceptance
- Collection of excreta and external secretions, including sweat
- Recording of data on subjects 18 years or older, using noninvasive procedures routinely employed in clinical practice
- Voice recordings
- Study of existing data, documents, records, pathological specimens, or diagnostic data

An expedited review does not automatically exempt the researcher from obtaining informed consent, and, most importantly, the department or agency head retains the final judgment as to whether or not a study may be exempt.

## Health Insurance Portability and Accountability Act of 1996 (HIPAA)

The subject's right to privacy is protected by the Health Insurance Portability and Accountability Act of 1996 (HIPAA), which describes federal standards to protect patients' medical records and other health information (DHHS, 2004 a,b). Compliance with these regulations (known as the Privacy Rule) has been required since 2003. The HIPAA Privacy Rule expanded a person's privacy to protect IIHI and described the ways in which covered entities can use or disclose this information. Covered entities include the person's (1) health provider, (2) health insurance plan, (3) employer, and (4) health care clearinghouse (public or private entity that processes or facilitates the processing of health information). According to the HIPAA Privacy Rule, IIHI is protected health information. Covered entities such as health care providers and health care agencies can allow researchers access to health care information if the information has been "de-identified," which involves removing the following 17 elements that could be used to identify a person, his or her employer, or his or her relatives.

- Names
- Geographic indicators smaller than a state
- All elements of dates (except year) for dates directly related to an individual (e.g., birth date, discharge date)
- Telephone numbers
- Facsimile (fax) numbers
- E-mail addresses
- Social Security numbers
- Health plan beneficiary numbers
- Account numbers
- Certificate/license numbers
- Vehicle identification and serial numbers
- Device identifiers and serial numbers
- Web universal resource locators (URLs)
- Internet protocol (IP) address numbers
- Biometric identifiers (e.g., fingerprints)
- Full-face photographic images
- Any other unique identifying number, characteristic, or code

As you can see, researchers are affected by the HIPAA Privacy Rule and must follow a protocol for accessing and communicating research subject information to protect patients' right to privacy.

IRBs can act on requests for a waiver or alteration of the authorization requirement for a research project. An altered authorization requirement occurs when an IRB approves a request that some, but not all, of the de-identification elements (e.g., name, address) be removed from the health information that is to be used in research. The researcher can also request a partial waiver of authorization, which allows the researcher to obtain PHI to contact and recruit potential subjects for a study. It is important to note that all institutions are guided by HIPAA guidelines in developing informed consent procedures.

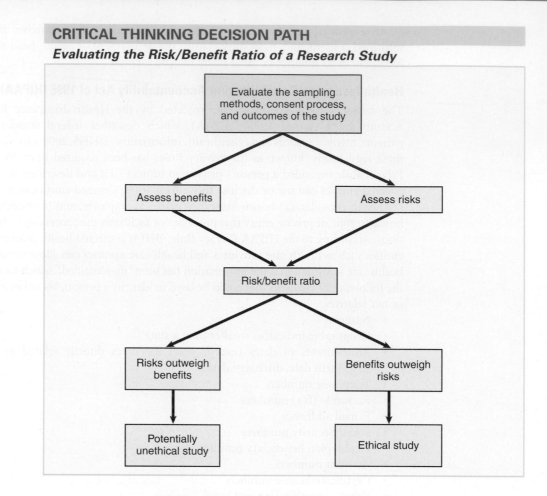

CRITICAL THINKING DECISION PATH

Evaluating the Risk/Benefit Ratio of a Research Study

Every researcher should consult an agency's research office to ensure that the application being prepared for IRB approval adheres to the most current requirements. Nurses who are critiquing published research should be conversant with current regulations to determine whether ethical standards have been met. The Critical Thinking Decision Path illustrates the ethical decision-making process an IRB might use in evaluating the risk/benefit ratio of a research study.

## Protecting Basic Human Rights of Vulnerable Groups

Researchers are advised to consult their agency's IRB for the most recent federal and state rules and guidelines when considering research involving vulnerable groups who may have diminished autonomy, such as the elderly, children, pregnant women, the unborn, those who are emotionally or physically disabled, prisoners, the deceased, students, and persons with AIDS. In addition, researchers should consult the IRB before planning research that potentially involves an oversubscribed research population, such as organ transplantation patients or AIDS patients, or "captive" and convenient populations, such as prisoners.

It should be emphasized that use of special populations does not preclude undertaking research; extra precautions must be taken, however, to protect their rights.

**Research with Children.** The age of majority differs from state to state, but there are some general rules for including children as subjects (Title 45, CFR46 Subpart D, DHHS, 2009). Usually a child can assent between the ages of 7 and 18 years. Research in children requires parental permission and child **assent**. Assent contains the following fundamental elements:

1. A basic understanding of what the child will be expected to do and what will be done to the child
2. A comprehension of the basic purpose of the research
3. An ability to express a preference regarding participation

In contrast to assent, **consent** requires a relatively advanced level of cognitive ability. Informed consent reflects competency standards requiring abstract appreciation and reasoning regarding the information provided. The issue of assent versus consent is interesting when one determines at what age children can make meaningful decisions about participating in research. There has been much discussion on the issue of child assent versus consent over the years. The Federal Guidelines have specific criteria and standards that must be met for children to participate in research. If the research involves more than minimal risk and does not offer direct benefit to the individual child, both parents must give permission. When individuals reach maturity, usually at age 18 years, they may render their own consent. They may do so at a younger age if they have been legally declared emancipated minors. Questions regarding this should be addressed by the IRB and/or research administration office and not left to the discretion of the researcher to answer.

**Research with Pregnant Women, Fetuses, and Neonates.** Research with pregnant women, fetuses, and neonates requires additional protection but may be conducted if specific criteria are met (HHS Code of Federal Regulations, Title 45, CFR46 Subpart B, 2009). Decisions are made relative to the direct or indirect benefit or lack of benefit to the pregnant woman and the fetus. For example, pregnant women may be involved in research if the research holds out the prospect of direct benefit to the pregnant women and fetus by providing data for assessing risks to pregnant women and fetuses. If the research holds out the prospect of direct benefit to the fetus solely, then both the mother and father must provide consent.

**Research with Prisoners.** The Federal Guidelines also provide guidance to IRBs regarding research with prisoners. These guidelines address the issues of allowable research, understandable language, adequate assurances that participation does not affect parole decisions, and risks and benefits (HHS Code of Federal Regulations, Title 45 Part 46, Subpart C, 2009).

**Research with the Elderly.** Elderly individuals were historically and are potentially vulnerable to abuse and as such require special consideration. There is no issue if the potential subject can supply legally effective informed consent. Competence is not a clear "black-or-white" issue. The complexity of the study may affect one's ability to consent to participate. The capacity to obtain informed consent should be assessed in each individual for each research protocol being considered. For example, an elderly person may be able to consent to participate in a simple observational study but not in a clinical drug trial. The issue of the necessity of requiring the elderly to provide consent often arises, and each situation must be evaluated for its potential to preserve the rights of this population.

---

**BOX 13-4    EXAMPLES OF LEGAL AND ETHICAL CONTENT IN PUBLISHED RESEARCH REPORTS FOUND IN THE APPENDICES**

- "The study was approved by the institutional review board, and research committee at each of the sites" (Thomas et al., 2012, p. 40).
- "Institutional Review Board approval was obtained prior to participant recruitment" (Alhusen et al, 2012, p. 115).
- "Approval from a university institutional Review Board was obtained prior to data collection" (Seiler & Moss, 2012, p. 306).

---

No vulnerable population may be singled out for study because it is convenient. For example, neither people with mental illness nor prisoners may be studied because they are an available and convenient group. Prisoners may be studied if the studies pertain to them; that is, studies concerning the effects and processes of incarceration. Similarly, people with mental illness may participate in studies that focus on expanding knowledge about psychiatric disorders and treatments. Students also are often a convenient group. They must not be singled out as research subjects because of convenience; the research questions must have some bearing on their status as students.

Researchers and patient caregivers involved in research with vulnerable populations are well advised to seek advice from their IRB. In all cases, the burden should be on the investigator to show the IRB that it is appropriate to involve vulnerable subjects in research.

**HELPFUL HINT**

Keep in mind that researchers rarely mention explicitly that the study participants were vulnerable subjects or that special precautions were taken to appropriately safeguard the human rights of this vulnerable group. Research consumers need to be attentive to the special needs of groups who may be unable to act as their own advocates or are unable to adequately assess the risk/benefit ratio of a research study.

## APPRAISING THE EVIDENCE
## LEGAL AND ETHICAL ASPECTS OF A RESEARCH STUDY

Research reports often do not contain detailed information regarding the ways in which the investigator adhered to the legal and ethical principles presented in this chapter. Space considerations in articles preclude extensive documentation of all legal and ethical aspects of a study. Lack of written evidence regarding the protection of human rights does not imply that appropriate steps were not taken.

The Critiquing Criteria box provides guidelines for evaluating the legal and ethical aspects of a study. When reading a study, due to space constraints, you will not see all areas explicitly addressed in the article; however, you should be aware of them and should determine that the researcher has addressed them before conducting the study. A nurse who is asked to serve as a member of an IRB will find the critiquing criteria useful in evaluating the legal and ethical aspects of the research proposal. Box 13-4 provides examples of statements in research articles that illustrate the brevity with which the legal and ethical component of a study is reported.

## CRITIQUING CRITERIA

### Legal and Ethical Issues

1. Was the study approved by an IRB or other agency committees?
2. Is there evidence that informed consent was obtained from all subjects or their representatives? How was it obtained?
3. Were the subjects protected from physical or emotional harm?
4. Were the subjects or their representatives informed about the purpose and nature of the study?
5. Were the subjects or their representatives informed about any potential risks that might result from participation in the study?
6. Is the research study designed to maximize the benefit(s) to human subjects and minimize the risks?
7. Were subjects coerced or unduly influenced to participate in this study? Did they have the right to refuse to participate or withdraw without penalty? Were vulnerable subjects used?
8. Were appropriate steps taken to safeguard the privacy of subjects? How have data been kept anonymous and/or confidential?

Information about the legal and ethical considerations of a study is usually presented in the methods section of an article. The subsection on the sample or data-collection methods is the most likely place for this information. The author most often indicates in a few sentences that informed consent was obtained and that approval from an IRB or similar committee was granted. It is likely that a paper will not be accepted for publication without such a discussion. This also makes it almost impossible for unauthorized research to be published. Therefore when an article provides evidence of having been approved by an external review committee, you can feel confident that the ethical issues raised by the study have been thoroughly reviewed and resolved.

To protect subject and institutional privacy, the locale of the study frequently is described in general terms in the sample subsection of the report. For example, the article might state that data were collected at a 1,000-bed tertiary care center in the Southwest, without mentioning its name. Protection of subject privacy may be explicitly addressed by statements indicating that anonymity or confidentiality of data was maintained or that grouped data were used in the data analysis.

When considering the special needs of vulnerable subjects, you should be sensitive to whether the special needs of groups, unable to act on their own behalf, have been addressed. For instance, has the right of self-determination been addressed by the informed consent protocol identified in the research report?

When qualitative studies are reported, verbatim quotes from informants often are incorporated into the findings section of the article. In such cases, you will evaluate how effectively the author protected the informant's identity, either by using a fictitious name or by withholding information such as age, gender, occupation, or other potentially identifying data (see Chapters 5, 6, and 7 for special ethical issues related to qualitative research).

It should be apparent from the preceding sections that although the need for guide-lines for the use of human and animal subjects in research is evident and the principles themselves are clear, there are many instances when you must use your best judgment both as a patient advocate and as a research consumer when evaluating the ethical nature of a research project. In any research situation, the basic guiding principle of protecting the patient's human rights must always apply. When conflicts arise, you must feel free to raise suitable questions with appropriate resources and personnel. In an institution these may include contacting the researcher first and then, if there is no resolution, the director of nursing research, and the chairperson of the IRB. In cases when ethical considerations in a research article are in question, clarification from a colleague, agency, or IRB is indicated. You should pursue your concerns until satisfied that the patient's rights and your rights as a professional nurse are protected.

## KEY POINTS

- Ethical and legal considerations in research first received attention after World War II during the Nuremberg Trials, from which developed the Nuremberg Code. This became the standard for research guidelines protecting the human rights of research subjects.
- The National Research Act, passed in 1974, created the National Commission for the Protection of Human Subjects of Biomedical and Behavioral Research. The findings, contained in the Belmont Report, discuss three basic ethical principles (respect for persons, beneficence, and justice) that underlie the conduct of research involving human subjects. Federal regulations developed in response to the Commission's report provide guidelines for informed consent and IRB protocols.
- The ANA's Commission on Nursing Research published *Human Rights Guidelines for Nurses in Clinical and Other Research* in 1985 for protection of human rights of research subjects. It is relevant to nurses as researchers as well as caregivers. The ANA's *Code for Nurses* (ANA, 2001) is integral with the research guidelines.
- The Health Insurance Portability and Accountability Act (HIPAA) implemented in 2003, includes privacy rules to protect an individual's health information that affect health care organizations and the conduct of research.
- Protection of human rights includes (1) right to self-determination, (2) right to privacy and dignity, (3) right to anonymity and confidentiality, (4) right to fair treatment, and (5) right to protection from discomfort and harm.
- Procedures for protecting basic human rights include gaining informed consent, which illustrates the ethical principle of respect, and obtaining IRB approval, which illustrates the ethical principles of respect, beneficence, and justice.
- Special consideration should be given to studies involving vulnerable populations, such as children, the elderly, prisoners, and those who are mentally or physically disabled.
- Nurses as consumers of research must be knowledgeable about the legal and ethical components of a research study so they can evaluate whether a researcher has ensured appropriate protection of human or animal rights.

## CRITICAL THINKING CHALLENGES

- A state government official interested in determining the number of infants infected with the human immunodeficiency virus (HIV) has approached your hospital to participate in a state-wide funded study. The protocol will include the testing of all newborns for HIV, but the mothers will not be told that the test is being done, nor will they be told the results. Using the basic ethical principles found in Box 13-2, defend or refute the practice. How will the findings of the proposed study be affected if the protocol is carried out?

- As a research consumer, what kind of information related to the legal and ethical aspects of a research study would you expect to see written about in a published research study? How does that differ from the data the researcher would have to prepare for an IRB submission?

- A randomized clinical trial (RCT) testing the effectiveness of a new Lyme disease vaccine is being conducted as a multi-site RCT. There are two vaccine intervention groups, each of which is receiving a different vaccine, and one control group that is receiving a placebo. Using the information in Table 13-2, identify the conditions under which the RCT is halted due to potential legal and ethical issues to subjects.

- What does risk/benefit ratio mean and how does it influence the strength and quality of evidence required for clinical decision making?

# REFERENCES

Alhusen, JL., Gross, D., Hayatt, MJ., Woods, AB(N)., & Sharps, PW. (2012). The influence of maternal-fetal attachment and health practices on neonatal outcomes in low-income women. *Research in Nursing & Health, 35*, 112–120.

Amdur, R. & Bankert, E. A. (2011). *Institutional Review Board: Member Handbook,* 3rd Ed. Boston, Jones & Bartlett

American Nurses Association. (1985). *Human rights guidelines for nurses in clinical and other research.* Kansas City, MO: Author.

American Nurses Association. (2001). *Code for nurses with interpretive statements.* Kansas City, MO: Author.

Brainard, J., & Miller, D. W. (2000). U.S. regulators suspend medical studies at two universities. *Chronicle of Higher Education,* A30.

French, H. W. (1997). AIDS research in Africa: juggling risks and hopes. *New York Times,* October 9, A1–A12.

Hershey, N., & Miller, R. D. (1976). *Human experimentation and the law.* Germantown, MD: Aspen.

Hilts, P. J. (1995). Agency faults a UCLA study for suffering of mental patients. *New York Times,* March 9, A1–A11.

Levine, R. J. (1986). Ethics and regulation of clinical research (2nd ed.). Baltimore, MD-Munich, Germany: Urban & Schwartzenberg.

National Commission for the Protection of Human Subjects of Biomedical and Behavioral Research. (1978). *Belmont report: ethical principles and guidelines for research involving human subjects, DHEW pub no 05.* Washington, DC: US Government Printing Office, 78-0012.

Reverby, S. M. (2000). History of an apology: from Tuskegee to the White House. *Research Practice,* (8), 1–12.

Rothman, D. J. (1982). Were Tuskegee and Willowbrook studies in nature? *Hastings Center Report, 12*(2), 5–7.

Seiler, A. J., & Moss, V. A. (2012). The experiences of nurse practitioners providing health care to the homeless. *Journal of the American Academy of Nurse Practitioners, 24*, 303–312.

Thomas, M. L., Elliott, J. E., Rao, S. M, et al. (2012). A randomized clinical trial of education or motivational-interviewing–based coaching compared to usual care to improve cancer pain management. *Oncology Nursing Forum, 39*(1), 39–49.

U. S. Department of Health and Human Services (USDHHS). (2009). 45 CFR 46. In *Code of Federal Regulations: protection of human subjects.*Washington, DC: Author.

U. S. Department of Health and Human Services (USDHHS). (2004a). Standards for privacy of individually identifiable health information: final rule. In *Code of Federal Regulations, title 45, parts 160 and 164*. Retrieved from www.hhs.gov/ocr/hipaa/finalreg.html.

U. S. Department of Health and Human Services (USDHHS). (2004b). *Institutional review boards and the HIPAA privacy rule: information for researchers*. Retrieved from http://privacy rule and research.nih.gov/irbandprivacyrule.asp.

U. S. Food and Drug Administration (FDA). (2012a). *A guide to informed consent, Code of Federal Regulations, Title 21, Part 50*. Retrieved from www.fda.gov/oc/ohrt/irbs/informedconsent.html.

U. S. Food and Drug Administration (FDA). (2012b). *Institutional review boards, Code of Federal Regulations, Title 21, Part 56*. Retrieved from www.fda.gov/oc/ohrt/irbs/appendixc.html.

Wheeler, D. L. (1997). Three medical organizations embroiled in controversy over use of placebos in AIDS studies abroad. *Chronicle of Higher Education*, A15–A16.

# ⊖volve WEBSITE

*Go to Evolve at http://evolve.elsevier.com/LoBiondo/ for review questions, critiquing exercises, and additional research articles for practice in reviewing and critiquing.*

# CHAPTER 14

# Data Collection Methods

*Susan Sullivan-Bolyai and Carol Bova*

## ℮volve WEBSITE

*Go to Evolve at http://evolve.elsevier.com/LoBiondo/ for review questions, critiquing exercises, and additional research articles for practice in reviewing and critiquing.*

## LEARNING OUTCOMES

*After reading this chapter, you should be able to do the following:*

- Define the types of data collection methods used in nursing research.
- List the advantages and disadvantages of each data collection method.
- Compare how specific data collection methods contribute to the strength of evidence in a research study.

- Identify potential sources of bias related to data collection.
- Discuss the importance of intervention fidelity in data collection.
- Critically evaluate the data collection methods used in published research studies.

## KEY TERMS

| | | | |
|---|---|---|---|
| anecdotes | field notes | observation | respondent burden |
| closed-ended questions | intervention | open-ended questions | scale |
| concealment | interview guide | operational definition | scientific observation |
| consistency | interviews | participant observation | self-report |
| content analysis | Likert scales | physiological data | systematic |
| debriefing | measurement | questionnaires | systematic error |
| demographic data | measurement error | random error | |
| existing data | objective | reactivity | |

Nurses are always collecting information (or data) from patients. We collect data on blood pressure, age, weight, height, and laboratory values as part of our daily work. Data collected for practice purposes and for research have several key differences. Data collection procedures in research must be objective and systematic. By **objective**, we mean that the data collected are free from the researchers' personal biases, beliefs, values, or attitudes. By **systematic**, we mean that the data are collected in a uniform, consistent, or standard way from each subject by everyone who is involved in the data collection process. When reading a study, the data collection methods should be identifiable and repeatable. Thus, when reading the research literature to inform your evidence-based practice, there are several issues to consider regarding study data collection descriptions.

It is important that researchers carefully define the *concept*s or *variables* they are interested in measuring. The process of translating a concept into a measurable variable for data collection requires the development of an **operational definition**. An operational definition is how the researcher will measure each variable. For example, Thomas and colleagues (2012) (see Appendix A) defined *quality of life* as including the four domains of physical, social, emotional, and functional well-being measured by the FACT-G, which is commonly used in cancer studies.

Ultimately, the degree to which the researcher is able to clearly define and measure study variables in an unbiased and consistent way is an important determinant of how useful the data will be to guide practice. The purpose of this chapter is to familiarize you with the various ways that researchers collect data from subjects. The chapter provides you with the tools for evaluating the types of data collection procedures commonly used in research publications, their strengths and weaknesses, how consistent data collection operations (a high level of fidelity) can increase study rigor and decrease bias that affects study internal and external validity, and how useful each technique is for providing evidence for nursing practice. This information will help you critique the research literature and decide whether the findings provide evidence that is applicable to your practice setting.

## MEASURING VARIABLES OF INTEREST

To a large extent, the success of a study depends on the *fidelity* (consistency and quality) of the data collection methods used. Researchers have many types of methods available for collecting information from subjects. Determining what **measurement** to use in a particular study may be the most difficult and time-consuming step in study design. Thus the process of evaluating and selecting the available instruments to measure variables of interest is of critical importance to the potential success of the study.

As you read research articles and the data collection techniques used, look for **consistency** with the study's aim, hypotheses, setting, and population. Data collection methods may be viewed as a two-step process. First, the researcher chooses the data collection method(s) for their study. In this chapter the selection of measures and the implementation of the data collection process are discussed. An algorithm that influences a researcher's choice of data collection methods is diagrammed in the Critical Thinking Decision Path. The second step is deciding if these methods are reliable and valid. Reliability and validity of instruments are discussed in detail in Chapter 15 (for quantitative research) and in Chapter 6 (for qualitative research).

**CRITICAL THINKING DECISION PATH**

*Consumer of Research Literature Review*

```
                        ┌──────────────────────────┐
                        │  Is the concept to be studied… │
                        └──────────────────────────┘
                                      │
        ┌─────────────────────────────┼─────────────────────────────┐
        │                             │                             │
 ┌──────────────────┐      ┌──────────────────────────┐      ┌──────────────────┐
 │ Physiological data? │      │ Complex environmental data? │      │  Self-report data? │
 └──────────────────┘      └──────────────────────────┘      └──────────────────┘
        │                             │                             │
 ┌──────────────────────┐      ┌──────────────────┐      ┌──────────────────┐
 │ Use physiological instrument │      │  Use observation  │      │  Discrete content? │
 └──────────────────────┘      └──────────────────┘      └──────────────────┘
                                      │                      ┌──────┴──────┐
                               ┌──────────────┐           ┌─────┐     ┌─────┐
                               │ Discrete content? │           │ Yes │     │ No  │
                               └──────────────┘           └─────┘     └─────┘
                               ┌──────┴──────┐              │           │
                            ┌─────┐     ┌─────┐    ┌──────────────┐  ┌──────────────┐
                            │ Yes │     │ No  │    │ Questionnaire │  │ Unstructured │
                            └─────┘     └─────┘    │ or structured │  │   interview   │
                               │           │       │   interview   │  └──────────────┘
                      ┌──────────────┐  ┌──────────┐└──────────────┘
                      │ Observational │  │ Field notes │
                      │     guide     │  └──────────┘
                      └──────────────┘
```

# DATA COLLECTION METHODS

When reading a research article, be aware that investigators must decide early in the research process whether they need to collect their own data or whether data already exist in the form of records or databases. This decision is based on a thorough literature review and the availability of existing data. If the researcher determines that no data exist, new data can be collected through **observation, self-report** (interviewing or questionnaires), or by collecting **physiological data** using standardized instruments or testing procedures (e.g., laboratory tests, x-rays). **Existing data** can be collected for research purposes by extracting data from medical records or state and national databases using standardized procedures. Each of these methods has a specific purpose, as well as pros and cons inherent in its use. It is also important to remember that all data collection methods rely on the ability of the researcher to standardize these procedures to increase data accuracy and reduce measurement error.

**Measurement error** is the difference between what really exists and what is measured in a given study. Every study has some amount of measurement error. Measurement error can be random or systematic (see Chapter 15). **Random error** occurs when scores vary in a random way. Random error occurs when data collectors do not use standard procedures to collect data consistently among all subjects in a study. **Systematic error** occurs when scores are incorrect but in the same direction. An example of systematic error occurs when all subjects were weighed using a weight scale that is under by 3 pounds for all subjects in the study. Researchers attempt to design data collection methods that will be consistently applied across all subjects and time points to reduce measurement error.

---

**HELPFUL HINT**

Remember that the researcher may not always present complete information about the way the data were collected, especially when established instruments were used. To learn about the instrument that was used in greater detail, you may need to consult the original article describing the instrument.

---

*Fidelity* means that data are collected from each subject in exactly the same manner with the same method by carefully trained data collectors (see Chapter 8). To help you decipher the quality of the data collection section in a research article, we will discuss the three main methods used for collecting data: observation, self-report, and physiological measurement.

---

**EVIDENCE-BASED PRACTICE TIP**

It is difficult to place confidence in a study's findings if the data collection methods are not consistent.

---

## Observational Methods

Observation is a method for collecting data on how people behave under certain conditions. Observation can take place in a natural setting (e.g., in the home, in the community, on a nursing unit) or laboratory setting and often includes collecting data on communication (verbal, nonverbal), behavior, and environmental conditions. Observation is also useful for collecting data that may have cultural or contextual influences. For example, if a nurse researcher wanted to understand the emergence of obesity among immigrants to the United States, it might be useful to observe food preparation, exercise patterns, and shopping practices among specific immigrant groups.

Although observing the environment is a normal part of living, **scientific observation** places a great deal of emphasis on the objective and systematic nature of the observation. The researcher is not merely looking at what is happening, but rather is watching with a trained eye for specific events. To be scientific, observations must fulfill the following four conditions:

1. Observations undertaken are consistent with the study's aims/objectives.
2. There is a standardized and systematic plan for observation and data recording.
3. All observations are checked and controlled.
4. The observations are related to scientific concepts and theories.

Observational methods may be structured or unstructured. Unstructured observation methods are not characterized by a total absence of structure, but usually involve collecting descriptive information about the topic of interest. In **participant observation**, the observer keeps **field notes** (a short summary of observations) to record the activities, as well as the observer's interpretations of these activities. *Field notes* usually are not restricted to any particular type of action or behavior; rather, they represent a narrative set of written notes intended to paint a picture of a social situation in a more general sense. Another type of unstructured observation is the use of anecdotes. **Anecdotes** are summaries of a particular observation that usually focus on the behaviors of interest and frequently add to the richness of research reports by illustrating a particular point (see Chapters 5 and 6 for more on data collection strategies). Structured observations involve specifying in advance

| | | Concealment | |
|---|---|---|---|
| | | Yes | No |
| **Intervention** | Yes | Researcher hidden<br><br>An intervention | Researcher open<br><br>An intervention |
| | No | Researcher hidden<br><br>No intervention | Researcher open<br><br>No intervention |

**FIGURE 14-1** Types of observational roles in research.

what behaviors or events are to be observed. Typically, standardized forms are used for record keeping and include categorization systems, checklists, or rating scales. Structured observation relies heavily on the formal training and standardization of the observers (see Chapter 15 for an explanation of interpreter reliability).

Observational methods can also be distinguished by the role of the observer. The observer's role is determined by the amount of interaction between the observer and those being observed. These methods are illustrated in Figure 14-1. Concealment refers to whether the subjects know they are being observed, and intervention deals with whether the observer provokes actions from those who are being observed. Box 14-1 describes the four basic types of observational roles implemented by the observer(s). These are distinguishable by the amount of concealment or intervention implemented by the observer.

Observing subjects without their knowledge may violate assumptions of informed consent, and therefore researchers face ethical problems with this approach. However, sometimes there is no other way to collect such data, and the data collected are unlikely to have negative consequences for the subject. In these cases, the disadvantages of the study are outweighed by the advantages. Further, the problem is often handled by informing subjects after the observation, allowing them the opportunity to refuse to have their data included in the study and discussing any questions they might have. This process is called debriefing.

When the observer is neither concealed nor intervening, the ethical question is not a problem. Here the observer makes no attempt to change the subjects' behavior and informs them that they are to be observed. Because the observer is present, this type of observation allows a greater depth of material to be studied than if the observer is separated from the subject by an artificial barrier, such as a one-way mirror. Participant observation is a commonly used observational technique in which the researcher functions as a part of a social group to study the group in question. The problem with this type of observation is reactivity (also referred to as the Hawthorne effect), or the distortion created when the subjects change behavior because they are being observed.

**EVIDENCE-BASED PRACTICE TIP**

When reading a research report that uses observation as a data collection method, you want to note evidence of consistency across data collectors through use of interrater reliability (see Chapter 15) data. When that is present, it increases your confidence that the data were collected systematically.

---

### BOX 14-1    BASIC TYPES OF OBSERVATIONAL ROLES

1. *Concealment without intervention.* The researcher watches subjects without their knowledge, and does not provoke the subject into action. Often such concealed observations use hidden television cameras, audio recording devices, or one-way mirrors. This method is often used in observational studies of children and their parents. You may be familiar with rooms with one-way mirrors in which a researcher can observe the behavior of the occupants of the room without being observed by them. Such studies allow for the observation of children's natural behavior and are often used in developmental research.

2. *Concealment with intervention.* Concealed observation with intervention involves staging a situation and observing the behaviors that are evoked in the subjects as a result of the intervention. Because the subjects are unaware of their participation in a research study, this type of observation has fallen into disfavor and rarely is used in nursing research.

3. *No concealment without intervention.* The researcher obtains informed consent from the subject to be observed and then simply observes his or her behavior. This was the type of observation done in a study by Aitken and colleagues (2009); nurses providing sedation management for a critically ill patient were observed and asked to think aloud during two occasions for 2 hours of care to examine the decision-making processes that nurses use when assessing and managing sedation needs of critically ill patients.

4. *No concealment with intervention.* No concealment with intervention is used when the researcher is observing the effects of an intervention introduced for scientific purposes. Because the subjects know they are participating in a research study, there are few problems with ethical concerns; however, *reactivity* is a problem in this type of study.

---

Scientific observation has several advantages, the main one being that observation may be the only way for the researcher to study the variable of interest. For example, what people say they do often may not be what they really do. Therefore, if the study is designed to obtain substantive findings about human behavior, observation may be the only way to ensure the validity of the findings. In addition, no other data collection method can match the depth and variety of information that can be collected when using these techniques. Such techniques also are quite flexible in that they may be used in both experimental and nonexperimental designs. As with all data collection methods, observation also has its disadvantages. Data obtained by observational techniques are vulnerable to observer bias. Emotions, prejudices, and values can influence the way behaviors and events are observed and recorded. In general, the more the observer needs to make inferences and judgments about what is being observed, the more likely it is that distortions will occur. Thus in judging the adequacy of observation methods, it is important to consider how observation forms were constructed and how observers were trained and evaluated.

Ethical issues can also occur if subjects are not fully aware that they are being observed. For the most part, it is best to fully inform subjects of the study's purpose and the fact that they are being observed. But in certain circumstances, informing the subjects will change behaviors (Hawthorne effect; see Chapter 8). For example, if a nurse researcher wanted to study hand-washing frequency on a nursing unit, telling the nurses that they were being observed for their rate of hand washing would likely increase the hand-washing rate and thereby make the study results less valid. Therefore researchers must carefully balance full disclosure of all research procedures with the ability to obtain valid data through observational methods.

## Self-Report Methods

Self-report methods require subjects to respond directly to either **interviews** or **questionnaires** (often called paper-and-pencil instruments) about their experiences, behaviors, feelings, or attitudes. Self-report methods are commonly used in nursing research and are most useful for collecting data on variables that cannot be directly observed or measured by physiological instruments. Some variables commonly measured by self-report in nursing research studies include quality of life, satisfaction with nursing care, social support, pain, uncertainty, and functional status.

The following are some considerations when evaluating self-report methods:

- *Social desirability.* There is no way to know for sure if a subject is telling the truth. People are known to respond to questions in a way that makes a favorable impression. For example, if a nurse researcher asks patients to describe the positive and negative aspects of nursing care received, the patient may want to please the researcher and respond with all positive responses, thus introducing bias into the data collection process. There is no way to tell whether the respondent is telling the truth or responding in a socially desirable way, so the accuracy of self-report measures is always open for scrutiny.
- *Respondent burden* is another concern for researchers who use self-report (Ulrich et al., 2012). **Respondent burden** occurs when the length of the questionnaire or interview is too long or the questions too difficult to answer in a reasonable amount of time considering respondents' age, health condition, or mental status. Respondent burden can result in incomplete or erroneous answers or missing data, jeopardizing the validity of the study findings.

## Interviews and Questionnaires

Interviews are a method of data collection where a data collector asks subjects to respond to a set of open-ended or closed-ended questions as described in Box 14-2. Interviews are used in both quantitative and qualitative research, but are best used when the researcher may need to clarify the task for the respondent or is interested in obtaining more personal information from the respondent.

Open-ended questions allow more varied information to be collected and require a qualitative or content analysis method to analyze responses (see Chapter 6). Content analysis is a method of analyzing narrative or word responses to questions and either counting similar responses or grouping the responses into themes or categories (also used in qualitative research). Interviews may take place face-to-face, over the telephone, or online via a Web-based format.

Questionnaires are paper-and-pencil instruments designed to gather data from individuals about knowledge, attitudes, beliefs, and feelings. Questionnaires, like interviews, may be open-ended or closed-ended as presented in Box 14-2. Questionnaires are most useful when there is a finite set of questions. Individual items in a questionnaire must be clearly written so that the intent of the question and the nature of the response options

> ### BOX 14-2    USES FOR OPEN-ENDED AND CLOSED-ENDED QUESTIONS
>
> - **Open-ended questions** are used when the researcher wants the subjects to respond in their own words or when the researcher does not know all of the possible alternative responses. Interviews that use open-ended questions often use a list of questions and probes called an **interview guide**. Responses to the interview guide are often audio-recorded to accurately capture the subject's responses. An example of an open-ended question is used for the interview in Appendix D.
> - **Closed-ended questions** are structured, fixed-response items with a fixed number of responses. Closed-ended questions are best used when the question has a finite number of responses and the respondent is to choose the one closest to the correct response. Fixed-response items have the advantage of simplifying the respondent's task but result in omission of important information about the subject. Interviews that use closed-ended questions typically record a subject's responses directly on the questionnaire. An example of a closed-ended item is found in Box 14-3.

are clear. Questionnaires may be composed of individual items that measure different variables or concepts (e.g., age, race, ethnicity, years of education) or scales. Survey researchers rely almost entirely on questionnaires for data collection.

Questionnaires can be referred to as instruments, measures, scales, or tools. When multiple items are used to measure a single concept, such as quality of life or anxiety, and the scores on those items are combined mathematically to obtain an overall score, the questionnaire or measurement instrument is called a scale. The important issue is that each of the items must be measuring the same concept or variable. An intelligence test is an example of a scale that combines individual item responses to determine an overall quantification of intelligence.

Scales can have subscales or total scale scores. For instance, in the study by Thomas and colleagues (2012) (see Appendix A), the FACT-G (with four separate domains measuring quality of life [QOL]), the "physical well-being" subscale has eight items that measure the single concept. Subjects responded to a five-point scale, ranging from 0 (not at all) to 5 (very much) for each of the seven physical well-being items; the eighth item had a range of 0-10 for how much physical well-being affects QOL. Thus the range of scores for that subscale would be 0 to 38. The total score range for the four domains combined is from 0-112. The response options for scales are typically lists of statements on which respondents indicate, for example, whether they "strongly agree," "agree," "disagree," or "strongly disagree." This type of response option is called a Likert-type scale. "True" or "False" may also be a response option.

### EVIDENCE-BASED PRACTICE TIP

Scales used in research should have evidence of adequate reliability and validity so that you feel confident that the findings reflect what the researcher intended to measure (see Chapter 15).

Box 14-3 shows three items from a survey of nursing job satisfaction. The first item is closed-ended and uses a Likert scale response format. The second item is also closed-ended, and it forces respondents to choose from a finite number of possible answers. The third item is open-ended and respondents use their own words to answer the question, allowing an unlimited number of possible answers. Often, researchers use a combination of Likert-type, closed-ended, and open-ended questions when collecting data in nursing research.

## BOX 14-3    EXAMPLES OF OPEN-ENDED AND CLOSED-ENDED QUESTIONS

**Open-Ended Questions**

Please list the three most important reasons why you chose to stay in your current job:

1. _____
2. _____
3. _____

**Closed-Ended Questions (Likert Scale)**

How satisfied are you with your current position?

| 1 | 2 | 3 | 4 | 5 |
|---|---|---|---|---|
| Very satisfied | Moderately satisfied | Undecided | Moderately dissatisfied | Very dissatisfied |

**Closed-Ended Questions**

On average, how many patients do you care for in 1 day?

1. 1 to 3
2. 4 to 6
3. 7 to 9
4. 10 to 12
5. 13 to 15
6. 16 to 18
7. 19 to 20
8. More than 20

Thomas and colleagues (2012; see Appendix A) used a self-report instrument to assess the intensity and interference of pain with daily function on a numeric score from 0 (does not interfere) to 10 (completely interferes). They also collected **demographic data.** Demographic data includes information that describes important characteristics about the subjects in a study (e.g., age, gender, race, ethnicity, education, marital status). It is important to collect demographic data in order to describe and compare different study samples so you can evaluate how similar the sample is to your patient population.

When reviewing articles with numerous questionnaires, remember (especially if the study deals with vulnerable populations) to assess if the author(s) addressed potential respondent burden such as:

- Reading level (eighth grade)
- Questionnaire font size (14-point font)
- Need to read and assist some subjects
- Time it took to complete the questionnaire (30 minutes)

This information is very important for judging the respondent burden associated with study participation. It is important to examine the benefits and caveats associated with using interviews and questionnaires as self-report methods. Interviews offer some advantages over questionnaires. The response rate is almost always higher with interviews and there are fewer missing data, which helps reduce bias.

Another advantage of the interview is that vulnerable populations such as children, the blind, and those with low literacy, may not be able to fill out a questionnaire. With

## HELPFUL HINT

Remember, sometimes researchers make trade-offs when determining the measures to be used. For example, a researcher may want to learn about an individual's attitudes regarding job satisfaction; however, practicalities may preclude using an interview, so a questionnaire may be used instead.

an interview, the data collector knows who is giving the answers. When questionnaires are mailed, for example, anyone in the household could be the person who supplies the answers. Interviews also allow for some safeguards such as clarifying misunderstood questions, and observing and recording the level of the respondent's understanding of the questions. In addition, the researcher has flexibility over the order of the questions.

With questionnaires, the respondent can answer questions in any order. Sometimes changing the order of the questions can change the response. Finally, interviews allow for richer and more complex data to be collected. This is particularly so when open-ended responses are sought. Even when closed-ended response items are used, interviewers can probe to understand why a respondent answered in a particular way.

Questionnaires also have certain advantages. They are much less expensive to administer than interviews that require hiring and thoroughly training interviewers. Thus if a researcher has a fixed amount of time and money, a larger and more diverse sample can be obtained with questionnaires. Questionnaires may allow for more confidentiality and anonymity with sensitive issues that participants may be reluctant to discuss in an interview. Finally, the fact that no interviewer is present assures the researcher and the reader that there will be no interviewer bias. *Interviewer bias* occurs when the interviewer unwittingly leads the respondent to answer in a certain way. This problem can be especially pronounced in studies that use open-ended questions. The tone used to ask the question and/or nonverbal interviewer responses such as a subtle nod of the head, could lead a respondent to change an answer to correspond with what the researcher wants to hear.

Finally, the use of Internet-based self-report data collection (both interviewing and questionnaire delivery) has gained momentum. The use of an online format is economical and can capture subjects from different geographic areas without the expense of travel or mailings. Open-ended questions are already typed and do not require transcription, and closed-ended questions can often be imported directly into statistical analysis software, and therefore reduce data entry mistakes. The main concerns with Internet-based data collection procedures involve the difficulty of ensuring informed consent (is checking a box indicating agreement to participate the same thing as signing an informed consent form?) and the protection of subject anonymity, which is difficult to guarantee with any Internet-based venue. In addition, the requirement that subjects have computer access limits the use of this method in certain age groups and populations. However, the advantages of increased efficiency and accuracy make Internet-based data collection a growing trend among nurse researchers.

## Physiological Measurement

Physiological data collection involves the use of specialized equipment to determine the physical and biological status of subjects. Such measures can be *physical,* such as weight or temperature; *chemical,* such as blood glucose level; *microbiological,* as with cultures; or *anatomical,* as in radiological examinations. What separates these data collection procedures from others used in research is that they require special equipment to make the observation.

Physiological or biological measurement is particularly suited to the study of many types of nursing problems. For example, examining different methods for taking a patient's temperature or blood pressure or monitoring blood glucose levels may yield important information for determining the effectiveness of certain nursing monitoring procedures or interventions. But it is important that the method be applied consistently to all subjects in the study. For example, nurses are quite familiar with taking blood pressure measurements. However, for research studies that involve blood pressure measurement, the process must be standardized (Bern et al., 2007; Pickering et al., 2005). The subject must be positioned (sitting or lying down) the same way for a specified period of time, the same blood pressure instrument must be used, and often multiple blood pressure measurements are taken under the same conditions to obtain an average value.

The advantages of using physiological data collection methods include the objectivity, precision, and sensitivity associated with these measures. Unless there is a technical malfunction, two readings of the same instrument taken at the same time by two different nurses are likely to yield the same result. Because such instruments are intended to measure the variable being studied, they offer the advantage of being precise and sensitive enough to pick up subtle variations in the variable of interest. It is also unlikely that a subject in a study can deliberately distort physiological information.

Physiological measurements are not without inherent disadvantages and include the following:

- Some instruments may be quite expensive to obtain and use.
- Physiological instruments often require specialized training to be used accurately.
- The variable of interest may be altered as a result of using the instrument. For example, an individual's blood pressure may increase just because a health care professional enters the room (called *white coat syndrome*).
- Although thought as being nonintrusive, the presence of some types of devices might change the measurement. For example, the presence of a heart rate monitoring device might make some patients anxious and increase their heart rate.
- All types of measuring devices are affected in some way by the environment. A simple thermometer can be affected by the subject drinking something hot or smoking a cigarette immediately before the temperature is taken. Thus it is important to consider whether the researcher controlled such environmental variables in the study.

## Existing Data

All of the data collection methods discussed thus far concern the ways that nurse researchers gather new data to study phenomena of interest. Sometimes existing data can be examined in a new way to study a problem. The use of records (e.g., medical records, care plans, hospital records, death certificates) and databases (e.g., U.S. Census, National Cancer Data Base, Minimum Data Set for Nursing Home Resident Assessment and Care Screening) are frequently used to answer research questions about clinical problems. Typically, this type of research design is referred to as *secondary analysis*.

The use of available data has certain advantages. First, data are already collected, thus eliminating subject burden and recruitment problems. Second, most databases contain large populations; therefore, sample size is rarely a problem and random sampling is possible. Larger samples allow the researcher to use more sophisticated analytic procedures, and random sampling enhances generalizability of findings. Some records and databases collect standardized data in a uniform way and allow the researcher to examine trends over time. Finally, the use of available records has the potential to save significant time and money.

On the other hand, institutions may be reluctant to allow researchers to have access to their records. If the records are kept so that an individual cannot be identified (known as de-identified data), this is usually not a problem. However, the Health Insurance Portability and Accountability Act (HIPAA), a federal law, protects the rights of individuals who may be identified in records (Bova et al., 2012; see Chapter 13). Recent interest in computerization of health records has led to discussion about the desirability of access to such records for research. Currently, it is not clear how much computerized health data will be readily available for research purposes.

Another problem that affects the quality of available data is that the researcher has access only to those records that have survived. If the records available are not representative of all of the possible records, the researcher may have to make an intelligent guess as to their accuracy. For example, a researcher might be interested in studying socioeconomic factors associated with the suicide rate. These data frequently are underreported because of the stigma attached to suicide, so the records would be biased.

---

### EVIDENCE-BASED PRACTICE TIP

Critical appraisal of any data collection method includes evaluating the appropriateness, objectivity, and consistency of the method employed.

---

## CONSTRUCTION OF NEW INSTRUMENTS

Sometimes researchers cannot locate an instrument with acceptable reliability and validity to measure the variable of interest (see Chapter 10). In this situation, a new instrument or scale must be developed. For example, Upton and Upton (2006) used instrument development procedures to develop a scale that measured nurses' knowledge, practice, and attitudes toward evidence-based practice.

Instrument development is complex and time consuming. It consists of the following steps:

- Define the concept to be measured
- Clarify the target population
- Develop the items
- Assess the items for content validity
- Develop instructions for respondents and users
- Pretest and pilot test the items
- Estimate reliability and validity

Defining the concept to be measured requires that the researcher develop an expertise in the concept, which includes an extensive review of the literature and of all existing measurements that deal with related concepts. The researcher will use all of this information to synthesize the available knowledge so that the construct can be defined.

Once defined, the individual items measuring the concept can be developed. The researcher will develop many more items than are needed to address each aspect of the concept. The items are evaluated by a panel of experts in the field to determine if the items measure what they are intended to measure (content validity) (see Chapter 15). Items will be eliminated if they are not specific to the concept. In this phase, the researcher needs to ensure consistency among the items, as well as consistency in testing and scoring procedures.

Finally, the researcher pilot tests the new instrument to determine the quality of the instrument as a whole (reliability and validity), as well as the ability of each item to discriminate individual respondents (variance in item response). Pilot testing can also yield important evidence about the reading level (too low or too high), length of the instrument (too short or too long), directions (clear or not clear), response rate (the percent of potential subjects who return a completed scale), and the appropriateness of culture or context. The researcher also may administer a related instrument to see if the new instrument is sufficiently different from the older one (construct validity). Instrument development and testing is an important part of nursing science because our ability to evaluate evidence related to practice depends on measuring nursing phenomena in a clear, consistent, and reliable way.

## APPRAISING THE EVIDENCE
## DATA COLLECTION METHODS

Assessing the adequacy of data collection methods is an important part of evaluating the results of studies that provide evidence for clinical practice. The data collection procedures provide a snapshot of how the study was conducted. From an evidence-based practice perspective you can judge if the data collection procedures would fit within your clinical environment and with your patient population. The manner in which the data were collected affects the study's internal and external validity. A well-developed methods section of a study decreases bias in the findings. A key element for evidence-based practice is if the procedures were consistently completed. Also consider the following:

- If observation was used, was an observation guide developed, and were the observers trained and supervised until there was a high level of interrater reliability? How was the training confirmed periodically throughout the study to maintain fidelity and decrease bias?
- Was a data collection procedure manual developed and used during the study?
- If the study tested an intervention, was there interventionist and data collector training?
- If a physiological instrument was used, was the instrument properly calibrated throughout the study, and were the data collected in the same manner from each subject?
- If there were missing data, how were the data accounted for?

Some of these details may be difficult to discern in a research article due to space limitations imposed by the journal. Typically, the interview guide, questionnaires, or scales are not available for review. However, research articles should indicate the following:

- Type(s) of data collection method used (self-report, observation, physiological, or existing data)
- Evidence of training and supervision for the data collectors and interventionists
- Consistency with which data collection procedures were applied across subjects
- Any threats to internal validity or bias related to issues of instrumentation or testing
- Any sources of bias related to external validity issues, such as the Hawthorne effect
- Scale reliability and validity discussed
- Interrater reliability across data collectors and time points (if observation was used)

When you review the data collection methods section of a study, it is important to think about the data strength and quality of the evidence. You should have confidence in the following:

- An appropriate data collection method was used
- Data collectors were appropriately trained and supervised

- Data were collected consistently by all data collectors
- Respondent burden, reactivity, and social desirability was avoided

You can critically appraise a study in terms of data collection bias being minimized, thereby strengthening potential applicability of the evidence provided by the findings. Because a research article does not always provide all of the details, it is not uncommon to contact the researcher to obtain added information that may assist you in using results in practice. Some helpful questions to ask are listed in the Critiquing Criteria box.

## CRITIQUING CRITERIA

### Data Collection Methods

1. Are all of the data collection instruments clearly identified and described?
2. Are operational definitions provided and clear?
3. Is the rationale for their selection given?
4. Is the method used appropriate to the problem being studied?
5. Were the methods used appropriate to the clinical situation?
6. Was a standardized manual used to guide data collection?
7. Were all data collectors adequately trained and supervised?
8. Are the data collection procedures the same for all subjects?

### Observational Methods

1. Who did the observing?
2. Were the observers trained to minimize bias?
3. Was there an observational guide?
4. Were the observers required to make inferences about what they saw?
5. Is there any reason to believe that the presence of the observers affected the behavior of the subjects?
6. Were the observations performed using the principles of informed consent?
7. Was interrater agreement between observers established?

### Self-Report: Interviews

1. Is the interview schedule described adequately enough to know whether it covers the topic?
2. Is there clear indication that the subjects understood the task and the questions?
3. Who were the interviewers, and how were they trained?
4. Is there evidence of interviewer bias?

### Self-Report: Questionnaires

1. Is the questionnaire described well enough to know whether it covers the topic?
2. Is there evidence that subjects were able to answer the questions?
3. Are the majority of the items appropriately closed-ended or open-ended?

### Physiological Measurement

1. Is the instrument used appropriate to the research question or hypothesis?
2. Is a rationale given for why a particular instrument was selected?
3. Is there a provision for evaluating the accuracy of the instrument?

### Existing Data: Records and Databases

1. Are the existing data used appropriately considering the research question and hypothesis being studied?
2. Are the data examined in such a way as to provide new information?
3. Is there any indication of selection bias in the available records?

# KEY POINTS

- Data collection methods are described as being both objective and systematic. The data collection methods of a study provide the operational definitions of the relevant variables.
- Types of data collection methods include observational, self-report, physiological, and existing data. Each method has advantages and disadvantages.
- Physiological measurement involves the use of technical instruments to collect data about patients' physical, chemical, microbiological, or anatomical status. They are suited to studying patient clinical outcomes and how to improve the effectiveness of nursing care. Physiological measurements are objective, precise, and sensitive. Expertise, training, and consistent application of these tests or procedures are needed to reduce measurement error associated with this data collection method.
- Observational methods are used in nursing research when the variables of interest deal with events or behaviors. Scientific observation requires preplanning, systematic recording, controlling the observations, and providing a relationship to scientific theory. This method is best suited to research problems that are difficult to view as a part of a whole. The advantages of observational methods are that they provide flexibility to measure many types of situations and they allow for depth and breadth of information to be collected. Disadvantages include: data may be distorted as a result of the observer's presence and observations may be biased by the person who is doing the observing.
- Interviews are commonly used data collection methods in nursing research. Either open-ended or closed-ended questions may be used when asking the subject questions. The form of the question should be clear to the respondent, free of suggestion, and grammatically correct.
- Questionnaires, or paper-and-pencil tests, are useful when there are a finite number of questions to be asked. Questions need to be clear and specific. Questionnaires are less costly in time and money to administer to large groups of subjects, particularly if the subjects are geographically widespread. Questionnaires also can be completely anonymous and prevent interviewer bias.
- Existing data in the form of records or large databases are an important source for research data. The use of available data may save the researcher considerable time and money when conducting a study. This method reduces problems with subject recruitment, access, and ethical concerns. However, records and available data are subject to problems of authenticity and accuracy.

# CRITICAL THINKING CHALLENGES

- When a researcher opts to use observation as the data collection method. What steps must be taken to minimize bias?
- In a randomized clinical trial investigating the differential effect of an educational video intervention in comparison to a telephone counseling intervention, data were collected at four different hospitals by four different data collectors. What steps should the researcher take to ensure intervention fidelity?
- What are the strengths and weaknesses of collecting data using existing sources such as records, charts, and databases?

- A journal club just finished reading the research report by Thomas and colleagues in Appendix A. As part of their critical appraisal of this study, they needed to identify the strengths and weaknesses of the data collection section of this research study. What might they list as part of their critique?
- How does a training manual decrease the possibility of introducing bias into the data collection process, thereby increasing intervention fidelity?

# REFERENCES

Aitken, L. M., Marshall, A. P., Elliott, R., et al. (2009). Critical care nurses decision making: sedation and management in intensive care. *Journal of Clinical Nursing, 18*(1), 36–45.

Bern, L., Brandt, M., Mbelu, N., et al. (2007). Differences in blood pressure values obtained with automated and manual methods in medical inpatients. *MEDSURG Nursing, 16*, 356–361.

Bova, C., Drexler, D., & Sullivan-Bolyai, S. (2012). Reframing the influence of HIPAA on research. *Chest, 141*, 782–786.

Pickering, T., Hall, J., Appel, L., et al. (2005). Recommendations for blood pressure measurement in humans and experimental animals: part 1: blood pressure measurement in humans: a statement for professionals from the Subcommittee of Professional and Public Education of the American Heart Association Council on High Blood Pressure Research. *Hypertension, 45*, 142–161.

Thomas, M. L., Elliott, J. E., Rao, S. M., et al. (2012). A randomized clinical trial of education or motivational-interviewing–based coaching compared to usual care to improve cancer pain management. *Oncology Nursing Forum, 39*(1), 39–49.

Ulrich, C. M., Knafl, K. A., Ratcliffe, S. J., et al. (2012). Developing a model of the benefits and burdens of research participation in cancer clinical trials. *American Journal of Bioethics Primary Research, 3*(2), 10–23.

Upton, D., & Upton, P. (2006). Development of an evidence-based practice questionnaire for nurses. *Journal of Advanced Nursing, 54*, 454–458.

**e**volve WEBSITE

*Go to Evolve at http://evolve.elsevier.com/LoBiondo/ for review questions, critiquing exercises, and additional research articles for practice in reviewing and critiquing.*

# CHAPTER 15

# Reliability and Validity

*Geri LoBiondo-Wood and Judith Haber*

## LEARNING OUTCOMES

*After reading this chapter, you should be able to do the following:*

- Discuss how measurement error can affect the outcomes of a research study.
- Discuss the purposes of reliability and validity.
- Define *reliability*.
- Discuss the concepts of stability, equivalence, and homogeneity as they relate to reliability.
- Compare and contrast the estimates of reliability.
- Define *validity*.
- Compare and contrast content, criterion-related, and construct validity.

- Identify the criteria for critiquing the reliability and validity of measurement tools.
- Use the critiquing criteria to evaluate the reliability and validity of measurement tools.
- Discuss how evidence related to reliability and validity contributes to the strength and quality of evidence provided by the findings of a research study and applicability to practice.

## KEY TERMS

| | | | |
|---|---|---|---|
| chance (random) errors | convergent validity | factor analysis | Kuder-Richardson |
| concurrent validity | criterion-related | homogeneity | (KR-20) coefficient |
| construct | validity | hypothesis-testing | Likert scale |
| construct validity | Cronbach's alpha | approach | multitrait-multimethod |
| content validity | divergent/discriminant | internal consistency | approach |
| content validity index | validity | interrater reliability | observed test score |
| contrasted-groups | equivalence | item to total | parallel or alternate |
| (known-groups) | error variance | correlations | form reliability |
| approach | face validity | kappa | predictive validity |

*Continued*

Measurement of nursing phenomena is a major concern of nursing researchers. Unless measurement instruments validly (accurately) and reliably (consistently) reflect the concepts of the theory being tested, conclusions drawn from a study will be invalid or biased and will not advance the development of evidence-based practice. Issues of reliability and validity are of central concern to researchers, as well as to an appraiser of research. From either perspective, the instruments that are used in a study must be evaluated. Researchers often face the challenge of developing new instruments and, as part of that process, establishing the reliability and validity of those instruments. The growing importance of measurement issues, instrument development, and related issues (e.g., reliability and validity) is evident in the *Journal of Nursing Measurement* and other nursing research journals.

Nurse investigators use instruments that have been developed by researchers in nursing and other disciplines. When reading studies, you must assess the reliability and validity of the instruments to determine the soundness of these selections in relation to the concepts (concepts are often called **constructs** in instrument development studies) or variables under study. The appropriateness of instruments and the extent to which reliability and validity are demonstrated have a profound influence on the strength of the findings and the extent to which bias is present. Invalid measures produce invalid estimates of the relationships between variables, thus introducing bias, which affects the study's internal and external validity. As such, the assessment of reliability and validity is an extremely important critical appraisal skill for assessing the strength and quality of evidence provided by the design and findings of a study and its applicability to practice.

Regardless of whether a new or already developed instrument is used in a study, evidence of reliability and validity is of crucial importance. This chapter examines the major types of reliability and validity and demonstrates the applicability of these concepts to the evaluation of instruments in nursing research and evidence-based practice.

## RELIABILITY, VALIDITY, AND MEASUREMENT ERROR

**Reliability** is the ability of an instrument to measure the attributes of a variable or construct *consistently*. **Validity** is the extent to which an instrument measures the attributes of a concept *accurately*. Each of these properties will be discussed later in the chapter. To understand reliability and validity, you need to understand potential errors related to instruments. Researchers may be concerned about whether the scores that were obtained for a sample of subjects were consistent, true measures of the behaviors and thus an accurate reflection of the differences between individuals. The extent of variability in test scores that is attributable to error rather than a true measure of the behaviors is the **error variance**. Error in measurement can occur in multiple ways.

An **observed test score** that is derived from a set of items actually consists of the true score plus error (Figure 15-1). The error may be either chance error or random error, or it

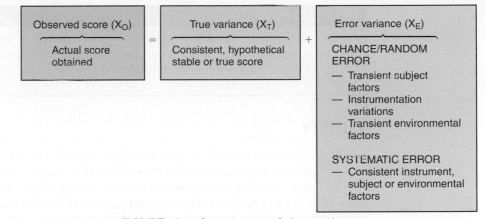

**FIGURE 15-1** Components of observed scores.

may be systematic or constant error. Validity is concerned with systematic error, whereas reliability is concerned with random error. **Chance** or **random errors** are errors that are difficult to control (e.g., a respondent's anxiety level at the time of testing). Random errors are unsystematic in nature. Random errors are a result of a transient state in the subject, the context of the study, or the administration of an instrument. For example, perceptions or behaviors that occur at a specific point in time (e.g., anxiety) are known as a state or transient characteristic and are often beyond the awareness and control of the examiner. Another example of random error is in a study that measures blood pressure. Random error resulting in different blood pressure readings could occur by misplacement of the cuff, not waiting for a specific time period before taking the blood pressure, or placing the arm randomly in relationship to the heart while measuring blood pressure.

Systematic or **constant error** is measurement error that is attributable to relatively stable characteristics of the study sample that may bias their behavior and/or cause incorrect instrument calibration. Such error has a systematic biasing influence on the subjects' responses and thereby influences the validity of the instruments. For instance, level of education, socioeconomic status, social desirability, response set, or other characteristics may influence the validity of the instrument by altering measurement of the "true" responses in a systematic way. For example, a subject is completing a survey examining attitudes about caring for elderly patients. If the subject wants to please the investigator, items may constantly be answered in a socially desirable way rather than how the individual actually feels, thus making the estimate of validity inaccurate. Systematic error occurs also when an instrument is improperly calibrated. Consider a scale that consistently gives a person's weight at 2 pounds less than the actual body weight. The scale could be quite reliable (i.e., capable of reproducing the precise measurement), but the result is consistently invalid.

The concept of error is important when appraising instruments in a study. The information regarding the instruments' reliability and validity is found in the instrument or measures section of a study, which can be separately titled or appear as a subsection of the methods section of a research report, unless the study is a psychometric or instrument development study (see Chapter 10).

> ### HELPFUL HINT
>
> Research articles vary considerably in the amount of detail included about reliability and validity. When the focus of a study is tool development, psychometric evaluation—including extensive reliability and validity data—is carefully documented and appears throughout the article rather than briefly in the "Instruments" or "Measures" section, as in articles reporting on the results of individual studies.

## VALIDITY

Validity is the extent to which an instrument measures the attributes of a concept accurately. When an instrument is valid, it truly reflects the concept it is supposed to measure. A valid instrument that is supposed to measure anxiety does so; it does not measure some other concept, such as stress. A measure can be reliable but not valid. Let us say that a researcher wanted to measure anxiety in patients by measuring their body temperatures. The researcher could obtain highly accurate, consistent, and precise temperature recordings, but such a measure may not be a valid indicator of anxiety. Thus the high reliability of an instrument is not necessarily congruent with evidence of validity. A valid instrument, however, is reliable. An instrument cannot validly measure the attribute of interest if it is erratic, inconsistent, or inaccurate. There are three types of validity that vary according to the kind of information provided and the purpose of the instrument (i.e., *content, criterion-related,* and *construct validity*). As you appraise research articles you will want to evaluate whether sufficient evidence of validity is present and whether the type of validity is appropriate to the study's design and instruments used in the study.

As you read the instruments or measures sections of studies, you will notice that validity data are reported much less frequently than reliability data. DeVon and colleagues (2007) note that adequate validity is frequently claimed, but rarely is the method specified. This lack of reporting, largely due to publication space constraints, shows the importance of critiquing the quality of the instruments and the conclusions (see Chapters 14 and 17).

> ### EVIDENCE-BASED PRACTICE TIP
>
> Selecting measurement instruments that have strong evidence of validity increases your confidence in the study findings—that the researcher actually measured what she or he intended to measure.

### Content Validity

Content validity represents the universe of content, or the domain of a given variable/construct. The universe of content provides the basis for developing the items that will adequately represent the content. When an investigator is developing an instrument and issues of content validity arise, the concern is whether the measurement instrument and the items it contains are representative of the content domain that the researcher intends to measure. The researcher begins by defining the concept and identifying the attributes or dimensions of the concept. The items that reflect the concept and its domain are developed.

When the researcher has completed this task, the items are submitted to a panel of judges considered to be experts about the concept. For example, researchers typically request that the judges indicate their agreement with the scope of the items and the extent to which the items reflect the concept under consideration. Box 15-1 provides an example of content validity.

## BOX 15-1   PUBLISHED EXAMPLES OF CONTENT VALIDITY AND CONTENT VALIDITY INDEX

The following text from various articles describes how content validity and content validity index can be determined in an article:

### Content Validity

"A panel of 13 experts evaluated content validity for the Perceived Self-Efficacy for Fatigue Self-Management. Experts were selected using selection criteria established by Grant and Davis and had experience in fatigue, clinical oncology, chronic illness, self-efficacy theory, research methods, statistics, or a combination of these. The expert panel were provided conceptual definitions, the measurement model, a description of the population and setting in which the instrument would be used. The panel identified items that were not stated clearly and commented on the items' representativeness and the instrument's comprehensiveness. Panel feedback was incorporated and concurrence achieved that the items were appropriate and relevant for persons with a chronic illness who were experiencing fatigue" (Hoffman et al., 2011, p. 169).

### Content Validity Index

"For the original Relationships with Health Care Provider Scale (RHCPS), the Item-level Content Validity Index (I-CVI) was calculated by a panel of five content experts rating each scale's item for its relevance to the construct of health care relationships. Experts were nurses with masters degrees or PhDs who were clinical providers or clinical researchers with experience with instrument development. The ratings were on a 4-point scale with a response format of 1 = *not relevant* to 4 = *highly relevant*. The I-CVI for each item was computed based on the percentage of experts giving a rating of 3 or 4, indicating item relevance . . . The content validity index for the total scale (S-CVI), calculated by averaging the I-CVI responses from the five experts and dividing by the number of items, was equal to .96. A rating of .90 is considered to be an acceptable standard for an S-CVI" (Anderson, et al., 2011, p. 7).

Another method used to establish content validity is the **content validity index** (CVI). The content validity index moves beyond the level of agreement of a panel of expert judges and calculates an index of interrater agreement or relevance. This calculation gives a researcher more confidence or evidence that the instrument truly reflects the concept or construct. When reading the instrument section of a research article, note that the authors will comment if a CVI was used to assess the content validity of an instrument. When reading a psychometric study that reports the development of an instrument, you will find great detail and a much longer section of how exactly the researchers calculated the CVI and the acceptable item cut-offs. In the scientific literature there has been discussion of accepting a CVI of .78 to 1.0 depending on the number of experts (DeVon et al., 2007; Lynn, 1986). An example from a study that used CVI is presented in Box 15-1. A subtype of content validity is **face validity**, which is a rudimentary type of validity that basically verifies that the instrument gives the appearance of measuring the concept. It is an intuitive type of validity in which colleagues or subjects are asked to read the instrument and evaluate the content in terms of whether it appears to reflect the concept the researcher intends to measure.

## EVIDENCE-BASED PRACTICE TIP

If face and/or content validity, the most basic types of validity, was (were) the only type(s) of validity reported in a research article, you would not appraise the measurement instrument(s) as having strong psychometric properties, which would negatively influence your confidence about the study findings.

---

### BOX 15-2    PUBLISHED EXAMPLES OF REPORTED CRITERION-RELATED VALIDITY

**Concurrent Validity**

Concurrent validity of the PTSD Checklist (PCL) has been supported by the statistically significant correlations between PCL scores and the Clinician-Administered PTSD Scale (Melvin et al., 2012; Appendix D).

**Predictive Validity**

In a study investigating family caregiving of older Chinese people with dementia, predictive validity of the Chinese version of the Attitudinal Familism Scale (AFS) was indicated by a significant positive correlation between familism and membership in an older cohort born in 1949 before China opened to the values of other countries (Liu et al., 2012).

---

## Criterion-Related Validity

Criterion-related validity indicates to what degree the subject's performance on the instrument and the subject's actual behavior are related. The criterion is usually the second measure, which assesses the same concept under study. For example, in a study by Sherman and colleagues (2012) investigating the effects of psychoeducation and telephone counseling on the adjustment of women with early-stage breast cancer, criterion-related validity was supported by correlating amount of distress experienced (ADE) scores measured by the Breast Cancer Treatment Response Inventory (BCTRI) and total scores from the Symptom Distress Scale ($r = .86$; $p < .000$). Two forms of criterion-related validity are concurrent and predictive.

Concurrent validity refers to the degree of correlation of one test with the scores of another more established instrument of the same concept when both are administered at the same time. A high correlation coefficient indicates agreement between the two measures and evidence of concurrent validity.

Predictive validity refers to the degree of correlation between the measure of the concept and some future measure of the same concept. Because of the passage of time, the correlation coefficients are likely to be lower for predictive validity studies. Examples of concurrent and predictive validity as they appear in research articles are illustrated in Box 15-2.

## Construct Validity

Construct validity is based on the extent to which a test measures a theoretical construct, attribute, or trait. It attempts to validate the theory underlying the measurement by testing of the hypothesized relationships. Testing confirms or fails to confirm the relationships that are predicted between and/or among concepts and, as such, provides more or less support for the construct validity of the instruments measuring those concepts. The establishment of construct validity is complex, often involving several studies and approaches. The hypothesis-testing, factor analytical, convergent and divergent, and contrasted-groups approaches are discussed below. Box 15-3 provides examples of different types of construct validity as it is reported in published research articles.

### Hypothesis-Testing Approach

When the hypothesis-testing approach is used, the investigator uses the theory or concept underlying the measurement instruments to validate the instrument. The investigator does this by developing hypotheses regarding the behavior of individuals with varying scores on the measurement instrument, collecting data to test the hypotheses, and making inferences

## BOX 15-3 PUBLISHED EXAMPLES OF REPORTED CONSTRUCT VALIDITY

The following examples from various articles describe how construct validity can be presented in an article.

**Contrasted Groups (Known Groups)**

Melvin and colleagues (2012; Appendix D) used the Revised Dyadic Adjustment Scale (RDAS), and reported that the RDAS showed a .97 correlation with the original scale and good discrimination between distressed and non-distressed couples in civilian population. In this study the RDAS was going to be used for the first time in a population of military couples and then the contrasted groups approach could be used to assess if the RDAS discriminated between distressed and non-distressed couples in a military population.

**Convergent Validity**

"**Convergent construct validity** of the Breast Cancer Treatment Response Inventory (BCTRI) was supported by correlating the amount of distress (ADE) score, measured by the BCTRI, and total scores from the Symptom Distress Scale (r = .86, p < .000)" (McCorkle & Young, 1978; Sherman et al, 2012).

**Divergent (Discriminant) Validity**

The Psychosocial Adjustment to Illness Scale (PAIS), a 46-item scale that assesses the impact of the illness on seven domains of adjustment, was used as a measure of social adjustment in a population of breast cancer patients. Findings confirmed discriminant validity with correlations between the total PAIS score of .81 for the Global Adjustment to Illness Scale, .60 for the SCL-90R General Severity Index, and .69 for the Affect Balance Scale (Sherman et al., 2012).

**Factor Analysis**

"In principal components factor analysis with varimax rotation, the scree plot suggested a one- or two-factor structure. The Kaiser-Meyer-Olkin (.96) and Barlett's tests (x2 [105, n = 431] = 5306.7, p < .001) indicated a high degree of common variance for items of the HCR Trust Scale" (Bova et al., 2012, p. 402).

**Hypothesis Testing**

In a study to identify predictors of caregiver strain and satisfaction associated with caring for veterans with chronic illness, construct validity of the Caregiver Strain Index (CSI) was supported by significant correlations between the physical and emotional health of the caregiver and subjective views of the caregiving situation. Positive responses to seven or more items indicate a high level of strain (Wakefield et al., 2012).

on the basis of the findings concerning whether the rationale underlying the instrument's construction is adequate to explain the findings and thereby provide support for evidence of construct validity.

### Convergent, Divergent, and Multitrait-Multimethod Approaches

Strategies for assessing construct validity include convergent, divergent, and multitrait-multimethod approaches. Convergent validity refers to a search for other measures of the construct. Sometimes two or more instruments that theoretically measure the same construct are identified, and both are administered to the same subjects. A correlational analysis (i.e., test of relationship; see Chapter 16) is performed. If the measures are positively correlated, convergent validity is said to be supported.

Divergent validity, sometimes called discriminant validity, uses measurement approaches that differentiate one construct from others that may be similar. Sometimes researchers search for instruments that measure the opposite of the construct. If the divergent measure is negatively related to other measures, validity for the measure is strengthened.

A specific method of assessing convergent and divergent validity is the **multitrait-multimethod approach**. This method, proposed by Campbell & Fiske (1959), also involves examining the relationship between instruments that should measure the same construct (convergent validity) and between those that should measure different constructs (discriminant validity). A variety of measurement strategies, however, are used. For example, anxiety could be measured by the following:

- Administering the State-Trait Anxiety Inventory
- Recording blood pressure readings
- Asking the subject about anxious feelings
- Observing the subject's behavior

The results of one of these measures should then be correlated with the results of each of the others in a multitrait-multimethod matrix (Waltz et al., 2010). The use of multiple measures of a concept decreases *systematic error*. A variety of data collection methods (e.g., self-report, observation, interview, collection of physiological data) will also diminish the effect of systematic error.

### Contrasted-Groups Approach

When the **contrasted-groups approach** (sometimes called the **known-groups approach**) is used to test construct validity, the researcher identifies two groups of individuals who are suspected to score extremely high or low in the characteristic being measured by the instrument. The instrument is administered to both the high-scoring and the low-scoring group, and the differences in scores are examined. If the instrument is sensitive to individual differences in the trait being measured, the mean performance of these two groups should differ significantly and evidence of construct validity would be supported. A *t* test or analysis of variance could be used to statistically test the difference between the two groups (see Chapter 16).

### Factor Analytical Approach

A final approach to assessing construct validity is **factor analysis**. This is a procedure that gives the researcher information about the extent to which a set of items measures the same underlying concept (variable) of a construct. Factor analysis assesses the degree to which the individual items on a scale truly cluster around one or more concepts. Items designed to measure the same concept should load on the same factor;

CHAPTER 15 Reliability and Validity 297

## CRITICAL THINKING DECISION PATH

*Determining the Appropriate Type of Validity and Reliability Selected for a Study*

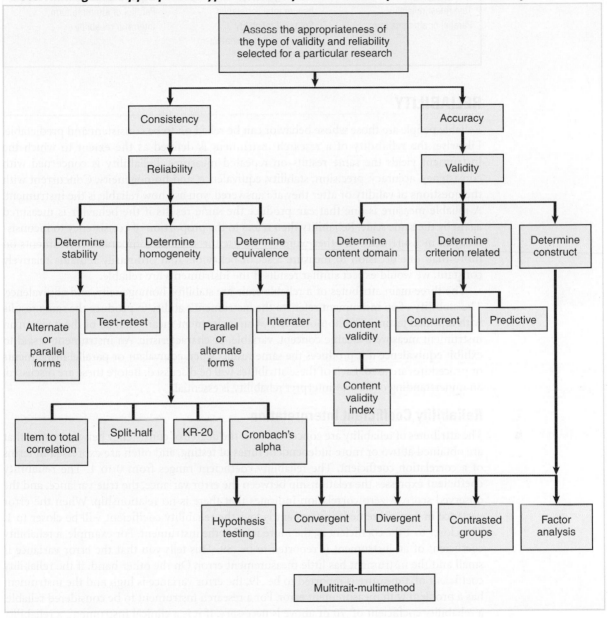

those designed to measure different concepts should load on different factors (Anastasi & Urbina, 1997; Furr & Bacharach, 2008; Nunnally & Bernstein, 1993). This analysis will also indicate whether the items in the instrument reflect a single construct or several constructs.

The Critical Thinking Decision Path will help you assess the appropriateness of the type of validity and reliability selected for use in a particular study.

---

> ### BOX 15-4    MEASURES USED TO TEST RELIABILITY
>
> | **Stability** | **Homogeneity** | **Equivalence** |
> |---|---|---|
> | Test-retest reliability | Item to total correlation | Parallel or alternate form |
> | Parallel or alternate form | Split-half reliability | Interrater reliability |
> | | Kuder-Richardson coefficient | |
> | | Cronbach's alpha | |

---

## RELIABILITY

Reliable people are those whose behavior can be relied on to be consistent and predictable. Likewise, the reliability of a research instrument is defined as the extent to which the instrument yields the same results on repeated measures. Reliability is concerned with consistency, accuracy, precision, stability, equivalence, and homogeneity. Concurrent with the questions of validity or after they are answered, you ask how reliable is the instrument. A reliable measure is one that can produce the same results if the behavior is measured again by the same scale. Reliability then refers to the proportion of consistency to inconsistency in measurement. In other words, if we use the same or comparable instruments on more than one occasion to measure a set of behaviors that ordinarily remains relatively constant, we would expect similar results if the instruments are reliable.

The three main attributes of a reliable scale are stability, homogeneity, and equivalence. The stability of an instrument refers to the instrument's ability to produce the same results with repeated testing. The homogeneity of an instrument means that all of the items in an instrument measure the same concept, variable, or characteristic. An instrument is said to exhibit equivalence if it produces the same results when equivalent or parallel instruments or procedures are used. Each of these attributes will be discussed. Before these are discussed, an understanding of how to interpret reliability is essential.

### Reliability Coefficient Interpretation

The attributes of reliability are concerned with the degree of consistency between scores that are obtained at two or more independent times of testing, and often are expressed in terms of a correlation coefficient. The reliability coefficient ranges from 0 to 1. The reliability coefficient expresses the relationship between the error variance, the true variance, and the observed score. A zero correlation indicates that there is no relationship. When the error variance in a measurement instrument is low, the reliability coefficient will be closer to 1. The closer to 1 the coefficient is, the more reliable the instrument. For example, a reliability coefficient of an instrument is reported to be .89. This tells you that the error variance is small and the instrument has little measurement error. On the other hand, if the reliability coefficient of a measure is reported to be .49, the error variance is high and the instrument has a problem with measurement error. For a research instrument to be considered reliable, a reliability coefficient of .70 or above is necessary. If it is a clinical instrument, a reliability coefficient of .90 or higher is considered to be an acceptable level of reliability. The interpretation of the reliability coefficient depends on the proposed purpose of the measure.

The tests of reliability used to calculate a reliability coefficient depends on the nature of the instrument. The tests are **test-retest, parallel or alternate form, item to total correlation, split-half, Kuder-Richardson (KR-20), Cronbach's alpha,** and **interrater reliability.** These tests as they relate to stability, equivalence, and homogeneity are listed in Box 15-4

---

## BOX 15-5 PUBLISHED EXAMPLES OF REPORTED RELIABILITY

### Reliability
#### Internal Consistency, Item Correlations, Inter-Item Correlations Reliability

"The standardized item alpha for the original Relationship with Health Care Provider Scale (RHCPS) was 0.64 for persons with HIV disease (Anderson et al., 2011). Inter-item correlation was highest ($r = .59$) between Item 1 ("How easy or difficult is it to talk with your primary care provider?") and Item 5 ("How satisfied are you with the care that you receive from your health care provider?"). Inter-item correlations are lowest ($r = 0.039$) between Item 2 ("How much do you trust that your health care provider is telling you the truth about your illness?") and Item 4 ("How comfortable do you feel in calling your health care provider to tell him or her that you have a new symptom or difficulty taking your medications?") Inspection of item-total statistics showed deletion of any one item would not improve the total scale alpha or increase the scale mean indicating the relevance of each item (Anderson et al., 2011)".

#### Test-Retest Reliability

In a study by de Man-van Ginkel and colleagues (2012) that screened for post-stroke depression using the Patient Health Questionnaire (PHQ-9), test-retest reliability was 0.84 as measured by the ICC.

#### Internal Consistency Reliability

In a study investigating combat-related post-traumatic stress symptoms (PTSS) and couple relationships in US Army combat veteran couples, PTSS symptoms were measured by the "Post-traumatic Stress Disorder Checklist (PCL; Weathers et al., 1993) . . . Cronbach's alpha reliabilities have ranged from 0.92 in civilians to 0.97 in military populations . . . Cronbach's alpha was 0.96 for the sample in this study (Melvin et al., 2012; Appendix D)".

#### Kuder-Richardson (KR-20) Internal Consistency Reliability

Internal consistency reliability of the HCR Trust Scale (Bova et al., 2012) was tested using the Kuder-Richardson KR-20 approach because the response format was binary; that is, "Yes" or "No." The KR-20 reliability coefficient was $r = .50$. The reason for the poor reliability for the HCR Trust scale in the study population of HIV-infected subjects was stated by the authors to be unknown.

#### Split-Half Reliability

The Geriatric Depression Scale (GDS-15) is used for assessing depression in older adults who have had a stroke and reports a split-half reliability of .75, which exceeds the reliability coefficient benchmark of $r = .70$ (de Man-van Ginkel et al., 2012).

#### Interrater Reliability and Kappa

In the Alhusen et al. (2012; Appendix B) study two undergraduate nursing students collected neonatal data on a random 25% sub-sample to assess inter-rater reliability. A kappa statistic of 1.0 was noted, indicating excellent agreement.

#### Item to Total Correlation

All of the corrected item to total correlations were higher than .40 for the 21 items on the questionnaire. Correlation coefficients ranged from .434 to .652 and achieved statistical significance ($p < .001$) (Chang, 2012).

---

and examples of types of reliability are in Box 15-5. There is no best means to assess reliability in relationship to stability, homogeneity, and equivalence. You should be aware that the reliability method that the researcher uses should be consistent with the study's aim and the instrument's format.

## Stability

An instrument is thought to be stable or to exhibit **stability** when the same results are obtained on repeated administration of the instrument. Researchers are concerned with stability when they expect the instrument to measure a concept consistently over a period of time. Measurement over time is important when an instrument is used in a longitudinal study and therefore used on several occasions. Stability is also a consideration when a researcher is conducting an intervention study that is designed to effect a change in a specific variable. In this case, the instrument is administered once and then again later, after the experimental intervention has been completed. The tests that are used to estimate stability are test-retest and parallel or alternate form.

## Test-Retest Reliability

Test-retest reliability is the administration of the same instrument to the same subjects under similar conditions on two or more occasions. Scores from repeated testing are compared. This comparison is expressed by a correlation coefficient, usually a Pearson *r* (see Chapter 16). The interval between repeated administrations varies and depends on the concept or variable being measured. For example, if the variable that the test measures is related to the developmental stages in children, the interval between tests should be short. The amount of time over which the variable was measured should also be recorded in the study. An example of an instrument that was assessed for test-retest reliability is Relationships with Health Care Provider Scale (RHCPS), an instrument that was developed for use with older adults to assess the type and quality of provider-patient health care relationship and how it impacts patient adherence (Anderson et al., 2011). In this case, test-retest reliability for a subsample of 72 persons from the total sample of 80 was .63 (p < .01) across 2 weeks. Consistent with the first test of RHCPS, the item with the highest mean was trust in the health care provider (M = 9.23; SD = 1.45) and the lowest was participation in health care decisions (M = 7.74); SD = 3.18). Although the interval was adequate (2 weeks) between testing, the coefficient was not above .70. As such, evidence of test-retest reliability was not at a satisfactory level (DeVon et al., 2007; Nunnally & Bernstein, 1993). Box 15-5 provides another example of test-retest reliability.

### HELPFUL HINT

When a longitudinal design with multiple data collection points is being conducted, look for evidence of test-retest or parallel form reliability.

## Parallel or Alternate Form

Parallel or alternate form reliability is applicable and can be tested only if two *comparable forms* of the *same* instrument exist. Not many instruments have a parallel form so it is unusual to find examples in the literature. It is similar to test-retest reliability in that the same individuals are tested within a specific interval, but it differs because a *different* form of the *same* test is given to the subjects on the second testing. **Parallel forms** or tests contain the same types of items that are based on the same concept, but the wording of the items is different. The development of parallel forms is desired if the instrument is intended to measure a variable for which a researcher believes that "test-wiseness" will be a problem (see Chapter 8). For example, the randomized controlled trial "Breast Cancer: Education, Counseling, and Adjustment" (Budin et al., 2008) studied the differential effect of a phase-specific standardized educational video intervention in comparison to a telephone counseling intervention on physical, emotional, and social adjustment

| TABLE 15-1 | EXAMPLES OF CRONBACH'S ALPHA FROM THE ALHUSEN STUDY (APPENDIX B) | | | |
|---|---|---|---|---|
| **DIMENSIONS** | **ORIGINAL** | **SAMPLE 1** | **SAMPLE 2** | **SAMPLE 3** |
| Negative Reactivity | .90 | .89 | .90 | .92 |
| Task Persistence | .90 | .89 | .91 | .92 |
| Approach/Withdrawal | .88 | .84 | .86 | .92 |
| Activity | .85 | .80 | .86 | .92 |

in women with breast cancer and their partners. The use of repeated measures over the four data collection points —"Coping with Your Diagnosis," "Recovering from Surgery," "Understanding Adjuvant Therapy," and "Ongoing Recovery"—made it appropriate to use two alternate forms of the Partner Relationship Inventory (Hoskins, 1988) to measure emotional adjustment in partners. An item on one scale ("I am able to tell my partner how I feel") is consistent with the paired item on the second form ("My partner tries to understand my feelings"). Practically speaking, it is difficult to develop alternate forms of an instrument when one considers the many issues of reliability and validity. If alternate forms of a test exist, they should be highly correlated if the measures are to be considered reliable.

## Internal Consistency/Homogeneity

Another attribute of an instrument related to reliability is the internal consistency or homogeneity. In this case, the items within the scale reflect or measure the same concept. This means that the items within the scale correlate or are complementary to each other. This also means that a scale is unidimensional. A unidimensional scale is one that measures one concept, such as self-efficacy. Box 15 5 provides several examples of how internal consistency is reported. Internal consistency can be assessed by using one of four methods: item to total correlations, split-half reliability, Kuder-Richardson (KR-20) coefficient, or Cronbach's alpha.

### EVIDENCE-BASED PRACTICE TIP

When the characteristics of a study sample differ significantly from the sample in the original study, check to see if the researcher has reestablished the reliability of the instrument with the current sample.

## Item to Total Correlations

Item to total correlations measure the relationship between each of the items and the total scale. When item to total correlations are calculated, a correlation for each item on the scale is generated (Table 15-1). Items that do not achieve a high correlation may be deleted from the instrument. Usually in a research study, all of the item to total correlations are not reported unless the study is a report of a methodological study. The lowest and highest correlations are typically reported.

## Cronbach's Alpha

The fourth and most commonly used test of internal consistency is Cronbach's alpha, which is used when a measurement instrument uses a Likert scale. Many scales used to measure

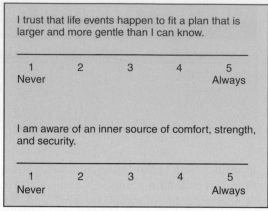

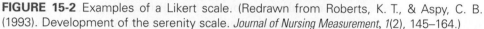

**FIGURE 15-2** Examples of a Likert scale. (Redrawn from Roberts, K. T., & Aspy, C. B. (1993). Development of the serenity scale. *Journal of Nursing Measurement*, 1(2), 145–164.)

psychosocial variables and attitudes have a Likert scale response format. A **Likert scale** format asks the subject to respond to a question on a scale of varying degrees of intensity between two extremes. The two extremes are anchored by responses ranging from "strongly agree" to "strongly disagree" or "most like me" to "least like me." The points between the two extremes may range from 1 to 4, 1 to 5, or 1 to 7. Subjects are asked to identify the response closest to how they feel. Alhusen and colleagues (2012; Appendix B) report the internal consistency for the Maternal-Fetal Attachment Scale (MFAS). "The MFAS is a 24-item measure that asks women to respond to questions or thoughts indicative of MFA. The scale contains 5-point Likert-type items with response options ranging from 1 (definitely no) to 5 (definitely yes). The total score ranges from 24 to 120 with higher scores indicative of higher levels of MFA. The Cronbach's alpha coefficient reported by Lindgren (2003) was .81 and for the current study was .90." Cronbach's alpha simultaneously compares each item in the scale with the others. A total score is then used in the data analysis as illustrated in Table 15-1. Alphas above .70 are sufficient evidence for supporting the internal consistency of the instrument. Figure 15-2 provides examples of items from an instrument that uses a Likert scale format.

## Split-Half Reliability

**Split-half reliability** involves dividing a scale into two halves and making a comparison. The halves may be odd-numbered and even-numbered items or may be a simple division of the first from the second half, or items may be randomly selected into halves that will be analyzed opposite one another. The split-half method provides a measure of consistency in terms of sampling the content. The two halves of the test or the contents in both halves are assumed to be comparable, and a reliability coefficient is calculated. If the scores for the two halves are approximately equal, the test may be considered reliable. See Box 15-5 for an example.

## Kuder-Richardson (KR-20) Coefficient

The **Kuder-Richardson (KR-20) coefficient** is the estimate of homogeneity used for instruments that have a dichotomous response format. A dichotomous response format is one in which the question asks for a "yes/no" or "true/false" response. The technique yields a correlation that is based on the consistency of responses to all the items of a single form of a test that is administered one time. The minimum acceptable KR-20 score is r = .70 (see Box 15-5).

---

**HELPFUL HINT**

If a research article provides information about the reliability of a measurement instrument but does not specify the type of reliability, it is probably safe to assume that internal consistency reliability was assessed using Cronbach's alpha.

---

## Equivalence

Equivalence either is the consistency or agreement among observers using the same measurement instrument or is the consistency or agreement between alternate forms of an instrument. An instrument is thought to demonstrate equivalence when two or more observers have a high percentage of agreement of an observed behavior or when alternate forms of a test yield a high correlation. There are two methods to test equivalence: interrater reliability and alternate or parallel form.

### Interrater Reliability

Some measurement instruments are not self-administered questionnaires but are direct measurements of observed behavior. Instruments that depend on direct observation of a behavior that is to be systematically recorded must be tested for interrater reliability. To accomplish interrater reliability, two or more individuals should make an observation or one observer should examine the behavior on several occasions. The observers should be trained or oriented to the definition and operationalization of the behavior to be observed. In the method of direct observation of behavior, the consistency or reliability of the observations between observers is extremely important. In the instance of interrater reliability, the reliability or consistency of the observer is tested rather than the reliability of the instrument. Interrater reliability is expressed as a percentage of agreement between scorers or as a correlation coefficient of the scores assigned to the observed behaviors.

In a study by deMan-van Ginkel and colleagues (2012) that investigated the reliability, validity, and clinical utility of the nine-item PHQ-9 and the two-item PHQ-2 patient health questionnaires in stroke patients in a clinical setting, interrater reliability was established based on the sum score level of the PHQ-9 and the PHQ-2, which showed similar results (ICC = .98, 95% CI[.96, .99]) demonstrating very good interrater reliability.

Kappa (K) expresses the level of agreement observed beyond the level that would be expected by chance alone. K ranges from +1 (total agreement) to 0 (no agreement). A K of .80 or better indicates good interrater reliability. K between .80 and .68 is considered acceptable/substantial agreement; less than .68 allows tentative conclusions to be drawn at times when lower levels are accepted (McDowell & Newell, 1996) (see Box 15-5).

### Parallel or Alternate Form

Parallel or alternate form was described in the discussion of stability in this chapter. Use of parallel forms is a measure of stability and equivalence. The procedures for assessing equivalence using parallel forms are the same.

## CLASSIC TEST THEORY VERSUS ITEM RESPONSE THEORY

The methods of reliability and validity described in this chapter are considered classical test theory (CTT) methods. There are newer methods that you will find described in research articles under the category of item response theory (IRT). The two methods share basic characteristics, but some feel that IRT methods are superior for discriminating test items. Several terms and concepts linked with IRT are: Rasch models and one (or two) parameter logistic models. The methodology of these methods are beyond the scope of this text, but several references are cited for future use (DeVellis, 2012; Furr & Bacharach, 2008).

## HOW VALIDITY AND RELIABILITY ARE REPORTED

When reading a research article, a lengthy discussion of how the different types of reliability and validity were obtained will not be found. What is found in the methods section is the instrument's title, a definition of the concept/construct that it measures, and a sentence or two about the data that support the reliability and validity assessed by previous researchers. This level of discussion is appropriate. Examples of what you will see include the following:
- "The Geriatric Depression Scale (GDS) has demonstrated a high degree of internal consistency (Cronbach's alpha = .94) and test-retest reliability of r = .85" (Wakefield et al., 2012).
- "Personality traits were assessed using the Big Five Inventory (BFI), a 44-item scale measuring agreeableness, openness to new experiences, conscientiousness, neuroticism, and extraversion. The BFI has a 5-point Likert response format. It has shown ample internal consistency, temporal stability, and convergent and divergent validity" (Williams et al., 2012).

## APPRAISING THE EVIDENCE
## RELIABILITY AND VALIDITY

Reliability and validity are two crucial aspects in the critical appraisal of a measurement instrument. Criteria for critiquing reliability and validity are presented in the Critiquing Criteria box. When reviewing a research article you need to appraise each instrument's level of reliability and validity. In a research article, the reliability and validity for each measure should be presented or a reference given where it was described in more detail. If these data have not been presented at all, you must seriously question the merit and use of the instrument and the evidence provided by the study's results.

## CRITIQUING CRITERIA

### Reliability and Validity

1. Was an appropriate method used to test the reliability of the instrument?
2. Is the reliability of the instrument adequate?
3. Was an appropriate method(s) used to test the validity of the instrument?
4. Is the validity of the measurement instrument adequate?
5. If the sample from the developmental stage of the instrument was different from the current sample, were the reliability and validity recalculated to determine if the instrument is appropriate for use in a different population?
6. Have the strengths and weaknesses related to the reliability and validity of each instrument been presented?
7. What kinds of threats to internal and/or external validity are presented by weaknesses in reliability and/or validity?
8. Are strengths and weaknesses of the reliability and validity appropriately addressed in the "Discussion," "Limitations," or "Recommendations" sections of the report?
9. How do the reliability and/or validity affect the strength and quality of the evidence provided by the study findings?

The amount of information provided for each instrument will vary depending on the study type and the instrument. In a psychometric study (an instrument development study) you will find great detail regarding how the researchers established the reliability and validity of the instrument. When reading a research article in which the instruments are used to test a research question or hypothesis, you may find only brief reference to the type of reliability and validity of the instrument. If the instrument is a well-known, reliable, and valid instrument, it is not uncommon that only a passing comment may be made, which is appropriate. For example, in the "Thomas and colleagues study (2012; Appendix A) the researchers noted, The FACT-G has been used in numerous studies of patients with cancer. The FACT-G has well established validity and reliability" (Cella, 1993). Sometimes, the authors will cite a reference that you can locate if you are interested in detailed data about the instrument's reliability or validity. For example, in the Thomas and colleagues study a number of references were cited in the instruments section for further information. If a study does not use reliable and valid questionnaires, you need to consider the sources of bias that may exist as threats to internal or external validity. It is very difficult to place confidence in the evidence generated by a study's findings if the measures used did not have established validity and reliability. The following discussion highlights key areas related to reliability and validity that should be evident to you as you read a research article.

Appropriate reliability tests should have been performed by the developer of the measurement instrument and should then have been included by the current researcher in the research report. If the initial standardization sample and the current sample have different characteristics (e.g., age, gender, ethnicity, race, geographic location), you would expect the following: (1) that a pilot study for the present sample would have been conducted to determine if the reliability was maintained, or (2) that a reliability estimate was calculated on the current sample. For example, if the standardization sample for an instrument that measures "satisfaction in an intimate heterosexual relationship" comprises undergraduate college students and if an investigator plans to use the instrument with married couples, it would be advisable to establish the reliability of the instrument with the latter group.

The investigator determines which type of reliability procedures are used in the study, depending on the nature of the measurement instrument and how it will be used. For example, if the instrument is to be administered twice, you would expect to read that test-retest reliability was used to establish the stability of the instrument. If an alternate form has been developed for use in a repeated-measures design, evidence of alternate form reliability should be presented to determine the equivalence of the parallel forms. If the degree of internal consistency among the items is relevant, an appropriate test of internal consistency should be presented. In some instances, more than one type of reliability will be presented, but as you assess the instruments section of a research report, you should determine whether all are appropriate. For example, the Kuder-Richardson formula implies that there is a single right or wrong answer, making it inappropriate to use with scales that provide a format of three or more possible responses. In the latter case, another formula is applied, such as Cronbach's coefficient alpha. Another important consideration is the acceptable level of reliability, which varies according to the type of test. Reliability coefficients of .70 or higher are desirable. The validity of an instrument is limited by its reliability; that is, less confidence can be placed in scores from tests with low reliability coefficients.

Satisfactory evidence of validity will probably be the most difficult item for you to ascertain. It is this aspect of measurement that is most likely to fall short of meeting the required criteria. Page count limitations often account for this brevity. Detailed validity data usually are only reported in studies focused on instrument development; therefore, validity data are mentioned only briefly or, sometimes, not at all. For example, in a study aiming to study barriers to meditation by gender and age among cancer family caregivers, the Caregiver Reaction Assessment (CRA) has been used extensively with cancer family caregiver populations with good internal consistency and content and construct validity testing (Nijboer et al., 1999; Stommel et al., 1992, Williams et al., 2012).

The most common type of reported validity is content validity. When reviewing a study, you want to find evidence of content validity. Once again, you will find the detailed reporting of content validity and the CVI in psychometric studies; Box 15-2 provides a good example of how content validity is reported in that kind of article. Such procedures provide you with assurance that the instrument is psychometrically sound and that the content of the items is consistent with the conceptual framework and construct definitions. In research studies where several instruments are used, the reporting of content validity is either absent or very brief.

Construct validity and criterion-related validity are some of the more precise statistical tests of whether the instrument measures what it is supposed to measure. Ideally, an instrument should provide evidence of content validity, as well as criterion-related or construct validity, before one invests a high level of confidence in the instrument. You can expect to see evidence that the reliability and validity of a measurement instrument are reestablished periodically, as Melvin and colleagues (2012; Appendix D) discuss when they indicate the Cronbach's alpha was .96 for the current sample of army couples.

You would also expect to see the strengths and weaknesses of instrument reliability and validity presented in the "Discussion," "Limitations," and/or "Recommendations" sections of an article. In this context, the reliability and validity might be discussed in terms of bias; that is, threats to internal and/or external validity that affect the study findings. For example, in the study by Melvin and colleagues in Appendix D, investigating combat-related post-traumatic stress symptoms (PTSS) and couple relationships in Army couples, the authors note that the findings related to low reliability of the Traumatic Events Questionnaire (TEQ) in this sample warrant further investigation in larger military couple samples. The authors indicate that they did not have a sufficient sample size to further explore the instrument using factor analysis, thus limiting the generalizability of the findings but more importantly suggesting the need for future research. The findings of any study in which the reliability and validity are limited does limit generalizability of the findings, but also adds to our knowledge regarding future research directions. This means that satisfactory reliability and validity that attest to the consistency and accuracy of the instruments used in a study must be evident and interpreted by the author(s) if the findings are to be applicable and generalizable. Finally, recommendations for improving future studies in relation to instrument reliability and validity should be proposed.

As you can see, the area of reliability and validity is complex. These aspects of research reports can be evaluated to varying degrees. You should not feel inhibited by the complexity of this topic; use the guidelines presented in this chapter to systematically assess the reliability and validity aspects of a research study. Collegial dialogue is also an approach to evaluating the merits and shortcomings of an existing, as well as a newly developed, instrument that is reported in the nursing literature. Such an exchange promotes the understanding of methodologies and techniques of reliability and validity, stimulates the acquisition of a basic knowledge of psychometrics, and encourages the exploration of alternative methods of observation and use of reliable and valid instruments in clinical practice.

## KEY POINTS

- Reliability and validity are crucial aspects of conducting and critiquing research.
- Validity is the extent to which an instrument measures the attributes of a concept accurately. Three types of validity are content validity, criterion-related validity, and construct validity.
- The choice of a method for establishing reliability or validity is important and is made by the researcher on the basis of the characteristics of the measurement device in question and its intended use.
- Reliability is the ability of an instrument to measure the attributes of a concept or construct consistently. The major tests of reliability are as follows: test-retest, parallel or alternate form, split-half, item to total correlation, Kuder-Richardson, Cronbach's alpha, and interrater reliability.
- The selection of a method for establishing reliability or validity depends on the characteristics of the instrument, the testing method that is used for collecting data from the sample, and the kinds of data that are obtained.
- Critical appraisal of instrument reliability and validity in a research report focuses on internal and external validity as sources of bias that contribute to the strength and quality of evidence provided by the findings.

## CRITICAL THINKING CHALLENGES

- Discuss the types of validity that must be established before you invest a high level of confidence in the measurement instruments used in a research study.
- What are the major tests of reliability? Why is it important to establish the appropriate type of reliability for a measurement instrument?
- A journal club just finished reading the research report by Thomas and colleagues in Appendix A. As part of their critical appraisal of this study, they needed to identify the strengths and weaknesses of the reliability and validity section of this research report. If you were a member of this journal club, how would you assess the reliability and validity of the instruments used in this study?

- How does the strength and quality of evidence related to reliability and validity influence applicability of findings to clinical practice?
- When a researcher does not report reliability or validity data, which threats to internal and/or external validity should you consider? How would these threats affect the strength and quality of evidence provided by the findings of the study?

## REFERENCES

Alhusen, J. L., Gross, D., Hayat, M. J., et al. (2012). The influence of maternal-fetal attachment and health practices on neonatal outcomes in low-income urban women. *Research in Nursing & Health, 35,* 112–120.

Anastasi, A., & Urbina, S. (1997). *Psychological testing* (7th ed.). New York, NY: Macmillan.

Anderson, E. H., Neafsey, P. J., & Peabody, S. (2011). Psychometrics of the computer-based relationships with health care provider scale in older adults. *Journal of Nursing Measurement, 19*(1), 3–16.

Bender, M., Connelly, C. D., Glaser, D., & Brown, C. (2012). Clinical nurse leader impact on microsystem care quality. *Nursing Research, 61*(5), 326–332.

Bova, C., Route, P. S., Fennie, K., et al. (2012). Measuring patient-provider trust in a primary care population: refinement of the health care relationship trust scale. *Research in Nursing and Health, 35,* 397–408.

Budin, W. C., Hoskins, C. N., Haber, J., et al. (2008). Education, counseling, and adjustment among patient and partners: a randomized clinical trial. *Nursing Research, 57,* 199–213.

Campbell, D., & Fiske, D. (1959). Convergent and discriminant validation by the matrix. *Psychological Bulletin, 53,* 273–302.

Chang, S. F. (2012). The development of an evaluation tool to measure nursing core curriculum teaching effectiveness: an exploratory factor analysis. *Journal of* Nursing Research, *20*(3), 228–235.

DeVon, F. A., Block, M. E., Moyle-Wright, P., et al. (2007). A psychometric toolbox for testing validity and reliability. *Journal of Nursing Scholarship, 39*(2), 155–164.

de Man-van Ginkel, J. M., Gooskens, F., Schepers, V. P. M., et al. (2012). Screening for poststroke depression using the patient health questionnaire. *Nursing Research, 61*(5), 333–341.

DeVellis, R. F. (2012). *Scale development: theory and applications.* Los Angeles, CA: Sage Publications.

Furr, M. R., & Bacharach, V. R. (2008). *Psychometrics: an introduction.* Los Angeles, CA: Sage Publications.

Hoffman, A. J., von Eye, A., Gift, A. G., et al. (2011). The development and testing of an instrument for perceived self-efficacy for fatigue-management. *Cancer Nursing, 34*(3), 167–175. doi: 10. 1097/NCC.ob013e31820f4ed1.

Hoskins, C. N. (1988). *The partner relationship inventory.* Palo Alto, CA: Consulting Psychologists Press.

Liu, Y., Insel, K. C., Reed, P. G., & Crist, J. D. (2012). Family caregiving of older Chinese people with dementia. *Nursing Research, 61*(1), 39–50.

Lynn, M. R. (1986). Determination and quantification of content validity. *Nursing Research, 35,* 382–385.

McDowell, I., & Newell, C. (1996). *Measuring health: a guide to rating scales and questionnaires.* New York, NY: Oxford Press.

Melvin, K. C., Gross, D., Hayat, M. J., et al. (2012). Couple functioning and post-traumatic stress symptoms in US Army: the role of resilience. *Nursing in Research & Health, 35,* 164–177.

Nunnally JC, Bernstein IH. (1993). *Psychometric theory* (3rd ed.). New York, NY: McGraw-Hill.

Sherman, D. W., Haber, J., Hoskins, C. N., et al. (2012). The effect of psychoeducation and telephone counseling on the adjustment of women with early-stage breast cancer. *Applied Nursing Research*, *25*, 3–16.

Thomas, M. L., Elliott, J. E., Rao, S. M., et al. (2012). A randomized clinical trial of education or motivational-interviewing–based coaching compared to usual care to improve cancer pain management. *Oncology Nursing Forum*, *39*(1), 39–49.

Wakefield, B. J., Hayes, J., Boren, S. A., et al. (2012). Strain and satisfaction in caregivers of veterans with chronic illness. *Research in Nursing & Health*, *35*, 55–69.

Waltz, C., Strickland, O., & Lenz, E. (2010). *Measurement in nursing research* (4th ed.). New York, NY: Springer.

Williams, A., Van Ness, P., Dixon, J., & McCorkle, R. (2012). Barriers to meditation by gender and age among cancer family caregivers, *Nursing Research*, *61*(1), 22–27.

# evolve WEBSITE

*Go to Evolve at http://evolve.elsevier.com/LoBiondo/ for review questions, critiquing exercises, and additional research articles for practice in reviewing and critiquing.*

# CHAPTER 16

# Data Analysis: Descriptive and Inferential Statistics

*Susan Sullivan-Bolyai and Carol Bova*

## evolve WEBSITE

*Go to Evolve at http://evolve.elsevier.com/LoBiondo/ for review questions, critiquing exercises, and additional research articles for practice in reviewing and critiquing.*

## LEARNING OUTCOMES

*After reading this chapter, you should be able to do the following:*

- Differentiate between descriptive and inferential statistics.
- State the purposes of descriptive statistics.
- Identify the levels of measurement in a research study.
- Describe a frequency distribution.
- List measures of central tendency and their use.
- List measures of variability and their use.
- Identify the purpose of inferential statistics.
- Explain the concept of probability as it applies to the analysis of sample data.

- Distinguish between a type I and type II error and its effect on a study's outcome.
- Distinguish between parametric and nonparametric tests.
- List some commonly used statistical tests and their purposes.
- Critically appraise the statistics used in published research studies.
- Evaluate the strength and quality of the evidence provided by the findings of a research study and determine their applicability to practice.

## KEY TERMS

| | | | |
|---|---|---|---|
| analysis of covariance | dichotomous variable | level of significance (alpha level) | modality |
| analysis of variance | factor analysis | mean | mode |
| categorical variable | Fisher's exact probability test | measures of central tendency | multiple analysis of variance |
| chi-square ($\chi^2$) | | | multiple regression |
| continuous variable | frequency distribution | measures of variability | multivariate statistics |
| correlation | inferential statistics | median | |
| degrees of freedom | interval measurement | measurement | |
| descriptive statistics | levels of measurement | | nominal measurement |

It is important for you to understand the principles underlying statistical methods used in quantitative nursing research. This understanding allows you to critically analyze the results of research that may be useful to practice. Researchers link the statistical analyses they choose with the type of research question, design, and level of data collected.

As you read a research article you will find a discussion of the statistical procedures used in both the methods and results sections. In the methods section, you will find the planned statistical analyses. In the results section, you will find the data generated from testing the hypotheses or research questions. These data are the analyses using both descriptive and inferential **statistics**.

Procedures that allow researchers to describe and summarize data are known as **descriptive statistics**. Descriptive statistics include measures of central tendency, such as mean, median, and mode; measures of variability, such as range and standard deviation (SD); and some correlation techniques, such as scatter plots. For example, Alhusen and colleagues (2012; Appendix B) used descriptive statistics to inform the reader about the subjects' personal characteristics (93% African American, 67% with less than a high school education) and clinical characteristics (84% initiated prenatal care by 14 weeks' gestation, and 32% were first pregnancies).

Statistical procedures that allow researchers to estimate how reliably they can make *predictions* and *generalize* findings based on the data are known as **inferential statistics**. Inferential statistics are used to analyze the data collected, test hypotheses, and answer the research questions in a research study. With inferential statistics, the researcher is trying to draw conclusions that extend beyond the immediate data of the study.

This chapter describes how researchers use descriptive and inferential statistics in nursing research studies. This will help you to determine the appropriateness of the statistics used and to interpret the strength and quality of the reported findings, as well as the clinical significance and applicability of the research results for your evidence-based practice.

## LEVELS OF MEASUREMENT

**Measurement** is the process of assigning numbers to variables or events according to rules. Every variable in a study that is assigned a specific number must be similar to every other variable assigned that number. In other words, if you decide to assign the number 1 to represent all male subjects in a sample and the number 2 to represent all female subjects, you must use this same numbering scheme throughout your study.

The measurement level is determined by the nature of the object or event being measured. Understanding the **levels of measurement** is an important first step when

## CRITICAL THINKING DECISION PATH

*Descriptive Statistics*

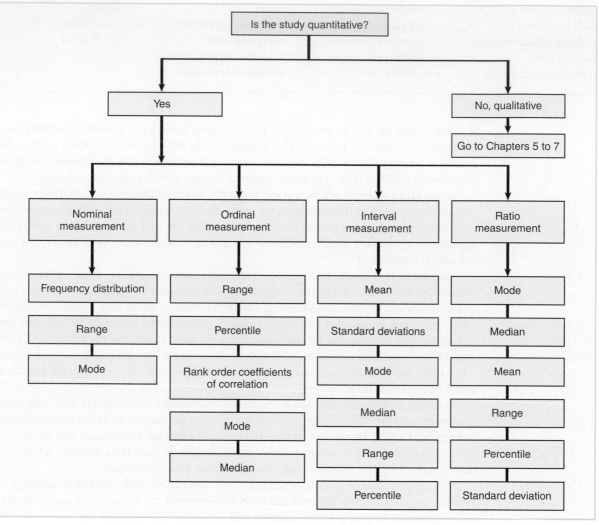

you evaluate the statistical analyses used in a study. There are four levels of measurement: nominal, ordinal, interval, and ratio (Table 16-1). The level of measurement of each variable determines the type of statistic that can be used to answer a research question or test a hypothesis. The higher the level of measurement, the greater the flexibility the researcher has in choosing statistical procedures. Every attempt should be made to use the highest level of measurement possible so that the maximum amount of information will be obtained from the data. The following Critical Thinking Decision Path illustrates the relationship between levels of measurement and appropriate choice of descriptive statistics.

| TABLE 16-1 | LEVEL OF MEASUREMENT SUMMARY TABLE | | |
|---|---|---|---|
| **MEASUREMENT** | **DESCRIPTION** | **MEASURES OF CENTRAL TENDENCY** | **MEASURES OF VARIABILITY** |
| Nominal | Classification | Mode | Modal percentage, range, frequency distribution |
| Ordinal | Relative rankings | Mode, median | Range, percentile, frequency distribution |
| Interval | Rank ordering with equal intervals | Mode, median, mean | Range, percentile, standard deviation |
| Ratio | Rank ordering with equal intervals and absolute zero | Mode, median, mean | All |

**Nominal measurement** is used to classify variables or events into categories. The categories are mutually exclusive; the variable or event either has or does not have the characteristic. The numbers assigned to each category are only labels; such numbers do not indicate more or less of a characteristic. Nominal-level measurement can be used to categorize a sample on such information as gender, marital status, or religious affiliation. For example, Alhusen and colleagues (2012; Appendix B) measured marital status using a nominal level of measurement. Nominal-level measurement is the lowest level and allows for the least amount of statistical manipulation. When using nominal-level variables, typically the frequency and percent are calculated. For example, Alhusen and colleagues (2012) found that among their sample of pregnant women 54% were single, 34% were partnered, and 10% were married.

A variable at the nominal level can also be categorized as either a ***dichotomous*** or ***categorical*** variable. A **dichotomous** (nominal) **variable** is one that has *only two true values*, such as true/false or yes/no. For example, in the Thomas and colleagues (2012; Appendix A) study the variable gender (male/female) is dichotomous because it has only two possible values. On the other hand, nominal variables that are **categorical** still have mutually exclusive categories but have *more than two true values*, such as marital status in the Alhusen and colleagues study (single, partnered/not married, married, other).

**Ordinal measurement** is used to show relative rankings of variables or events. The numbers assigned to each category can be compared, and a member of a higher category can be said to have more of an attribute than a person in a lower category. The intervals between numbers on the scale are not necessarily equal, and there is no absolute zero. For example, ordinal measurement is used to formulate class rankings, where one student can be ranked higher or lower than another. However, the difference in actual grade point average between students may differ widely. Another example is ranking individuals by their level of wellness or by their ability to carry out activities of daily living. Alhusen and colleagues used an ordinal variable to measure the household income of pregnant women in their study and found that 46% ($n = 76$) of the study participants had household incomes under $10,000. Ordinal-level data are limited in the amount of mathematical manipulation possible. Frequencies, percentages, medians, percentiles, and rank order coefficients of correlation can be calculated for ordinal-level data.

**Interval measurement** shows rankings of events or variables on a scale with equal intervals between the numbers. The zero point remains arbitrary and not absolute. For example, interval measurements are used in measuring temperatures on the Fahrenheit scale. The distances between degrees are equal, but the zero point is arbitrary and does not represent the absence of temperature. Test scores also represent interval data. The differences between test scores represent equal intervals, but a zero does not represent the total absence of knowledge.

In many areas in the social sciences, including nursing, the classification of the level of measurement of scales that use Likert-type response options to measure concepts such as quality of life, depression, functional status, or social support is controversial, with some regarding these measurements as ordinal and others as interval. You need to be aware of this controversy and look at each study individually in terms of how the data are analyzed. Interval-level data allow more manipulation of data, including the addition and subtraction of numbers and the calculation of means. This additional manipulation is why many argue for classifying behavioral scale data as interval level. For example, Alhusen and colleagues (2012) used the Maternal-Fetal Attachment Scale (MFAS), which rates 24 items related to attachment on a 5-point Likert scale from 1 (definitely no) to 5 (definitely yes) with higher scores indicating greater maternal-fetal attachment. They reported the mean MFAS score as 84.1 with a standard deviation (SD) of 14.2.

**Ratio measurement** shows rankings of events or variables on scales with equal intervals and absolute zeros. The number represents the actual amount of the property the object possesses. Ratio measurement is the highest level of measurement, but it is most often used in the physical sciences. Examples of ratio-level data that are commonly used in nursing research are height, weight, pulse, and blood pressure. All mathematical procedures can be performed on data from ratio scales. Therefore the use of any statistical procedure is possible as long as it is appropriate to the design of the study.

## DESCRIPTIVE STATISTICS

### Frequency Distribution

One way of organizing descriptive data is by using a frequency distribution. In a **frequency distribution** the number of times each event occurs is counted. The data can also be grouped and the frequency of each group reported. Table 16-2 shows the results of an examination given to a class of 51 students. The results of the examination are reported in several ways. The columns on the left give the raw data tally and the frequency for each grade, and the columns on the right give the grouped data tally and grouped frequencies.

When data are grouped, it is necessary to define the size of the group or the interval width so that no score will fall into two groups and each group will be mutually exclusive.

| TABLE 16-2 | FREQUENCY DISTRIBUTION | | | | |
|---|---|---|---|---|---|
| **INDIVIDUAL** | | | **GROUP** | | |
| **SCORE** | **TALLY** | **FREQUENCY** | **SCORE** | **TALLY** | **FREQUENCY** |
| 90 | I | 1 | >89 | I | 1 |
| 88 | I | 1 | | | |
| 86 | I | 1 | 80-89 | IIIII IIIII IIIII | 15 |
| 84 | IIIII I | 6 | | | |
| 82 | II | 2 | 70-79 | IIIII IIIII IIIII IIIII III | 23 |
| 80 | IIIII | 5 | | | |
| 78 | IIIII | 5 | | | |
| 76 | I | 1 | 60-69 | IIIII IIIII | 10 |
| 74 | IIIII II | 7 | | | |
| 72 | IIIII IIII | 9 | <59 | II | 2 |
| 70 | I | 1 | | | |
| 68 | III | 3 | | | |
| 66 | II | 2 | | | |
| 64 | IIII | 4 | | | |
| 62 | I | 1 | | | |
| 60 | | 0 | | | |
| 58 | I | 1 | | | |
| 56 | | 0 | | | |
| 54 | I | 1 | | | |
| 52 | | 0 | | | |
| 50 | | 0 | | | |
| Total | | 51 | | | 51 |

Mean, 73.1; standard deviation, 12.1; median, 74; mode, 72; range, 36 (54-90).

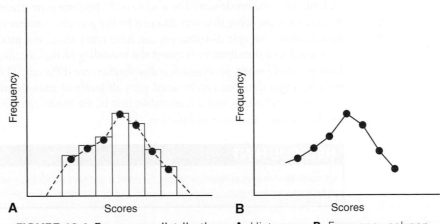

**A**  Scores    **B**  Scores

**FIGURE 16-1** Frequency distributions. **A,** Histogram. **B,** Frequency polygon.

The grouping of the data in Table 16-2 prevents overlap; each score falls into only one group. The grouping should allow for a precise presentation of the data without serious loss of information.

Information about frequency distributions may be presented in the form of a table, such as Table 16-2, or in graphic form. Figure 16-1 illustrates the most common graphic forms:

the histogram and the frequency polygon. The two graphic methods are similar in that both plot scores, or percentages of occurrence, against frequency. The greater the number of points plotted, the smoother the resulting graph. The shape of the resulting graph allows for observations that further describe the data.

## Measures of Central Tendency

Measures of central tendency are used to describe the pattern of responses among a sample. Measures of central tendency include the mean, median, and mode. They yield a single number that describes the middle of the group and summarize the members of a sample. Each measure of central tendency has a specific use and is most appropriate to specific kinds of measurement and types of distributions.

The mean is the arithmetical average of all the scores (add all of the values in a distribution and divide by the total number of values) and is used with interval or ratio data. The mean is the most widely used measure of central tendency. Most statistical tests of significance use the mean. The mean is affected by every score and can change greatly with extreme scores, especially in studies that have a limited sample size. The mean is generally considered the single best point for summarizing data when using interval- or ratio-level data. You can find the mean in research reports by looking for the symbols $M =$ or $\bar{x}$.

The median is the score where 50% of the scores are above it and 50% of the scores are below it. The median is not sensitive to extremes in high and low scores. It is best used when the data are skewed (see Normal Distribution in this chapter), and the researcher is interested in the "typical" score. For example, if age is a variable and there is a wide range with extreme scores that may affect the mean, it would be appropriate to also report the median. The median is easy to find either by inspection or by calculation and can be used with ordinal-, interval-, and ratio-level data.

The mode is the most frequent value in a distribution. The mode is determined by inspection of the frequency distribution (not by mathematical calculation). For example, in Table 16-2 the mode would be a score of 72 because nine students received this score and it represents the score that was attained by the greatest number of students. It is important to note that a sample distribution can have more than one mode. The number of modes contained in a distribution is called the modality of the distribution. It is also possible to have no mode when all scores in a distribution are different. The mode is most often used with nominal data but can be used with all levels of measurement. The mode cannot be used for calculations, and it is unstable; that is, the mode can fluctuate widely from sample to sample from the same population.

### HELPFUL HINT

Of the three measures of central tendency, the mean is the most stable, the least affected by extremes, and the most useful for other calculations. The mean can only be calculated with interval and ratio data.

When you examine a research study, the measures of central tendency provide you with important information about the distribution of scores in a sample. If the distribution is symmetrical and unimodal, the mean, median, and mode will coincide. If the distribution is skewed (asymmetrical), the mean will be pulled in the direction of the long tail of the distribution and will differ from the median. With a skewed distribution, all three statistics should be reported. It is also helpful to report the mean and median for interval- and ratio-level data so the reader knows whether or not the distribution was symmetrical.

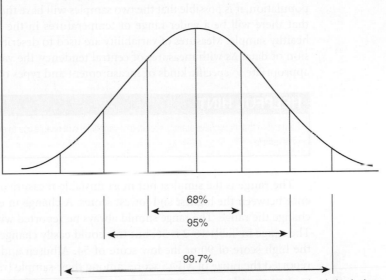
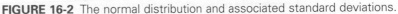

**FIGURE 16-2** The normal distribution and associated standard deviations.

## Normal Distribution

The concept of the **normal distribution** is based on the observation that data from repeated measures of interval- or ratio-level data group themselves about a midpoint in a distribution in a manner that closely approximates the normal curve illustrated in Figure 16-2. The **normal curve** is one that is symmetrical about the mean and is uni-modal. The mean, median, and mode are equal. An additional characteristic of the normal curve is that a fixed percentage of the scores falls within a given distance of the mean. As shown in Figure 16-2, about 68% of the scores or means will fall within 1 SD of the mean, 95% within 2 SD of the mean, and 99.7% within 3 SD of the mean. The presence or absence of a normal distribution is a fundamental issue when examining the appropriate use of inferential statistical procedures.

## Interpreting Measures of Variability

Variability or dispersion is concerned with the spread of data. **Measures of variability** answer questions such as the following: "Is the sample homogeneous or heterogeneous?" "Is the sample similar or different?" If a researcher measures oral temperatures in two samples, one sample drawn from a healthy population and one sample from a hospitalized population, it is possible that the two samples will have the same mean. However, it is likely that there will be a wider range of temperatures in the hospitalized sample than in the healthy sample. Measures of variability are used to describe these differences in the dispersion of data. As with measures of central tendency, the various measures of variability are appropriate to specific kinds of measurement and types of distributions.

---

**HELPFUL HINT**

Remember that descriptive statistics related to variability will enable you to evaluate the homogeneity or heterogeneity of a sample.

---

The **range** is the simplest but most unstable measure of variability. Range is the difference between the highest and lowest scores. A change in either of these two scores would change the range. The range should always be reported with other measures of variability. The range in Table 16-2 is 36, but this could easily change with an increase or decrease in the high score of 90 or the low score of 54. Alhusen and colleagues (2012; Appendix B) reported the range of MFAS scores among their sample (range = 52-116).

A **percentile** represents the percentage of cases a given score exceeds. The median is the 50% percentile, and in Table 16-2 it is a score of 74. A score in the 90th percentile is exceeded by only 10% of the scores. The zero percentile and the 100th percentile are usually dropped.

The **standard deviation (SD)** is the most frequently used measure of variability, and it is based on the concept of the normal curve (see Figure 16-2). It is a measure of average deviation of the scores from the mean and as such should always be reported with the mean. The SD takes all scores into account and can be used to interpret individual scores. The SD is used in the calculation of many inferential statistics.

---

**HELPFUL HINT**

Many measures of variability exist. The SD is the most stable and useful because it helps you to visualize how the scores disperse around the mean.

---

## INFERENTIAL STATISTICS

Inferential statistics combine mathematical processes and logic and allow researchers to test hypotheses about a population using data obtained from probability samples. Statistical inference is generally used for two purposes: to estimate the probability that the statistics in the sample accurately reflect the population parameter and to test hypotheses about a population.

A **parameter** is a characteristic of a *population,* whereas a **statistic** is a characteristic of a *sample.* We use statistics to estimate population parameters. Suppose we randomly sample 100 people with chronic lung disease and use an interval-level scale to study their knowledge of the disease. If the mean score for these subjects is 65, the mean represents the sample statistic. If we were able to study every subject with chronic lung disease, we could calculate an average knowledge score and that score would be the parameter for the population. As you know, a researcher rarely is able to study an entire population, so inferential

## CRITICAL THINKING DECISION PATH

*Inferential Statistics—Difference Questions*

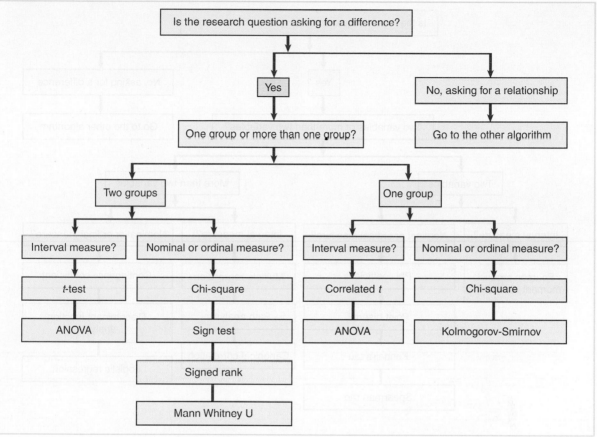

statistics provide evidence that allows the researcher to make statements about the larger population from studying the sample.

The example given alludes to two important qualifications of how a study must be conducted so that inferential statistics may be used. First, it was stated that the sample was selected using probability methods (see Chapter 12). Because you are already familiar with the advantages of probability sampling, it should be clear that if we wish to make statements about a population from a sample, that sample must be representative. All procedures for inferential statistics are based on the assumption that the sample was drawn with a known probability. Second, the scale used has to be at either an interval or a ratio level of measurement. This is because the mathematical operations involved in doing inferential statistics require this higher level of measurement. It should be noted that in studies that use nonprobability methods of sampling, inferential statistics are also used. To compensate for the use of nonprobability sampling methods, researchers use techniques such as sample size estimation using power analysis. The following two Critical Thinking Decision Paths examine inferential statistics and provide matrices that researchers use for statistical decision making.

## CRITICAL THINKING DECISION PATH

### *Inferential Statistics—Relationship Questions*

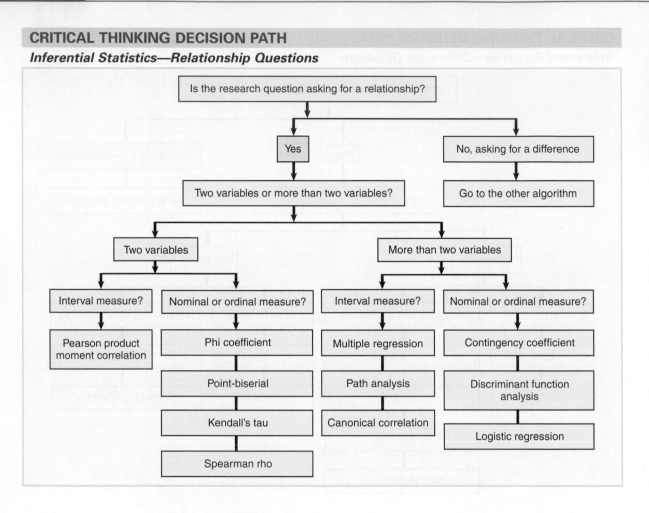

## Hypothesis Testing

Inferential statistics are used for hypothesis testing. Statistical hypothesis testing allows researchers to make objective decisions about the outcome of their study. The use of statistical hypothesis testing answers questions such as the following: "How much of this effect is a result of chance?" "How strongly are these two variables associated with each other?" "What is the effect of the intervention?"

The procedures used when making inferences are based on principles of negative inference. In other words, if a researcher studied the effect of a new educational program for patients with chronic lung disease, the researcher would actually have two hypotheses: the scientific hypothesis and the null hypothesis. The research or **scientific hypothesis** is that which the researcher believes will be the outcome of the study. In our example, the scientific hypothesis would be that the educational intervention would have a marked impact on the outcome in the experimental group beyond that in the control group. The **null hypothesis**, which is the hypothesis that actually can be tested by statistical methods, would state that there is no difference between the groups. Inferential statistics use the null hypothesis to test the validity of a scientific hypothesis. The null hypothesis states that there is no relationship between the variables and that any observed relationship or difference is merely a function of chance.

**HELPFUL HINT**

Remember that most samples used in clinical research are samples of convenience, but often researchers use inferential statistics. Although such use violates one of the assumptions of such tests, the tests are robust enough to not seriously affect the results unless the data are skewed in unknown ways.

## Probability

Probability theory underlies all of the procedures discussed in this chapter. The **probability** of an event is its long-run relative frequency (0% to 100%) in repeated trials under similar conditions. In other words, what are the chances of obtaining the same result from a study that can be carried out many times under identical conditions? It is the notion of repeated trials that allows researchers to use probability to test hypotheses.

Statistical probability is based on the concept of **sampling error**. Remember that the use of inferential statistics is based on random sampling. However, even when samples are randomly selected, there is always the possibility of some error in sampling. Therefore the characteristics of any given sample may be different from those of the entire population. The tendency for statistics to fluctuate from one sample to another is known as sampling error.

**EVIDENCE-BASED PRACTICE TIP**

Remember that the strength and quality of evidence are enhanced by repeated trials that have consistent findings, thereby increasing generalizability of the findings and applicability to clinical practice.

## Type I and Type II Errors

Statistical inference is always based on incomplete information about a population, and it is possible for errors to occur. There are two types of errors in statistical inference—type I and type II errors. A **type I error** occurs when a researcher rejects a null hypothesis when it is actually true (i.e., accepts the premise that there is a difference when actually there is no difference between groups). A **type II error** occurs when a researcher accepts a null hypothesis that is actually false (i.e., accepts the premise that there is no difference between the groups when a difference actually exists). The relationship of the two types of errors is shown in Figure 16-3.

When critiquing a study to see if there is a possibility of a type I error having occurred (rejecting the null hypothesis when it is actually true), one should consider the reliability and validity of the instruments used. For example, if the instruments did not accurately measure the intervention variables, one could conclude that the intervention made a difference when in reality it did not. It is critical to consider the reliability and validity of all

| Conclusion of test of significance | REALITY | |
|---|---|---|
| | Null hypothesis is true | Null hypothesis is not true |
| Not statistically significant | Correct conclusion | Type II error |
| Statistically significant | Type I error | Correct conclusion |

**FIGURE 16-3** Outcome of statistical decision making.

the measurement instruments reported (see Chapter 15). For example, Alhusen and colleagues (2012) reported the reliability of the Maternal-Fetal Attachment Scale (MFAS) in their sample and found it was reliable as evidenced by a Cronbach's alpha of .88 (refer to Chapter 15 to review scale reliability). This gives the reader greater confidence in the results of the study.

In a practice discipline, type I errors usually are considered more serious because if a researcher declares that differences exist where none are present, the potential exists for patient care to be affected adversely. Type II errors (accepting the null hypothesis when it is false) often occur when the sample is too small, thereby limiting the opportunity to measure *the treatment effect,* a true difference between two groups. A larger sample size improves the ability to *detect the treatment effect,* that is, differences between two groups. If no significant difference is found between two groups with a large sample, it provides stronger evidence (than with a small sample) not to reject the null hypothesis.

## Level of Significance

The researcher does not know when an error in statistical decision making has occurred. It is possible to know only that the null hypothesis is indeed true or false if data from the total population are available. However, the researcher can control the risk of making type I errors by setting the level of significance before the study begins (a priori).

The level of significance (alpha level) is the probability of making a type I error, the probability of rejecting a true null hypothesis. The minimum level of significance acceptable for most research is .05. If the researcher sets alpha, or the level of significance, at .05, the researcher is willing to accept the fact that if the study were done 100 times, the decision to reject the null hypothesis would be wrong 5 times out of those 100 trials. If, as is sometimes done, the researcher wants to have a smaller risk of rejecting a true null hypothesis, the level of significance may be set at .01. In this case the researcher is willing to be wrong only once in 100 trials.

The decision as to how strictly the alpha level should be set depends on how important it is to not make an error. For example, if the results of a study are to be used to determine whether a great deal of money should be spent in an area of nursing care, the researcher may decide that the accuracy of the results is so important that an alpha level of .01 is needed. In most studies, however, alpha is set at .05.

Perhaps you are thinking that researchers should always use the lowest alpha level possible to keep the risk of both types of errors at a minimum. Unfortunately, decreasing the risk of making a type I error increases the risk of making a type II error. Therefore the researcher always has to accept more of a risk of one type of error when setting the alpha level.

## Clinical and Statistical Significance

It is important for you to realize that there is a difference between statistical significance and clinical significance. When a researcher tests a hypothesis and finds that it is statistically significant, it means that the finding is unlikely to have happened by chance. For example, if a study was designed to test an intervention to help a large sample of patients lose weight, and the researchers found that a change in weight of 1.02 pounds was statistically significant, one might find this questionable because few would say that a change in weight of just over 1 pound would represent a clinically significant difference. Therefore as a consumer of research it is important for you to evaluate the clinical significance as well as the statistical significance of findings.

Some people believe that if findings are not statistically significant, they have no practical value. However, knowing that something does not work is important information to share with the scientific community. Nonsupported hypotheses provide as much information about the intervention as do supported hypotheses. Nonsignificant results (sometimes called negative findings) force the researcher to return to the literature and consider alternative explanations for why the intervention did not work as planned.

## Parametric and Nonparametric Statistics

Tests of significance may be parametric or nonparametric. **Parametric statistics** have the following attributes:

1. They involve the estimation of at least one population parameter.
2. They require measurement on at least an interval scale.
3. They involve certain assumptions about the variables being studied.

One important assumption is that the variable is normally distributed in the overall population.

In contrast to parametric tests, **nonparametric statistics** are not based on the estimation of population parameters, so they involve less restrictive assumptions about the underlying distribution. Nonparametric tests usually are applied when the variables have been measured on a nominal or ordinal scale or when the distribution of scores is severely skewed.

| TABLE 16-3 | **TESTS OF DIFFERENCES BETWEEN MEANS** | | | |
|---|---|---|---|---|
| | | **TWO GROUPS** | | |
| **LEVEL OF MEASUREMENT** | **ONE GROUP** | **RELATED** | **INDEPENDENT** | **MORE THAN TWO GROUPS** |
| **Nonparametric** | | | | |
| Nominal | Chi-square | Chi-square Fisher exact probability | Chi-square | Chi-square |
| Ordinal | Kolmogorov-Smirnov | Sign test Wilcoxon matched pairs Signed rank | Chi-square Median test Mann-Whitney U | Chi-square |
| **Parametric** | | | | |
| Interval or ratio | Correlated $t$ ANOVA (repeated measures) | Correlated $t$ | Independent $t$ ANOVA | ANOVA ANCOVA MANOVA |

| TABLE 16-4 | **TESTS OF ASSOCIATION** | |
|---|---|---|
| **LEVEL OF MEASUREMENT** | **TWO VARIABLES** | **MORE THAN TWO VARIABLES** |
| **Nonparametric** | | |
| Nominal | Phi coefficient Point-biserial | Contingency coefficient |
| Ordinal | Kendall's tau Spearman rho | Discriminant function analysis |
| **Parametric** | | |
| Interval or ratio | Pearson $r$ | Multiple regression Path analysis Canonical correlation |

There has been some debate about the relative merits of the two types of statistical tests. The moderate position taken by most researchers and statisticians is that nonparametric statistics are best used when data are not at the interval level of measurement, when the sample is small and data do not approximate a normal distribution. However, most researchers prefer to use parametric statistics whenever possible (as long as data meet the assumptions) because they are more powerful and more flexible than nonparametric statistics.

Tables 16-3 and 16-4 list the commonly used inferential statistics. The test used depends on the level of the measurement of the variables in question and the type of hypothesis being studied. Basically, these statistics test two types of hypotheses: that there is a difference between groups (see Table 16-3) or that there is a relationship between two or more variables (see Table 16-4).

**EVIDENCE-BASED PRACTICE TIP**

Try to discern whether the test chosen for analyzing the data was chosen because it gave a significant *p* value. A statistical test should be chosen on the basis of its appropriateness for the type of data collected, not because it gives the answer that the researcher hoped to obtain.

## Tests of Difference

The type of test used for any particular study depends primarily on whether the researcher is examining differences in one, two, or three or more groups and whether the data to be analyzed are nominal, ordinal, or interval (see Table 16-3). Suppose a researcher has conducted an experimental study using an after-only design (see Chapter 9). What the researcher hopes to determine is that the two randomly assigned groups are different after the introduction of the experimental treatment. If the measurements taken are at the interval level, the researcher would use the *t* test to analyze the data. If the *t* statistic was found to be high enough as to be unlikely to have occurred by chance, the researcher would reject the null hypothesis and conclude that the two groups were indeed more different than would have been expected on the basis of chance alone. In other words, the researcher would conclude that the experimental treatment had the desired effect.

**EVIDENCE-BASED PRACTICE TIP**

Tests of difference are most commonly used in experimental and quasi-experimental designs that provide Level II and Level III evidence.

The *t* **statistic** is commonly used in nursing research. This statistic tests whether two group means are different. Thus this statistic is used when the researcher has two groups, and the question is whether the mean scores on some measure are more different than would be expected by chance. To use this test, the dependent variable must have been measured at the interval or ratio level, and the two groups must be independent. By independent we mean that nothing in one group helps determine who is in the other group. If the groups are related, as when samples are matched, and the researcher also wants to determine differences between the two groups, a paired or correlated *t* test would be used. The **degrees of freedom** (represents the freedom of a score's value to vary given what is known about the other scores and the sum of scores; often $df = N - 1$) that are reported with the *t* statistic and the probability value *(p)*. Degrees of freedom is usually abbreviated as *df*.

The *t* statistic illustrates one of the major purposes of research in nursing—to demonstrate that there are differences between groups. Groups may be naturally occurring collections, such as gender, or they may be experimentally created, such as the treatment and control groups. Sometimes a researcher has more than two groups, or measurements are taken more than once, and then **analysis of variance** (ANOVA) is used. ANOVA is similar to the *t* test. Like the *t* statistic, ANOVA tests whether group means differ, but rather than testing each pair of means separately, ANOVA considers the variation between groups and within groups.

**HELPFUL HINT**

A research report may not always contain the test that was done. You can find this information by looking at the tables. For example, a table with *t* statistics will contain a column for "*t*" values, and an ANOVA table will contain "*F*" values.

Analysis of covariance (ANCOVA) is used to measure differences among group means, but it also uses a statistical technique to equate the groups under study on an important variable. Another expansion of the notion of analysis of variance is **multiple analysis of variance** (MANOVA), which also is used to determine differences in group means, but it is used when there is more than one dependent variable.

## Nonparametric Statistics

When data are at the nominal level and the researcher wants to determine whether groups are different, the researcher uses the **chi-square** $(\chi^2)$. Chi-square is a nonparametric statistic used to determine whether the frequency in each category is different from what would be expected by chance. As with the $t$ test and ANOVA, if the calculated chi-square is high enough, the researcher would conclude that the frequencies found would not be expected on the basis of chance alone, and the null hypothesis would be rejected. Although this test is quite robust and can be used in many different situations, it cannot be used to compare frequencies when samples are small and expected frequencies are less than 6 in each cell. In these instances the **Fisher's exact probability test** is used.

When the data are ranks, or are at the ordinal level, researchers have several other nonparametric tests at their disposal. These include the *Kolmogorov-Smirnov test,* the *sign test,* the *Wilcoxon matched pairs test,* the *signed rank test for related groups,* the *median test,* and the *Mann-Whitney U test for independent groups.* Explanation of these tests is beyond the scope of this chapter; those readers who desire further information should consult a general statistics book.

---

**HELPFUL HINT**

Chi-square is the test of difference commonly used for nominal level demographic variables such as gender, marital status, religion, ethnicity, and others.

---

## Tests of Relationships

Researchers often are interested in exploring the *relationship* between two or more variables. Such studies use statistics that determine the **correlation**, or the degree of association, between two or more variables. Tests of the relationships between variables are sometimes considered to be descriptive statistics when they are used to describe the magnitude and direction of a relationship of two variables in a sample and the researcher does not wish to make statements about the larger population. Such statistics also can be inferential when they are used to test hypotheses about the correlations that exist in the target population.

---

**EVIDENCE-BASED PRACTICE TIP**

You will often note that in the Results or Findings section of a research study parametric (e.g., *t*-tests, ANOVA) and nonparametric (e.g., chi-square, Fisher's exact probability test) will be used to test differences between and among variables depending on their level of measurement. For example, chi-square may be used to test differences between nominal level demographic variables, *t*-tests will be used to test the hypotheses or research questions about differences between two groups, and ANOVA will be used to test differences between and among groups when there are multiple comparisons.

---

Null hypothesis tests of the relationships between variables assume that there is no relationship between the variables. Thus when a researcher rejects this type of null hypothesis, the conclusion is that the variables are in fact related. Suppose a researcher is interested in the relationship between the age of patients and the length of time it takes them to recover from surgery. As with other statistics discussed, the researcher would design a study to collect the appropriate data and then analyze the data using measures of association. In this example, age and length of time until recovery would be considered interval-level measurements. The researcher would use a test called the **Pearson correlation coefficient, Pearson** $r$, or **Pearson product moment correlation coefficient.** Once the Pearson $r$ is calculated, the researcher consults the distribution for this test to determine whether the value obtained is likely to have occurred by chance. Again, the research reports both the value of the correlation and its probability of occurring by chance.

Correlation coefficients can range in value from $-1.0$ to $+1.0$ and also can be zero. A zero coefficient means that there is no relationship between the variables. *A perfect positive correlation* is indicated by a $+1.0$ coefficient, and a *perfect negative correlation* by a $-1.0$ coefficient. We can illustrate the meaning of these coefficients by using the example from the previous paragraph. If there were no relationship between the age of the patient and the time required for the patient to recover from surgery, the researcher would find a correlation of zero. However, if the correlation was $+1.0$, it would mean that the older the patient, the longer the recovery time. A negative coefficient would imply that the younger the patient, the longer the recovery time.

Of course, relationships are rarely perfect. The magnitude of the relationship is indicated by how close the correlation comes to the absolute value of 1. Thus a correlation of $-.76$ is just as strong as a correlation of $+.76$, but the direction of the relationship is opposite. In addition, a correlation of .76 is stronger than a correlation of .32. When a researcher tests hypotheses about the relationships between two variables, the test considers whether the magnitude of the correlation is large enough not to have occurred by chance. This is the meaning of the probability value or the $p$ value reported with correlation coefficients. As with other statistical tests of significance, the larger the sample, the greater the likelihood of finding a significant correlation. Therefore researchers also report the degrees of freedom *(df)* associated with the test performed.

Nominal and ordinal data also can be tested for relationships by nonparametric statistics. When two variables being tested have only two levels (e.g., male/female; yes/no), the *phi coefficient* can be used to test relationships. When the researcher is interested in the relationship between a nominal variable and an interval variable, the *point-biserial correlation* is used. *Spearman rho* is used to determine the degree of association between two sets of ranks, as is *Kendall's tau.* All of these correlation coefficients may range in value from $-1.0$ to $+1.0$.

## EVIDENCE-BASED PRACTICE TIP

Tests of relationship are usually associated with nonexperimental designs that provide Level IV evidence. Establishing a strong statistically significant relationship between variables often lends support for replicating the study to increase the consistency of the findings and provide a foundation for developing an intervention study.

## Advanced Statistics

Nurse researchers are often interested in health problems that are very complex and require that we analyze many different variables at once using advanced statistical procedures called

**multivariate statistics.** Computer software has made the use of multivariate statistics quite accessible to researchers. When researchers are interested in understanding more about a problem than just the relationship between two variables, they often use a technique called **multiple regression,** which measures the relationship between one interval-level–dependent variable and several independent variables. Multiple regression is the expansion of correlation to include more than two variables, and it is used when the researcher wants to determine what variables contribute to the explanation of the dependent variable and to what degree. For example, a researcher may be interested in determining what factors help women decide to breast-feed their infants. A number of variables, such as the mother's age, previous experience with breast-feeding, number of other children, and knowledge of the advantages of breast-feeding, might be measured and analyzed to see whether they, separately and together, predict the length of breast-feeding. Such a study would require the use of multiple regression.

Another advanced technique often used in nursing research is **factor analysis.** There are two types of factor analysis, exploratory and confirmatory factor analysis. Exploratory factor analysis is used to reduce a set of data so that it may be easily described and used. It is also used in the early phases of instrument development and theory development. Factor analysis is used to determine whether a scale actually measured the concepts that it is intended to measure. Confirmatory factor analysis resembles structural equation modeling and is used in instrument development to examine construct validity and reliability and to compare factor structures across groups (Plichta & Kelvin, 2012).

Many nursing studies use statistical modeling procedures to answer research questions. Causal modeling is used most often when researchers want to test hypotheses and theoretically derived relationships. *Path analysis, structured equation modeling (SEM),* and *linear structural relations analysis (LISREL)* are different types of modeling procedures used in nursing research.

Many other statistical techniques are available to nurse researchers. It is beyond the scope of this chapter to review all statistical analyses available. You should consider having several statistical texts available to you as you sort through the evidence reported in studies that are important to your clinical practice (e.g., Field, 2005; Plichta & Kelvin, 2012).

## APPRAISING THE EVIDENCE
## DESCRIPTIVE AND INFERENTIAL STATISTICS

Nurses are challenged to understand the results of research studies that use sophisticated statistical procedures. Understanding the principles that guide statistical analysis is the first step in this process. Statistics are used to describe the samples of studies and to test for hypothesized differences or associations in the sample. Knowing the characteristics of the sample of a study allows you to determine whether the results are potentially useful for your patients. For example, if a study sample was primarily white with a mean age of 42 years (SD 2.5), the findings may not be applicable if your patients are mostly elderly and African American. Cultural, demographic, or clinical factors of an elderly population of a different ethnic group may contribute to different results. Thus understanding the descriptive statistics of a study will assist you in determining the applicability of findings to your practice setting.

Statistics are also used to test hypotheses. Inferential statistics used to analyze data and the associated significance level ($p$ values) indicates the likelihood that the association or

## CRITIQUING CRITERIA

### Descriptive and Inferential Statistics

1. Were appropriate descriptive statistics used?
2. What level of measurement is used to measure each of the major variables?
3. Is the sample size large enough to prevent one extreme score from affecting the summary statistics used?
4. What descriptive statistics are reported?
5. Were these descriptive statistics appropriate to the level of measurement for each variable?
6. Are there appropriate summary statistics for each major variable, for example, demographic variables, and any other relevant data?
7. Does the hypothesis indicate that the researcher is interested in testing for differences between groups or in testing for relationships? What is the level of significance?
8. Does the level of measurement permit the use of parametric statistics?
9. Is the size of the sample large enough to permit the use of parametric statistics?
10. Has the researcher provided enough information to decide whether the appropriate statistics were used?
11. Are the statistics used appropriate to the hypothesis, the research question, the method, the sample, and the level of measurement?
12. Are the results for each of the research questions or hypotheses presented clearly and appropriately?
13. If tables and graphs are used, do they agree with the text and extend it, or do they merely repeat it?
14. Are the results understandable?
15. Is a distinction made between clinical significance and statistical significance? How is it made?

difference found in a study is due to chance or to a true difference between groups. The closer the $p$ value is to zero, the less likely the association or difference of a study is due to chance. Thus inferential statistics provide an objective way to determine if the results of the study are likely to be a true representation of reality. However, it is still important for you to judge the clinical significance of the findings. Was there a big enough effect (difference between the experimental and control groups) to warrant changing current practice?

The Cochrane Report by Murphy and colleagues (2012; Appendix E) provides an excellent example of the summarization of many studies (meta-analysis) that can help direct an evidence-based practice for improving psychological well being for women after miscarriage.

### EVIDENCE-BASED PRACTICE TIP

A basic understanding of statistics will improve your ability to think about the effect of the independent variable (IV) on the dependent variable (DV) and related patient outcomes for your patient population and practice setting.

There are a few steps to follow when critiquing the statistics used in nursing studies (see Critiquing Criteria box). Before a decision can be made as to whether the statistics that were used make sense, it is important to return to the beginning of the research study and review the purpose of the study. Just as the hypotheses or research questions should flow from the purpose of a study, so should the hypotheses or research questions suggest the type of analysis that will follow. The hypotheses or the research questions should indicate the major variables that are expected to be tested and presented in the "Results" section. Both the summary descriptive statistics and the results of the inferential testing of each of the variables should be in the "Results" section with appropriate information.

After reviewing the hypotheses or research questions, you should proceed to the "Methods" section. Next, try to determine the level of measurement for each variable. From this information it is possible to determine the measures of central tendency and variability that should be used to summarize the data. For example, you would not expect to see a mean used as a summary statistic for the nominal variable of gender. In all likelihood, gender would be reported as a frequency distribution. But you would expect to find a mean and SD for a variable that used a questionniare. The means and SD should be provided for measurements performed at the interval level. The sample size is another aspect of the "Methods" section that is important to review when evaluating the researcher's use of descriptive statistics. The sample is usually described using descriptive summary statistics. Remember, the larger the sample, the less chance that one outlying score will affect the summary statistics. It is also important to note whether the researchers indicated that they did a power analysis to estimate the sample size needed to conduct the study.

If tables or graphs are used, they should agree with the information presented in the text. Evaluate whether the tables and graphs are clearly labeled. If the researcher presents grouped frequency data, the groups should be logical and mutually exclusive. The size of the interval in grouped data should not obscure the pattern of the data, nor should it create an artificial pattern. Each table and graph should be referred to in the text, but each should add to the text—not merely repeat it.

The following are some simple steps for reading a table:

1. Look at the title of the table and see if it matches the purpose of the table.
2. Review the column headings and assess whether the headings follow logically from the title.
3. Look at the abbreviations used. Are they clear and easy to understand? Are any nonstandard abbreviations explained?
4. Evaluate whether the statistics contained in the table are appropriate to the level of measurement for each variable.

After evaluating the descriptive statistics, inferential statistics can then be evaluated. The place to begin appraising the inferential statistical analysis of a research study is with the hypothesis or research question. If the hypothesis or research question indicates that a relationship will be found, you should expect to find tests of correlation. If the study is experimental or quasi-experimental, the hypothesis or research question would indicate that the author is looking for significant differences between the groups studied, and you would expect to find statistical tests of differences between means that test the effect of the intervention. Then as you read the "Methods" section of the paper, again consider what level of measurement the author has used to measure the important variables. If the level of measurement is interval or ratio, the statistics most likely will be parametric statistics. On the other hand, if the variables are measured at the nominal or ordinal level, the statistics used should be nonparametric. Also consider the size of the sample, and remember that samples have to be large enough to permit the assumption of normality. If the sample is quite small, for example, 5 to 10 subjects, the researcher may have violated the assumptions necessary for inferential statistics to be used. Thus the important question is whether the researcher has provided enough justification to use the statistics presented.

Finally, consider the results as they are presented. There should be enough data presented for each hypothesis or research question studied to determine whether the researcher actually examined each hypothesis or research question. The tables should accurately reflect the procedure performed and be in harmony with the text. For example, the text should not indicate that a test reached statistical significance while the tables indicate that the probability value of the test was above .05. If the researcher has used analyses that are not discussed in this text, you may want to refer to a statistics text to decide whether the analysis was appropriate to the hypothesis or research question and the level of measurement.

There are two other aspects of the data analysis section that you should appraise. The results of the study in the text of the article should be clear. In addition, the author should attempt to make a distinction between clinical and statistical significance of the evidence related to the findings. Some results may be statistically significant, but their clinical importance may be doubtful in terms of applicability for a patient population or clinical setting. If this is so, the author should note it. Alternatively, you may find yourself reading a research study that is elegantly presented, but you come away with a "so what?" feeling. From an evidence-based practice perspective, a significant hypothesis or research question should contribute to improving patient care and clinical outcomes. The important question to ask is "What is the strength and quality of the evidence provided by the findings of this study and their applicability to practice?"

Note that the critical analysis of a research paper's statistical analysis is not done in a vacuum. It is possible to judge the adequacy of the analysis only in relationship to the other important aspects of the paper: the problem, the hypotheses, the research question, the design, the data collection methods, and the sample. Without consideration of these aspects of the research process, the statistics themselves have very little meaning.

## ▎ KEY POINTS

- Descriptive statistics are a means of describing and organizing data gathered in research.
- The four levels of measurement are nominal, ordinal, interval, and ratio. Each has appropriate descriptive techniques associated with it.
- Measures of central tendency describe the average member of a sample. The mode is the most frequent score, the median is the middle score, and the mean is the arithmetical average of the scores. The mean is the most stable and useful of the measures of central tendency and, combined with the standard deviation, forms the basis for many of the inferential statistics.
- The frequency distribution presents data in tabular or graphic form and allows for the calculation or observations of characteristics of the distribution of the data, including skew symmetry, and modality.
- In nonsymmetrical distributions, the degree and direction of the off-center peak are described in terms of positive or negative skew.
- The range reflects differences between high and low scores.
- The standard deviation is the most stable and useful measure of variability. It is derived from the concept of the normal curve. In the normal curve, sample scores and the means of large numbers of samples group themselves around the midpoint in the distribution, with a fixed percentage of the scores falling within given distances of the mean. This tendency of means to approximate the normal curve is called the sampling distribution of the means.
- Inferential statistics are a tool to test hypotheses about populations from sample data.

- Because the sampling distribution of the means follows a normal curve, researchers are able to estimate the probability that a certain sample will have the same properties as the total population of interest. Sampling distributions provide the basis for all inferential statistics.
- Inferential statistics allow researchers to estimate population parameters and to test hypotheses. The use of these statistics allows researchers to make objective decisions about the outcome of the study. Such decisions are based on the rejection or acceptance of the null hypothesis, which states that there is no relationship between the variables.
- If the null hypothesis is accepted, this result indicates that the findings are likely to have occurred by chance. If the null hypothesis is rejected, the researcher accepts the scientific hypothesis that a relationship exists between the variables that is unlikely to have been found by chance.
- Statistical hypothesis testing is subject to two types of errors: type I and type II.
- A type I error occurs when the researcher rejects a null hypothesis that is actually true.
- A type II error occurs when the researcher accepts a null hypothesis that is actually false.
- The researcher controls the risk of making a type I error by setting the alpha level, or level of significance; however, reducing the risk of a type I error by reducing the level of significance increases the risk of making a type II error.
- The results of statistical tests are reported to be significant or nonsignificant. Statistically significant results are those whose probability of occurring is less than .05 or .01, depending on the level of significance set by the researcher.
- Commonly used parametric and nonparametric statistical tests include those that test for differences between means, such as the *t* test and ANOVA, and those that test for differences in proportions, such as the chi-square test.
- Tests that examine data for the presence of relationships include the Pearson *r*, the sign test, the Wilcoxon matched pairs, signed rank test, and multiple regression.
- The most important aspect of critiquing statistical analyses is the relationship of the statistics employed to the problem, design, and method used in the study. Clues to the appropriate statistical test to be used by the researcher should stem from the researcher's hypotheses. The reader also should determine if all of the hypotheses have been presented in the paper.
- A basic understanding of statistics will improve your ability to think about the level of evidence provided by the study design and findings and their relevance to patient outcomes for your patient population and practice setting.

## CRITICAL THINKING CHALLENGES

- When reading a research study, what is the significance of applying findings if a nurse researcher made a type I error in statistical inference?
- What is the relationship between the level of measurement a researcher uses and the choice of statistics used? As you read a research study, identify the statistics, level of measurement, and the associated level of evidence provided by the design.
- When reviewing a study you find the sample size provided does not seem adequate. Before you make this final decision, think about how the design type (e.g., pilot study, intervention study), data-collection methods, the number of variables, and the sensitivity of the data-collection instruments can affect your decision.
- When reading a study you find that the findings were not significant statistically. Consider what the application of such findings could possibly offer your practice.

## REFERENCES

Alhusen, J. L., Gross, D., Hayat, M. J., et al. (2012).The influence of maternal-fetal attachment and health practices on neonatal outcomes in low-income, urban women. *Research in Nursing & Health, 35,* 112–120. doi: 10.1002/nur.21464.

Field, A. (2005). *Discovering statistics using SPSS* (2nd ed.). Thousand Oaks, CA: Sage.

Murphy, F. A., Lipp, A., Powles, D. L. (2012). Follow-up for improving psychological well being for women after a miscarriage (Review). *The Cochrane Collaboration*, John Wiley & Sons, Ltd. doi: 10.1002/14651858.CD008679.pub2.

Plichta, S. B., Kelvin, E. (2012). *Munro's Statistical Methods for Health Care Research* (6th ed.). Philadelphia, PA: Lippincott Williams & Wilkins.

Thomas, M. L., Elliott, J. E., Rao, S. M., et al. (2012). A randomized, clinical trial of education or motivational-interviewing–based coaching compared to usual care to improve cancer pain management. *Oncology Nursing Forum, 39,* 39–49. doi:10.1188/12.ONF.39-49.

## ℮volve WEBSITE

*Go to Evolve at http://evolve.elsevier.com/LoBiondo/ for review questions, critquing exercises, and additional research articles for practice in reviewing and critiquing.*

# 17

# Understanding Research Findings

*Geri LoBiondo-Wood*

**evolve** WEBSITE

Go to Evolve at *http://evolve.elsevier.com/LoBiondo/* for review questions, critiquing exercises, and additional
research articles for practice in reviewing and critiquing.

## LEARNING OUTCOMES

*After reading this chapter, you should be able to do the following:*

- Discuss the difference between the "Results" and the "Discussion" sections of a research article.
- Identify the format and components of the "Results" section.
- Determine if both statistically supported and statistically unsupported findings are appropriately discussed.
- Determine whether the results are objectively reported.
- Describe how tables and figures are used in a research report.
- List the criteria of a meaningful table.

- Identify the format and components of the "Discussion" section.
- Determine the purpose of the "Discussion" section.
- Discuss the importance of including generalizability and limitations of a study in the report.
- Determine the purpose of including recommendations in the study report.
- Discuss how the strength, quality, and consistency of evidence provided by the findings are related to a study's results, limitations, generalizability, and applicability to practice.

## KEY TERMS

confidence interval          generalizability          limitations          recommendations
findings

The ultimate goal of nursing research is to develop nursing knowledge that advances evidence-based nursing practice and quality patient care. From a clinical application perspective, analysis, interpretation, discussion, and generalizability of the results of a study become highly important pieces of the research study. After the analysis of the data, the researcher puts the final pieces of the jigsaw puzzle together to view the total picture with a critical eye. This process is analogous to evaluation, the last step in the nursing process. You may view these last sections as an easier step for the investigator, but it is here that a most critical and creative process comes to the forefront. In the final sections of the report, after the statistical procedures have been applied, the researcher relates the findings to the research question, hypotheses, theoretical framework, literature, methods, and analyses; reviews the study and its findings for any potential bias; and makes an evidence-informed decision about the application of the study's findings to practice.

The final sections of published research studies are generally titled "Results" and "Discussion," but other topics, such as conclusions, limitations of findings, recommendations, and implications for future research and nursing practice, may be separately addressed or subsumed within these sections. The presentation format of these areas is a function of the author's and the journal's stylistic considerations. The function of these final sections is to integrate all aspects of the research process, as well as to discuss, interpret, and identify the limitations, the threats related to bias, and generalizability relevant to the investigation, thereby furthering evidence-based practice. The process that both an investigator and you use to assess the results of a study is depicted in the Critical Thinking Decision Path.

The goal of this chapter is to introduce the purpose and content of the final sections of a research study where data are presented, interpreted, discussed, and generalized. An understanding of what an investigator presents in these sections will help you to critically analyze an investigator's findings.

## FINDINGS

The **findings** of a study are the results, conclusions, interpretations, recommendations, and implications for future research and nursing practice, which are addressed by separating the presentation into two major areas. These two areas are the results and the discussion of the results. The "Results" section focuses on the results or statistical findings of a study, and the "Discussion" section focuses on the remaining topics. For both sections, the rule applies—as it does to all other sections of a report—that the content must be presented clearly, concisely, and logically.

---

### EVIDENCE-BASED PRACTICE TIP

Evidence-based practice is an active process that requires you to consider how, and if, research findings are applicable to your patient population and practice setting.

---

### Results

The "Results" section of a research study is considered to be the data-bound section of the report and is where the quantitative data or numbers generated by the descriptive and inferential statistical tests are presented. Other headings that may be used for the results

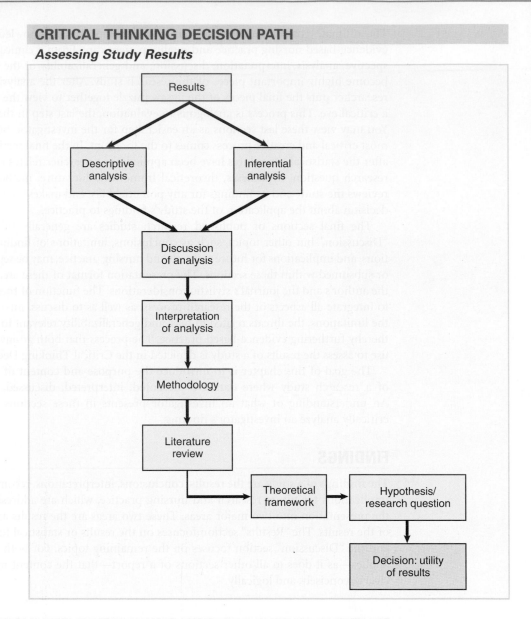

CRITICAL THINKING DECISION PATH

*Assessing Study Results*

Results

Descriptive analysis

Inferential analysis

Discussion of analysis

Interpretation of analysis

Methodology

Literature review

Theoretical framework

Hypothesis/ research question

Decision: utility of results

section are "Statistical Analyses," "Data Analysis," or "Analysis." The results of the data analysis set the stage for the interpretations or discussion and the limitations sections that follows the results. The "Results" section should reflect analysis of each research question and/or hypothesis tested. The information from each hypothesis or research question should be sequentially presented. The tests used to analyze the data should be identified. If the exact test that was used is not explicitly stated, the values obtained should be noted. The researcher does this by providing the numerical values of the statistics and stating the specific test value and probability level achieved (see Chapter 16). Examples of these statistical results can be found in Table 17-1. These numbers and their signs should not frighten you.

| TABLE 17-1 | **EXAMPLES OF REPORTED STATISTICAL RESULTS** |
|---|---|
| **STATISTICAL TEST** | **EXAMPLES OF REPORTED RESULTS** |
| Mean | $m = 118.28$ |
| Standard deviation | $SD = 62.5$ |
| Pearson correlation | $r = .49, P < .01$ |
| Analysis of variance | $F = 3.59, df = 2, 48, P < .05$ |
| $t$ test | $t = 2.65, P < .01$ |
| Chi-square | $\chi^2 = 2.52, df = 1, P < .05$ |

The numbers are important, but there is much more to the research process than the numbers. They are one piece of the whole. Chapter 16 conceptually presents the meanings of the numbers found in studies. Whether you only superficially understand statistics or have an in-depth knowledge of statistics, it should be obvious that the results are clearly stated, and the presence or lack of statistically significant results should be noted.

**HELPFUL HINT**

In the "Results" section of a research report, the descriptive statistics results are generally presented first; then the inferential results of each hypothesis or research question that was tested are presented.

At times the researchers will begin the "Results" or "Data Analysis" section by identifying the name of the statistical software program they used to analyze the data. This is not a statistical test but a computer program specifically designed to analyze a variety of statistical tests. For example, Alhusen and colleagues (2012; Appendix B) state that "data were analyzed using PASW Statistics 18, Release Version 18.00." PASW Statistics 18 was the statistical program, and the statistical tests used were Pearson correlations and point biserial coefficient and logistic regression (see Chapter 16).

The researcher will present the data for all of the hypotheses tested or research questions asked (e.g., whether the hypotheses were accepted, rejected, supported, or partially supported). If the data supported the hypotheses, you may be tempted to assume that the hypotheses were *proven;* however, this is not true. It only means that the hypotheses were supported and the results suggest that the relationships or differences tested, which were derived from the theoretical framework, were statistically significant and probably logical in that study's sample. You may think that if a researcher's results are not supported statistically or are only partially supported, the study is irrelevant or possibly should not have been published, but this also is not true. If the data are not supported, you should not expect the researcher to bury the work in a file. It is as important for you to review and understand unsupported studies as it is for the researcher. Information obtained from unsupported studies can often be as useful as data obtained from studies with supported hypotheses and research questions.

Studies that have findings that do not support one or more hypotheses or research questions can be used to suggest **limitations** (problems with the study's validity, bias, or study

---

**BOX 17-1    EXAMPLES OF RESULTS SECTION**

- "After controlling for average pain at baseline, no differences were found among the three groups in average pain intensity scores at the end of the study (p = .08)" (Thomas et al., 2012).
- "Resilience remained significant after controlling for couple effects (z = 2.9, p = .04), with resilience acting inversely on the relationship" (Melvin et al., 2012).

---

weaknesses) of particular aspects of a study's design and procedures. Findings from studies with data that do not support the hypotheses or research questions may suggest that current modes of practice or current theory in an area may not be supported by research evidence and therefore must be reexamined, researched further, and not be used at this time to support changes in practice. Data help generate new knowledge and evidence, as well as prevent knowledge stagnation. Generally, the results are interpreted in a separate section of the report. At times, you may find that the "Results" section contains the results and the researcher's interpretations, which are generally found in the "Discussion" section. Integrating the results with the discussion in a report is the author's or journal editor's decision. Both sections may be integrated when a study contains several segments that may be viewed as fairly separate subproblems of a major overall problem.

The investigator should also demonstrate objectivity in the presentation of the results. For example, the following quote by Alhusen and colleagues (2012; Appendix B) is an appropriate way to express results: "As hypothesized, there was a significant negative relationship between MFA and adverse neonatal outcomes supporting our first hypothesis." The investigators would be accused of lacking objectivity if they had stated the results in the following manner: "The results were not surprising as we found that the mean scores were significantly different in the comparison group, as we expected." Opinions or reactionary statements about the data in the "Results" section are therefore avoided. Box 17-1 provides examples of objectively stated results. As you appraise a study, you should consider the following points when reading the "Results" section:

- Investigators responded objectively to the results in the discussion of the findings.
- The investigator interpreted the evidence provided by the results, with a careful reflection on all aspects of the study that preceded the results.
- The data presented are summarized. Much data are generated, but only the critical summary numbers for each test are presented. Examples of summarized demographic data are the means and standard deviations of age, education, and income. Including all data is too cumbersome. The results can be viewed as a summary.
- The reduction of data is in both the written text and through the use of tables and figures. Tables and figures facilitate the presentation of large amounts of data.
- Results for the descriptive and inferential statistics for each hypothesis or research question are presented. No data should be omitted even if they are not significant.
- Any untoward events during the course of the study should be reported.

In their study, Alhusen and colleagues (2012) developed tables to present the results visually. Table 17-2 provides a portion of the descriptive results about the subjects' demographics. Table 17-3 provides the correlations among the study's variables. Tables allow researchers to provide a more visually thorough explanation and discussion of the results. If tables and figures are used, they must be concise. Although the article's text is the major mode of communicating the results, the tables and figures serve a

## TABLE 17-2 DEMOGRAPHIC CHARACTERISTICS OF PARTICIPANTS

| VARIABLE | N | % |
|---|---|---|
| **Race** | | |
| African American | 155 | 93 |
| White non-Hispanic | 9 | 5 |
| Other | 2 | 2 |
| **Education** | | |
| Less than high school | 110 | 67 |
| High school graduate/GED | 45 | 27 |
| Some college/trade school | 5 | 3 |
| College/trade school graduate | 6 | 3 |
| **Marital Status** | | |
| Single | 90 | 54 |
| Partnered/not married | 56 | 34 |
| Married | 17 | 10 |
| Other | 3 | 2 |
| **Employment Status** | | |
| Unemployed | 127 | 77 |
| Employed full-time | 25 | 15 |
| Employed part-time | 14 | 8 |

Alhusen, J.L., et al.: The influence of maternal-fetal attachment and health practices on neonatal outcomes in low-income urban women, *Res Nurs Health* 35:112-120, 2012.

## TABLE 17-3 CORRELATIONS AMONG THE MAIN STUDY VARIABLES (N = 166)

| VARIABLE | 1 | 2 | 3 | 4 |
|---|---|---|---|---|
| **1.** MFA | — | | | |
| **2.** Health Practices | .86* | — | | |
| **3.** Adverse Neonatal Outcome[a] | −.52* | −.63* | — | |
| **4.** Pregnancy Wantedness[b] | −.28* | −.34* | .19* | — |
| **5.** Income[c] | .25* | .31* | −.23* | −.18* |

MFA, maternal-fetal attachment.
[a]Referent group was no adverse outcome.
[b]Referent group was pregnancy was wanted.
[c]Referent group was income <$10,000/year.
*p < .05.
Alhusen, J.L., et al.: The influence of maternal-fetal attachment and health practices on neonatal outcomes in low-income urban women, *Res Nurs Health* 35:112-120, 2012.

supplementary but independent role. The role of tables and figures is to report results with some detail that the investigator does not explore in the text. This does not mean that tables and figures should not be mentioned in the text. The amount of detail that an author uses in the text to describe the specific tabled data varies according to the needs of the author. A good table is one that meets the following criteria:

- Supplements and economizes the text
- Has precise titles and headings
- Does not repeat the text

Tables are found in each of the studies in the Appendices. Each of these tables helps to economize and supplement the text clearly with precise data that help you to visualize the variables quickly and to assess the results.

---

### EVIDENCE-BASED PRACTICE TIP

As you reflect on the results of a study, think about how the results fit with previous research on the topic and the strength and quality of available evidence on which to base clinical practice decisions.

---

## Discussion

In the "Discussion" section, the investigator interprets and discusses the study's results. The researcher makes the data come alive and gives the numbers in quantitative studies or the concepts in qualitative studies meaning and interpretation. The "Discussion" section will contain the discussion of the findings, the study's **limitations**, and **recommendations** for practice and future research. At times these topics are separated as stand-alone sections of the research report, or they may be integrated under the title of "Discussion." You may ask where the investigator extracted the meaning that is applied in this section. If the researcher does the job properly, you will find a return to the beginning of the study. The researcher returns to the earlier points in the study where a purpose, objective, and research question and/or a hypothesis was identified and independent and dependent variables were related on the basis of a theoretical framework and literature review (see Chapters 3 and 4). It is in this section that the researcher discusses

- Both the supported and nonsupported data
- The limitations or weaknesses (threats to internal or external validity) of a study in light of the design, sample, instruments, data collection procedures, and intervention fidelity
- How the theoretical framework was supported or not supported
- How the data may suggest additional or previously unrealized findings
- The strength and quality of the evidence provided by the study and its findings interpreted in relation to its applicability to practice and future research

Even if the data are supported, it is not the final word. Statistical significance is not the endpoint of a researcher's thinking; statistically significant but low $p$ values may not be

---

### HELPFUL HINT

A well-written "Results" section is systematic, logical, concise, and drawn from all of the analyzed data. All that is written in the "Results" section should be geared to letting the data reflect the testing of the research questions and hypotheses. The length of this section depends on the scope and breadth of the analysis.

indicative of research breakthroughs. It is important to think beyond statistical significance to clinical significance. This means that statistical significance in a study does not always indicate that the results of a study are clinically significant. As the body of nursing research grows, so does the profession's ability to critically analyze beyond the test of significance and assess a research study's applicability to practice. Chapters 19 through 21 review methods used to analyze the usefulness and applicability of research findings. Within nursing and health care literature, discussion of clinical significance, evidence-based practice and quality improvement has become a focal point (Gold & Taylor, 2007; Titler, 2012). As indicated throughout this text, many important pieces in the research puzzle must fit together for a study to be evaluated as a well-done study. The evidence generated by the findings of a study is appraised in order to validate current practice or support the need for a change in practice. Results of nonsupported hypotheses or research questions do not require the investigator to go on a fault-finding tour of each piece of the study—this can become an overdone process. All research studies have weaknesses. The final discussion is an attempt to identify the strengths as well as the weaknesses or bias of the study.

Therefore, researchers and appraisers should accept statistical significance with prudence. Statistically significant findings are not the sole means of establishing a study's merit. Remember that accepting statistical significance means accepting that the sample mean is the same as the population mean. Statistical significance is a measure of assessment that if true does not automatically give merit to a study, and if untrue does not necessarily negate the value of a study (see Chapter 12). Another method to assess the merit of a study and determine whether the findings from one study can be generalized is to calculate a **confidence interval**. A confidence interval quantifies the uncertainty of a statistic or the probable value range within which a population parameter is expected to lie (see Chapter 19). The process used to calculate a confidence interval is beyond the scope of this text, but references are provided for further explanation (Altman, 2005; Altman, Machin et al., 2005; Kline, 2004; Wright, 1997). Other aspects, such as the sample, instruments, data collection methods, and fidelity, must also be considered.

Whether the results are or are not statistically supported, in the "Discussion" section, the researcher returns to the conceptual/theoretical framework and analyzes each step of the research process to accomplish a discussion of the following issues:

- Suggest what the possible or actual problems were in the study.
- Whether findings are supported or not supported, the researcher is obliged to review the study's processes.
- Was the theoretical thinking correct? (see Chapters 3 and 4)
- Was the design chosen correct? (see Chapters 9 and 10)
- Sampling methods (see Chapter 12): Was the sample size adequate? Were the inclusion and exclusion criteria delineated well?
- Did any bias arise during the conduct of the study; that is, threats to internal and external validity? (see Chapter 8)
- Was data collection consistent and did it exhibit fidelity? (see Chapter 14)
- Instruments: Were they sensitive to what was being testing? Were they reliable and valid? (see Chapters 14 and 15)
- Discuss the analysis choices. (see Chapter 16)

Whether the results are or are not supported, the investigator attempts to go on a fact-finding tour rather than a fault-finding one. The purpose of the "Discussion" section, then, is not to show humility or one's technical competence but rather to enable you to judge the

validity of the interpretations drawn from the data and the general worth of the study. It is in the "Discussion" section of the report that the researcher ties together all the loose ends of the study and returns to the beginning to assess if the findings support, extend, or counter the theoretical framework of the study. It is from this point that you can begin to think about clinical relevance, the need for replication, or the germination of an idea for further research. The researcher also includes generalizability and recommendations for future research, as well as a summary or a conclusion.

Generalizations (generalizability) are inferences that the data are representative of similar phenomena in a population beyond the study's sample. Reviewers of research findings are cautioned not to generalize beyond the population on which a study is based. Rarely, if ever, can one study be a recommendation for action. Beware of research studies that may overgeneralize. Generalizations that draw conclusions and make inferences for a specific group within a particular situation and at a particular time are appropriate. An example of such a limitation is drawn from the study conducted by Alhusen and colleagues (2012; Appendix B). The researchers appropriately noted the following:

> "This study has two important limitations. First, MFA and health practices were collected via self-report measures in a cross-sectional manner making inference about their causal relationships impossible. Tobacco use and substance use, factors known to contribute to poor neonatal outcomes, may have been underreported. Second, these results are based on a convenience sample and therefore cannot be generalized beyond this group of women."

This type of statement is important for reviewers of research. It helps to guide thinking in terms of a study's clinical relevance and also suggests areas for further research. One study does not provide all of the answers, nor should it. In fact, the risk versus the benefit of the potential change in practice must be considered in terms of the strength and quality of the evidence (see Chapter 19). The greater the risk involved in making a change in practice, the stronger the evidence needs to be to justify the merit of implementing a practice change. The final steps of evaluation are critical links to the refinement of practice and the generation of future research. Evaluation of research, like evaluation of the nursing process, is not the last link in the chain but a connection between the strength of the evidence that may serve to improve nursing care and inform clinical decision making and support an evidence-based practice.

---

**HELPFUL HINT**

It has been said that a good study is one that raises more questions than it answers. So you should not view an investigator's review of limitations, generalizations, and implications of the findings for practice as lack of research skills, but as the beginning of the next step in the research process.

---

The final area that the investigator integrates into the "Discussion" is the recommendations. The recommendations are the investigator's suggestions for the study's application to practice, theory, and further research. This requires the investigator to reflect on the following questions:

- What contribution to clinical practice does this study make?
- What are the strength, quality, and consistency of the evidence provided by the findings?
- Does the evidence provided in the findings validate current practice or support the need for change in practice?

BOX 17-2   EXAMPLES OF RESEARCH RECOMMENDATIONS
AND PRACTICE IMPLICATIONS

**Research Recommendations**

- "Future studies should compare a coaching intervention with different types of controls to ensure that the specific effect of the intervention can be better distinguished from those of other controlled factors, such as time, attention, motivation, expectations, and experience" (Thomas et al., 2012).
- "Future researchers should test culturally relevant interventions aimed at improving the maternal-fetal relationship" (Alhusen et al., 2012).
- "Investigation of other post-combat problems, such as depression and traumatic brain injury, and their potential for affecting the couple relationship would be a logical next step in the dyadic exploration of combat veteran couples" (Melvin et al., 2012).

**Practice Implications**

- "Using motivational interviewing, APNs and patients can jointly develop an appropriate plan of care to decrease those symptoms. Motivational interviewing is a skill that can be mastered by an APN with sufficient training" (Thomas et al., 2012).
- "This study provides an important contribution to understanding the influence of MFA on health practices during pregnancy, and ultimately neonatal outcomes, in a sample of urban, low-income, predominantly African-American women" (Alhusen et al., 2012).
- "Investigation of other post-combat problems, such as depression and other traumatic brain injury, and their potential for affecting the couple relationship would be a logical step. In the meantime, nurses can best serve military and civilian couples by asking both military and civilian couples about combat and other trauma exposures" (Melvin et al., 2012).

Box 17-2 provides examples of recommendations for future research and implications for nursing practice. This evaluation places the study into the realm of what is known and what needs to be known before being used. Nursing knowledge and evidence-based practice have grown tremendously over the last century through the efforts of many nurse researchers and scholars.

# APPRAISING THE EVIDENCE
## RESEARCH FINDINGS

The "Results" and the "Discussion of the Results" sections are the researcher's opportunity to examine the logic of the hypothesis(es) or research question(s) posed, the theoretical framework, the methods, and the analysis (see the Critiquing Criteria box). This final section requires as much logic, conciseness, and specificity as employed in the preceding steps of the research process. You should be able to identify statements of the type of analysis that was used and whether the data statistically supported the hypothesis(es) or research question(s). These statements should be straightforward and should not reflect bias (see Tables 17-2 and 17-3). Auxiliary data or serendipitous findings also may be presented. If such auxiliary findings are presented, they should be as dispassionately presented as were the hypothesis and research question data.

The statistical test(s) used should also be noted. The numerical value of the obtained data should also be presented (see Tables 17-1, 17-2, and 17-3). The presentation of the

## CRITIQUING CRITERIA
### *Research Findings*

1. Are the results of each of the hypotheses presented?
2. Is the information regarding the results concisely and sequentially presented?
3. Are the tests that were used to analyze the data presented?
4. Are the results presented objectively?
5. If tables or figures are used, do they meet the following standards?
   a. They supplement and economize the text.
   b. They have precise titles and headings.
   c. They are not repetitious of the text.
6. Are the results interpreted in light of the hypotheses and theoretical framework and all of the other steps that preceded the results?
7. If the data are supported, does the investigator provide a discussion of how the theoretical framework was supported?
8. How does the investigator attempt to identify the study's weaknesses; that is, threats to internal and external validity, and strengths, as well as suggest possible solutions for the research area?
9. Does the researcher discuss the study's clinical relevance?
10. Are any generalizations made, and if so, are they within the scope of the findings or beyond the findings?
11. Are any recommendations for future research stated or implied?
12. What is the study's strength of evidence?

tests, the numerical values found, and the statements of support or nonsupport should be clear, concise, and systematically reported. For illustrative purposes that facilitate readability, the researchers should present extensive findings in tables. If the findings were not supported, you should—as the researcher did—attempt to identify, without finding fault, possible methodological problems (e.g., sample too small to detect a treatment effect).

From a consumer perspective, the "Discussion" section at the end of a research report is very important for determining potential application to practice. The "Discussion" section should interpret the study's data for future research and implications for practice, including its strength, quality, gaps, limitations, and conclusions of the study. Statements reflecting the underlying theory are necessary, whether or not the hypotheses were supported. Included in this discussion are the limitations for practice. This discussion should reflect each step of the research process and potential threats to internal validity or bias and external validity or generalizability.

This last presentation can help you begin to rethink clinical practice, provoke discussion in clinical settings (see Chapters 19 and 20), and find similar studies that may support or refute the phenomena being studied to more fully understand the problem.

One study alone does not lead to a practice change. Evidence-based practice and quality improvement requires you to critically read and understand each study; that is, the quality of the study, the strength of the evidence generated by the findings and its consistency with other studies in the area, and the number of studies that were conducted in the area. This assessment along with the active use of clinical judgment and patient preference leads to evidence-based practice.

## KEY POINTS

- The analysis of the findings is the final step of a research study. It is in this section that the consumer will find the results printed in a straightforward manner.
- All results should be reported whether or not they support the hypothesis. Tables and figures may be used to illustrate and condense data for presentation.
- Once the results are reported, the researcher interprets the results. In this presentation, usually titled "Discussion," the consumer should be able to identify the key topics being discussed. The key topics, which include an interpretation of the results, are the limitations, generalizations, implications, and recommendations for future research.
- The researcher draws together the theoretical framework and makes interpretations based on the findings and theory in the section on the interpretation of the results. Both statistically supported and unsupported results should be interpreted. If the results are not supported, the researcher should discuss the results, reflecting on the theory as well as possible problems with the methods, procedures, design, and analysis.
- The researcher should present the limitations or weaknesses of the study. This presentation is important because it affects the study's generalizability. The generalizations or inferences about similar findings in other samples also are presented in light of the findings.
- Be alert for sweeping claims or overgeneralizations that a researcher may state. An overextension of the data can alert the consumer to possible researcher bias.
- The recommendations provide the consumer with suggestions regarding the study's application to practice, theory, and future research. These recommendations furnish the critiquer with a final perspective from the researcher on the utility of the investigation.
- The strength, quality, and consistency of the evidence provided by the findings are related to the study's limitations, generalizability, and applicability to practice.

## CRITICAL THINKING CHALLENGES

- Do you agree or disagree with the statement that "a good study is one that raises more questions than it answers"? Support your perspective with examples.
- As the number of resources such as the Cochrane Library, meta-analysis, systematic reviews, and evidence-based reports in journals grow, why is it necessary to be able to critically read and appraise the studies within the reports yourself? Justify your answer.
- Defend or refute this statement. "All results should be reported and interpreted whether or not they support the hypothesis." If all findings are not reported, would this affect the applicability to the patient population and practice setting?
- How does a clear understanding of a study's discussion of the findings and implications for practice help you to rethink your practice?

## REFERENCES

Alhusen, J. L., Gross, D., Hayatt, M. J., et al. (2012). The influence of maternal-fetal attachment and health practices on neonatal outcomes in low-income women. *Research in Nursing & Health, 35,* 112–120.

Altman, D. G. (2005).Why we need confidence intervals. *World Journal of Surgery, 29,* 554–556.

Altman, D. G., Machin, D., Bryant, T., & Gardener, S. (2005). *Statistics with confidence: confidence intervals and statistical guidelines* (2nd ed.). London, UK: BMJ Books.

Gold, M., & Taylor, E. F. (2007). Moving research into practice: lessons from the US Agency for Healthcare Research and Quality's IDSRN program. *Implementation Science, 2*, 9.

Kline, R. B. (2004). *Beyond significance testing: reforming data analysis methods in behavioral research* (1st ed.). Washington, DC: American Psychological Association.

Melvin, K. C., Gross, D., Hayat, M. J., et al. (2012). Couple functioning and post-traumatice stress symptoms in US army couples: the role of resilience. *Research in Nursing & Health, 35,* 164–177.

Thomas, M. L., Elliott, J. E., Rao, S. M., et al. (2012). A randomized clinical trial of education or motivational-interviewing–based coaching compared to usual care to improve cancer pain management. *Oncology Nursing Forum, 39*(1), 39–49.

Titler, M. G. (2012). Nursing science and evidence-based practice. *Western Journal of Nursing Research, 33*(3), 291–295.

Wright, D. B. (1997). *Understanding statistics: an introduction for the social sciences.* London, UK: Sage.

# ꗋVOLVE WEBSITE

*Go to Evolve at http://evolve.elsevier.com/LoBiondo/ for review questions, critiquing exercises, and additional research articles for practice in reviewing and critiquing.*

# CHAPTER 18

# Appraising Quantitative Research

*Nancy E. Kline*

## ⊖volve WEBSITE

*Go to Evolve at http://evolve.elsevier.com/LoBiondo/ for additional research articles for review questions, critiquing exercises, and practice in reviewing and critiquing.*

## LEARNING OUTCOMES

*After reading this chapter, you should be able to do the following:*

- Identify the purpose of the critical appraisal process.
- Describe the criteria for each step of the critical appraisal process.
- Describe the strengths and weaknesses of a research report.

- Assess the strength, quality, and consistency of evidence provided by a quantitative research report.
- Discuss applicability of the findings of a research report for evidence-based nursing practice.
- Conduct a critique of a research report.

Critical appraisal and interpretation of the findings of a research article is an acquired skill that is important for nurses to master as they learn to determine the usefulness of the published literature. As we strive to make recommendations to change or support nursing practice, it is important for you to be able to assess the strengths and weaknesses of a research report.

Critical appraisal is an evaluation of the strength and quality, as well as the weaknesses, of the study, not a "criticism" of the work, per se. It provides a structure for reviewing the sections of a research study. This chapter presents critiques of two quantitative studies, a randomized controlled trial (RCT) and a descriptive study, according to the critiquing criteria shown in Table 18-1. These studies provide Level II and Level IV evidence.

As reinforced throughout each chapter of this book, it is not only important to conduct and read research, but to actively use research findings to inform evidence-based practice. As nurse researchers increase the depth (quality) and breadth (quantity) of studies, the data to support evidence-informed decision making regarding applicability of clinical interventions that contribute to quality outcomes are more readily available. This chapter presents

| TABLE 18-1 | SUMMARY OF MAJOR CONTENT SECTIONS OF A RESEARCH REPORT AND RELATED CRITICAL APPRAISAL GUIDELINES |
|---|---|
| **SECTION** | **CRITICAL APPRAISAL QUESTIONS TO GUIDE EVALUATION** |
| Background and Significance (see Chapters 2 and 3) | Does the background and significance section make it clear why the proposed study is being done? |
| Research Question and Hypothesis (see Chapter 2) | 1. What research question(s) or hypothesis(es) are stated and are they appropriate to express a relationship between an independent and a dependent variable? <br> 2. Has the research question(s) or hypothesis(es) been placed in the context of an appropriate theoretical framework? <br> 3. Has the research question(s) or hypothesis(es) been substantiated by adequate experiential and scientific background material? <br> 4. Has the purpose, aim(s), or goal(s) of the study been substantiated? <br> 5. Is each research question or hypothesis specific to one relationship so that each can be either supported or not supported? <br> 6. Given the level of evidence suggested by the research question, hypothesis, and design, what is the potential applicability to practice? |
| Review of the Literature (see Chapters 3 and 4) | 1. Does the search strategy include an appropriate and adequate number of databases and other resources to identify key published and unpublished research and theoretical resources? <br> 2. Is there an appropriate theoretical/conceptual framework that guides development of the research study? <br> 3. Are both primary source theoretical and research literature used? <br> 4. What gaps or inconsistencies in knowledge or research does the literature uncover so that it builds on earlier studies? <br> 5. Does the review include a summary/critique of each study that includes the strengths and weakness or limitations of the study? <br> 6. Is the literature review presented in an organized format that flows logically? <br> 7. Is there a synthesis summary that presents the overall strengths and weaknesses and arrives at a logical conclusion that generates hypotheses or research questions? |
| **Methods** | |
| Internal and External Validity (see Chapter 8) | 1. What are the controls for the threats to internal validity? Are they appropriate? <br> 2. What are the controls for the threats to external validity? Are they appropriate? <br> 3. What are the sources of bias and are they dealt with appropriately? <br> 4. How do the threats to internal and external validity contribute to the strength and quality of evidence? <br> 5. Was the fidelity of the intervention maintained, and if so, how? |
| Research Design (see Chapters 9 and 10) | 1. What type of design is used in the study? <br> 2. Is the rationale for the design appropriate? <br> 3. Does the design used seem to flow from the proposed research question(s) or hypothesis(es), theoretical framework, and literature review? <br> 4. What types of controls are provided by the design that increase or decrease bias? |
| Sampling (see Chapter 12) | 1. What type of sampling strategy is used? Is it appropriate for the design? <br> 2. How was the sample selected? Was the strategy used appropriate for the design? <br> 3. Does the sample reflect the population as identified in the research question or hypothesis? <br> 4. Is the sample size appropriate? How is it substantiated? Was a power analysis necessary? <br> 5. To what population may the findings be generalized? |
| Legal-Ethical Issues (see Chapter 13) | 1. How have the rights of subjects been protected? <br> 2. What indications are given that institutional review board approval has been obtained? <br> 3. What evidence is given that informed consent of the subjects has been obtained? |

| TABLE 18-1 | SUMMARY OF MAJOR CONTENT SECTIONS OF A RESEARCH REPORT AND RELATED CRITICAL APPRAISAL GUIDELINES—cont'd |
|---|---|
| **SECTION** | **CRITICAL APPRAISAL QUESTIONS TO GUIDE EVALUATION** |
| Data Collection Methods and Procedures (see Chapter 14) | 1. Physiological measurement: <br>    a. Is a rationale given for why a particular instrument or method was selected? If so, what is it? <br>    b. What provision is made for maintaining accuracy of the instrument and its use, if any? <br> 2. Observation: <br>    a. Who did the observing? <br>    b. How were the observers trained and supervised to minimize bias? <br>    c. Was there an observation guide? <br>    d. Was interrater reliability calculated? <br>    e. Is there any reason to believe that the presence of observers affected the behavior of the subjects? <br> 3. Interviews: <br>    a. Who were the interviewers? How were they trained and supervised to minimize bias? <br>    b. Is there any evidence of interview bias, and if so, what is it? How does it affect the strength and quality of evidence? <br> 4. Instruments: <br>    a. What is the type and/or format of the instruments (e.g., Likert scale)? <br>    b. Are the operational definitions provided by the instruments consistent with the conceptual definition(s)? <br>    c. Is the format appropriate for use with this population? <br>    d. What type of bias is possible with self-report instruments? <br> 5. Available data and records: <br>    a. Are the records or data sets used appropriate for the research question(s) or hypothesis(es)? <br>    b. What sources of bias are possible with use of records or existing data sets? <br> 6. Overall, how was intervention fidelity maintained? |
| Reliability and Validity (see Chapter 15) | 1. Was an appropriate method used to test the reliability of the instrument(s)? <br> 2. Was the reliability of the instrument(s) adequate? <br> 3. Was the appropriate method(s) used to test the validity of the instrument(s)? <br> 4. Have the strengths and weaknesses related to reliability and validity of each instrument been presented? <br> 5. What kinds of threats to internal and external validity are presented as weaknesses in reliability and/or validity? <br> 6. How do the reliability and/or validity affect the strength and quality of evidence provided by the study findings? |
| Data Analysis (see Chapter 16) | 1. Were the descriptive or inferential statistics appropriate to the level of measurement for each variable? <br> 2. Are the inferential statistics appropriate for the type of design, research question(s) or hypothesis(es)? <br> 3. If tables or figures are used, do they meet the following standards? <br>    a. They supplement and economize the text. <br>    b. They have precise titles and headings. <br>    c. They do not repeat the text. <br> 4. Did testing of the research question(s) or hypothesis(es) clearly support or not support each research question or hypothesis? |

*Continued*

| TABLE 18-1 | SUMMARY OF MAJOR CONTENT SECTIONS OF A RESEARCH REPORT AND RELATED CRITICAL APPRAISAL GUIDELINES—cont'd |
|---|---|
| **SECTION** | **CRITICAL APPRAISAL QUESTIONS TO GUIDE EVALUATION** |
| Conclusions, Implications, and Recommendations (see Chapter 17) | 1. Are the results of each research question or hypothesis presented objectively? <br> 2. Is the information regarding the results concisely and sequentially presented? <br> 3. If the data are supportive of the hypothesis or research question, does the investigator provide a discussion of how the theoretical framework was supported? <br> 4. How does the investigator attempt to identify the study's weaknesses and limitations (e.g., threats to internal and external validity) and strengths and suggest possible research solutions in future studies? <br> 5. Does the researcher discuss the study's relevance to clinical practice? <br> 6. Are any generalizations made and, if so, are they made within the scope of the findings? <br> 7. Are any recommendations for future research stated or implied? |
| Applicability to Nursing Practice (see Chapter 17) | 1. What are the risks/benefits involved for patients if the findings are applied in practice? <br> 2. What are the costs/benefits of applying the findings of the study? <br> 3. Do the strengths of the study outweigh the weaknesses? <br> 4. What is the strength, quality, and consistency of evidence provided by the study findings? <br> 5. Are the study findings applicable in terms of feasibility? <br> 6. Are the study findings generalizable? <br> 7. Would it be possible to replicate this study in another clinical setting? |

critiques of two studies, each of which tests research questions reflecting different quantitative designs. Criteria used to help you in judging the relative merit of a research study are found in previous chapters. An abbreviated set of critical appraisal questions presented in Table 18-1 summarize detailed criteria found at the end of each chapter and are used as a critical appraisal guide for the two sample research critiques in this chapter. These critiques are included to illustrate the critical appraisal process and the potential applicability of research findings to clinical practice, thereby enhancing the evidence base for nursing practice.

For clarification, you are encouraged to return to earlier chapters for the detailed presentation of each step of the research process, key terms, and the critiquing criteria associated with each step of the research process. The criteria and examples in this chapter apply to quantitative studies using experimental and nonexperimental designs that provided Levels II and IV evidence.

## STYLISTIC CONSIDERATIONS

When you are reading research, it is important to consider the type of journal in which the article is published. Some journals publish articles regarding the conduct, methodology, or results of research studies (e.g., *Nursing Research*). Other journals (e.g., *Journal of Obstetric, Gynecologic, and Neonatal Research*) publish clinical, educational, and research articles. The author decides where to submit the manuscript based on the focus of the particular journal. Guidelines for publication, also known as "Information for Authors," are journal-specific and provide information regarding style, citations, and formatting. Typically, research articles include the following:

- Abstract
- Introduction

- Background and significance
- Literature review (sometimes includes theoretical framework)
- Methodology
- Results
- Discussion
- Conclusions

If the article is *scientifically rigorous,* there is a decreased likelihood that the results occurred by chance alone, or owing to extraneous conditions. Critical appraisal is the process of identifying the methodological flaws or omissions that may lead the reader to question the outcome(s) of the study or, conversely, to document the strengths and limitations and objectively judging that the work is sound and provides consistent, quality evidence that supports applicability to practice. Such judgments are the hallmark of promoting a sound evidence base for quality nursing practice.

# CRITIQUE OF A QUANTITATIVE RESEARCH STUDY

## THE RESEARCH STUDY

The study "The Effects of Psychoeducation and Telephone Counseling on the Adjustment of Women with Early-Stage Breast Cancer," by Deborah Witt Sherman and colleagues, published in *Applied Nursing Research,* is critiqued. The article is presented in its entirety and followed by the critique.

### The Effects of Psychoeducation and Telephone Counseling on the Adjustment of Women with Early-Stage Breast Cancer

*Deborah Witt Sherman, Judith Haber, Carol Noll Hoskins, Wendy C. Budin, Greg Maislin, Shilpa Shukla, Frances Cartwright-Alcarese, Christina Beyer McSherry, Renee Feurbach, Mildred Ortu Kowalski, Mary Rosedale, Annie Roth*

#### ABSTRACT

**Background:** Throughout the illness trajectory, women with breast cancer experience issues that are related to physical, emotional, and social adjustment. Despite a general consensus that state-of-the-art treatment for breast cancer should include educational and counseling interventions to reduce illness or treatment-related symptoms, there are few prospective, theoretically based, phase-specific, randomized controlled trials that have evaluated the effectiveness of such interventions in promoting adjustment.

**Purpose:** The aim of this study is to examine the physical, emotional, and social adjustment of women with early-stage breast cancer who received psychoeducation by videotapes, telephone counseling, or psychoeducation plus telephone counseling as interventions that address the specific needs of women during the diagnostic, postsurgery, adjuvant therapy, and ongoing recovery phases of breast cancer.

**Design:** Primary data from a randomized controlled clinical trial.

**Setting:** Three major medical centers and one community hospital in New York City.

**Methods:** A total of 249 patients were randomly assigned to either the control group receiving usual care or to one of the three intervention groups. The interventions were administered at the diagnostic, postsurgery, adjuvant therapy, and ongoing recovery phases. Analyses were based on a mixed model analysis of variance.

**Main Research Variables and Measurement:** Physical adjustment was measured by the side effects incidence and severity subscales of the Breast Cancer Treatment Response Inventory (BCTRI) and the overall health status score of the Self-Rated Health Subscale of the Multilevel Assessment Instrument. Emotional adjustment was measured using the psychological well-being subscale of the Profile of Adaptation to Life Clinical Scale and the side effect distress subscale of BCTRI. Social adjustment was measured by the domestic, vocational, and social environments subscales of the Psychosocial Adjustment to Illness Scale.

**Findings:** Patients in all groups showed improvement over time in overall health, psychological well-being, and social adjustment. There were no significant group differences in physical adjustment, as measured by side effect incidence, severity, or overall health. There was poorer emotional adjustment over time in the usual care (control) group as compared to the intervention groups on the measure of side effect distress. For the telephone counseling group, there was a marked decline in psychological well-being from the adjuvant therapy phase through the ongoing recovery phase. There were no significant group differences in the dimensions of social adjustment.

**Conclusion:** The longitudinal design of this study has captured the dynamic process of adjustment to breast cancer, which in some aspects and at various phases has been different for the control and intervention groups. Although patients who received the study interventions improved in adjustment, the overall conclusion regarding physical, emotional, and social adjustment is that usual care, which was the standard of care for women in both the usual care (control) and intervention groups, supported their adjustment to breast cancer, with or without additional interventions.

**Implications for Nursing:** The results are important to evidence-based practice and the determination of the efficacy and cost-effectiveness of interventions in improving patient outcomes. There is a need to further examine adjustment issues that continue during the ongoing recovery phase.

**Key Points:** Psychoeducation by videotapes and telephone counseling decreased side effect distress and side effect severity and increased psychological well-being during the adjuvant therapy phase. All patients in the control and intervention groups improved in adjustment. Adjustment issues are still present in the ongoing recovery phase.

## 1. Introduction

The American Cancer Society (2007) estimated that 178,480 women in the United States will be diagnosed with invasive breast cancer and 62,032 women would be diagnosed with noninvasive breast cancer. Early-stage breast cancer includes (a) tumors up to 2 cm that have spread to axillary lymph nodes; (b) tumors 2 and 5 cm that have or have not spread to axillary lymph nodes; or (c) tumors greater than 5 cm but have not spread outside the breast (National Cancer Institute, 2007). Although early diagnosis and successful medical interventions have improved longterm prognosis, women often experience uncertainty about their future (ACS, 2007). Because adjustment to breast cancer does not end with the completion of medical treatment, it is important to examine physical, psychological, and social adjustment as an ongoing process (Iscoe, Williams, Szalai, & Osoba, 1991; Varricchio, 1990).

Based on an earlier descriptive study (Hoskins et al., 1996a), four phases of the breast cancer experience were identified: diagnosis (biopsy results obtained), postsurgery (2 days following definitive surgery), adjuvant therapy (postdiscussion with oncologist of the need for chemotherapy or radiation therapy), and ongoing recovery (2 weeks following completion of chemotherapy or radiation or 6 months after surgery if no chemotherapy or radiation was received). At each of these four phases, health-relevant information and social support were key coping strategies in promoting physical, social, and emotional adjustment. Based on findings and an extensive review of the literature, Hoskins et al. (2001) developed and pilot tested a series of four phase-specific, 30-minute videotapes to provide a standardized evidence-based psychoeducational intervention, as well as a phase-specific telephone counseling intervention that focused on physical, emotional, and social needs of women and their partners.

A randomized clinical trial was conducted to examine the physical, emotional, and social adjustment of women with early-stage breast cancer who received the standardized psychoeducation by video, telephone counseling, or psychoeducation by video with telephone counseling, as interventions. The purpose of the interventions was to address the specific needs of women during the diagnostic, postsurgery, adjuvant therapy, and recovery phases of breast cancer. The primary hypotheses related to patient's adjustment were the following: (a) physical adjustment would be greater in each of the study intervention groups as compared to the control group who received usual care; (b) emotional adjustment would be greater in each of the study intervention groups as compared to the control group who received usual care; and (c) social adjustment would be greater in each of the study intervention groups as compared to the control group who received usual care. A previously published article by the research team (Budin, Cartwright, & Hoskins, 2008; Budin, Hoskin, et al., 2008) provides an overview of a randomized trial with a primary focus on the methodology and general results of the trial. The purpose of this article is to focus, specifically, on the primary data related to the adjustment of patients with early-stage breast cancer, with an emphasis on the implications for evidence-based practice and future research.

## 2. Background Literature

Over the last 30 years, there has been a proliferation of studies regarding the impact of breast cancer on a woman's well-being. Loveys and Klaich (1991) reported that as a chronic disease, the acceptance of a breast cancer diagnosis, treatment decisions, emotional distress related to physical change and loss, alterations in lifestyle, uncertainty, and need for information and support are ongoing issues. In general, it was agreed that the broad domains of adjustment to breast cancer may be conceptualized as psychological (Walker, Nail, & Croyle, 1999), physical (Cohen, Kahn, & Steeves, 1998; Wyatt & Friedman, 1998), and social (Northhouse, Dorris, & Charron-Moore, 1995). Adjustment has also been commonly conceptualized as role performance (Derogatis, 1983), self-esteem and body image (Kemeny, Wellisch, & Schain, 1988), psychosexual and psychosocial adjustment (Capone, Good, Westie, & Jacobson, 1980; Hasida, Gilbar, & Lev, 2001; Wimberly, Carver, Laurenceau, Harris, & Antonia, 2005), emotional symptoms (Hoskins et al., 1996a; Pasacreta, 1997), symptom experiences and distress (Boehmke & Dickerson, 2005), and quality of life (Badger et al., 2005; Sammarco, 2001).

Based on their research, Sklalla, Bakitas, Furstenberg, Ahles, and Henderson (2004) identified the informational needs of patients and their spouses to be the treatment process, specifically information regarding chemotherapy or radiation therapy, specific side effects, and the implication for their lives. Ahles et al. (2006) studied patients ($n = 644$) who were randomized to a control group receiving usual care and an intervention group, which received information regarding problem solving and pain management skills by telephone intervention. Patients in the intervention group reported less pain, improved physical and emotional vitality, and improved functional status when compared with patients receiving usual care at 6 months.

Several randomized controlled trials of women with breast cancer have supported the use of psychoeducation and telephone counseling in promoting adjustment. Based on the Roy Adaptation Model, Samarel, Tulman, and Fawcett (2002) randomized 125 women with early-stage breast cancer to either the intervention group, which received 13 months of combined individual telephone and in-person group support and education, or to Control Group 1, which received 13 months of telephone-only individual support and education, or Control Group 2, which received one-time mailed educational material. The results indicated that the intervention group and Control Group 1 reported less mood disturbance, loneliness, and higher quality relationships than Control Group 2. There were no group differences in cancer-related worry or well-being. The results suggest that telephone support may provide an alternative to support groups.

Rawl et al. (2002), based on a randomized controlled trial of 109 patients diagnosed with breast, lung, and colon cancer receiving chemotherapy, reported that those who received four telephone interventions and five in-person clinic visits had significantly less depression and improved quality of life midway through chemotherapy and 1 month post-chemotherapy. It was concluded that this nurse-directed intervention improved psychological symptoms for patients with cancer.

Badger et al. (2005) examined the effectiveness of telephone counseling compared to usual care on symptom management and quality of life for women ($n = 48$) with breast cancer. Findings indicated that women in the intervention group had decreased depression, fatigue, and stress over time and increases in positive affect. Ahles et al. (2006) randomized patients ($n = 644$) with pain and psychological problems to a control group receiving usual care and an intervention group, which received information regarding problem solving and pain management skills by telephone intervention. Patients in the intervention group reported improved pain, physical and emotional vitality, and functional status verses when compared with patients receiving usual care at 6 months.

Samdgrem and McCaul (2006) also tested interventions involving health education and emotional expression provided through a telephone intervention for women ($n = 218$) with Stage 1, 2, and 3 breast cancer. Oncology advanced practice nurses conducted the telephone intervention, with the results indicating that patients receiving telephone therapy had less perceived stress and better knowledge; however, there was no significant difference in quality of life or mood. The results indicate that telephone therapy is a viable intervention that promoted the retention of patients, but it was concluded that both the control and intervention groups showed improvement in quality of life and mood over time. Badger, Segrin, Dorros, Meek and Lopez (2007) conducted a randomized control trial of 96 women and their partners who were randomly assigned to either 6-week programs of telephone interpersonal counseling, self-managed exercise, or attention control. The results indicated that depression scores decreased over time for all groups and that women in the telephone counseling and exercise groups had lower anxiety scores.

### 3. Theoretical Framework

The theoretical framework that guided the development of the study's interventions, mediating/moderating, and outcome variables included the Stress and Coping Model (Lazarus & Folkman, 1984), the Crisis Intervention Model (Morely, Messick, & Aguilera, 1967), findings of the preliminary descriptive study (Hoskins et al., 1996a, 1996b), and the pilot study to test the feasibility of a randomized controlled trial (Hoskins et al., 2001; refer to Fig. 1). According to the framework, cancer can be appraised as harm, loss, threat, challenge, or some combination of these (Lazarus & Folkman, 1984). As such, stress and its appraisal are assumed to be inherent dimensions of the breast cancer experience (Folkman & Greer, 2000). According to Lazarus and Folkman's Stress and Coping Model (1984), the concept of adaptation refers to an individual's adjustment in relation to their appraisal of

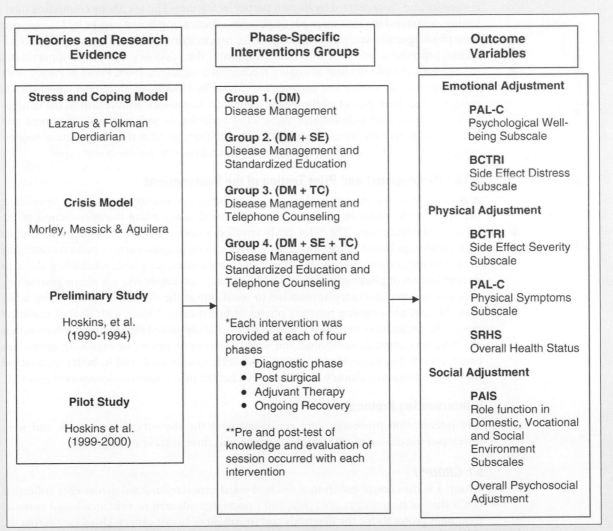

**FIGURE 1** Phase-specific breast cancer intervention study—theoretical framework.

support resources and coping skills. Lazarus and Folkman (1984) and Derdiarian (1986, 1987a, 1987b, 1989) view information seeking as a primary mode of coping, which permits the individual to appraise the harms, threats, and challenges imposed by the diagnosis and treatment. Cohen and Lazarus (1979) contend that informational interventions help patients see how they can assume an active role in treatment and thus maintain some control. The hypothesis of this study was that information by psychoeducational videotape would promote emotional, physical, and social adjustment.

The intervention model of this study also focuses on crisis prevention by maximizing physical adjustment and emotional adjustment, role performance, perceived social support, and overall health status. As a crisis intervention, telephone counseling is based on the notion that each phase of the breast cancer experience, that is, diagnosis, postsurgery, adjuvant therapy, and ongoing recovery (Blutz, Speca, Brasher, Geggie, & Page, 2000; Hoskins et al., 1996a; Northouse, & Swain, 1987; Sadeh-Tessa, Drory, Ginzburg, & Stadler, 1999), is stressful and characterized by its own particular features. The telephone counseling intervention addressed the unique needs of patients experiencing breast cancer by (a) assessing their phase-specific perceptions and emotions; (b) clarifying questions about medical treatments, procedures, and side effects; (c) exploring the adequacy of social supports; and (d) assessing the effectiveness of coping mechanisms (Aguilera, 1998; Parad & Parad, 1990; Sadeh-Tessa et al., 1999). The preliminary studies by Hoskins et al. (1996a, 1996b, 2001) enhanced the development of the extant theoretical framework with regard to the conceptual and operational definition of the studies variables, as well as the development and implementation of the intervention protocols. The findings related to the potential moderating variables and adjustment outcomes will be addressed in a subsequent paper.

## 4. The Development and Pilot Testing of the Interventions

A pilot study of the randomized trial was conducted by Hoskins et al. (2001) to evaluate the intervention protocols and obtain preliminary data regarding the effectiveness of the proposed interventions. The pilot study enrolled a nonprobability sample of 12 women with early-stage breast cancer and their partners. Four patient–partner pairs received one of three interventions: psychoeducational videotapes alone, telephone counseling alone, or a combination of phase-specific psychoeducational videotapes and telephone counseling, which were complementary approaches to usual care at the diagnostic, postsurgery, adjuvant therapy, and ongoing recovery phases of breast cancer. Even with limited statistical power, the preliminary results of the feasibility study supported the proposed interventions as promoting physical, emotional, and social adjustment among women with early-stage breast cancer. The value of conducting a full-scale randomized trial to better understand the relative treatment efficacy and differential benefit of the interventions was supported.

## 5. Intervention Protocols

The intervention protocols were consistent with the theoretical framework and were developed for the usual care (control) group and three intervention groups.

### 5.1. GROUP 1

Group 1 is the control group that received usual care standardized across data collection (DC) sites as surgeons, radiologists, and oncologists adhered to evidence-based national treatment protocols for the diagnosis and treatment of breast cancer. Usual care across the phases of breast cancer consisted of office visits or inpatient visits in which the patient was seen by the respective physician and nursing staff; educational information was made available relative to the specific phases of the breast cancer experience including breast cancer diagnosis, surgical, and adjuvant treatments; and information was provided regarding breast cancer support groups or if necessary referrals were made for psychological support. Phase-specific videotapes or telephone counseling were not interventions offered as a part of usual care. In this study, usual care was given to the control and intervention groups.

### 5.2. GROUP 2

Group 2 is an intervention group that received usual care plus four phase-specific psychoeducational videos: (a) Coping With Your Diagnosis, (b) Recovering From Surgery, (c) Understanding Adjuvant Therapy, and (d) Your Ongoing Recovery. Patients viewed the videotapes either in the institutional setting or in their homes. The content of each video was organized under three topics: (a) Health Relevant Information, (b) Information for Skill Development, and (c) Psychosocial Support.

### 5.3. GROUP 3

Group 3 is an intervention group that received usual care plus a telephone counseling intervention, which was individualized based on the Crisis Intervention Model. The telephone counseling intervention protocol consisted of four phase-specific telephone-counseling sessions. The objectives of the telephone counseling intervention were to (a) reduce anxiety, (b) shape reality-based appraisals, (c) facilitate attainment of support, (d) process information, (e) encourage adaptive behavioral change, (f) promote functional communication, and (g) promote reintegration of a holistic concept of self. The sessions were conducted by a nurse interventionist trained and supervised in individualized telephone counseling approaches. The setting for the telephone intervention was the patient's home.

### 5.4. GROUP 4

Group 4 is an intervention group that received usual care plus phase-specific psychoeducational videotapes and telephone counseling as described above.

## 6. Methods

### 6.1. STUDY SAMPLE AND SETTING

A purposive sample of 249 patients was enrolled from three major medical centers and one community hospital in New York City. Analyses of pilot data were used to determine a reasonable expectation for group differences in mean changes among primary measures to sample size determination. These were expressed in terms of a mean change for the usual care, plus psychoeducational videos and telephone counseling groups that was one-fourth standard deviation above the grand mean, one-fourth standard deviation below the grand mean for the usual care group, and at the grand mean for the usual care plus psychoeducational videos, and usual care plus telephone counseling groups. This corresponds to two group standardized effect size of $d = 0.50$ between the extremes. This profile corresponds to a median effect size of $f = 0.25$ as defined by Cohen (1988). A target sample of 61 per group was selected to achieve a power of at least 80% for detecting group differences in mean change scores, assuming $\alpha = .01$ and $f \geq .25$. At the planning stage, the effect of reduced sample size from 61 per group to the sample sizes actually obtained (roughly 40 per group) in the study would serve to increase the minimum detectable effect sizes between group means at the extremes by about 26% (i.e., from $d = 0.50$ to $d = 0.63$).

Patients met the following inclusion criteria: (a) a confirmed diagnosis of early-stage breast cancer as per the National Cancer Institute Guidelines, (b) was enrolled in one of the four oncology services that were part of the study, (c) had no previous history of cancer, (d) had identified a person most intimately involved in the breast cancer experience who was named their "partner," (e) was able to read and understand English, (f) had no concurrent, uncontrolled, chronic medical illness as recorded on the Primary Medical Data Form and verified by the medical record, and (g) had no history of psychiatric hospitalization or drug abuse. Although breast cancer occurs among men, the percentage is small compared to women. Because of the complexity of factors that may differ from those experienced by women, men were excluded from the sample.

## 6.2. DESIGN AND DC

A randomized block design was used to assign patients to either the usual care (control group) or one of three intervention groups. The study was approved by the review boards of four participating institutions.

### 6.2.1. RECRUITMENT ACTIVITIES

The procedure for recruiting patients consisted of the following: (a) the project director at each site reviewed the preadmission schedule weekly with the Oncology Coordinator to identify new patients who potentially met the inclusion criteria; (b) the surgeon obtained the patient's permission for referral to the project director for a recruitment interview; and (c) patients were screened by the project director during the recruitment interview to verify that they met the inclusion criteria.

### 6.2.2. ENROLLMENT PROCEDURES

If the patient met the inclusion criteria, the study was explained to the patient. All patients who agreed to enroll in the study signed an informed consent form and completed the study questionnaires as baseline data and a demographic data form. Medical data were recorded by the project director on the Primary Medical Data Form based on patient's self-report and documentation from the patient's medical record. Upon completion of the informed consent, the project director disclosed the patient's random assignment to the control group or one of the intervention groups. Random assignments (using a block size of four) were computer generated for each site and were provided to each site in sealed, individually numbered envelopes. The assignment remained unknown to the project director, physician, and patient. Each intervention was administered by a trained nurse interventionist who used a standardized manual of phase-specific protocols and scripts to insure intervention fidelity across DC sites. Training and supervision of the nurse interventionist were conducted by a coinvestigator who was an advanced practice psychiatric nurse. The nurse interventionist distributed the study's instruments at the time of the intervention. The participant mailed the completed packet of instruments in a prestamped envelope to the project office. The site project director administered the packet of five inventories to participants in the control group. Confidentiality was maintained through the use of code numbers. Completed questionnaires were maintained in locked files and computer data was protected.

In addition to the baseline data obtained upon enrollment in the study (DC Point 0), there were four DC points: DC 1—within 1 week following biopsy but prior to surgery; DC 2—within 72 hours following surgery either in hospital or postdischarge; DC 3—during discussions of adjuvant therapy within 72 hours of patient's appointment with the medical and/or radiation oncologist; and DC 4—within 14 days of the patient's completion of adjuvant therapy or 6-month surgery anniversary date.

### 6.3. INSTRUMENTS

At each DC point, participants completed a packet of the following instruments:

The *Profile of Adaptation to Life Clinical Scale* (PAL-C; Ellsworth, 1981) is a 41-item self-report inventory that is designed to measure variations in adjustment and functioning over time. Evidence of discriminant validity was provided by the subscales of psychological well-being and physical symptoms. In the preliminary descriptive study (Hoskins, 1990–1994), coefficient alphas were .75 for psychological well-being and .83 for physical symptoms. Test-Retest reliabilities were .80 and greater. The psychological well-being subscale addresses enjoyment in talking with others, finding work interesting, feelings of trust, involved, and feelings of being needed and useful. Scores for psychological well-being range from 5 to 20, with a higher score reflecting higher levels of psychological wellbeing. Physical symptoms subscale scores range from 7 to 28, with a higher score reflecting a higher level of physical symptoms experienced.

The *Self-Report Health Scale* (SRHS; Lawton, Moss, Fulcomer, & Kleban, 1982) is a four-item subscale of the Multilevel Assessment Instrument (MAI), which assesses perceived health status. Construct validity was supported by a correlation of .67 between the summary domain for physical health and the SRHS and by a correlation of .63 between the ratings by the MAI interviewer and a clinician (Lawton et al., 1982). Factor analytic evaluation of the SRHS in the preliminary descriptive study (Hoskins et al., 1996a) revealed two factors, each consisting of two items and a reliability coefficient of .76 and test–retest of .92 at 3 weeks. The reliability estimate from the interitem correlation coefficient between perceived health status and Factor 1 (better health) was .60 and 0.69 for Factor 2 (no problems; Hoskins & Merrifield, 1993), indicating that each factor contributed substantially to the variance in perceived health status. Scores for overall health status range from 4 to 13, with a higher score reflecting better overall perceived health status.

*Psychosocial Adjustment to Illness Scale* (PAIS; Derogatis, 1983) is a 46-item scale that assesses the impact of the illness on seven domains of adjustment. Scores for role function in the domestic, vocational, and social environments were used in this study as the measures of social adjustment. Studies of discriminant validity among patients with breast cancer yielded correlations between the total PAIS score of .81 for the Global Adjustment to Illness Scale, .60 for the SCL-90-R General Severity Index, and .69 for the Affect Balance Scale (Hoskins, 1990–1994). The ranges in alpha coefficients in a preliminary, descriptive study by Murphy (1994) were .66 to .77 for domestic environment, 64 to .75 for vocational environment, and .83 to .85 for the social environment.

The domestic environment domain reflects difficulties that arise primarily in the home or family environment due to illness. The eight items measure a number of aspects of family living, including financial impact of the illness, quality of relationships, family communications, and effects of physical disabilities. Scores for domestic environment range from 0 to 24, with a higher score reflecting poorer adjustment or more problems. The vocational environment subscale reveals the impact of an illness on vocational adjustment related to work, school, or home, as appropriate. Six items measure perceived quality of job performance, job satisfaction, lost time, job interest, and a number of other variables that are associated with the nature of vocational adjustment. Scores for vocational environment range from 0 to 18, with a higher score reflecting poorer adjustment or more problems. Social environment reflects the status of the patient's current social and leisure time activities and the degree to which the patient has suffered impairment or constriction of these activities as a result of the current illness and/or its residual effects. Scores for social environment range from 0 to 18, with a higher score reflecting poorer adjustment or more problems.

The *Breast Cancer Treatment Response* Inventory (BCTRI; Budin, Cartwright-Alcarese, et al., 2008) provides a multidimensional assessment of the incidence, severity, and degree of distress of 19 side effects of breast cancer treatment. The BCTRI was pilot tested among 105 women with breast cancer from the time of diagnosis throughout treatment and ongoing recovery. Internal consistency was demonstrated with Cronbach's alpha coefficients of .64 for symptom incidence or occurrence, .77 for severity of symptoms, and .72 for amount of distress (ADE) experienced (Budin, Cartwright, & Hoskins, in press). Discriminant validity was supported by comparing the mean score for ADE reported by those receiving chemotherapy and those who were not ($t = 4.4$, $p < .000$). Criterion validity was supported by correlating ADE scores, measured by the BCTRI, and total scores from the Symptom Distress Scale ($r = .86$, $p < .000$; McCorkle & Young, 1978).

Side effect incidence is the sum of the number of side effects reported ranging from 0 to 19, with higher scores indicating greater side effect incidence. Side effect severity is the sum of ratings for severity (or intensity) for each of the 19 side effects associated with breast cancer treatment. Scores for side effect severity range from 1 to 57 depending on the number of side effects experienced, with a higher score reflecting a higher degree of side effect severity. Side effect distress is the sum of the ratings for how distressful each of 19 side effects experienced were. Scores for side effect distress range from 0 to 57 depending on the number of side effects experienced with a higher score reflecting higher degree of side effect distress.

*Primary Medical Data Form* was completed upon entry into the study and provided results of previous mammography, history of breast cancer, previous surgical procedures, results of lymph node dissection, and staging of the cancer.

*Demographic Data Form* was completed upon entry into the study and included characteristics such as age, marital and parental status, ethnicity, occupation, income, how the breast lesion was detected, the patient's understanding of the breast lesion, presence of any chronic illness, family history of breast cancer, and psychiatric problems.

### 6.4. STATISTICAL ANALYSES

The primary outcomes consisted of mean changes in emotional, physical, and social adjustment for patients with early-stage breast cancer. An initial analysis examined whether there were any differences among the four groups (usual care, usual care plus psychoeducational videos, usual care plus telephone counseling or usual care plus psychoeducational videos and telephone counseling) for any demographic and baseline characteristics. A Wilcoxon rank sum test indicated differences among the groups for continuous measures such as age and overall health status and chi-square-assessed baseline differences among groups for categorical measures such as ethnicity.

For each outcome measure, descriptive statistics including mean, standard deviation, median, and mean difference from baseline were computed for each of the four periods (baseline, postsurgery, adjuvant therapy, and ongoing recovery); a composite period endpoint was constructed by averaging scores over postsurgery, adjuvant therapy, and ongoing recovery phases. Because there were a number of missing values at the baseline and diagnostic periods, a last observation carried forward algorithm was used to construct a composite baseline/diagnostic score. If the diagnostic period had missing data, then the value from the baseline period was carried forward to the diagnostic period.

For the main efficacy analyses, a mixed model analysis of variance (ANOVA; PROC MIXED in SAS software) was used to analyze the mean changes over time (from baseline to postsurgery, adjuvant therapy, and ongoing recovery) for each of the outcome measures. The model included terms for the four groups (usual care plus three intervention groups), site (three medical centers and one community hospital in New York City), time (postsurgery, adjuvant therapy, and ongoing recovery), and Group $\times$ Time interaction. In addition, the baseline score for each outcome measure was included as a covariate in the model (except for measures of side effects). Inclusion of the baseline score served to model the outcome measures as change scores (specifically the change from baseline).

The mixed model ANOVA used an autoregressive covariance structure for the random (time) effect in the model, which accounts for the fact that measures that are closer in time are generally more correlated. If the main effect of group was statistically significant, further multiplicity-adjusted post hoc tests were conducted to determine pairwise differences. The $p$ value for the test of interaction was set to $p = .100$ to maximize the chances of picking up a true difference among groups over time. If the interaction of time and group was statistically significant (at $p < .100$), a closed testing procedure for simultaneous confidence intervals was performed to compute the adjusted p values for simple effects of group within each period and changes over time within each group. This method allows control of family-wise Type I error for a given set of simultaneous comparisons for a mixed model so that the overall alpha level does not exceed $p < 0.5$. Least square means, which are the predicted means derived from the ANOVA model, are presented to summarize the effects in the model. These means reflect the model-derived change scores from baseline, adjusting for intervention group differences at the baseline/diagnostic assessment period, as well as any differences among clinical sites.

## 7. Results

### 7.1. DEMOGRAPHIC AND BASELINE CHARACTERISTICS

Demographic and baseline characteristics of the sample are summarized in Table 1. The usual care (control) group and the three intervention groups were similar in terms of baseline sociodemographic characteristics. Subjects ranged in age from 51.8 to 54.1 across the four groups. With regard to ethnicity, Caucasians ranged from 67% to 71% across groups, and the percentages of African American subjects ranged from 10% to 22% across groups. Most of the participants across all groups were Christian (Protestant or Catholic). Greater than 70% of participants in all groups had children. More than half of the subjects in each of the four groups were living with a partner or spouse, and approximately three quarters of each group had at least some college education. The full-time employment rate ranged from 48% to 63% across groups. Most of the sample found the breast lesion by routine mammography (47.2%) or self-breast examination (26.9%), with 53% having a lumpectomy or partial mastectomy (20%) and lymph node dissection (74%; refer to Table 2 for medical variables). The only statistically significant difference ($p = .003$) among the groups was for "length of time known about lump." A significant difference was found between the psychoeducational videotape group and the telephone counseling group, with respective means of 11.5 and 5.6 months.

| VARIABLE | PATIENTS | |
|---|---|---|
| | *n* | % |
| Age in years, *M* (*SD*), range | 53.8 (11.7), 33–98 | |
| Marital status | | |
|    Single, never married | 28 | 13.5 |
|    Single, living with partner | 8 | 3.8 |
|    Married, living with partner | 117 | 56.3 |
|    Divorced/Separated | 27 | 12.9 |
|    Widowed | 24 | 11.5 |
|    Other | 4 | 1.9 |
|    (missing) | (41) | |
| Race | | |
|    White | 148 | 69.2 |
|    African American | 33 | 15.5 |
|    Latino/Hispanic | 19 | 8.9 |
|    Asian or Pacific Islander | 11 | 5.1 |
|    Other | 3 | 1.4 |
|    (missing) | (35) | |
| Religious preference | | |
|    Protestant | 43 | 21.1 |
|    Catholic | 85 | 41.7 |
|    Jewish | 42 | 20.6 |
|    Islam | 2 | 1.0 |
|    Other | 3 | 1.4 |
|    (missing) | (35) | (51) |
| Level of education | | |
|    Some high school | 10 | 4.7 |
|    High school graduate | 38 | 17.9 |
|    Partial college | 51 | 24.1 |
|    College graduate | 56 | 26.4 |
|    Graduate degree | 42 | 19.8 |
|    Postgraduate degree | 7 | 3.3 |
|    Other | 8 | 3.8 |
|    (missing) | (37) | (47) |
| Employment status | | |
|    Unemployed | 22 | 10.4 |
|    Part-time | 26 | 12.3 |
|    Full-time | 112 | 52.8 |
|    Retired | 34 | 16.0 |
|    Medical disability | 3 | 1.4 |
|    Other | 14 | 7.1 |
|    (missing) | (37) | (47) |
| Work change | | |
|    No | 124 | 67.0 |
|    Yes | 61 | 33.0 |
|    (missing) | (64) | (69) |

**TABLE 1    DEMOGRAPHIC VARIABLES FOR PATIENTS (*N* = 249)**

| TABLE 1 | DEMOGRAPHIC VARIABLES FOR PATIENTS (*N* = 249)—cont'd | | |
|---|---|---|---|
| **VARIABLE** | **PATIENTS** | | |
| | | *n* | **%** |
| Working less | | 33 | 55.9 |
| Working more | | 2 | 3.4 |
| On disability | | 3 | 5.1 |
| Leave of absence | | 8 | 13.6 |
| Other | | 13 | 22.0 |
| (missing) | | (190) | |
| Combined annual income | | | |
| Below $19,000 | | 20 | 9.9 |
| $19,000–$29,999 | | 17 | 8.4 |
| $30,000–$39,999 | | 20 | 9.9 |
| $40,000–$49,999 | | 20 | 9.9 |
| More than $50,000 | | 126 | 62.1 |
| (missing) | | (46) | (59) |
| Children | | | |
| No | | 52 | 24.5 |
| Yes | | 160 | 75.5 |
| (missing) | | (37) | (46) |

*Note.* Values are expressed as numbers (percentages) unless otherwise indicated.

### 7.2. PHYSICAL, EMOTIONAL, AND SOCIAL ADJUSTMENT

For all measures with a baseline score, pretest baseline scores were significantly related to subsequent posttest scores (postsurgery, adjuvant therapy, and ongoing recovery) at $p < .001$.

### 7.2.1. PHYSICAL ADJUSTMENT

Physical adjustment, defined as expected health status and absence or presence of physical problems or symptoms at a given phase of illness, was measured by the side effects incidence and severity subscales of the BCTRI and the Overall Health Status score of the SRHS of the MAI. The results are cited below.

### 7.2.2. SIDE EFFECT INCIDENCE

The results of a mixed model ANOVA showed a statistically significant effect for time ($p < .0001$), indicating that all four groups reported fewer side effects over time from postsurgery to ongoing recovery. The mean number of reported side effects decreased from a mean of 6–7 during immediate postsurgery to a mean of 4–5 during ongoing recovery. There were no significant group differences or group by time interactions.

### 7.2.3. SIDE EFFECT SEVERITY

Results for side effect severity showed only a significant main effect for time, $F(2, 146) = 5.86$, $p = .004$, for the model. There was no significant group or Group × Time interactions. In general, for all groups, it appeared that side effect severity increased slightly from postsurgery (mean range = 27.6–30.1, with higher scores indicating poorer outcomes) to adjuvant

## TABLE 2　MEDICAL VARIABLES FOR PATIENTS (*N* = 249)

| VARIABLE | PATIENTS | |
|---|---|---|
| | *n* | % |
| How breast lesion was found | | |
| By self-casual examination | 57 | 26.9 |
| Routine breast self-examination | 4 | 1.9 |
| Clinical breast examination | 15 | 7.1 |
| Routine mammogram | 100 | 47.2 |
| Diagnostic follow-up examination | 26 | 12.3 |
| Other | 10 | 4.7 |
| (missing) | (37) | |
| Personal history of breast problems | | |
| No | 150 | 71.1 |
| Yes | 61 | 28.9 |
| (missing) | (38) | |
| Family history of breast cancer | | |
| No | 106 | 50.2 |
| Yes | 105 | 49.8 |
| (missing) | 38 | |
| Surgical procedure | | |
| Wide excision/Lumpectomy | 110 | 53.4 |
| Partial mastectomy | 42 | 20.4 |
| Total mastectomy | 18 | 8.7 |
| Modified radical mastectomy | 36 | 17.5 |
| (missing) | (43) | |
| Lymph node dissection | | |
| No | 54 | 25.8 |
| Yes | 155 | 74.2 |
| (missing) | (40) | |
| Lymph node status | | |
| Positive | 53 | 34.6 |
| Negative | 100 | 65.4 |
| (missing) | (96) | |
| Sentinel node biopsy | | |
| No | 154 | 79.0 |
| Yes | 41 | 21.0 |
| (missing) | (54) | |
| Sentinel node results | | |
| Positive | 5 | 16.1 |
| Negative | 26 | 83.9 |
| Stage of disease | | |
| Stage 0 | 43 | 22.9 |
| Stage I | 75 | 39.9 |
| Stage II | 57 | 30.3 |
| Stage III | 11 | 5.9 |
| Information not available | 2 | 1.1 |
| (missing) | (61) | |

therapy (range = 25.7–28.3). Side effect severity then increased from adjuvant therapy to ongoing recovery (range = 25.7–31.7).

### 7.2.4. OVERALL HEALTH STATUS

The results of the ANOVA for patients' overall health showed only a significant main effect for time ($p < .0001$). There was no significant group or Group × Time differences. Overall health ratings for all four groups showed similar improvement from postsurgery through ongoing recovery. The means at baseline ranged from 8.5 to 8.9, and the means for ongoing recovery ranged from 9.4 to 10.4, with higher scores representing better overall perceived health.

## 7.3. EMOTIONAL ADJUSTMENT

Emotional adjustment was defined as positive or negative adjustment to conditions related to the illness. Emotional adjustment was measured using the psychological well-being subscale of the PAL-C (Ellsworth, 1981) and the side effect distress subscale of the BCTRI (Budin, Cartwright-Alcarese, Hoskins, in press).

### 7.3.1. PSYCHOLOGICAL WELL-BEING

The results of the ANOVA revealed a statistically significant main effect of time, $F(2, 313)$ = 3.44, $p = .033$, reflecting an increase over time in scores for psychological well-being (from postsurgery to ongoing recovery) pooling over all groups. However, this was modified by a significant group by time interaction, $F(6, 315) = 2.85, p = .010$, which indicated that the change over time in psychological wellbeing was not the same among the four groups. For the telephone counseling group, there was an improvement from baseline to adjuvant therapy, followed by a decrease in psychological well-being from the adjuvant therapy phase to the ongoing recovery phase ($p = .002$), whereas the other groups did not show a significant change over time, $F(3, 400) = 3.28, p = .063$.

### 7.3.2. SIDE EFFECT DISTRESS

Although there was no significant main effect for group or time for side effect distress, there was a trend for a statistically significant Group × Time interaction, $F(6, 135) = 1.95$, $p = .077$. Adjusted post hoc tests showed that side effect distress increased over time only for the control group ($p = .012$), whereas scores for the other three treatment groups remained relatively constant from postsurgery to ongoing recovery. Although side effect distress increased during ongoing recovery in the control group ($M = 27.0$) relative to the other groups, with means of 23.0, 22.5, and 18.8, respectively, for the telephone counseling, psychoeducational videotapes, and videotapes plus telephone counseling groups, this difference was not statistically significant ($p = .132$).

## 7.4. SOCIAL ADJUSTMENT

Social adjustment defined as the impact of illness on the ability to function in the domestic, vocational, and social environments was measured by the domestic, vocational, and social environments subscales of the PAIS (Derogatis & Derogatis, 1990).

### 7.4.1. VOCATIONAL ENVIRONMENT

The ANOVA results indicated a significant main effect for time, $F(2, 265) = 3.80, p = .024$ (log transformed), with scores for vocational well-being improving over time (lower scores denote better outcome). Mean scores ranged from 4.4 to 6.0 at postsurgery and improved (decreased) to a range of 4.3 to 5.0 by the ongoing recovery phase. There were no significant group or Group $\times$ Time interactions.

### 7.4.2. DOMESTIC ENVIRONMENT

Results of the ANOVA indicated no statistically significant main effect for time, group, or Group $\times$ Time interactions.

### 7.4.3. SOCIAL ENVIRONMENT

Results of the ANOVA indicated a statistically significant main effect for time, $F(2, 309) = 13.0$, $p < .0001$, but no significant group or Group $\times$ Time differences. There was improvement in patients' social environment scores for all groups from postsurgery to ongoing recovery (with lower scores denoting better social environment scores). Patients' scores improved by about 2 points from postsurgery to ongoing recovery for all four groups. Scores ranged from 5.2 to 6.0 immediately postsurgery and improved (decreased) to a range of 3.5 to 4.2 by ongoing recovery.

## 8. Discussion and implications

Although breast cancer affects women of all ethnic and sociodemographic backgrounds, approximately 70% of this sample were Caucasian women in their 50s who lived with a partner or spouse and had other characteristics reflecting a relatively homogeneous group of women. The sample at baseline, by virtue of demographics and adjustment scores, was a fairly well-adjusted group. In general, this sample of women was self-selected and motivated to participate in a research study. Irrespective of the interventions, all groups showed improvement in their adjustment scores over time. There was a subset of women who did not adjust as well, and the question remains as to how to identify such patients and meet their needs. Given the homogeneity of the sample, there is a lack of generalizability of the findings to the general population. However, this sample was more heterogeneous than the 89% Caucasian sample reported by Samarel et al. (2002) and the 85% Caucasian sample reported by Badger et al. (2007). Although the medical centers who participated in this study were located in an urban environment and served an ethnically and socioeconomically diverse population, further research is needed to understand factors related to minority participation in breast cancer research.

### 8.1. PHYSICAL ADJUSTMENT

As a primary hypothesis, it was predicted that patients enrolled in any one of the three intervention groups would have great physical adjustment compared to the usual care (control) group. As a component of physical adjustment, results indicated that there were no significant differences between the usual care (control) group and the intervention groups with respect to the incidence of side effects or side effect severity. As the groups were randomly assigned, the expectation was that each group would be similar with regard to number of women with each stage of breast cancer (I or II), type of surgery, and type of adjuvant therapy and therefore similar in the incidence and severity of side effects. There was the diminution of the number of side effects for all groups from postsurgery to ongoing recovery, indicating that even without interventions, the incidence of side effects diminished over time. For all groups, side effect severity improved slightly from postsurgery to adjuvant therapy and then increased from adjuvant therapy to ongoing recovery. It was expected that during the adjuvant therapy phase, side effects of chemotherapy or radiation therapy would increase in severity and last for several weeks to months.

Although this study did not provide physiological interventions, all groups received usual care, which involved attention to physiological needs of patients by the physician and nursing staff. It was thought that information and support regarding physical changes and issues, as offered by psychoeducational videotapes and telephone counseling, would enhance physical adjustment beyond the interventions offered through usual care. However, psychological interventions had no effect on physical adjustment. The fact that the incidence of side effects diminished for all groups over time may reflect the body's capacity to heal itself over time with or without additional interventions. Prior studies by Ell et al. (1989) and Iscoe et al. (1991) indicated that adjustment does not end with completion of treatment but that indeed, the ongoing recovery may be fraught with continued physical issues such as chronic pain issues, lymphedema, or persistent sensory changes from chemotherapy or radiation therapy. Our study also indicated the persistence of physical issues during the ongoing recovery phase. The results regarding "overall health" further indicates that individuals in all groups had increased overall health from postsurgery through ongoing recovery and that baseline scores regarding overall health were predictive of overall health during all phases of the illness experience. In general, changes in the treatment of breast cancer not only improved the morbidity and mortality rates but also improved the overall health of women with breast cancer (ACS, 2007).

### 8.2. EMOTIONAL ADJUSTMENT

As a primary hypothesis, it was predicted that patients enrolled in any one of the three intervention groups would have great emotional adjustment compared to the usual care (control) group. The results related to emotional adjustment indicated a significant increase in psychological well-being over time for both the usual care (control) and intervention groups from postsurgery to ongoing recovery. Interestingly, although the control group had lower psychological wellbeing scores from postsurgery through the adjuvant therapy phase, their scores did improve during ongoing recovery. In a study on the effectiveness of telephone delivered psychosocial interventions in reducing depression and anxiety of women with breast cancer, Badger et al. (2007) reported that irrespective of group assignment, there were effects of time such that depression and anxiety generally decreased with time. Using the Lazarus and Folkmans's conceptual model, Maeda, Kurihara, Morishima, and Munakata (2008) reported, based on a sample of 28 women with early-stage breast cancer ($n = 14$ control group; $n = 14$ experimental group), that a three-session intervention of medical and psychological information and counseling using a structured association techniques resulted in no significant Group $\times$ Time interaction on psychological status but that the experimental group showed significant improvement in anxiety at 3 months following surgery and depression over time. Based on crisis theory, it suggests for better or worse, crises are resolved within 4 to 8 weeks (Aguilera, 1998). With the experience of cancer, there are a series of crises that occur in relation to the diagnosis, surgical treatment, and adjuvant treatment phases of the experience, which continue into the ongoing recovery phase (Hoskins et al., 1996a, 1996b). Each phase of the breast cancer experience provides health professionals with an opportunity to promote adjustment. The Stress and Coping Model by Lazarus and Folkman (1984) suggests that information on the initiation of treatment and expected side effects in the adjuvant therapy phase would promote emotional adjustment. The fact that there were no significant group differences in terms of emotional adjustment suggests that the information and support offered as usual care to both the control and intervention groups was sufficient to promote emotional adjustment. This may further explain why the control group's psychological well-being also increased during the ongoing recovery phase, as well as explaining why those in the intervention groups had improved psychological well-being during the adjuvant therapy phase.

Interestingly, the group who received the telephone counseling alone had an increase in psychological wellbeing from baseline to the adjuvant therapy phase; however, their psychological well-being scores decreased during the ongoing recovery phase. As proposed by the study's theoretical framework, the adaptational needs and demands are specific to each phase of the breast cancer experience. Crisis intervention, offered through telephone counseling, assists patients in coping with the varying intensity and regulation of emotional responses, influencing the phase-specific adjustment process (Aguilera, 1998; Lazarus & Folkman, 1984). Studies by Chamberalin et al. (2006), Rawl et al. (2002), Badger et al. (2005), and Seigel, Mesagno, Karus, and Christ (1992) indicate that telephone interventions improve the psychological well-being of patients with cancer. In our study, it is possible that the individualized, personal discussion offered to the telephone intervention group keeps the health related issues at the forefront in their minds, providing an emotional outlet to express ongoing concerns, yet not allowing the opportunity to forget their worries. It is not clear, however, why the results were not similar for those receiving both the telephone intervention and the psychoeducational videotape intervention. Samarel et al. (2002) found that the telephone-only support group was equally effective in promoting adaptation to early-stage breast cancer when compared to a combined telephone and psychoeducation intervention or an education intervention alone. In our study, further analysis of the patient's evaluation data regarding the videotapes and telephone counseling interventions may provide further insights in understanding these results. As with other variables, the results indicate that baseline psychological well-being is highly correlated with psychological well-being during subsequent phases of the breast cancer experience, which is consistent with the findings of our preliminary study (Hoskins et al., 1996a). This suggests that the initial assessment of psychological well-being may identify those at high risk for emotional distress and allow early and ongoing interventions to promote psychological well-being. Yet, researchers must consider this in light of the findings of a study of 708 Australian women diagnosed with nonmetastatic breast cancer (Phillips et al., 2008) in which psychological coping was examined at 11 months postdiagnosis. The results indicated that greater anxiety was predictive of poorer distant disease-free survival and overall survival. The authors concluded that although psychological support may improve quality of life, interventions for adverse psychological factors may not improve survival.

As a dimension of emotional adjustment, it was found that group differences did exist with regard to side effect distress as predicted. The analyses indicated that the control group reported more side effect distress during ongoing recovery than subjects in the intervention groups. Without additional support, as in the case of the control group, the ongoing recovery phase may be associated with increasing concerns regarding the effects of chemotherapy or radiation therapy indicating poorer emotional adjustment.

### 8.3. SOCIAL ADJUSTMENT
As a primary hypothesis, it was predicted that patients enrolled in any one of the three intervention groups would have great social adjustment compared to the usual care (control) group. With regard to social adjustment in the domestic, vocational, and social

environments, the results indicate that social adjustment of women at baseline was associated with posttest scores for all groups during all phases. Simply stated, women who have greater social adjustment before the diagnosis and treatment of breast cancer experience better social adjustment during the breast cancer experience. Results further indicated that there were no significant differences between the control and intervention groups in terms of their domestic, vocational, or social environment adjustment. In what may be considered a related concept, Samarel, Fawcett, and Tulman (1997) reported no significant difference in functional status in the combined telephone counseling and psychoeducational intervention group or for those who received telephone counseling or psychoeducation alone.

Although there was no significant change in domestic environment adjustment over time, vocational environment adjustment increased over time. This may be explained by changes in surgical procedures and improved symptom management, which has improved the functional status of women following breast cancer surgery and during the adjuvant therapy phase. Current treatments with a decreased side effect profile may enable women in both the control and intervention groups to continue many of their domestic and vocational roles. Many women in our study discussed their social adjustment. If they stayed at home as mothers, they were able to generally maintain their role responsibilities with support of the family (Lewis, 1990). If they were working outside of the home, many had a rapid return to work within weeks after surgery, and many coped with chemotherapy by taking only 1 or 2 days off from work immediately after each treatment or shortened their workday when receiving radiation therapy. Further research regarding vocational adjustment is important because there is an expectation of rapid recovery given the effectiveness of modern medicine and an expectation by patients and employers of an early return to their jobs despite a lifethreatening condition. Research of the ongoing recovery may provide insight into work-related expectations and an understanding of how persistent side effects affect adjustment during the ongoing recovery period. Although there were no significant differences between groups with regard to social environment adjustment and all groups demonstrated improvement from postsurgery to ongoing recovery, further research may promote a further understanding of social adjustment for women diagnosed with breast cancer.

The relative homogeneity of the sample and attrition rates was a limitation of this study. Although recruitment of minority participants was a priority, additional strategies to enroll minority participants need further consideration. The lack of significant findings in this study may have occurred due to the underpowering of the study as a result of the attrition rate. Because this study was a phase-specific intervention study, the DC points of the diagnosis, postsurgery, and adjuvant therapy phases were often extremely close in time. There may not have been sufficient time from baseline to other time points to detect a differentiated treatment effect. Given that the adjuvant therapy phase was identified as the time of discussion of options for chemotherapy or radiation therapy rather than a time point during the adjuvant therapy phase, a differentiated treatment effect may not have been detected. With regard to the telephone intervention, perhaps a more intense intervention with more frequent intervention points or a longer telephone intervention would have produced significant effects. In Badger et al.'s study (2007), the 30-minute telephone counseling intervention was offered weekly for 6 weeks and found to significantly lower depression and anxiety. Bennett, Lyons, Winters-Stone, Nail, and Scherer (2007) also considered, in their study of motivational interviewing to increase physical activity in long-term cancer survivors, that perhaps a more intense intervention such as a more frequent telephone calls would produce significant effects on outcomes in future studies. As such, we recommend that further consideration should be given to the "dose" and "frequency" of the intervention to obtain a treatment effect.

## 9. Conclusion

The longitudinal design of this study has captured the dynamic process of adjustment to breast cancer. Each phase of breast cancer is an opportunity for nurses to provide information about physical, emotional, and social changes associated with the breast cancer experience and to provide support in their adjustment to illness. Nurses can emphasize, based on the conclusions of this study, that physical, emotional, and social adjustment occurs over time with or without additional interventions, as the body and spirit have a natural capacity to heal. Overall, the results suggest that the information and support offered as usual care to both the control and intervention groups was sufficient to promote adjustment. However, the study identified a subset of women who did not adjust well. Given that baseline physical, emotional, and social adjustment scores predict adjustment during the various phases of the breast cancer experience, baseline may be an important time point to identify those at risk for problems with adjustment and allow early and ongoing interventions to promote overall health and emotional well-being. The results of this study also indicated that adjustment issues continue in the ongoing recovery phase. Because individuals who received telephone counseling demonstrated lower emotional adjustment, the personal discussion regarding their cancer experience, although providing an outlet for their concerns, may not allow the opportunity to move health-related concerns to the background. Further research is therefore needed to understand the long-term physical, emotional, and social issues experienced as women enter the phase termed *survivorship* and the value added or effects of various interventions in promoting ongoing adjustment. On a clinical level, nurses may assess how work- and family-related expectations relate to a woman's adjustment; from a research perspective, additional insights can be gained through qualitative studies. This study informs evidence-based practice and highlights practice and research considerations in the care of women with early-stage breast cancer.

## Acknowledgment

We would like to thank the following physician colleagues who supported the study: Dr. Roy Ashikari, Dr. Andrew Ashikari (The Community Hospital at Dobbs Ferry, NY); Dr. Sheldon Feldman, Dr. Ronald Blum, Dr. Stewart Fleishman (Beth Israel Medical Center, NY); Dr. Amber Guth, Dr. Richard Shapiro, Dr. Deborah Axelrod, Dr. Karen Hiotis (New York University Medical Center, NY).

## REFERENCES

Aguilera, D. C. (1998). *Crisis intervention: theory and methodology* (8th ed.) St. Louis: C.V. Mosby.

Ahles, T., Wasson, J., Seville, J., Johnson, D., Cole, B., Hanscom, B., et al. (2006). A controlled trial of methods for managing pain in primary care patients with or without co-occurring psychosocial problems. *Annals of Family Medicine, 4*(4), 341–350.

American Cancer Society. (2007). *Cancer facts and figures 2007.* Atlanta, GA: American Cancer Society.

Badger, T., Segrin, C., Dorros, S., Meek, P., & Lopez, A. (2007). Depression and anxiety in women with breast cancer and their partners. *Nursing Research, 56*(10), 44–53.

Badger, T., Segrin, C., Meek, P., Lopez, A., Bonham, E., & Sieger, A. (2005). Telephone\Interpersonal counseling with women with breast cancer: Symptom management and quality of life. *Oncology Nursing Forum, 32*(2), 273–279.

Bennett, J., Lyons, K., Winters-Stone, K., Nail, L., & Scherer, J. (2007). Motivational interviewing to increase physical activity in long-term cancer survivors. *Nursing Research*, *56*(1), 18–27.

Blutz, B. D., Specca, M., Brasher, P. M., Geggie, P. H., & Page, S. A. (2000). A randomized trial of a brief psychoeducation support group for partners of early stage breast cancer patients. *Psycho-oncology*, *9*, 303–313.

Boehmke, M. M., & Dickerson, S. S. (2005). Symptoms, symptom experiences, and symptoms encountered by women with breast cancer undergoing current treatment modalities. *Cancer Nursing*, *28*(5), 382–389.

Budin, W., Cartwright-Alcarese, F., & Hoskins, C. N. (In press). The Breast Cancer Treatment Response Inventory: development, psychometric testing and refinement in practice. *Oncology Nursing Forum*.

Budin, W., Cartwright, F., & Hoskins, C. (2008). The Breast Cancer Treatment Response Inventory: development, psychometric testing and utility for use in clinical practice. *Oncology Nursing Forum*, *35*(2), 209–215.

Budin, W., Hoskin, C. N., Haber, J., Sherman, D. W., Mailsin, G., Cater, J. R., Cartwright-Alcarese, F., Kowalski, M., McSherry, C., Feurback, R., & Shulka, S. (2008). Breast cancer: education, counseling and adjustment among patients and partners: a randomized controlled trial. *Journal of Nursing Research*, *57*(3), 199–213.

Capone, M. A., Good, R. S., Westie, K. S., & Jacobson, A. F. (1980). Psychosocial rehabilitation of gynecologic oncology patients. *Archives of Physical Medicine and Rehabilitation*, *61*, 128–132.

Chamberalin, M., Wilmoth, M., Tulman, L., Coleman, E., Stewart, C., & Samarel, N. (2006). Women's perceptions of the effectiveness of telephone support and education on their adjustment to breast cancer. *Oncology Nursing Forum*, *33*(1), 138–144.

Cohen, F., & Lazarus, R. C. (1979). Coping with the stress of illness. In G. C. Stone, F. Cohen, & N. E. Adler (Eds.), *Health psychology* (pp. 247–254). San Francisco, CA: Jossey-Bass.

Cohen, J. (1988). *Statistical power for behavioral sciences* (2nd ed.). Hillsdale, NJ: Lawrence Erlbaum Associates.

Cohen, M. Z., Kahn, D. L., & Steeves, R. H. (1998). Beyond body image: the experience of breast cancer. *Oncology Nursing Forum*, *25*(5), 835–841.

Derdiarian, A. K. (1986). Informational needs of recently diagnosed cancer patients. *Nursing Research*, *35*(5), 278–281.

Derdiarian, A. K. (1987a). Informational needs of recently diagnosed cancer patients. Part I: A theoretical framework. *Cancer Nursing*, *10*(2), 107–115.

Derdiarian, A. K. (1987b). Informational needs of recently diagnosed cancer patients. Part II: Method and description. *Cancer Nursing*, *10*(3), 156–163.

Derdiarian, A. K. (1989). Effects of information on recently diagnosed cancer patients' and spouses' satisfaction with care. *Cancer Nursing*, *12*, 285–292.

Derogatis, L. R. (1983). *The psychosocial adjustment to illness scale*. Baltimore, MD: Clinical Psychometric Research.

Derogatis, L. R., & Derogatis, M. F. (1990). *PAIS and PAIS-SR administration, scoring and procedures manual*. Towson, MD: Clinical Psychometrics Research, Inc.

Ellsworth, R. (1981). *Profile of adaptation to life clinical scale*. Palo Alto, CA: Consulting Psychologists Press.

Folkman, S., & Greer, S. (2000). Promoting psychological well-being in the face of serious illness: when theory, research and practice inform each other. *Psycho-oncology*, *7*(9), 11–19.

Hasida, B., Gilbar, O., & Lev, S. (2001). Coping with breast cancer: patient, spouse, and dyad models. *Psychomatic Medicine*, *63*, 32–39.

Hoskins, C. N. (1995). Patterns of adjustment among women with breast cancer and their partners. *Psychological Reports, 77*, 1017–1018.

Hoskins, C. N., Baker, S., Bohlander, J., Bookbinder, M., Budin, W., Ekstrom, D., et al. (1996a). Social support and patterns of adjustment to breast cancer. *Journal of Scholarly Inquiry for Nursing Practice: An International Journal*, *10*(2), 99–123.

Hoskins, C. N., Baker, S., Bohlander, J., Bookbinder, M., Budin, W., Ekstrom, D., et al. (1996b). Adjustment among spouses of women with breast cancer. *Journal of Psychosocial Oncology*, 14(1), 41−69.

Hoskins, C. N., Haber, J., Budin, W., Cartwright-Alcarese, F., Kowalski, M., Panke, J., et al. (2001). Breast cancer: education, counseling, and adjustment—a pilot study. *Psychological Reports*, 89, 677−704.

Hoskins, C. N., & Merrifield P. (1993). Factor analyses and reliability estimates for the self-rated health scale (Unpublished data).

Iscoe, N., Williams, J., Szalai, J., & Osoba, H. (1991). Prediction of psychosocial distress in patients with breast cancer. *British Journal of Cancer*, 64, 353−356.

Kemeny, M. M., Wellisch, D. K., & Schain, W. S. (1988). Psychosocial outcomes in a randomized surgical trial for treatment of primary breast cancer. *Cancer*, 62, 1231−1237.

Lawton, M. P., Moss, M. S., Fulcomer, M., & Kleban, M. H. (1982). A research and service oriented multilevel assessment instrument. *Journal of Gerontology*, 37, 91−99.

Lazarus, R., & Folkman, S. (1984). *Stress, appraisal, and coping*. New York, NY: Springer.

Lewis, F. M. (1990). Strengthening family supports. *Cancer*, 65, 752−759.

Loveys, B. J., & Klaich, K. (1991). Breast cancer: demands of illness. *Oncology Nursing*, 18, 75−79.

Maeda, T., Kurihara, H., Morishima, I., & Munakata, T. (2008). The effect of psychological intervention on personality change, coping, psychological distress of Japanese primary breast cancer patients. *Cancer Nursing*, 31(4), 27−35.

McCorkle, R., & Young, K. (1978). Development of a symptom distress scale. *Cancer Nursing*, 1, 373−378.

Morely, W. E., Messick, J. M., & Aguilera, D. C. (1967). Crisis: paradigms of intervention. *Journal of Psychiatric Nursing Mental Health Services*, 5, 531–44.

Murphy, G. (1994). Psychosocial adjustment to illness: an examination of measures (Unpublished Doctoral Dissertation. New York, NY: New York University).

National Cancer Institute. (2007). *Staging of breast cancer*. Retrieved from http://www.cancer.gov.

Northhouse, L. L., Dorris, G., & Charron-Moore, C. (1995). Factors affecting couples' adjustment to recurrent breast cancer. *Social Science Medicine*, 41(1), 69−76.

Northouse, L. L., & Swain, M. A. (1987). Adjustment of patients and husbands to the initial impact of breast cancer. *Nursing Research*, 36, 221−225.

Parad, H. J., & Parad, L. G. (1990). Crisis intervention: an introductory overview. In H. J. Parad, & L. G. Parad (Eds.), *Crisis intervention: the practitioner's sourcebook for brief therapy* (pp. 1−66). Milwaukee, WI: Family Service America.

Pasacreta, J. V. (1997). Depressive phenomena, physical symptom distress, and functional status among women with breast cancer. *Nursing Research*, 46(4), 214−221.

Phillips, K., Osborne, R., Giles, G., Dite, G., Apicella, C., Hopper, J., et al. (2008). Psychological factors and survival of young women with breast cancer: a population-based prospective cohort study. *Journal of Clinical Oncology*, 26(28), 4666−4671.

Rawl, S., Given, B., Given, C., Champion, V., Kozachik, S., Barton, D., et al. (2002). Intervention to improve psychological functioning for newly diagnosed patients with cancer. *Oncology Nursing Forum*, 29(6), 967−975.

Sadeh-Tessa, D., Drory, M., Ginzburg, K., & Stadler, J. (1999). Stages of breast cancer: an Israeli psychosocial intervention model. *Journal of Psychosocial Oncology*, 17(3–4), 63−83.

Samarel, N., Fawcett, J., & Tulman, L. (1997). Effect of support groups with coaching on adaptation to early stage breast cancer. *Research in Nursing & Health*, 20, 15−26.

Samarel, N., Tulman, L., & Fawcett, J. (2002). Effects of two types of social support and education on adaptation to early-stage breast cancer. *Research in Nursing & Health*, 25, 459−470.

Samdgrem, A., & McCaul, K. (2006). Long-term telephone therapy outcomes for breast cancer patients. *Psycho-oncology, 24*, 1038−1048.

Sammarco, A. (2001). Psychosocial stages and quality of life of women with breast cancer. *Cancer Nursing, 24*(4), 272−277.

Seigel, K., Mesagno, P., Karus, D. G., & Christ, G. (1992). Reducing the prevalence of unmet needs for concrete services of patients with cancer. *Cancer, 69*, 1873−1883.

Sklalla, K. A., Bakitas, M., Furstenberg, C. T., Ahles, T., & Henderson, J. V. (2004). Patients' need for information about cancer therapy. *Oncology Nursing Forum, 31*(1), 316−323.

Varricchio, C. (1990). Relevance of quality of life to clinical nursing practice. *Seminars in Oncology Nursing, 6*, 255−259.

Walker, B. L., Nail, L. M., & Croyle, R. T. (1999). Does emotional expression make a difference in reactions to breast cancer? *Oncology Nursing Forum, 26*(6), 1025−1032.

Wimberly, S. R., Carver, J., Laurenceau, J., Harris, S. D., & Antonia, M. H. (2005). Perceived partner reactions to diagnosis and treatment of breast cancer: impact on psychosocial and psychosexual adjustment. *Journal of Counseling and Clinical Psychology, 73*, 300−311.

Wyatt, G. K., & Friedman, L. L. (1998). Physical and psychosocial outcomes of midlife and older women following surgery and adjuvant therapy for breast cancer. *Oncology Nursing Forum, 25*(4), 761−768.

# THE CRITIQUE

This is a critical appraisal of the article "The effects of psychoeducation and telephone counseling on the adjustment of women with early-stage breast cancer" (Sherman et al., 2012) to determine its usefulness for nursing practice.

## PROBLEM AND PURPOSE

The purpose of this study, to focus on "primary data related to adjustment of patients with early-stage breast cancer," is concise and clearly stated. The independent variables are disease management, standardized education, and telephone counseling, and the dependent variables are physical, emotional, and social adjustment. The population under study is clearly defined, and the results "are important to evidence-based practice and the determination of the efficacy and cost-effectiveness of interventions in improving patient outcomes."

## REVIEW OF THE LITERATURE

From the time of diagnosis of breast cancer, and throughout treatment and recovery, women are faced with issues related to physical, emotional, and social adjustment. Although it is widely accepted that these women should receive educational and counseling interventions to manage these issues, there have been few studies to evaluate the effectiveness of these programs to promote adjustment.

Prior studies have concluded that the use of psychoeducation and telephone counseling in promoting adjustment are effective interventions. Previously published work by members of this research team (Budin, Cartwright et al., 2008; Budin, Hoskin et al., 2008) reported details of the methodology and general results when disease management, standardized education and telephone counseling are used to increase physical, emotional, and social adjustment in this population. The identified gap in the literature is to specifically examine these interventions in women with early-stage breast cancer.

Several theoretical frameworks were used to guide the development of the interventions, including the Stress and Coping Model (Lazarus & Folkman, 1984) and the Crisis Intervention Model (Morely et al., 1967). In addition, prior work by one of the authors led to a pilot study to test the feasibility of the intervention (Hoskins et al., 2001). Despite limited statistical power, the results of the pilot study supported the use of the interventions and further study testing the effectiveness of the interventions in promoting physical, emotional, and social adjustment in women with early-stage breast cancer. Figure 1 presents the theoretical framework that provides a visual description of the structure of the study.

### RESEARCH QUESTIONS

Three hypotheses were identified in the study: (1) physical adjustment would be greater in each of the study intervention groups as compared to the control group who received usual care; (2) emotional adjustment would be greater in each of the study intervention groups as compared with the control group who received usual care; and (3) social adjustment would be greater in each of the study intervention groups as compared with the control group who received usual care.

The directional hypotheses are appropriate for this study because the relationships between the variables have been previously tested in a pilot study.

### SAMPLE

The convenience sample consisted of 249 women from three major medical centers and one community hospital in New York City. The sample size appropriately was justified by power analysis, as 61 participants per group were needed to achieve a power of 80% using an $\alpha = .01$ and $f \geq .25$. The effect size was determined by using analyses of pilot data to determine a difference in group means of the primary measures.

Inclusion criteria were clearly defined, in terms of ensuring that all women had the same diagnosis and had no history of cancer, other chronic illness, psychiatric hospitalization, or drug abuse. Men were appropriately excluded because, although they can be diagnosed with breast cancer, it is a very rare occurrence, and their emotional, physical, and social adjustment may likely be very different from that of women. Patients were identified by the site project director each week in collaboration with the oncology coordinator, the then surgeon obtained the patient's permission for referral for a recruitment interview. Patients were subsequently screened by the program director.

Although the sample was not randomly selected, there was random assignment to intervention or control groups. There were no significant demographic differences between the four groups in terms of age, ethnicity, religion, education, employment, how the lump was identified, or definitive surgical procedures. The variable "length of time known about lump" was significantly different ($p = .003$) between the psychoeducational videotape group and the telephone counseling group ($M = 11.5$ and $5.6$ months, respectively). Although the groups were largely equivalent at baseline, this one factor needs to be acknowledged when the study results are interpreted.

### RESEARCH DESIGN

The three required elements of an RCT are present in this study, which provides Level II evidence. Participants were randomly assigned to a comparison group (disease management) or one of three intervention groups (disease management + standardized education; disease management + telephone counseling; disease management + standardized education + telephone counseling). A randomized block design was used to allocate participants to treatment group.

### THREATS TO INTERNAL VALIDITY

Potential subjects were screened and, if they met inclusion criteria, were asked to participate. Selection bias may be an issue in studies that use convenience sampling, and in this study the site project director did not have initial contact with the subjects; the surgeon did. It is not known whether the surgeon may have avoided mentioning the study to certain patients who he or she may have thought were not appropriate for the study. To minimize this potential bias, consenting participants were then randomized to one of the four groups, and other than the variable "length of time known about lump" the groups were equivalent at baseline in terms of other important categorical variables. Data were collected by patient report at four timepoints, which may lead participants to remember items, causing test-retest effect.

### THREATS TO EXTERNAL VALIDITY

The investigators appropriately minimized threats to external validity by maximizing control of extraneous variables. As mentioned previously, subjects were randomized by a computer for each site and provided in sealed, individually numbered envelopes. The project director, physician, and patient were blinded to group assignment. Nurse interventionists were trained by a coinvestigator who was an advanced practice psychiatric nurse. Each nurse interventionist used a standardized manual of protocols to ensure intervention fidelity. All of these factors minimize threats to external validity and maximize generalizability.

### RESEARCH METHODOLOGY

Data collection was by patient self-report at four timepoints: 1 week after biopsy (but before surgery), 72 hours after surgery, 72 hours after discussion regarding radiation and/or chemotherapy, and 6 months after surgery.

### LEGAL-ETHICAL ISSUES

The study was reviewed and approved by the appropriate institutional review board, and informed consent was obtained from all participants before study initiation.

### INSTRUMENTS

Acceptable reliability and validity data were reported for the Profile of Adaptation to Life Clinical Scale (PAL-C), the Self-Report Health Scale (SRHS), the Psychosocial Adjustment to Illness Scale (PAIS), and the Breast Cancer Treatment Response Inventory (BCTRI).

### DATA ANALYSIS

Demographic variables were appropriately summarized using descriptive statistics, which is the appropriate analysis of categorical variables. For dependent variables, descriptive statistics used to calculate mean difference from baseline were computed for each timepoint. A "last-observation carried forward algorithm" was used to account for missing data in the intent-to-treat analysis. ANOVA was appropriately used for the main efficacy analyses, and post-hoc testing was conducted as needed. Two tables are used to visually display the data.

### CONCLUSIONS, IMPLICATIONS, AND RECOMMENDATIONS

The authors reported that all four groups reported fewer side effects over time ($p = .0001$), although side effect severity increased slightly after surgery and also from adjuvant therapy to recovery. Overall health ratings improved over time as well. In terms of psychological well-being, the telephone counseling group improved from baseline to adjuvant therapy, but declined from adjuvant therapy to ongoing recovery ($p = .002$). The other groups did not show a significant difference over time. Only the control group demonstrated a significant increase in side effect distress over time ($p = .012$). In regard to social environment, scores for all groups improved over time ($p = .0001$). The fact that there were no significant group differences in terms of emotional adjustment suggests that the information and support offered as usual care to both control and intervention groups was sufficient to promote emotional adjustment.

The Level II RCT design, when including all required elements (i.e., randomization, intervention and control groups, and manipulation of the independent variable), is what allows the investigator to determine cause-and-effect relationships. In this case, minimizing threats to internal validity strengthens the study. By ensuring a relatively homogenous sample, maintaining consistency in data collection, manipulating the independent variables, and randomly assigning patients to groups, the threat to external validity is minimized.

Limitations of the study, as clearly described by the investigator, included generalizability; although this sample was more heterogeneous than prior studies and although this study was conducted in an urban environment, there was minimal minority participation.

### IMPLICATIONS FOR NURSING PRACTICE

This is a well-designed and well-conducted RCT that provides Level II evidence. The interventions pose minimal risk. Although the initial cost for training the nurse interventionists may be an issue, the strengths in the study design, data collection methods, and measures to minimize threats to internal and external validity make this strong Level II evidence that demonstrates that physical, emotional, and social adjustment improve over time with or without additional intervention. Baseline may be an important time to identify those at risk for adjustment and target this group for intervention.

# CRITIQUE OF A QUANTITATIVE RESEARCH STUDY

## THE RESEARCH STUDY

The study "Asthma Severity in Children and the Quality of Life of Their Parents" by Noelle S. Cerdan and colleagues, published in *Applied Nursing Research,* is critiqued. The article is presented in its entirety and followed by the critique.

## Asthma Severity in Children and the Quality of Life of their Parents

*Noelle S. Cerdan, Patricia T. Alpert, Sheniz Moonie, Dianne Cyrkiel, Shona Rue*

### Abstract

This study examines the effect of asthma severity of children aged 7–17 years and sociodemographic characteristics on the caregiver's quality of life. For parents of asthmatic children, there was a negative correlation between overall asthma severity and quality-of-life score. Measuring parental quality of life enables the development of effective asthma programs. Published by Elsevier Inc.

### 1. Introduction

Quality of life (QOL) can be described as general satisfaction with everyday living (Vila et al., 2004) and is closely related to health status. Along with asthma symptoms and other clinical indicators, QOL measurements are important when assessing asthmatic children and their caregivers holistically (Juniper, Guyatt, Feeny, Ferrie, & Townsend, 1996). This descriptive, cross-sectional study examines the effect of asthma severity on caregivers' QOL using the Paediatric Asthma Caregiver's Quality of Life Questionnaire (PACQLQ) of Juniper et al. (1996), which considers activity limitation and emotional function. The PACQLQ also examines the relationship between caregivers' QOL and caregiver sociodemographic characteristics.

### 2. Background

Asthma is one of the most common chronic diseases in the United States, affecting about 22.2 million people, 6.5 million of which were children, in 2005 (National Center for Health Statistics [NCHS], 2007). School-age children with asthma are affected by the frequency and severity of episodes, hospital admissions, side effects of medications, morbidity and mortality, and costs of hospitalizations (Vila et al., 2004). Asthma also affects other aspects of life, such as school attendance, physical activity, family dynamic, coping style, psychological functioning, and sleep (Marsac, Funk, & Nelson, 2006; Moonie, Sterling, Figgs, & Castro, 2006).

Parents as caregivers are responsible for many aspects of their children's care, including symptom observation, medication administration, and transportation to health care services (Halterman et al., 2004). Because asthma is a chronic condition, parents can experience long-term stressors that impact work productivity, medical decision-making, and overall care and discipline issues (Halterman et al., 2004; Laforest et al., 2004).

In addition, other sociodemographic factors such as marital status, smoking status, educational level and income, presence of family and support systems, presence of other children in the household, and the parents being diagnosed with asthma themselves can contribute to changes in parental QOL. Many studies show that childhood morbidity and mortality related to asthma are associated with being low-income families, being a minority, and living in the inner city (NCHS, 2007).

To date, research results relating asthma characteristics including clinical measures and or symptoms and PACQLQ-measured QOL are inconsistent. Developed in Canada by Juniper et al. (1996), the PACQLQ showed acceptable levels of correlation between asthma status and parental QOL. Results showed that the PACQLQ was able to detect QOL changes over time ($p < .001$) and detect stability in those who did not change ($p < .0001$). Following school-age children through the school year in the United States, Halterman et al. (2004) showed that baseline asthma severity measured by asthma severity symptoms (i.e., daytime and nighttime symptoms, the need for rescue inhaler use, and the number of symptom-free days) significantly correlated with the PACQLQ score (range $r = .23–.51$, all $p < .1$). The highest correlation was between symptom-free days and parental QOL ($r = .51$, $p < .001$). At the end of the school year, significant correlations were found with all measures of asthma severity, except for rescue inhaler use. An increase in symptom-free days over time correlated with an improvement in PACQLQ scores ($r = .30$, $p < .001$). Conversely, an increase in daytime ($r = −.27$, $p < .001$) and nighttime ($r = −.22$, $p = .005$) symptoms correlated with lower PACQLQ scores.

Over a 3-month period, Osman, Baxter-Jones, and Helms (2001) showed a significant correlation between a change in children's asthma symptoms and PACQLQ scores ($r = .54–.57$, $p < .001$) even if the PACQLQ scores were not clinically significant. This suggests that other social and or psychological factors, in addition to asthma severity, may influence PACQLQ scores (Vila et al., 2004).

Many studies relate children's asthma prevalence to sociodemographic characteristics such as minority families living in low-income urban neighborhoods (Akinbami & Schoendorf, 2002). One study suggests that the prevalence and severity of asthma are associated with being African American or Hispanic and to poverty-related factors such as young maternal age, secondhand exposure to cigarette smoke, low birth weight, and living in crowded inner cities (Williams, Sternthal, & Wright, 2009).

Erickson et al. (2002) showed that household income and lower perceived asthma severity were statistically significant predictors of QOL as measured by the PACQLQ. Longer length of time diagnosed with asthma, longer length of time enrolled in a specialty clinic, fewer siblings living in the household, and greater convenience of seeing the physician were all related to higher QOL. Using Carstair's deprivation scores to describe the sociodemographics of the families in their study, Osman et al. (2001) found that younger mothers, those who come from less affluent families, and those with greater social deprivation had lower PACQLQ scores. Parental work absenteeism related to the child's illness can have economical implications for parents (Dean, Calimlim, Kindermann, Khandker, Tinkelman, 2009; Laforest et al., 2004).

This study is different from other studies that utilized the PACQLQ because this study used the current National Asthma Education and Prevention Program (NAEPP) guidelines in diagnosing asthma severity in children. The guidelines categorize patients based on worsening physical symptoms such as increased nighttime awakenings, increased use of rescue medication for symptom control, interference with normal activity, and decreased lung function. Very few studies have documented asthma severity using NAEPP guidelines, and for those that did, they have had inadequate sample sizes. In addition, this study uses several measurement tools and clinical indices such as pulmonary function tests (PFTs), whereas other studies depended solely on self-reported asthma severity or administrative records, which can underestimate asthma prevalence. Lastly, the current QOL literature for asthma is conflicted and not highly abundant, so this study lends greater insight to the current research literature.

This study is important to nursing because it offers a more holistic focus when addressing asthmatic children and their parents in the clinical setting. Operationalizing parental QOL measures as functional limitations and emotional dimensions allows nurse researchers to quantify the degree of burden that parents experience so that more effective asthma programs can be developed (Halterman et al., 2004). In addition, being familiar with the NAEPP (2007) guidelines in daily practice, nurses can better identify at-risk parents of asthmatic children to more quickly implement appropriate care. QOL has been shown to be an important outcome measure, and being aware of its effect on the individual is important for adherence to medical treatment (Marsac et al., 2006). The objective of this study was to examine the effect of children's asthma severity and sociodemographic factors on parental QOL measured through the PACQLQ.

## 3. Research Design and Methodology

This correlational study utilized a convenience sample of parents of children and adolescents, aged 7 to 17 years, with medical diagnoses of mild intermittent to severe persistent asthma. This study was reviewed and approved by the institutional review board at the University of Nevada, Las Vegas. From August 2008 to February 2009, participants were chosen from a pediatric pulmonology outpatient clinic located in Las Vegas, Nevada. Parents of children aged from 7 to 17 years were targeted because parents with children in this age range were used to validate the PACQLQ (Juniper et al., 1996). Parents surveyed were legal guardians of the asthmatic children. The clinic was chosen by the investigators because the clinic had patients with a greater variety of asthma severity (i.e., mild, moderate, or severe) and sociodemographic factors (i.e., health insurance coverage, parental age and ethnicity, and other variables). Children with a diagnosis of other chronic conditions such as depression, cerebral palsy, diabetes, hypothyroidism, and cancer were excluded from the study. Because most children with asthma also have atopic conditions such as eczema, allergy, and rhinoconjunctivitis, patients with atopy were not excluded from this study (Reichenberg & Broberg, 2001).

One of the researchers reviewed the charts of all scheduled patients to verify asthma diagnosis and age. Those deemed to be eligible to participate were approached in the waiting room by the researcher as patients and parents came in for their scheduled appointments. All potential participants were told that the researcher was not an employee of the clinic. They were also told that their participation was voluntary and declining participation would not jeopardize their relationship with their doctor or office staff. Those who agreed to participate completed the informed consent and their children offered assent. Participants were asked to confirm the age of their children and their children's asthma diagnosis. They were also asked their relationship to the children and were excluded if they were not the biological parents, adoptive parents, stepparents, legal guardians, or foster parents. Only one set of questionnaires were completed for each family.

Prior to completing the three questionnaires, the researcher gave parents explicit instructions on how to answer the items for each questionnaire, including the option not to answer questions that made them feel uncomfortable. If participants had questions after they started completing the questionnaires, they were told to choose the answer that they most strongly agreed with. To maintain participant confidentiality, participant questionnaires were assigned numbers, and participant names or any other identifying information such as address, telephone number, or birth date were not recorded. The parents returned the questionnaires to the researcher in an unmarked manila envelope to further ensure confidentiality.

The three questionnaires utilized were as follows: (1) the PACQLQ (Juniper et al., 1996), (2) the asthma severity questionnaire, and (3) the sociodemographic factors questionnaire. The PACQLQ, a 13-item questionnaire, measures activity limitation and emotional function. This tool is frequently utilized to measure the burden that parents experience in caring for their asthmatic children (aged 7 to 17 years). Specifically, this tool measures how a child's asthma interferes with the parent's daily activities (activity limitation) and the emotions generated (emotional function). The questionnaire contains four items addressing activity limitations and nine items addressing emotional function, with all questions being weighed equally. Parents respond to this questionnaire using a 7-point Likert-type scale, where 1 represents *severe impairment* and 7 represents *no impairment*. Examples of questions include the following: "How often did your child's asthma interfere with your job or work around the house?" and "How often were you bothered because your child's asthma interfered with family relationships?" The PACQLQ score produced a mean activity limitation score, a mean emotional function score, and a total mean score (Juniper et al., 1996). The questionnaire has been studied to be reliable and valid in certain populations. The PACQLQ has good reliability, with an intraclass correlation coefficient for overall QOL = .85, emotional function = .80, and activity limitation = .84 (Juniper et al., 1996).

The Asthma Severity Questionnaire was developed by the researchers for use in this study and includes 18 questions to categorize the child's asthma severity, which mirrors the 2007 NAEPP asthma classification guidelines. The NAEPP asthma classifications include intermittent asthma, mild persistent asthma, moderate persistent asthma, and severe persistent asthma. The NAEPP guidelines to classify asthma severity were turned into questions. Examples of questions included the following: "In the past 30 days, how often has your child had asthma symptoms such as wheezing, coughing, and shortness of breath during the day?" and "In the past 30 days, how often did your child wake up during the night due to asthma symptoms such as wheezing, coughing, and shortness of breath?" Participants were also asked about medication use within the past week to verify appropriate classification severity-specific treatment based on NAEPP guidelines. Other questions (not specific to the NAEPP guidelines), such as the number of days of school the child has missed, the number of days spent in the emergency room (ER) or hospital, and parental perception of asthma severity and control, were included based on findings of a literature review. The questionnaire was reviewed by two content experts but was not piloted prior to use in this study. In addition, spirometry readings, including forced expiratory volume in one second (FEV1) and forced expiratory volume in one second/forced vital capacity ration (FEV1/FVC) ratios, were obtained from the children's medical records with the permission of the pediatric pulmonologist and informed consent from the parents to further categorize the children's asthma severity based on the NAEPP guidelines.

The Sociodemographic Factor Questionnaire, developed by this study's investigators, was based on literature identification of the demographic variables associated with asthma morbidity and mortality. This questionnaire asked 18 questions on age, ethnicity, income, education level, place of residence, employment, health insurance coverage, social support, and other variables.

### 3.1. DATA ANALYSIS

Data entry and analyses were performed utilizing the Statistical Package for the Social Sciences Version 17.0. To assess the relationship between asthma severity and parental QOL, Spearman's correlation ($\rho$), analysis of variance (ANOVA), and linear and multivariate regressions were performed. To determine the relationship between sociodemographic factors and parental QOL, Spearman's correlation ($\rho$), chi-square, and independent $t$ tests were performed.

## 4. Results

A total of 112 parents who met the study criteria were invited to participate in the study. Ten parents were not interested in participating in the study and one parent did not return the survey to the researcher. Of the original 114 parents invited, 101 (88.59%) participated in the study. Tables 1 and 2 show the demographic characteristics of the participants. The Cronbach alpha coefficient for the PACQLQ was .89 of the total score, which suggests good internal consistency.

Before correlation analyses on the data were performed, scatterplots were generated and checked for violation of assumptions of normality, linearity, and homoscedasticity. Using Spearman's correlation ($\rho$), significant negative correlations were found between overall asthma severity and mean activity limitation scores ($\rho = -.400$, $p < .001$), mean emotional function scores ($\rho = -.258$, $p < .001$), and mean total PACQLQ scores ($\rho = -.342$, $p < .001$). Significant moderate, negative correlations were found between PACQLQ scores and asthma day symptoms, asthma night symptoms, and asthma exercise symptoms. As asthma severity and other asthma factors increased, PACQLQ scores decreased, indicating poorer QOL. No significant relationships were found between PFT scores and PACQLQ scores.

In addition, significant positive correlations were found between employment income and mean activity limitation scores (moderate correlation, $\rho = .363$, $p < .001$), mean emotional function scores (small correlation, $\rho = .291$, $p < .05$), and mean total PACQLQ scores (moderate correlation, $\rho = .346$, $p < .001$). This indicates that parents with higher incomes experience increased QOL. Table 3 provides the details of these analyses.

ANOVA was used to compare mean PACQLQ scores for each asthma severity group. Participants were divided based on asthma severity rating prescribed according to NAEPP guidelines. The assumption of homogeneity of variance was not violated. The overall PACQLQ scores were statistically significant for the four asthma severity groups, $F(2, 101) = 4.942$, $p = .003$. The effect size, calculated using eta squared, was .132. Post hoc comparisons using Tukey's honestly significant different (HSD) test indicated that the mean score for the mild intermittent group ($M = 5.25$, $SD = 1.18$) was significantly different from that of the moderate persistent group ($M = 4.31$, $SD = 1.21$) and that of the severe persistent group ($M = 4.11$, $SD = 1.49$). Table 4 provides the details of these analyses.

ANOVAs to compare activity limitation scores showed statistical significance in overall PACQLQ scores for the four asthma severity groups, $F(3, 101) = 7.56$, $p = .0005$. The effect size, calculated using eta squared, was .189. Post hoc comparisons using Tukey's HSD test indicated that the mean score for the mild intermittent group ($M = 5.37$, $SD = 1.31$) was significantly different from that of the moderate persistent group ($M = 4.02$, $SD = 1.75$) and that of the severe persistent group ($M = 3.55$, $SD = 1.91$). The mild persistent group ($M = 5.13$, $SD = 1.25$) was significantly different from the severe persistent group ($M = 3.55$, $SD = 1.91$).

ANOVA comparisons of emotional function scores showed statistical significance in PACQLQ scores for the four asthma severity groups, $F(3, 101) = 2.855$, $p = .041$. The effect

| TABLE 1 | DEMOGRAPHIC CHARACTERISTICS BY MEANS ($N = 101$) | | |
|---|---|---|---|
| **CAREGIVER OR CHILD CHARACTERISTICS** | | *M* | *SD* |
| Child | | | |
| Age (years) | | 10.26 | 2.78 |
| Length of diagnosis (years) | | 6.49 | 3.90 |
| ER visits in the past year | | 1.01 | 1.98 |
| Hospitalizations in the past year | | 0.25 | 0.79 |
| School days missed in the past year | | 5.85 | 9.24 |
| Caregiver | | | |
| Age (years) | | 39.34 | 7.71 |
| Workdays missed in the past year | | 4.46 | 7.43 |
| Number of people living in home | | 3.67 | 1.78 |
| Number of children living in home | | 2.63 | 1.21 |

size, calculated using eta squared, was .08. Post hoc comparisons using Tukey's HSD test showed no significant differences among the four groups of asthma severity.

Univariate linear regression was used to determine which asthma severity and sociodemographic factors predicted parental QOL scores. Prior to performing linear regression, the data set was assessed for multicollinearity, singularity, outliers, normality, linearity, homoscedasticity, and independence of residuals. Predictor of better QOL included increased income. Factors predicting poor QOL included increased hospitalization days, increased ER visits, and increased school days and workdays missed (Table 5). The significant variables (i.e., income, ER visits, hospitalization days, school days missed, and workdays missed) were further tested using multiple linear regression. Relationships between ER visits and mean total PACQLQ scores, mean activity limitation scores, and mean emotional function scores were significant. The correlation between the mean activity limitation score and workdays missed ($\beta = -.069, p < .043, r^2 = .317$) was also significant (Table 6).

Independent t tests were performed to compare the mean PACQLQ scores between different paired groups of sociodemographic factors (i.e., male vs female, owning a home vs renting, and other groups). Prior to performing the data analyses, the samples were checked for normal distribution, homogeneity of variance, independence of observations, and level of measurement. Parents who were not Black or African, owned a car, were able to pay health costs, owned a home, and perceived their children's asthma as under control had higher mean total, mean activity limitation, and mean emotional function PACQLQ scores.

## 5. Discussion

The main finding in this study is that higher levels of asthma severity reflected decreased PACQLQ scores, or decreased parental QOL. This current study affirms findings by Williams et al. (2000), who also found a negative correlation between PACQLQ scores for parents and their children's asthma severity scores over a period of 4 months ($r = -.39, p < .001$). They also found that PACQLQ scores were correlated negatively with the number of days missed from school ($r = -.24, p < .001$), which this study supports. One explanation may be that parental QOL is affected by concerns of rising medical expenses with increasing asthma

| TABLE 2 | DEMOGRAPHIC CHARACTERISTICS BY PERCENTAGES ($N = 101$) | | |
|---|---|---|---|
| **CAREGIVER OR CHILD CHARACTERISTICS** | **%** | **CAREGIVER OR CHILD CHARACTERISTICS** | **%** |
| Child | | Parent with medically diagnosed | 38.6 |
| Male | 55.4 | asthma | |
| Female | 44.6 | Family history of asthma | 73.3 |
| Caregiver | | Smokers | 9.9 |
| Male | 20.8 | Employed | 69.3 |
| Female | 79.2 | Work hours per week[a] | |
| Age | | <40 | 24.5 |
| ≤30 years | 11.9 | ≥40 | 42.1 |
| >30 years | 87.1 | Education | |
| Martial status | | High school | 32.7 |
| Single | 12.9 | College | 58.4 |
| Married | 64.4 | Graduate school | 8.9 |
| Separated/Divorced | 18.8 | Annual income[a] | |
| Living with significant other | 4.0 | Less than $30,000 | 15.8 |
| Ethnicity | | $30,000 to $45,000 | 18.8 |
| White/Caucasian | 58.4 | $45,000 to $60,000 | 10.9 |
| Hispanic | 20.8 | $60,000 to $75,000 | 9.9 |
| Black/African | 15.8 | Greater than $75,000 | 12.0 |
| Other | 5.0 | Insurance | |
| Caregiver type | | No insurance | 5.0 |
| Mother | 75.2 | Medicaid | 16.8 |
| Father | 18.8 | Private insurance | 78.2 |
| Other | 6.0 | Ability to pay for health expenses | 86.1 |
| Parent perception of control | 74.3 | Residence type | |
| Owning a vehicle | 95 | Own | 68.3 |
| Language | | Rent | 29.7 |
| English | 89.1 | Family or friend support | 88.1 |
| Spanish | 4.0 | | |
| English and Spanish | 5.9 | | |

[a] $n = 72$.

severity, stress related to the disease process, availability of social support, access to medical care and appropriate medication, and the impact of asthma on daily activities in the home (Annett, Bender, DuHamel, & Lapidus, 2003; Erickson et al., 2002).

Participants grouped by asthma severity according to NAEPP guidelines showed significant differences in PACQLQ scores. As asthma severity increased, mean parental PACQLQ scores decreased, indicating decreased QOL ($df = 3$, $F = 7.56$, $p = .0005$, $\eta^2 = .189$). This finding indicates that parents of children with mild asthma claimed better QOL. This suggests that children with higher asthma severity require levels of care that place greater activity restriction and emotional responsibility on parents.

In this current study, several sociodemographic factors were shown to influence parental QOL, some of which do not support current findings in the literature. For example, increased ER visits were significantly related to decreased overall QOL in this study. This is contrary to findings by Halterman et al. (2004), who identified increased symptom-free

### TABLE 3 CORRELATION BETWEEN ASTHMA SEVERITY RATING AND PACQLQ SCORES

| ASTHMA SEVERITY MEASURE | ACTIVITY LIMITATION SUBSCALE ($\rho$) | EMOTIONAL FUNCTION SUBSCALE ($\rho$) | PACQLQ SUMMARY SCORES ($\rho$) |
|---|---|---|---|
| Asthma severity | −.40** | −.26** | −.34** |
| Day symptoms | −.43** | −.29** | −.37** |
| Exercise symptoms | −.44** | −.30** | −.39** |
| Night symptoms | −.48** | −.33** | −.43** |
| Rescue inhaler use | −.31** | ns | ns |
| ER visits | −.45** | −.41** | −.46** |
| Hospitalization days | −.22* | −.20* | −.24* |
| Parental perception of asthma severity | −.58** | −.49** | −.58** |
| Parental perception of control | −.37** | −.28** | −.34** |
| School days missed | −.36** | −.24** | −.31** |
| Workdays missed | −.49** | −.24* | −.37** |
| Annual income | .36** | .29* | .35** |

*Note.* $\rho$ = Spearman $\rho$; *ns* = not significant.
* $p < 0.05$.
** $p < 0.001$.

### TABLE 4 PACQLQ SCORES AND RESEARCHER RATING OF ASTHMA SEVERITY

| ASTHMA SEVERITY RATING BY CAREGIVER | ACTIVITY LIMITATION SUBSCALE, *M (SD)*[a] | EMOTIONAL FUNCTION SUBSCALE, *M (SD)*[b] | PACQLQ SUMMARY SCORES, *M (SD)*[c] |
|---|---|---|---|
| Mild intermittent | 5.37 (1.31) | 5.20 (1.22) | 5.25 (1.18) |
| Mild persistent | 5.13 (1.25) | 4.68 (1.14) | 4.82 (0.95) |
| Moderate persistent | 4.02 (1.75) | 4.43 (1.14) | 4.31 (1.21) |
| Severe persistent | 3.55 (1.91) | 4.36 (1.51) | 4.11 (1.49) |

[a] $df = 3$, $F = 7.56$, $p = .0005$, $\eta^2 = .189$.
[b] $df = 3$, $F = 2.855$, $p = .041$, $\eta^2 = .08$.
[c] $df = 2$, $F = 4.942$, $p = .003$, $\eta^2 = .132$.

days and the parental perceptions of asthma control. They did not find ER visits to be a significant factor associated with parental QOL. Instead, their predictive factors of worse QOL included Hispanic ethnicity, use of daily maintenance medication, and secondhand smoke exposure in the home. Research by Erickson et al. (2002) and Annett et al. (2003) were more closely aligned with findings from this study.

Several studies suggested that the prevalence and severity of asthma are associated with ethnicity and poverty-related factors such as young maternal age, maternal cigarette smoking, low birth weight, and living in crowded conditions in the inner city (Williams et al., 2009). This study supported the idea that sociodemographic factors also influence parental perception of QOL. A family history of asthma; being single, divorced, or widowed; and perceived poor asthma control yielded significantly lower PACQLQ scores.

| TABLE 5 | UNIVARIATE REGRESSION MODEL PREDICTING QOL | | | | | |
|---|---|---|---|---|---|---|
| **PREDICTOR** | **ACTIVITY LIMITATION SUBSCALE** | | **EMOTIONAL FUNCTION SUBSCALE** | | **PACQLQ SUMMARY SCORES** | |
| | *B* | $R^2$ | *B* | $R^2$ | *B* | $R^2$ |
| Annual income | .23 | .08*** | ns | ns | .11 | .05* |
| Hospitalization days | −.57 | .06* | ns | ns | −.30 | .03** |
| ER visits | −.33 | .15** | −.20 | .09** | −.24 | .13** |
| School days missed | −.08 | .18** | −.03 | .04* | −.05 | .10*** |
| Workdays missed | −.11 | .21** | −.04 | .05* | −.06 | .12* |

Note. *B* = unstandardized beta coefficient; $R^2$ = adjusted $r^2$; ns = not significant.
* $p < 0.05$.
** $p < 0.005$.
*** $p < 0.001$.

| TABLE 6 | MULTIPLE REGRESSION MODELS PREDICTING QOL | | | | | |
|---|---|---|---|---|---|---|
| **PREDICTOR** | **ACTIVITY LIMITATION SUBSCALE** | | **EMOTIONAL FUNCTION SUBSCALE** | | **PACQLQ SUMMARY SCORES** | |
| | *B* | $R^2$ | *B* | $R^2$ | *B* | $R^2$ |
| ER visits | −.25 | .32* | −.18 | .08* | −.20 | .19* |
| Workdays missed | −.07 | .32* | ns | ns | ns | ns |

Note. *B* = unstandardized beta coefficient; $R^2$ = adjusted $r^2$; ns = not significant.
* $p < 0.05$.

Correlational analyses of mean PACQLQ scores and sociodemographic factors revealed different findings from other studies. For example, Osman et al. (2001) found sociodemographic factors such as being a young mother, being from less affluent families, and having increased socioeconomic deprivation scores also scored lower on the PACQLQ. Dalheim-Englund, Rydstrom, Rasmussen, Moller, and Sandman (2004) found another set of sociodemographic factors; place of residence, age of the child, and severity of the child's asthma impacted PACQLQ scores. These findings suggest that many factors in addition to asthma severity can influence parental QOL, which is similar to this study's findings.

The strengths of this study included the close timing of actual events and responses to the questionnaires. The PACQLQ and asthma severity questionnaires ask questions within the past week and past month, respectively. Because parents would better remember important events related to their children's asthma within these time frames, this reduced the risk of recall error and improved accuracy of reporting the data (Reichenberg & Broberg, 2001). The PACQLQ was studied to be both reliable and responsive with moderate validity (Juniper et al., 1996), which strengthened the results obtained. Many studies used the PACQLQ showing reliability and validity (Dalheim-Englund et al., 2004; Laforest et al., 2004; Osman et al., 2001; Reichenberg et al., 2001).

This study had several limitations. First, utilizing a cross-sectional study design provides a snapshot of the lives of children with asthma and their parents at a specific point in time, and answers to the questionnaires could have been different if a longer period or a different period (seasonal influence of certain types of asthma) was used (Dalheim-Englund et al., 2004; Reichenberg et al., 2001). Ideally, a longitudinal research study would provide ongoing changes in QOL as related to changes in life events related to asthma. Another limitation is selection bias because some parents were more willing to participate in the study due to the manifestation of their children's asthma severity.

## 6. Conclusion and Recommendations

The evidence presented in this study supports the idea that numerous factors such as asthma severity and sociodemographic factors are capable of influencing QOL. Measuring parental QOL can help to develop more effective asthma programs that take the experiences of parents into consideration (Halterman et al., 2004), an important component for successful medical and nursing care.

One area for future research is to test a larger number of participants over a longer period in multiple settings. Examining a larger number of participants in different settings allows assessment for study consistency, and the longitudinal design may account for changing sociodemographic and asthma severity on QOL. Several other measures such as parents' own physical disabilities, coping abilities, psychological health, family context, and other unknown factors may be revealed in a longitudinal study design. Recent studies suggest that psychological factors and parents' mental health influence PACQLQ scores and health care utilization for their asthmatic children (Dalheim-Englund et al., 2004; Vila et al., 2004). Thus, another area for future research should be to examine other factors besides asthma severity and sociodemographic factors that may influence QOL. To determine if other factors influence QOL, instrumentation research to develop other measurement tools aside from the PACQLQ needs to occur.

Supporting previous research findings, this current study helped affirm the idea that nurses working with families of asthmatic children need to aggressively provide care through patient education and vigilant monitoring. This study showed that asthma severity is closely aligned with parental QOL. Understanding this relationship, nurses can positively influence care by assuring tight control of asthma severity, and even reversing the asthma severity category of patients has the potential to elevate QOL for both parents and asthmatic children especially in families that are the most vulnerable.

## REFERENCES

Akinbami, L. J., & Schoendorf, K. C. (2002). Trends in childhood asthma: prevalence, health care utilization, and mortality. *Pediatrics, 110,* 315–322.

Annett, R. D., Bender, B. G., DuHamel, T. R., & Lapidus, J. (2003). Factors influencing parent reports on quality of life for children with asthma. *Journal of Asthma, 40,* 577–587.

Dalheim-Englund, A., Rydstrom, I., Rasmussen, B. H., Moller, C., & Sandman, P. (2004). Having a child with asthma—quality of life for Swedish parents. *Journal of Clinical Nursing, 13,* 386–395.

Dean, B. B., Calimlim, B. M., Kindermann, S. L., Khandker, R. K., & Tinkelman, D. (2009). The impact of uncontrolled asthma on absenteeism and health-related quality of life. *Journal of Asthma, 46,* 861–866.

Erickson, S. R., Munzenberger, P. J., Plante, M. J., Kirking, D. M., Hurwitz, M., & Vanuya, R. Z. (2002). Influence of sociodemographic factors on the health-related quality of life of pediatric patients with asthma and their caregivers. *Journal of Asthma, 39,* 107–117.

Halterman, J. S., Yoos, H. L., Conn, K. M., Callahan, P. M., Montes, G., & Neely, T. L., et al. (2004). The impact of childhood asthma on parental quality of life. *Journal of Asthma, 41*, 645–653.

Juniper, E. F., Guyatt, G. H., Feeny, P. J., Ferrie, L. E., & Townsend, M. (1996). Measuring quality of life in the parents of children with asthma. *Quality of Life Research, 5*, 27–34.

Laforest, L., Yin, D., Kocevar, V. S., Pacheco, Y., Dickson, N., & Gormand, F, et al. (2004). Association between asthma control in children and loss of workdays by caregivers. *Annals of Allergy, Asthma, and Immunology, 93*, 265–271.

Marsac, M. L., Funk, J. B., & Nelson, L. (2006). Coping styles, psychological functioning and quality of life in children with asthma. *Child: Care, Health and Development, 33*, 360–367.

Moonie, S., Sterling, D. A., Figgs, L. W., & Castro, M. (2006). Asthma status and severity affects missed school days. *Journal of School Health, 76*, 18–24.

National Asthma Education and Prevention Program (NAEPP). (2007). *Guidelines for the diagnosis and management of asthma (EPR-3)*. Retrieved from http://www.nhlbi.nih.gov/guidelines/asthma/index.htm

National Center for Health Statistics (NCHS). (2007). *Asthma prevalence, health care use and mortality: United States, 2003–2005*. Retrieved from http://www.cdc.gov/nchs/products/pubs/pubd/hestats/ashtma03-05/asthma03-05.htm

Osman, L. M., Baxter-Jones, A. D. G., & Helms, P. J. (2001). Parents' quality of life and respiratory symptoms in young children with mild wheeze. *European Respiratory Journal, 17*, 254–258.

Reichenberg, K., & Broberg, A. G. (2001). The paediatric asthma caregiver's quality of life questionnaire in Swedish parents. *Acta Paediatrica, International Journal of Paediatrics, 90*, 45–50.

Vila, G., Hayder, R., Bertrand, C., Falissard, B., De Blic, J., & Mouren-Simeoni, M., et al. (2004). Psychopathology and quality of life for adolescents with asthma and their parents. *Psychosomatics, 44*, 319–328.

Williams, D. R., Sternthal, M., & Wright, R. J. (2009). Social determinants: taking the social context of asthma seriously. *Pediatrics, 123*, S174–S184.

Williams, S., Sehgal, M., Falter, K., Dennis, R., Jones, D., Boudreaux, J., et al. (2000). Effect of asthma on the quality of life among children and their caregivers in the Atlanta Empowerment Zone. *Journal of Urban Health: Bulletin of the New York Academy of Medicine, 77*, 268–279.

## THE CRITIQUE

This is a critical appraisal of the article, "Asthma severity in children and the quality of life of their parents" (Cerdan et al., 2012) to determine its usefulness for nursing practice.

### PROBLEM AND PURPOSE

Quality of life (QOL) is related to health status of an individual, and when assessing patients with chronic illness, it is important to assess how the illness is affecting the child and family. The purpose of this study is clearly stated as follows: "This descriptive, cross-sectional study examines the effect of asthma severity on caregivers' QOL."

### REVIEW OF THE LITERATURE

The introduction of the article explains that asthma is one of the most common chronic diseases in the US, affecting more than 6.5 million children. The review of the literature describes how asthma affects the child in terms of time needed for medical visits, hospitalizations, school attendance, and family dynamics, among others. Parents have to care for the child and may also be at risk for functional limitations that may be affected by impairment in quality of life.

This study fills a gap in the nursing literature owing to the holistic focus when addressing asthmatic children and their parents in the clinical setting. Operationalizing parental QOL measures as functional limitations and emotional dimensions allows nurse researchers to quantify the degree of burden that parents experience so that more effective asthma programs can be developed (Halterman et al., 2004). In addition, being familiar with the NAEPP (2007) guidelines in daily practice, nurses can better identify at-risk parents of asthmatic children to more quickly implement appropriate care. QOL has been shown to be an important outcome measure, and being aware of its effect on the individual is important for adherence to medical treatment (Marsac et al., 2006).

### RESEARCH QUESTIONS
The objective of this study was to examine the effect of children's asthma severity and sociodemographic factors on parental QOL. It would not be appropriate to use hypotheses to guide this study because of the exploratory, nonexperimental design.

### SAMPLE
A convenience sample of parents of 101 children (age 7 to 17 years) with mild to intermittent to severe asthma were recruited from a pediatric pulmonology clinic. A strength of the study is that parents of children age 7 to 17 years were targeted for sample recruitment because they were similar to the parents and children who were used to validate the QOL instrument used in the study. The clinic was chosen by the investigators because the clinic had patients with a greater variety of asthma severity (i.e., mild, moderate, or severe) and a diverse set of sociodemographic factors (e.g., health insurance coverage, parental age and ethnicity). The sample size was not justified with use of power analysis. Given the exploratory nature of the study, the sampling procedure is adequate, but the results must be interpreted cautiously because of limited generalizability.

### RESEARCH DESIGN
A descriptive, correlational design was used providing Level IV evidence. Data were collected at one time point (cross-sectional). This is a nonexperimental study because no randomization was done and there is no manipulation of the independent variables, nor is there a control group. The relationship of the variables can be explored, but no causality can be inferred. It is important to note that although this study provides a lower level of evidence than an RCT, as long as the design is sound and appropriate for the research questions, it may provide preliminary data to support future intervention studies. Since there is a gap in the literature, the findings of this study may provide the best available evidence.

### THREATS TO INTERNAL VALIDITY
No threats from history, mortality (or attrition), or maturation affect this study. The instruments used to measure QOL and asthma severity do not have adequate psychometric properties, which may affect the ability to adequately measure the outcome variables. This is discussed further in the "Instruments" section.

### THREATS TO EXTERNAL VALIDITY
As this is a convenience sample, potential bias may unknowingly be introduced, limiting generalizability of the results. The sample is predominantly Caucasian (58%); however,

there is representation from Latino (21%) and African-American (16%) participants. The authors specifically chose this clinic for its ethnic diversity, which is a strength.

### RESEARCH METHODS

One researcher reviewed the charts of scheduled patients to ensure asthma diagnosis and age, and approached parents or legal guardians in the waiting room. It appears that data collection methods were carried out consistently with each participant, although there was no mention of training or supervision of the data collectors to ensure systematic collection of data.

### LEGAL-ETHICAL ISSUES

The protocol was approved by the appropriate institutional review board. Those who agreed to participate completed the informed consent, and their children offered assent.

### INSTRUMENTS

The Pediatric Asthma Caregiver's Quality of Life Questionnaire (PACQLQ), a 13-item questionnaire, measures activity limitation and emotional function in children and adolescents with asthma (Juniper et al., 1996). Reliability data are acceptable with an intraclass correlation coefficient for overall QOL = .85, emotional function = .80, and activity limitation = .84, but no validity data are reported. The Asthma Severity Questionnaire was developed by the researchers for use in this study, and the content was based on the National Asthma Education and Prevention Program (NAEPP) Guidelines for the diagnosis and management of asthma (2007). The questionnaire was reviewed by two content experts but not piloted before use in this study.

### RELIABILITY AND VALIDITY

That the instruments used in this study do not demonstrate adequate psychometric properties is a weakness and leads to questions about the accuracy with which the tools measure the variables.

### DATA ANALYSIS

To assess the relationship between asthma severity and parental QOL, Spearman's correlation, ANOVA, and linear and multivariate regressions were appropriately calcuated. To determine the relationship between sociodemographic factors and parental QOL, Spearman's correlation, chi-square, and independent t tests were performed. Although not specifically stated, it appears that significance was set at .05. Three tables appropriately were used to visually display the data.

### CONCLUSIONS, IMPLICATIONS, AND RECOMMENDATIONS

For parents of asthmatic children, there was a negative correlation between overall asthma severity and QOL score. As asthma severity and other asthma factors increased, PACQLQ scores decreased, indicating poorer QOL. This finding indicates that parents of children with mild asthma claimed better QOL. This suggests that children with higher asthma severity require levels of care that place greater activity restriction and emotional responsibility on parents.

### APPLICATION TO NURSING PRACTICE

This nonexperimental, correlational study provides data that may eventually lead to an intervention study. The findings support the association between overall asthma severity in children and QOL score in parents. The strengths outweigh the weaknesses, although the results must be interpreted with caution because of limited generalizability. The risks are minimal, and there are no potential benefits to the individual subjects, but there may be a benefit to the greater society by the dissemination of findings in the literature and applicability to future studies. Further longitudinal studies would be useful to confirm this.

## ■ CRITICAL THINKING CHALLENGES

- Discuss how the stylistic considerations of a journal affect the researcher's ability to present the research findings of a quantitative report.
- Discuss how the limitations of a research study affect generalizability of the findings.
- Discuss how you differentiate the "critical appraisal" process from simply "criticizing" a research report.
- Analyze how threats to internal and external validity affect the strength and quality of evidence provided by the findings of a research study.
- How would a staff nurse who has just critically appraised the study by Sherman and colleagues determine whether the findings of this study were applicable to practice?

## REFERENCES

Cerdan, N. S., Alpert, P. T., Moonie, S., et al. (2012). Asthma severity in children and the quality of life of their parents. *Applied Nursing Research*, 25, 131–137.

Sherman, D. W., Haber, J., Hoskins, C. N., et al. (2012). The effects of psychoeducation and telephone counseling on the adjustment of women with early-stage breast cancer. *Applied Nursing Research*, 25, 3–16.

# ℮volve WEBSITE

*Go to Evolve at http://evolve.elsevier.com/LoBiondo/ for review questions, critiquing exercises, and additional research articles for practice in reviewing and critiquing.*

# PART IV

# Application of Research: Evidence-Based Practice

**Research Vignette: Ann Kurth**

# RESEARCH VIGNETTE

## INCORPORATING INFORMATION AND COMMUNICATION TECHNOLOGY TOOLS FOR HIV INTO PRACTICE

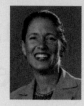

**Ann Kurth, RN, PhD, FAAN**
**Professor and Executive Director**
**New York University College of Nursing, Global Division**
**New York, New York**

As the largest cadre of health providers globally, nursing has been on the frontlines of human immunodeficiency virus (HIV) prevention, care, and research. However, even in resource-rich settings like the United States, there is often not enough staff time or resources to provide evidence-based counseling to reduce secondary HIV transmission (prevention with positives) or to prevent primary HIV infection. The literature consistently shows that many providers, including nurses, do not routinely assess sexual risks of their patients—even in HIV clinics—leading to missed opportunities to improve the sexual health of persons living with HIV (PLWH) and their partners. Providing evidence-based support for adherence to life-saving antiretroviral therapy (ART) is inconsistently provided, especially in low-income countries such as sub-Saharan Africa, where two thirds of all PLWH globally reside, yet which has fewer than 3% of the world's health care workers and less than 1% of all global health expenditures.

I was in nursing school in the mid-1980s when the HIV epidemic was burgeoning in New York City. Before that I had been conducting research in Malawi, East Africa, when awareness of HIV as an etiologic agent and social decimator was not yet widespread. With more ART availability in sub-Saharan Africa and with leaders calling for an end to perinatal HIV transmission, and other "getting to zero [incident infection]" targets, the survival of men, women and children is increasing.[1]

These inspiring goals make addressing health provider constraints more urgent. It was this recognition of unmet patient counseling needs that has driven much of my research focus. How can we expand the support options for people at risk for, or already living with, HIV without overburdening strained health systems? One avenue to explore was the use of self-administered counseling, specifically using computers and handheld devices to deliver tailored, interactive counseling elements shown to work in randomized trials (Kamb et al., 1998; O'Donnell et al., 1998). My goal was a scalable intervention that minimizes implementation and maintenance costs, providing an option for patients without access to best-practice counseling or an adjunct to those receiving high-quality support from providers for HIV prevention and ART adherence.

While a doctoral student at University of Washington, I worked with an interprofessional team that included medicine, psychology, and software design to submit a grant to the Centers for Disease Control and Prevention (CDC) to develop a computerized counseling software tool. The resultant CARE (Computer Assessment and Risk Reduction Education) counseling software has now evolved through a scientific sequence applied to a range

---

[1] See http://www.un.org/en/events/aidsday/ for 2015 goals. Accessed 2/1/2013.

of clinical content, target populations, and languages. Our studies have evaluated using the tool to facilitate rapid HIV testing (Test CARE) and to address ART adherence and prevention with PLWH (CARE+). CARE/CARE+ content has been modified for delivery to populations in the U. S. and in Kenya in languages including English, Spanish, and Kiswahili, and a version has been used to conduct field surveys of pesticide exposure among migrant workers (Hofmann et al., 2010).

Leveraging our interprofessional expertise and user-centered design (Kurth et al., 2006), we first built a general HIV/STI risk reduction tool using literature review, expert input, and iterative testing of the software user interface in street intercept reviews (Hendry et al., 2005). The beta version of CARE underwent "think aloud" usability testing with male and female patients (ages 18 to 64 years; 60% nonwhite) and then feasibility testing in five clinics in three U.S. cities. That mixed-method evaluation using participant observation and interviews and staff focus groups found that participants (58% nonwhite) used CARE with minimal to no assistance even among non–computer-literate users. CARE usefulness was rated an average of 8.2 on an ascending utility scale of 0 to 10. Honesty, reduced time constraints, privacy, and lack of judgment associated with CARE appeared to enhance self-evaluation, which can be important in moving patients toward behavior change. Clinic staff felt that this tool could help expand services, standardize education, and support behavioral priming (Mackenzie et al., 2007).

Our team then developed a version to expand access to rapid HIV testing, given that knowledge of HIV infection is the portal to life-saving treatment and can in itself result in behavioral risk reduction. I received an NIAID New Investigator award to modify the CARE platform to add elements of HIV consent and data elements that the CDC required HIV test sites to report. We assessed feasibility and acceptability of the Test CARE tool in emergency departments (EDs) in Seattle and Baltimore. Nearly all respondents at both sites rated the tool as useful, with 90% rating the tool >7 (0-10 ascending scale). When asked about HIV/STI counseling preferences, 58% preferred a computer and 24% a person (Spielberg et al., 2011a). We went on to assess the tool in a randomized comparison of the Test CARE session with rapid HIV testing, compared with what was then standard at the public tertiary care hospital ED in Seattle (i.e., HIV testing only if patient was symptomatic or requested a test). Results regarding acceptability and costs were promising (Kurth et al., 2013). Test CARE also was used by a mobile HIV testing van and was found to double the number of HIV tests staff were able to do and to shorten the program reporting-reimbursement cycle for the agency (Spielberg et al., 2011b). Test CARE is now being used in a HIV testing study among high-risk heterosexuals in NYC, among drug court attendees in Philadelphia and New York City, and among returning citizens released from Rikers Island Prison.

I received a K01 award from the CDC to create and evaluate the CARE+ tool focusing on positive prevention and ART adherence among PLWH. I added a pharmacist, a psychologist, and several infectious disease/HIV physicians to this team to help modify the content using formative research and the evidence base for ART adherence (Amico et al., 2006; Simoni et al., 2006) and secondary transmission risk reduction (Richardson et al., 2004; Fisher et al, 2006). Usability testing documented that participants felt they were able to get information, that the computer modality reduced social desirability and human counselor variability, and that non–computer-literate persons found the tablet computer accessible. Average time for session completion suggested a rapid learning curve; psychometric performance of key variables was reasonable. We undertook a randomized controlled trial (RCT) in two sites in Seattle (Kurth et al, 2007). This 9-month RCT showed an intervention effect in terms of HIV-1 viral load reduction, ART adherence improvement, and declines in some key self-reported HIV transmission sexual risk behaviors (article under submission).

Based on previous work, as well as work carried out in Kenya with PLWH, nurses, and other providers, we have now codified a cultural contextualization methodology for adapting the software with new clinical and sociobehavioral content, languages, or target user groups (Kurth et al, 2010). There are now several RCTs of CARE+ intervention versions underway or just completed, several of which include economic evaluations: in New York City for Spanish-speaking Latinos; in Kenya; a Washington, DC version focusing on linkage to HIV care for returning citizens recently released from correctional facilities; and Bronx and DC versions focusing on positive prevention. From these studies we will learn about the utility of computerized counseling in the real world—where every person with HIV disease, and every nurse partner, can promote healthy lives.

# REFERENCES

Amico, K. R., Harman, J. J., & Johnson, B. T. (2006). Efficacy of antiretroviral therapy adherence interventions: a research synthesis of trials, 1996 to 2004. *Journal of Acquired Immune Deficiency Syndromes, 41*(3), 285–297.

Fisher, J. D., Fisher, W. A., Cornman, D. H., et al. (2006). Clinician-delivered intervention during routine clinical care reduces unprotected sexual behavior among HIV-infected patients. *Journal of Acquired Immune Deficiency Syndromes, 41*(1), 44–52. (See also Fisher, J. D., Cornman, D. H., Osborn, C. Y., et al. (2004). Clinician-initiated HIV risk reduction intervention for HIV-positive persons: formative research, acceptability, and fidelity of the options project. *Journal of Acquired Immune Deficiency Syndromes, 37*, S78–S87.)

Hendry, D. G., Mackenzie, S., Kurth, A., et al. (2005). Evaluating paper prototypes on the street. In G. C. van der Veer, & C. Gale (Eds.), *Extended Abstract Proceedings of the 2005 Conference on Human Factors in Computing Systems* (pp. 1447–1450). New York, NY: ACM Press. Available at http://doi.acm.org/10.1145/1056808.1056938

Hofmann, J. N., Checkoway, H., Borges, O., et al. (2010). Development of a computer-based survey instrument for organophosphate and N-methyl-carbamate exposure assessment among agricultural pesticide handlers. *Annals of Occupational Hygiene, 54*(6), 640–650.

Kamb, M. L., Fishbein, M., Douglas, J. M., Jr., et al. for the Project RESPECT Study Group. (1998). Efficacy of risk-reduction counseling to prevent human immunodeficiency virus and sexually transmitted diseases: a randomized controlled trial. *Journal of the American Medical Association, 280*(13), 1161–1167.

Kurth, A., Baliddawa, J., Were, M., et al. (2010, November). User-centered design for mobile health intervention content in a low-income setting. 3rd Annual National Institute of Health Summit, Washington, DC..

Kurth, A., Clausen, M., Severynen, A., et al. (2007, April). A randomized clinical trial of a computer counseling intervention to support antiretroviral therapy adherence and HIV transmission risk reduction: baseline findings. 2nd Annual International Conference on HIV Treatment and Adherence, Jersey City, NJ.

Kurth, A., Severynen, A., & Spielberg, F. (2013). Addressing unmet need for HIV testing in emergency care settings: a role for computer-facilitated rapid HIV testing. [In Press.]

Kurth, A., Spielberg, F., Mackenzie, S., et al. (2006, May). Development and software usability testing of an interactive computer counseling tool to reduce STI risk. National STD Prevention Conference, Jacksonville, FL.

Mackenzie, S. L., Kurth, A. E., Spielberg, F., et al. (2007). Patient and staff perspectives on the use of a computer counseling tool for HIV and sexually transmitted infection risk reduction. *Journal of Adolescent Health, 40*(6), 572.e9–572.e16.

O'Donnell, C. R., O'Donnell, L., San Doval, A., et al. (1998). Reductions in STD infections subsequent to an STD clinic visit: using video-based patient education. *Sexually Transmitted Diseases, 25*(3), 161–168.

Richardson, J. L., Milam, J., McCutchan, A., et al. (2004). Effect of brief safer-sex counseling by medical providers to HIV-1 seropositive patients: a multi-clinic assessment. *Journal of Acquired Immune Deficiency Syndromes, 18*(8), 1179–1186.

Simoni, J., Pearson, C., Pantalone, D., et al. (2006). Efficacy of interventions in improving highly active antiretroviral therapy adherence and HIV-1 RNA viral load: a meta-analytic review of randomized controlled trials. *Journal of Acquired Immune Deficiency Syndromes, 43*(Suppl 1), S23–35.

Spielberg, F., Kurth, A., Severynen, A., et al. (2011a). Computer-facilitated rapid HIV testing in emergency care settings: provider and patient usability and acceptability. *AIDS Education & Prevention, 23*(3), 206–221.

Spielberg, F., Kurth, A., Reidy, W., et al. (2011b). Iterative evaluation in a mobile counseling and testing program to reach people of color at risk for HIV: new strategies improve program acceptability, effectiveness, and evaluation capabilities. *AIDS Education & Prevention, 23*(Suppl 3), 110–116.

# CHAPTER 19

# Strategies and Tools for Developing an Evidence-Based Practice

*Carl A. Kirton*

## ℮volve WEBSITE

*Go to Evolve at http://evolve.elsevier.com/LoBiondo/ for review questions, critiquing exercises, and additional research articles for practice in reviewing and critiquing.*

## LEARNING OUTCOMES

*After reading this chapter, you should be able to do the following:*

- Identify the key elements of a focused clinical question.
- Discuss the use of databases to search the literature.
- Screen a research article for relevance and validity.
- Critically appraise study results and apply the findings to practice.
- Make clinical decisions based on evidence from the literature combined with clinical expertise and patient preferences.

## KEY TERMS

absolute risk reduction
confidence interval
control event rate
electronic index
experimental event rate
information literacy

likelihood ratio
negative likelihood
  ratio
negative predictive
  value
null value

number needed to treat
odds ratio
positive likelihood
  ratio
positive predictive
  value

prefiltered evidence
relative risk
relative risk reduction
sensitivity
specificity

In today's environment of knowledge explosion, new investigations are published at a frequency with which even seasoned practitioners have a hard time keeping pace. With so much new information, maintaining a clinical practice that is based on new evidence can be challenging. However, the development of evidence-based nursing practice is contingent on applying new and important evidence to clinical practice. A few simple techniques will help you move to a practice that is evidence oriented. This chapter will assist you in becoming a more efficient and effective reader of the professional literature. Through a few important tools and a crisp understanding of the important components of a study, you will be able to use an evidence base to determine the merits of a study for your practice and for your patients.

Consider the case of a nurse who uses evidence from the literature to support her practice:

> Nancy Sanchez is a staff registered nurse who works on a general medical unit; she is also a member of her hospital's clinical practice committee. The committee is revising its fall protocol and wants to use best practices supported by the literature for each specific nursing intervention. It has been recommended to purchase bed alarms as part of the hospital's fall prevention program. Nancy decides to consult the literature to evaluate the effectiveness of bed alarms to prevent falls on a general medical unit.

## EVIDENCE-BASED TOOL #1: ASKING A FOCUSED CLINICAL QUESTION

Developing a focused clinical question will help Nancy to focus on the relevant issue and prepare her for subsequent steps in the evidence-based practice process (see Chapters 1, 2, and 3). A focused clinical question using the PICO format (see Chapters 2 and 3) is developed by answering the following four questions:

1. What is the *population* I am interested in?
2. What is the *intervention* I am interested in?
3. What will this intervention be *compared* to? (Note: depending on the study design, this step may or may not apply.)
4. How will I know if the intervention makes things better or worse (identify an *outcome* that is measurable)?

As you recall from Chapters 1, 2, and 3, most evidence-based practitioners use the simple mnemonic **PICO** to help recall all of the requirements for a well-designed clinical question (Table 19-1).

> Because Nancy is familiar with the evidence-based practice approach for developing clinical questions, she identifies the four important components and develops the following clinical question: On a general medical unit, does the use of a bed alarm help reduce the incidence of falls in adult patients?

Once a clinical question has been framed, it can be organized into one of four fundamental types of commonly used clinical categories:

1. **Therapy category:** When you want to answer a question about the effectiveness of a particular treatment or intervention, you will select studies that have the following characteristics:
   - Experimental or quasi-experimental study design (see Chapter 9)
   - Outcome known or of probable clinical importance observed over a clinically significant period of time

   When studies are in this category, you use a therapy appraisal tool to evaluate the article. A therapy tool can be accessed at: http://www.casp-uk.net/wp-content/uploads/2011/11/CASP_RCT_Appraisal_Checklist_14oct10.pdf.

| TABLE 19-1 | **USING PICO TO FORMULATE CLINICAL QUESTIONS** | |
|---|---|---|
| **P**atient population | What group do you want information on? | Adults with common warts |
| **I**ntervention (or exposure) | What event do you want to study the effect of? | Duct tape |
| **C**omparison | Compared to what? Better or worse than no intervention at all, or than another intervention? | Physical methods (e.g., cryotherapy) or no intervention at all (e.g., placebo) |
| **O**utcomes | What is the effect of the intervention? | Wart resolution |

Data from Wenner R, Askari SK, Cham PMH, et al: Duct tape for the treatment of common warts in adults: a double-blind randomized controlled trial, *Arch Dermatol* 143(3):309–313, 2007.

2. **Diagnosis category:** When you want to answer a question about the usefulness, accuracy, selection, or interpretation of a particular measurement instrument or laboratory test, you will select studies that have the following characteristics:
   - Cross-sectional study design (see Chapter 10) with people suspected to have the condition of interest
   - Administration to the patient of both the new instrument or diagnostic test and the accepted "gold standard" measure
   - Comparison of the results of the new instrument or test and the "gold standard"
   
   When studies are in this category, you use a diagnostic test appraisal tool to evaluate the article. A diagnostic tool can be accessed at http://www.casp-uk.net/wp-content/uploads/2011/11/CASP_Diagnostic_Appraisal_Checklist_14oct10.pdf.

3. **Prognosis category:** When you want to answer a question about a patient's likely course for a particular disease state or identify factors that may alter the patient's prognosis, you will select studies that have the following characteristics:
   - Nonexperimental, usually longitudinal study of a particular group (cohort) for a particular outcome or disease (see Chapter 10)
   - Follow-up for a clinically relevant period of time (time is the exposure)
   - Determination of factors in those who do and do not develop a particular outcome
   
   When studies are in this category, you use a prognosis appraisal tool (sometimes called a cohort tool) to evaluate the article. A prognosis tool can be accessed at http://www.casp-uk.net/wp-content/uploads/2011/11/CASP_Cohort_Appraisal_Checklist_14oct10.pdf.

4. **Harm category:** When you want to determine whether or not one variable is related to or caused by another, you will select studies that have the following characteristics:
   - Nonexperimental, usually longitudinal or retrospective (ex post facto or case control) study designs over a clinically relevant period of time (see Chapter 10)
   - Assessment of whether or not the patient has been exposed to the independent variable
   
   When studies are in this category, you use a harm appraisal tool (sometimes called a case-control tool) to evaluate the article. A harm tool can be accessed at http://www.casp-uk.net/wp-content/uploads/2011/11/CASP_Case-Control_Appraisal_Checklist_14oct10.pdf.

There are two important reasons for applying clinical categories to the professional literature. First, knowing to which category a clinical question belongs helps you search the literature efficiently (see Chapter 3). Second, these structured tools, based on study research design, help you to systematically appraise the strength and quality of evidence provided in research articles.

## EVIDENCE-BASED TOOL #2: SEARCHING THE LITERATURE

All the skills that Nancy needs to consult the literature and answer a clinical question are conceptually defined as **information literacy**. Your librarian is the best person to help you develop the necessary skills to become information literate. Part of being information literate is having the skills necessary to electronically search the literature to obtain the best evidence for answering your clinical question.

The literature is organized into **electronic indexes** or *databases*. Chapter 3 discusses the differences among databases and how to use these databases to search the literature. One or two sessions with a librarian will help you focus your search to your clinical question. You can also learn how to effectively search databases through a Web-based tutorial located at www.nlm.nih.gov/bsd/disted/pubmed.html#qt.

Using the PubMed database (www.pubmed.gov), Nancy uses the search function and enters the term "bed alarms." This strategy provides her with 92 articles. She does a quick scan and realizes that many of the articles do not answer her clinical question, many are not research studies, and some articles are about alarms other than bed alarms to prevent falls. She recalls that the PubMed database has a clinical queries filter option that finds citations that correspond to a specific clinical category. She reenters the search term "bed alarm" and selects the therapy option (which will only yield articles that use an experimental study design). Her search yields four individual articles with a controlled study design. A careful perusal of the list of articles and a well-designed clinical question help Nancy to select the key articles.

---

### EVIDENCE-BASED PRACTICE TIP

Prefiltered sources of evidence can be found in journal format and electronic format. **Prefiltered evidence** is evidence in which an editorial team has already read and summarized articles on a topic and appraised its relevance to clinical care. Prefiltered sources include *Clinical Evidence,* available online at http://clinicalevidence.com/x/index.html and in print; *Evidence-Based Nursing* is available online at http://ebn.bmjjournals.com and in print.

---

## EVIDENCE-BASED TOOL #3: SCREENING YOUR FINDINGS

Once you have searched and selected the potential articles, how do you know which articles are appropriate to answer your clinical question? This is accomplished by screening the articles for quality, relevance, and credibility by answering the following questions (D'Auria, 2007; Miser, 2000):

1. Is each article from a peer-reviewed journal? Articles published in peer-reviewed journals have had an extensive review and editing process (see Chapter 3).
2. Are the setting and sample of each study similar to mine so that results, if valid, would apply to my practice or to my patient population (see Chapter 12)?
3. Are any of the studies sponsored by an organization that may influence the study design or results (see Chapter 13)?

Your responses to these questions help you decide to what extent you want to appraise an individual article. For example, if the study population is markedly different from the one to which you will apply the results, you may want to consider selecting a more appropriate study. If an article is worth evaluating, you should use the category-specific tool URLs identified in Evidence-Based Tool #1 to critically appraise the article.

Nancy reviews the abstract of the articles retrieved from her PubMed citation lists and selects the following article: "Effects of an Intervention to Increase Bed Alarm Use to Prevent Falls in Hospitalized Patients: A Cluster Randomized Trial" (Schorr et al., 2012). This study was published in 2012 in Annals of Internal Medicine, a peer-reviewed journal. This is a clinical intervention trial that has an experimental design and is a therapy category study. Nancy reads the abstract and finds that the objective of the study was to investigate whether an intervention aimed at increasing bed alarm use decreases hospital falls on one unit compared to usual care (the placebo). The setting of the study was in an urban academically affiliated community hospital. The study authors received funding for this investigation from the National Institute on Aging, and Nancy finds that there were no funding or conflict of interest issues noted. Nancy decides that this study is worth evaluating and selects the therapy category tool.

### HELPFUL HINT

When appraising studies obtained in a search, consider both studies with significant findings (treatment is better) and studies with non significant findings (treatment is worse or there is no difference). Studies reporting non significant findings are more difficult to find but are equally important.

## EVIDENCE-BASED TOOL #4: APPRAISE EACH ARTICLE'S FINDINGS

Applying study results to individual patients or to a specific patient population and communicating study findings to patients in a meaningful way are the hallmark of evidence-based practice. Common evidence-based practice conventions that researchers and research consumers use to appraise and report study results in clinical practice are identified by four different types of clinical categories: therapy, diagnosis (sensitivity and specificity), prognosis, and harm. The language common to meta-analysis was discussed in Chapter 11. Familiarity with these evidence-based practice clinical categories will help Nancy, as well as you, to search for, screen, select, and appraise articles appropriate for answering clinical questions.

### Therapy Category

In articles that belong to the therapy category (experimental, randomized controlled trials [RCTs], or intervention studies), investigators attempt to determine if a difference exists between two or more interventions. The evidence-based language used in a therapy article depends on whether the numerical values of the study variables are *continuous* (a variable that measures a degree of change or a difference on a range, such as blood pressure) or *discrete*, also known as dichotomous (measuring whether or not an event did or did not occur, such as the number of people diagnosed with type 2 diabetes) (Table 19-2).

Generally speaking, therapy studies measure outcomes using discrete variables and present results as measures of association as illustrated in Table 19-3. Understanding these measures is challenging but particularly important because they are used by nurses and other health care providers to communicate to each other and to patients the risks and benefits or lack of benefits of a treatment (or treatments). They are particularly useful to nurses because they inform decision making that validates current practice or provides evidence that supports the need for change in clinical practice.

| TABLE 19-2 | DIFFERENCE BETWEEN CONTINUOUS AND DISCRETE VARIABLES | |
|---|---|---|
| **RESEARCHER OBJECTIVE** | **VARIABLE** | **HOW THE OUTCOME IS DESCRIBED IN THE RESEARCH ARTICLE** |
| **CONTINUOUS VARIABLES** | | |
| Researcher is interested in degree of change after exposure to an intervention | Pain score, levels of psychological distress, blood pressure, weight | Measures of central tendency (e.g., mean, median, or standard deviation) |
| **DISCRETE VARIABLES** | | |
| Researcher is interested in whether or not an "event" occurred or did not occur | Death, diarrhea, pressure ulcer, pregnancy: "Yes" or "No" | Measures of event probability (e.g., relative risk or odds ratio) |

For example, patients with heart failure (HF) generally have a poor quality of life because they often require frequent hospital admissions to manage the worsening of their disease; in fact, it is the most common diagnosis in patients older than 65 years admitted to hospitals, and it is estimated that more than $39.2 billion is spent annually on the management of HF (American Heart Association, 2012). One of the HF management goals is to reduce the number of inpatient admissions to the hospital. Investigators asked the following focused clinical question: "In patients with chronic heart failure, does a telephone intervention by nurses reduce admission for worsening HF?" (GESICA Investigators, 2005).

In this RCT, participants with HF were randomized to receive usual HF care (the *control group*) or an intervention that consisted of a phone call every 2 weeks to monitor patients and make therapeutic recommendations as to medications, diet, or physical activity. The data for the primary study endpoint is described in Table 19-4. From the calculated study data in Table 19-4, it can be concluded that a telephone intervention by nurses is effective in reducing hospitalization for worsening HF. But with so many calculated values (e.g., relative risk [RR], relative risk reduction [RRR], absolute risk reduction [ARR]), it could be difficult for you to know which one of these numerical variables is most important (see Table 19-3 for definitions).

The RR and the RRR, although useful for statistical purposes, tend to overestimate treatment effects because these measures do not take into account the baseline risk for the event, in this case hospitalization, and therefore do not provide a useful measure for how the information applies to your individual patient. The ARR (see Table 19-3) is a better value because it does take into account the baseline risk; however, armed with the absolute risk reduction, how does the nurse know whether or not that ARR is clinically useful? In our example the ARR was 5%; it is difficult to determine if this value is impressive or not.

Two other measures can help you determine if the reported or calculated measures are clinically meaningful. They are the **number needed to treat** (NNT) and the **confidence interval** (CI). These measures allow you to make inferences about how realistically the results about the effectiveness of an intervention can be generalized to individual patients and to a population of patients with similar characteristics in the research study.

The NNT is a useful measure for determining the effectiveness of the intervention and its application to individual patients. It is defined as the number of people who need to receive a treatment (or the intervention) in order for one patient to receive any benefit. The NNT may or may not be reported by the study researchers but is easily calculated from the ARR; NNT = 1/ARR. Interventions with a high NNT require considerable expense and human resources to provide any benefit or to prevent a single episode of the outcome,

**TABLE 19-3    MEASURES OF ASSOCIATION FOR TRIALS THAT REPORT DISCRETE OUTCOMES**

| MEASURE OF ASSOCIATION | DEFINITION | COMMENT |
|---|---|---|
| Control event rate (CER) | Proportion of patients in control group in which an event is observed | The CER is calculated by dividing the number of patients who experienced the outcome of interest by the total number of patients in the control group. |
| Experimental event rate (EER) | Proportion of patients in experimental treatment groups in which an event is observed | The EER is calculated by dividing the number of patients who experienced the outcome of interest by the total number of patients in the experimental group. |
| Absolute risk reduction (ARR), also called risk difference or attributable risk reduction | This value tells us the reduction of risk in absolute terms. The ARR is considered the "real" reduction because it is the difference between the risk observed in those who did and did not experience the event. | Arithmetic difference in risk of outcome between patients who have had the event and those who have not had the event, calculated as EER − CER |
| Relative risk (RR), also called risk ratio | Risk of event after experimental treatment as a percentage of original risk | The RR is calculated by dividing the EER/CER. If CER and EER are the same, the RR = 1 (this means there is no difference between the experimental and control group outcomes). If the risk of the event is reduced in EER compared with CER, RR < 1. *The further to the left of 1 the RR is, the greater the event, the less likely the event is to occur.* If the risk of an event is greater in EER compared with CER, RR > 1. *The further to the right of 1 the RR is, the greater the event is likely to occur.* |
| Relative risk reduction (RRR) | This value tells us the reduction in risk in relative terms. The relative risk reduction is an estimate of the percentage of baseline risk that is removed as a result of the therapy; it is calculated as the ARR between the treatment and control groups divided by the absolute risk among patients in the control group. | Percent reduction in risk that is removed after considering the percent of risk that would occur anyway (the control group's risk), calculated as EER − CER/CER |

Note: When the experimental treatment *increases* the probability of a *good outcome* (e.g., satisfactory hemoglobin $A_{1c}$ levels), there is a **benefit increase** rather than a risk reduction. The calculations remain the same.

whereas a low NNT is desirable because it means that more individuals will benefit from the intervention. In a hypothetical situation we would be more likely to implement an intervention where the NNT = 5 versus an intervention where the NNT = 200.

Using the data from Table 19-4 we can calculate the NNT. Recall that the calculation is 1/AAR, which is 1/5 (or 100/0.05) = 20. The interpretation for the NNT is that we would have to provide 20 patients with the telephone nursing intervention for one of them to benefit from not being hospitalized. In other words, 1 in 20 patients will benefit from the nursing intervention. This gives us a very different and patient-level perspective of the intervention.

The second clinically useful measure is the confidence interval (CI). The CI is a range of values, based on a random sample of the population that often accompanies measures of

## TABLE 19-4   INTERPRETATION OF MEASURES OF ASSOCIATION

*Clinical question:* In patients with chronic heart failure, does a telephone intervention by nurses reduce admission for worsening heart failure (HF)?

| TREATMENT | TOTAL NUMBER OF PATIENTS | NUMBER OF PATIENTS WHO WERE ADMITTED | NUMBER WHO WERE NOT ADMITTED |
|---|---|---|---|
| Nurse intervention group | 760 | 200 | 560 |
| Usual care group | 758 | 235 | 523 |
| **TOTALS** | **1518** | **435** | **1083** |

### Calculations Made from Study Results

| | |
|---|---|
| Experimental event rate (EER) | 200/760 = 0.26 or 26%<br>*Interpretation:* The EER is the proportion of patients in the experimental group who experienced the primary outcome, hospitalization. The interpretation is that 26% of the patients who received the nurse intervention were hospitalized. |
| Control event rate (CER) | 235/758 = 0.31 or 31%<br>*Interpretation:* The EER is the proportion of patients in the control group who experienced the primary outcome, hospitalization. The interpretation is that 31% of the patients who received the usual care were hospitalized. |
| Absolute risk reduction (ARR) | 31% − 26% = 5%<br>*Interpretation:* The RR is helpful in telling us if the risk of an event is reduced or increased. It is helpful to know by how much the event is reduced given that we now know that hospitalization occurs in those who do and do not receive the intervention. In this case 5% of the patients who received the intervention are spared hospitalization. |
| Relative risk (RR) | EER/CER<br>*Interpretation:* We can easily calculate the relative risk, but the study authors have already provided that information. The RR for hospitalization is 0.80. Recall from Table 19-3 that if the RR < 1.0, the risk of an event is reduced. In this case the intervention *reduces* the risk of hospitalization. The actual interpretation is that the risk of hospitalization is 0.80 times less than for participants who did not receive the intervention. |
| Relative risk reduction (RRR) | RRR = 1.0 − RR<br>1.0 − 0.80 = 0.20 or 20%<br>*Interpretation:* The RRR is helpful in telling us how much of the baseline risk (the control group event rate) is removed as a result of having the intervention. In this case the nurse intervention reduced hospitalization by 20% relative to the control group. |

central tendency and measures of association and provides you with a measure of precision or uncertainty about the sample findings. Typically, investigators record their CI results as a 95% degree of certainty; at times you may also see the degree of certainty recorded as 99%. Professional journals often require investigators to include CIs as one of the statistical methods used to interpret study findings. Even when CIs are not reported, they can be easily calculated from study data. The method for performing these calculations is widely available in statistical texts.

Returning to the GESICA (2005) study, it was learned that the RR for hospitalization for study participants who received the intervention was 0.80. The authors accompanied this data with a 95% CI so that the RR with CI is reported as 0.80 (0.66–.097). The CI, the number in parentheses, helps us to place the study results in context for all patients similar to those in the study (generalizability).

As a result of the calculated CI for the GESICA study, it can be stated that in adults with HF (the study population) we can be 95% certain that when a nurse provides biweekly telephone interventions, the risk of hospitalization will be reduced anywhere from 0.66 times less likely (*or a 34% reduction in hospitalization*) to 0.97 times less likely (*or a 3% reduction in hospitalization*). Although the study authors did not calculate the NNT, we now know how to do this, and when researchers report the NNT typically they also calculate the CI for the NNT. In the GESICA study, the calculated CI for the NNT of 20 is (10 to 108). With this information we now can state that the nursing intervention, when applied to our entire patient population, not just the sample, will successfully reduce hospitalization, but we would have to apply the intervention anywhere between 10 and 108 times before one patient gets any benefit. With such a large range, we might think twice about whether or not we want to implement this intervention. We would think differently about the intervention if the CI for the NNT were much narrower, say, 10 to 15 versus 10 to 108.

Another unique feature of the confidence interval is that it can tell us whether or not the study results are statistically significant. When an experimental value is obtained that indicates there is no difference between the treatment and control groups, we label that value "the value of no effect," or the **null value**. The value of no effect varies according to the outcome measure.

When examining a CI, if the interval does not include the null value, the effect is said to be statistically significant. When the CI does contain the null value, the results are said to be nonsignificant because the null value represents the value of no difference; that is, there is no difference between the treatment and control groups. In studies of equivalence (e.g., a study to determine if two treatments are similar) this is a desired finding, but in studies of superiority or inferiority (e.g., a study to determine if one treatment is better than the other) this is not the case.

The null value varies depending on the outcome measure. For numerical values determined by proportions/ratio (e.g., relative risk, odds ratio) the null value is "1." That is, if the CI does not include the value "1," the finding is statistically significant. If the CI does include the value "1," the finding is not statistically significant. If we examine an actual table from the GESICA study we can see an excellent demonstration of this concept (Figure 19-1).

For numerical values determined by a mean difference between the score in the intervention group and the control group (usually with continuous measures), the null value is "0." In this case if the CI includes the null value of "0," the result is not statistically significant. If the CI does not include the null value of "0," the result is statistically significant as illustrated in Figure 19-2, *A* to *D*.

Pittler and colleagues (2007) reviewed nine trials in which the use of magnets in the control of pain compared to a placebo was evaluated. Figure 19-3 summarizes the results from these nine studies. Because the difference in pain score is the outcome of analysis, the null value is "0." Looking at the table you can see that only one out of nine studies achieved statistical significance, leading this author to conclude that the evidence for use of magnets to control pain is not supported by the majority of research studies.

## Diagnosis Articles

In articles that answer clinical questions of diagnosis, investigators study the ability of screening or diagnostic tests, or components of the clinical examination to detect (or not detect) disease when the patient has (or does not have) the particular disease of interest. The accuracy of a test, or technique, is measured by its sensitivity and specificity (Table 19-5).

| Endpoint | Intervention (n = 760) | Control (n = 758) | Relative risk (95% CI) | P value |
|---|---|---|---|---|
| Primary endpoint | 200 (26.3) | 235 (31.0) | 0.80 (0.66 to 0.97) | 0.026 |
| Heart failure admission | 128 (16.8) | 169 (22.3) | 0.71 (0.56 to 0.91) | 0.005 |
| All cause mortality | 116 (15.3) | 122 (16.1) | 0.95 (0.73 to 1.23) | 0.690 |
| All cause admission | 261 (34.3) | 296 (39.1) | 0.85 (0.72 to 0.99) | 0.049 |
| Cardiovascular admission | 183 (24.1) | 228 (30.1) | 0.76 (0.62 to 0.93) | 0.006 |
| All cause admission and/or all cause mortality | 299 (39.3) | 339 (44.7) | 0.86 (0.73 to 1.00) | 0.057 |
| Cardiovascular admission and/or all cause mortality | 239 (31.4) | 288 (38.0) | 0.79 (0.65 to 0.95) | 0.01 |

The relative risk is determined by a proportion between intervention and the control group. Therefore the null value is "1." Any confidence interval that includes the null value means that the endpoint finding is not a statistically significant finding.

These confidence intervals contain the null value of "1" and as a result these endpoints are not statistically significant.

FIGURE 19-1 Summary of primary and secondary endpoints showing the effect of a telephone nursing intervention in patients with heart failure. Values are numbers (percentages) unless stated otherwise. (From GESICA Investigators: Randomised trial of telephone intervention in chronic heart failure: DIAL trial, *BMJ* 331:425, 2005.)

Sensitivity is the proportion of those with disease who test positive; that is, sensitivity is a measure of how well the test detects disease when it is really there—a highly sensitive test has few false negatives. Specificity is the proportion of those without disease who test negative. It measures how well the test rules out disease when it is really absent; a specific test has few false positives. Sensitivity and specificity have some deficiencies in clinical use, primarily because sensitivity and specificity are merely characteristics of the performance of the test.

Describing diagnostic tests in this way tells us how good the test is, but what is more useful is how well the test performs in a particular population with a particular disease prevalence. This is important because in a population in which a disease is quite prevalent, there are fewer incorrect test results (false positives) as compared with populations with low disease prevalence for which a positive test may truly be a false positive. Predictive values are a measure of accuracy that accounts for the prevalence of a disease. As illustrated in Table 19-5, a positive predictive value (PPV) expresses the proportion of those with positive test results who truly have disease, and a negative predictive value (NPV) expresses the proportion of those with negative test results who truly do not have disease. Let us observe how these characteristics of diagnostic tests are used in nursing practice.

A study was conducted to evaluate a new method of on-site appraisal of bacteriuria in adult patients with incontinence who reside in nursing homes. Researchers compared a new method of pressing a urine dipstick into a wet incontinence pad and compared this method with the gold standard of sending a clean-catch specimen to a laboratory for

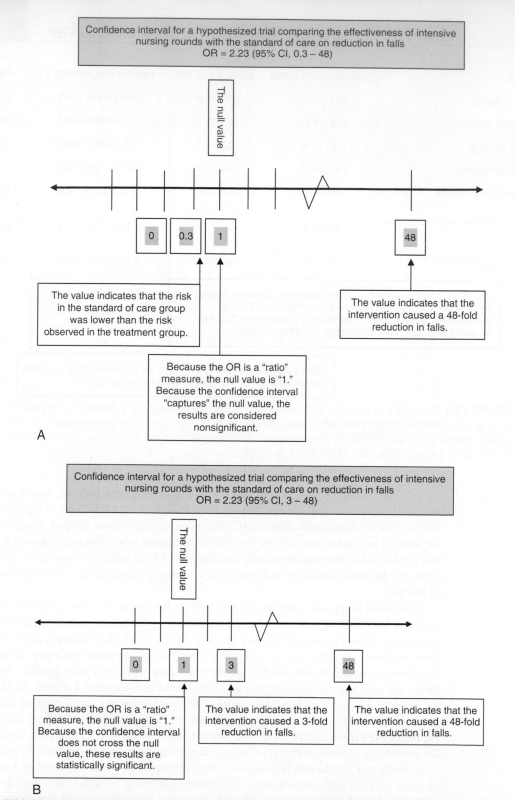

Confidence interval for a hypothesized trial comparing the effectiveness of intensive nursing rounds with the standard of care on reduction in falls
OR = 2.23 (95% CI, 0.3 – 48)

The null value

0   0.3   1                48

The value indicates that the risk in the standard of care group was lower than the risk observed in the treatment group.

The value indicates that the intervention caused a 48-fold reduction in falls.

Because the OR is a "ratio" measure, the null value is "1." Because the confidence interval "captures" the null value, the results are considered nonsignificant.

A

Confidence interval for a hypothesized trial comparing the effectiveness of intensive nursing rounds with the standard of care on reduction in falls
OR = 2.23 (95% CI, 3 – 48)

The null value

0   1   3                48

Because the OR is a "ratio" measure, the null value is "1." Because the confidence interval does not cross the null value, these results are statistically significant.

The value indicates that the intervention caused a 3-fold reduction in falls.

The value indicates that the intervention caused a 48-fold reduction in falls.

B

**FIGURE 19-2  A,** Confidence interval (nonsignificant) for a hypothesized trial comparing the ratio of events in the experimental group and control group. **B,** Confidence interval (significant) for a hypothesized trial comparing the ratio of events in the experimental group and control group.

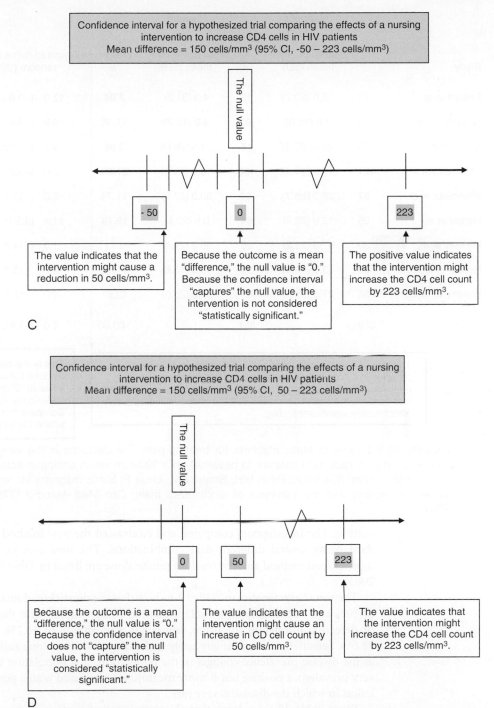

Confidence interval for a hypothesized trial comparing the effects of a nursing intervention to increase CD4 cells in HIV patients
Mean difference = 150 cells/mm³ (95% CI, -50 – 223 cells/mm³)

The null value

- 50

0

223

The value indicates that the intervention might cause a reduction in 50 cells/mm³.

Because the outcome is a mean "difference," the null value is "0." Because the confidence interval "captures" the null value, the intervention is not considered "statistically significant."

The positive value indicates that the intervention might increase the CD4 cell count by 223 cells/mm³.

C

Confidence interval for a hypothesized trial comparing the effects of a nursing intervention to increase CD4 cells in HIV patients
Mean difference = 150 cells/mm³ (95% CI, 50 – 223 cells/mm³)

The null value

0

50

223

Because the outcome is a mean "difference," the null value is "0." Because the confidence interval does not "capture" the null value, the intervention is considered "statistically significant."

The value indicates that the intervention might cause an increase in CD cell count by 50 cells/mm³.

The value indicates that the intervention might increase the CD4 cell count by 223 cells/mm³.

D

**FIGURE 19-2—cont'd C,** Confidence interval (nonsignificant) for a hypothesized control trial comparing the difference between two treatments. **D,** Confidence interval (significant) for a hypothesized control trial comparing the difference between two treatments.

| Study | n | Magnets Pain score, mm, mean (SD) | n | Placebo Pain score, mm, mean (SD) | Weight, % | Weighted mean difference, random (95% CI) |
|---|---|---|---|---|---|---|
| Colbert et al. | 13 | 16.0 (23.7) | 12 | 4.0 (31.2) | 2.94 | 12.0 (−9.8 to 33.8) |
| Collacott et al. | 20 | 4.9 (16.0) | 20 | 4.0 (18.0) | 11.46 | 0.9 (−9.6 to 11.4) |
| Carter et al. | 15 | 24.0 (27.0) | 15 | 24.0 (26.0) | 3.86 | 0.0 (−19.0 to 19.0) |
| Weintraub et al. | 121 | 17.0 (27.6) | 106 | 15.0 (28.2) | 21.28 | 2.0 (−5.3 to 9.3) |
| Winemiller et al. | 57 | 28.0 (25.7) | 44 | 30.0 (27.0) | 11.79 | −2.0 (−12.4 to 8.4) |
| Harlow et al. | 65 | 12.0 (23.4) | 64 | 0.6 (22.4) | 18.73 | 11.4 (3.5 to 19.3) |
| Mikesky et al. | 20 | 57.6 (22.2) | 20 | 56.3 (27.4) | 5.71 | 1.3 (−14.2 to 16.8) |
| Reeser et al. | 23 | 13.0 (18.0) | 23 | 15.6 (18.6) | 11.42 | −2.6 (−13.2 to 8.0) |
| Winemiller et al. | 36 | 27.0 (21.0) | 47 | 31.0 (25.0) | 12.81 | −4.0 (−13.9 to 5.9) |
| *Overall* | 370 | | 351 | | 100.00 | 2.0 (−1.8 to 5.8) |

The statistics is the calculated mean difference in pain score between the intervention (magnets) and the control group (placebo). Therefore the null value is "0." Any confidence interval that includes the null value means that the endpoint finding is not a statistically significant finding.

This is the only study where the CI does not contain the null value of "0" and is considered statistically significant. Compare this to all studies where the CI contains the null.

**FIGURE 19-3** Effects of static magnets for treating pain. The outcome is the weighted mean difference in pain reduction (relative to baseline) on a 100-mm visual analogue scale with 95% confidence interval *(CI)*. (From Pitter MH, Brown EM, Ernst E: Static magnets for reducing pain: systematic review and meta-analysis of randomized trials, *Can Med Assoc J* 177(7):736–742, 2007.)

culture. The investigators compared and contrasted the new method with the gold standard using several different data combinations. The measures of accuracy using the dipstick/pad method and the result of nitrite alone are listed in Table 19-6 (Midthun et al., 2003).

The test characteristics in Table 19-6 show that the dipstick/pad method has a sensitivity of 70% and a specificity of 97%. This method compares well with the laboratory method of detecting nitrates in the urine, which has a sensitivity of 66.7% and a specificity of 98.6%. Sensitivity and specificity apply to the diagnostic test alone and do not change even as the disease prevalence changes in the population. In a population in which a disease is very prevalent, a positive test is more meaningful compared with a positive test in a population in which the disease is very rare.

From Table 19-6 we learn that the prevalence of bacteriuria in an elderly, primarily female population is 28%. Combining this information with sensitivity and specificity, we find that the PPV is 90%; this means that 90% of primarily elderly female nursing home residents with a positive dipstick/pad method will have bacteriuria.

| TABLE 19-5 | REPORTING THE OUTCOME RESULTS OF DIAGNOSTIC TRIALS | |
|---|---|---|
| **MEASURE OF ACCURACY** | **DEFINITION** | **COMMENTS** |
| Sensitivity | A characteristic of a diagnostic test. It is the ability of the test to detect the proportion of people with the disease or disorder of interest. For a test to be useful in ruling out a disease, it must have a high sensitivity. | Formula for sensitivity: $TP/(TP + FN)$, where TP and FN are number of true positive and false negative results, respectively |
| Specificity | A characteristic of a diagnostic test. It is the ability of the test to detect the proportion of people without the disease or disorder of interest. For a test to be useful at confirming a disease, it must have a high specificity. | Formula for specificity: $TN/(TN + FP)$, where TN and FP are number of true negative and false positive results, respectively |
| *Positive predictive value (PPV) and negative predictive value (NPV) are closely related to sensitivity and specificity (how well the test performs) but differ in that sensitivity and specificity are fixed characteristics of a diagnostic test whereas PPV and NPV consider how well the test performs in populations with difference prevalence of the disease it is testing.* | | |
| Positive predictive value | This is the proportion of people with a positive test who have the target disorder. | Formula for positive predictive value: $PPV = TP/(TP + FP)$ |
| Negative predictive value | This is the proportion of people with a negative test who do not have the target disorder. | Formula for negative predictive value: $NPV = TN/(TN + FN)$ |
| ***Likelihood ratio (LR):*** *A likelihood ratio is a measure that a given test result would be expected in a patient with the target disorder compared to the likelihood that the same result would be expected in a patient without the target disorder. It measures the power of a test to change the pretest into the* ***posttest probability*** *of a disease being present.* | | |
| Positive likelihood ratio | The LR of a positive test tells us how well a positive test result does by comparing its performance when the disease is present to that when it is absent. The best test to use for ruling in a disease is the one with the largest likelihood ratio of a positive test. | Formula for positive likelihood ratio: $\text{Sensitivity}/(1 - \text{Specificity})$ |
| Negative likelihood ratio | The LR of a negative test tells us how well a negative test result does by comparing its performance when the disease is absent to that when it is present. The better test to use to rule out disease is the one with the smaller likelihood ratio of a negative test. | Formula for negative likelihood ratio: $(1 - \text{Sensitivity})/\text{Specificity}$ |

Combining sensitivity, specificity, PPV, NPV, and prevalence to make clinical decisions based on the results of testing is cumbersome and complex. Fortunately, all of these measures can be described by one number, the likelihood ratio (LR). This value tells us how many more times a positive test (or negative test) distinguished between those who have the disorder and those who do not have the disorder. As you can see from Table 19-5, the LR is calculated from the test's sensitivity and specificity, and with more training in determining disease prevalence you could actually state the numerical probability that a patient might have a disease based on the test's LR.

As illustrated in Table 19-7, a test with a large positive likelihood ratio (e.g., greater than 10), when applied, provides the clinician with a high degree of certainty that the patient has the suspected disorder. Conversely, tests with a very low positive likelihood ratio (e.g., less than 2), when applied, provide you with little to no change in the degree of certainty that the patient has the suspected disorder.

| TABLE 19-6 | NITRITE RESULTS INDICATIVE FOR BACTERIURIA USING THE DIPSTICK/PAD METHOD | | | |
|---|---|---|---|---|
| | | **(GOLD STANDARD) CULTURE RESULTS** | | |
| **METHOD** | **TEST RESULT** | **POSITIVE** | **NEGATIVE** | **TOTALS** |
| Dipstick/pad (new test) | Positive | **19** (a) | **2** (b) | 21 |
| | Negative | **8** (c) | **69** (d) | 77 |
| Totals | | **27** | **71** | 98 |

**Calculations Made from Study Results**

Sensitivity = a/(a + c)     19/27 = 0.70 or 70%
*Interpretation:* The dipstick/pad method is 70% accurate in detecting the proportion of patients with positive tests as having bacteriuria.

Specificity = d/(b + d)     69/71 + 0.972 or 97%
*Interpretation:* The dipstick/pad method is 97% accurate in detecting the proportion of patients with negative tests as not having bacteriuria.

Prevalence of bacteriuria in this population (elderly, primarily female nursing home residents) = (a + c)/Total population     27/98 = 0.275
*Interpretation:* The prevalence of bacteriuria in an elderly female population is 28%.

Positive predictive value = a/(a + b)     19/21 = 0.90 or 90%
*Interpretation:* 90% of primarily elderly female nursing home residents with a positive dipstick/pad method will have bacteriuria. 10% will not have bacteriuria.

Negative predictive value = d/(c + d)     69/77 = 0.896 or 90%
*Interpretation:* 90% of primarily elderly female nursing home residents with a negative dipstick/pad method will not have bacteriuria. 10% will have bacteriuria.

Likelihood ratio (LR+) = Sensitivity/ (1 − Specificity)     0.70/(1 − 0.972) = 0.70/0.028 = 25
*Interpretation:* Female elderly nursing home residents with a positive dipstick/pad method test are 25 times more likely to have a urinary tract infection (UTI) than patients without bacteriuria (i.e., a positive test is very useful for ruling in UTI).

Likelihood ratio (LR−) = (1 − Sensitivity)/ Specificity     1 − 0.72/0.97 = 0.29
*Interpretation:* Female elderly nursing home residents with a negative dipstick/pad method test are 0.29 times more likely to have a UTI than patients without bacteriuria (i.e., a negative test is moderately useful for ruling out UTI; this actually is the false-negative rate. It means that we will have more false-negative tests, and this may not be so good in this population).

When a test has a likelihood ratio of "1" (the null value), the test will not contribute to decision making in any meaningful way and should not be used. A test with a large **negative likelihood ratio** provides the clinician with a high degree of certainty that the patient does not have the disease. The further away from "1" the negative LR is, the better the test will be for its use in ruling out disease (i.e., there will be few false negatives). More and more journal articles require authors to provide test LRs; they may also be available in secondary sources.

| TABLE 19-7 | **HOW MUCH DO LIKELIHOOD RATIO CHANGES AFFECT PROBABILITY OF DISEASE?** | |
|---|---|---|
| **LIKELIHOOD RATIO POSITIVE** | **LIKELIHOOD RATIO NEGATIVE** | **PROBABILITY THAT PATIENT HAS (LR) OR DOES NOT HAVE (LR)** |
| LR > 10 | LR < 0.1 | Large |
| LR 5-10 | LR 0.1-0.2 | Moderate |
| LR 2-5 | LR 0.2-0.5 | Small |
| LR < 2 | LR > 0.5 | Tiny |
| LR = 1.0 | | Test provides no useful information |

## Prognosis Articles

In articles that answer clinical questions of prognosis, investigators conduct studies in which they want to determine the outcome of a particular disease or condition. Prognosis studies can often be identified by their longitudinal cohort design (see Chapter 10). At the conclusion of a longitudinal study, investigators statistically analyze data to determine which factors are strongly associated with the study outcomes, usually through a technique called multivariate regression analysis or simply multiple regression (see Chapter 16).

From this advanced statistical analysis, several factors are usually identified that predict the probability of developing the outcome or a particular disease. The probability is called an **odds ratio**. The odds ratio (Table 19-8) indicates how much more likely certain independent variables (factors) predict the probability of developing the dependent variable (outcome or disease).

A prospective cohort, longitudinal study was carried out for 1.8 years to identify predictors of the development of pressure ulcers in a population of surgical patients. The investigators examined several patient characteristics and operating room care characteristics and the subsequent development of a hospital acquired pressure ulcer. The study predictors are presented in Table 19-9, with their respective CIs.

The interpretation of the odds ratios is similar to and interpreted in the same way as the risk ratio (see Table 19-3). A higher odds ratio indicates a greater probability of the development of the outcome. An odds ratio below one indicates that the probability of developing the outcome is reduced. Also recall from our discussion that whenever we are appraising CIs (to determine statistical significance) we have to appraise the null value. Because we are evaluating a "ratio," the null value is equal to 1. Thus any odds ratio CI interval that contains a null value of 1 is not a significant finding.

A quick review of Table 19-9 indicates that for this group, the number of surgeries and a higher risk mortality score are the strongest predictors of pressure ulcer development.

Using prognostic information with an evidence-based lens helps the nurse and patient focus on reducing factors that may lead to disease or disability. It also helps the nurse with providing education and information to patients and their families regarding the course of the condition.

---

**HELPFUL HINT**

When evaluating whether or not you should spend time reviewing an article, examine the article's tables. The information you need to answer your clinical question should be contained in one or more of the tables.

| TABLE 19-8 | MEASURES OF ASSOCIATION FOR TRIALS THAT REPORT DISCRETE OUTCOMES | |
|---|---|---|
| **MEASURE OF ASSOCIATION** | **DEFINITION** | **COMMENT** |
| **Reporting events in terms of the probability of it occurring (good or bad):** | | |
| Odds ratio (OR) | We could estimate the odds of an event occurring. The OR is usually the measure of choice in the analysis of nonexperimental design studies. It is the probability of a given event occurring to the probability of the event not occurring. | If the OR = 1.0, this means there is no difference in the probablity of an event occurring between the experimental and control group outcomes. If the probability of the event is reduced between groups, the OR is < 1.0 (i.e., the event is less likely in the treatment group than the control group). If the odds of an event is increased between groups, the OR > 1.0 (i.e., the event is more likely to occur in the treatment group than the control group). |

| TABLE 19-9 | PREDICTORS OF DEVELOPMENT OF A HOSPITAL-ACQUIRED PRESSURE ULCER (*N* = 3225) | | |
|---|---|---|---|
| **PREDICTOR** | **ODDS RATIO** | **95% CONFIDENCE INTERVAL** | **$P$ VALUE** |
| Body mass index (BMI)* | 0.97 | 0.95-0.98 | <.001 |
| History of diabetes | 1.49 | 1.14-1.95 | <.001 |
| Use of vasopressors | 1.33 | 1.03-1.73 | .03 |
| Number of surgeries | 2.23 | 1.45-3.44 | <.001 |
| Total time in operating room | 1.07 | 1.03-1.11 | <.001 |
| Braden Score at admission** | .089 | 0.86-0.93 | <.001 |
| Risk of mortality | | | <.001 |
| 1 | Reference | 1.49-3.62 | |
| 2 | 2.32 | 3.58-8.45 | |
| 3 | 5.50 | 7.1-17.5 | |
| 4 | 11.15 | | |

*The OR indicates that each additional point increase in BMI reduced the risk for pressure ulcer by 0.97.

**The OR indicates that for each additional point in the Braden Score, the patient was 0.98 less likely to acquire a pressure ulcer. Data fromTschannen, D., Bates, O., Talsma, A, Guo, Y. (2012). Patient-specific and surgical characteristics in the development of pressure ulcers. *American Journal of Critical Care, 21*, 116–125.

### Harm Articles

In articles that answer clinical questions of harm, investigators want to determine if an individual has been harmed by being exposed to a particular event. Harm studies can be identified by their case-control design (see Chapter 10). In this type of study, investigators select the outcome they are interested in (e.g., pressure ulcers), and they examine if any one factor explains those who have and do not have the outcome of interest. The measure of association that best describes the analyzed data in case-control studies is the odds ratio.

Hopcia and colleagues (2012) used a case-control study design to determine if consecutive or cumulative shift work by registered nurses increased the odds for occupational injuries. Table 19-10 presents the consecutive shift data.

The interpretation of this data is relatively straightforward. You can see from the table that most of the odds ratios are greater than one. If you were to interpret this data using

| TABLE 19-10 | ODDS RATIOS FOR CONSECUTIVE SHIFTS (NUMBER OF SHIFTS WORKED IN A ROW) PRIOR TO INJURY | | | | |
|---|---|---|---|---|---|
| **EXPOSURE— CONSECUTIVE SHIFTS** | **NUMBER OF SHIFTS** | **CASES (N = 502)** | **CONTROLS (N = 502)** | **OR (95% CI)** | **p** |
| Any shifts ≥ 4 hours (days, evenings, nights, or rotating) | 0 | 299 (59.6%) | 306 (61.0%) | 1* | |
| | 1 to 2 | 190 (37.8%) | 190 (37.8%) | 0.81 (0.60–1.08) | .16 |
| | 3 to 11 | 13 (2.6%) | 6 (1.2%) | 1.19 (0.39–3.65) | .75 |
| 12-hour (or longer) shifts (days, evenings, nights, or rotating) | 0 | 297 (59.2%) | 373 (74.3%) | 1* | |
| | 1 to 2 | 189 (37.6%) | 124 (24.7%) | 1.77 (1.30–2.44) | .000 |
| | 3 to 6 | 16 (3.2%) | 5 (1.0%) | 1.30 (0.70–2.43) | .402 |
| 12-hour (or longer) night shifts | 0 | 336 (72.1%) | 362 (77.7%) | 1* | |
| | 1 to 2 | 115 (24.7%) | 91 (19.5%) | 1.09 (0.76–1.57) | .64 |
| | 3 to 6 | 15 (3.2%) | 13 (2.8%) | 1.19 (0.71–2.01) | .50 |

Note. *OR = odds ratio; CI = confidence interval. *Referent category.*
Data from Hopcia, K., Dennerlein, JT., Hashimoto, D., et al. (2012). Occupational injuries for consecutive and cumulative shifts among hospital registered nurses and patient care associates: a case-control study. *Workplace Health Safety,* 60(10),437–44.

the odds ratio alone you would be correct in concluding that the greater the number of consecutive days a registered nurse works, the greater the probability that he or she will sustain an occupational injury. Based on the previous discussion of confidence intervals you know that the confidence interval indicates how well the study findings can be generalized to the population of registered nurses. A quick review of all of the confidence intervals, except for one, includes the null value and, as such, the study findings as it relates to consecutive shift work are not statistically significant findings.

Harm data with its measure of probabilities help you to identify factors that may or may not contribute to an adverse or beneficial outcome. This information will be useful for the nursing plan of care, program planning, or patient and family education.

## Meta-Analysis

Meta-analysis statistically combines the results of multiple studies (usually RCTs) to answer a focused clinical question through an objective appraisal of carefully synthesized research evidence. The strength of a meta-analysis lies in its use of statistical analysis to summarize studies. As discussed in Chapter 11:

- A clinical question is used to guide the process
- All relevant studies, published and unpublished, on the question are gathered using preestablished inclusion and exclusion criteria to determine the studies to be used in the meta-analysis
- At least two individuals independently assess the quality of each study based on preestablished criteria
- Statistically combine the results of individual studies, and present a balanced and impartial quantitative and narrative evidence summary of the findings that represents a "state-of-the-science" conclusion about the strength, quality, and consistency of evidence supporting benefits and risks of a given health care practice (Liberati et al., 2009; Moher et al., 2009).

A methodologically sound meta-analysis is more likely than an individual study to be successful in identifying the true effect of an intervention because it limits bias. A relative risk or, more commonly, the odds ratio is the statistic of choice for use in a meta-analysis (see Tables 19-3 and 19-8). Meta-analysis can also report on continuous data, typically the mean difference in outcomes will be reported.

The usual manner of displaying data in a meta-analysis is by a pictorial representation known as a *blobbogram,* accompanied by a summary measure of effect size in relative risk, odds ratio or mean difference (see Chapter 11). Let us see how blobbograms and relative risk ratios are used to summarize the studies in a systematic review by practicing with the data from the Cochrane Review to determine the benefit of psychological follow-up in detecting psychological complications after a woman has experienced a miscarriage (see Appendix E). The table "Analysis 1.1" compares the effect of one counseling session versus no counseling sessions on psychological well being. In the first column, the first outcome listed is anxiety. The reviewers identified two studies: Lee, 1996 and Nikcevic, 2007. The next four columns tell you about the sample size in each of the groups and their mean score (and standard deviation) on a measure of anxiety. In the center of the table, you see that a horizontal line represents each trial in the analysis. The findings from each individual study are represented as a blob or square (the measured effect) on the vertical line. You will also note that the blob or square is a bit different in size. This size reflects the weight the study has on the overall analysis. This is determined by the sample size and the quality of the study. The width of the horizontal line represents the 95% confidence interval. The vertical line is the line of no effect (i.e., the null value), and we know that when the statistic is the relative risk ratio, the null value is "1." When the statistic is the mean difference, the null value is "0."

---

**HELPFUL HINT**

When appraising the different types of reviews, it is important to be able to distinguish a meta-analysis that analytically assesses studies from a systematic review that appraises the literature with or without an analytic approach to an integrative review that also appraises and synthesizes the literature but without an analytic process (see Chapter 10).

---

When the confidence interval of the result (horizontal line) touches or crosses the line of no effect (vertical line), we can say that the study findings did not reach statistical significance. If the confidence interval does not cross the vertical line, we can say that the study results reached statistical significance.

In examining the blobbogram in Analysis 1.1 "Anxiety," it is clear that both studies cross the line of no effect. Because the analysis crosses the line of no effect, these studies have statistically insignificant findings. To the far right of the blobbogram, the investigators have also provided the numerical equivalent of each blobbogram.

You will also notice other important information and additional statistical analyses that may accompany the blobbogram table, such as a test to determine how well the results of each of the individual trials are mathematically compatible (heterogeneity) and a test for overall effect. The reader is referred to a book of advanced research methods for discussion of these topics.

A diamond represents the summary ratio for the two studies combined. There is a subtotal diamond for the effect of one counseling session on anxiety after a miscarriage. In this case, after statistically pooling the results of each of the controlled trials, it shows that these studies, statistically combined, overall favor the treatment (one counseling session). Because the total diamond touches the line of no effect, the overall interpretation is that one counseling session at four months does not significantly impact anxiety after a miscarriage.

If this is a methodologically sound review (and Cochrane reviews are), it can be used to support or change nursing practice or specific nursing interventions. A simple tool to help determine whether or not a systematic review is methodologically sound can be found at www.casp-uk.net/wp-content/uploads/2011/11/CASP_Systematic_Review_Appraisal_Checklist_14oct10.pdf.

As Nancy evaluates the literature, she determines that the article, "Effects of an Intervention to Increase Bed Alarm Use to Prevent Fall in Hospitalized Patients: A Cluster Randomized Trial" is a clinical intervention trial that has an experimental study design and is a therapy category study. Nancy selects a therapy critical appraisal tool and answers the critical appraisal questions.

---

### EVIDENCE-BASED PRACTICE TIP

When answering a clinical question, check to see if a Cochrane review has been performed. This will save you time searching the literature. A Cochrane review is a systematic review that primarily uses meta-analysis to investigate the effects of interventions for prevention, treatment, and rehabilitation in a health care setting or on health-related disorders. Most Cochrane reviews are based on RCTs, but other types of evidence may also be taken into account, if appropriate. If the data collected in a review are of sufficient quality and similar enough, they are summarized statistically in a meta-analysis. You should always check the Cochrane Web site, www.cochrane.org, to see if a review has been published on the topic of interest.

---

## EVIDENCE-BASED TOOL #5: APPLYING THE FINDINGS

Evidence-based practice is about integrating individual clinical expertise and patient preferences with the best external evidence to guide clinical decision making (Sackett et al, 1996). With a few simple tools (see the Web links listed earlier in this chapter) and some practice, your day-to-day practice can be more evidence based. We know that using evidence in clinical decision making by nurses and all other health care professionals interested in matters associated with the care of individuals, communities, and health systems is increasingly important to achieving quality patient outcomes and cannot be ignored. Let us see how Nancy uses evidence to make a clinically effective decision and perhaps make a practice change.

Nancy critically appraises the article, and she learns that the control unit had 408 falls (or 4.56 falls per 1000 patient days) and in the intervention group there were 315 falls (or 5.62 falls per 1000 patient days). Examining the changes in pre-intervention and post-intervention falls rate, she notes that the study authors calculated a relative risk of 1.09 with a confidence of 0.55 to 1.53. Nancy knows that a relative risk greater than 1 means that there was an increase in the outcome (falls) in the intervention group relative to the control. She also examines the confidence intervals and notes that the range includes the null value of "1" making this finding not statistically significant. Nancy is surprised by the study findings and plans to examine other studies on this subject and will report back to the clinical practice committee that this randomized trial did not find any benefit in the use of bed alarms in reducing falls rate and should be considered supportive rather than an essential part of the falls prevention program.

## KEY POINTS

- Asking a focused clinical question using the PICO approach is an important evidence-based practice tool.
- Several types of evidence-based practice clinical categories used by nurses and other clinicians are the following: therapy, diagnosis, prognosis, and harm. These categories focus development of the clinical question, the literature search, and critical appraisal of research studies.
- An efficient and effective literature search, using information literacy skills, is critical in locating evidence to answer the clinical question.
- Sources of evidence (e.g., articles, evidence-based practice guidelines, evidence-based practice protocols) must be screened for relevance and credibility.
- Appraising the evidence generated by research studies using an accepted critiquing tool is essential in determining the strength, quality, and consistency of evidence offered by a research study.
- Articles that belong to the therapy category are designed to determine if a difference exists between two or more treatments.
- Articles that belong to the diagnosis category are designed to investigate the ability of screening or diagnostic tests, tools, or components of the clinical examination to detect whether or not the patient has a particular disease using likelihood ratios.
- Articles in the prognosis category are designed to determine the outcomes of a particular disease or condition.
- Articles in the harm category are designed to determine if an individual has been harmed by being exposed to a particular event.
- Meta-analysis is a research method that statistically combines the results of multiple studies (usually RCTs) and is designed to answer a focused clinical question through objective appraisal of synthesized evidence.

## CRITICAL THINKING CHALLENGES

- How would you use the PICO format to formulate a clinical question? Provide a clinical example.
- How can the nurse determine if reported or calculated measures in a research study are clinically significant enough to inform evidence-based clinical decisions?
- How can a nurse in clinical practice determine whether the strength and quality of evidence provided by a diagnostic tool is sufficient to justify ordering it as a diagnostic test? Provide an example of a diagnostic test used to diagnose a specific illness.
- Choose a research article and identify the study's main (or primary) and secondary outcomes. Identify whether these outcomes are measured as discrete and continuous variables.

- Choose a meta-analysis from a peer-reviewed journal and describe how you as a nurse would use the findings of this meta-analysis in making a clinical decision about applicability of a nursing intervention for your specific patient population and clinical setting.

## REFERENCES

American Heart Association. (2012). *Heart disease and stroke statistics* [Data file]. Retrieved from http://circ.ahajournals.org/content/early/2012/12/12/CIR.0b013e31828124ad.citation.

D'Auria, J. P. (2007). Using an evidence-based approach to critical appraisal. *Journal of Pediatric Health Care, 2,* 343–346.

GESICA Investigators. (2005). Randomised trial of telephone intervention in chronic heart failure: DIAL trial. *British Medical Journal, 331,* 425–430.

Hopcia, K., Dennerlein, J. T., Hashimoto, D., et al. (2012). Occupational injuries for consecutive and cumulative shifts among hospital registered nurses and patient care associates: a case-control study. *Workplace Health Safety, 60*(10), 437–444.

Liberati, A. Altman, D. G, Tetzlaff, J., et al. (2009). The PRISMA statement for reporting systematic reviews and meta-analyses of studies that evaluate health care interventions: explanation and elaboration. *Annuals of Internal Medicine, 151*(4), w65–w94.

Moher, D., Liberati, A., Tetzlaff, J., & Altman, D. G. (2009). Preferred reporting items for systematic reviews and meta-analyses: the PRISMA statement. *PLOS Medical,* e1000097.

Midthun, S. J., Paur, R. A., Lindseth, G., et al. (2003). Bacteriuria detection with a urine dipstick applied to incontinence pads of nursing home residents. *Geriatric Nursing, 24*(4), 206–209.

Miser, W. F. (2000). Critical appraisal of the literature: how to assess an article and still enjoy life. In J. P. Geyman, R. A. Deyo, & S. D. Ramsey, (Eds.), *Evidence based clinical practice: concepts and approaches* (pp. 41–56). Boston, MA: Butterworth-Heinemann.

Pittler, M. H., Brown, E. M., & Ernst, E. (2007). Static magnets for reducing pain: systematic review and meta-analysis of randomized trials. *Canadian Medical Association Journal, 177*(7), 736–742.

Sackett, D. L., Rosenberg, W. M. C., Gray, J. A. M., et al. (1996). Evidence based medicine: what it is and what it isn't. *British Medical Journal, 312,* 71–72.

Schorr, R. I., Chandler, A. M., Mon, L. C., et al. (2012). Effects of an intervention to increase bed alarm use to prevent falls in hospitalized patients: a cluster randomized trial. *Annals of Internal Medicine, 157,* 692–699.

Tschannen, D., Bates, O., Talsma, A., & Guo, Y. (2012). Patient-specific and surgical characteristics in the development of pressure ulcers. *American Journal of Critical Care, 21,* 116–125.

## evolve WEBSITE

*Go to Evolve at http://evolve.elsevier.com/LoBiondo/ for review questions, critiquing exercises, and additional research articles for practice in reviewing and critiquing.*

# CHAPTER

# 20

# Developing an Evidence-Based Practice

*Marita Titler*

## ⓔvolve WEBSITE

*Go to Evolve at http://evolve.elsevier.com/LoBiondo/ for review questions, critiquing exercises, and additional research articles for practice in reviewing and critiquing.*

## LEARNING OUTCOMES

*After reading this chapter, you should be able to do the following:*

- Differentiate among conduct of nursing research, research utilization, and evidence-based practice.
- Describe the steps of evidence-based practice.
- Identify barriers to implementing evidence-based practice.
- Describe strategies for implementing evidence-based practice changes.

- Identify steps for evaluating an evidence-based change in practice.
- Use research findings and other forms of evidence to improve the quality of care.

## KEY TERMS

conduct of research
dissemination
evaluation

evidence-based practice
evidence-based practice
   guidelines

knowledge-focused
   triggers
opinion leaders

problem-focused
   triggers
research utilization

Evidence-based health care practices are available for a number of conditions. However, these practices are not always implemented in care delivery settings. Variation in practices abound, and availability of high-quality research does not ensure that the findings will be used to affect patient outcomes (Centers for Medicare and Medicaid Services, 2008; Institute of Medicine, 2001). The use of evidence-based practices is now an expected standard as demonstrated by recent regulations from the Centers for Medicare and Medicaid Services (CMS) regarding not paying for nosocomial events such as injury from falls, Foley catheter-associated urinary tract infections, and stage 3 and 4 pressure ulcers. These practices all have a strong evidence base and when enacted, can prevent these nosocomial events. However, implementing such evidence-based safety practices is a challenge and requires use of strategies that address the systems of care, individual practitioners, senior leadership, and, ultimately, changing health care cultures to be evidence-based practice environments (Leape, 2005).

Translation of research into practice (TRIP) is a multifaceted, systemic process of promoting adoption of evidence-based practices in delivery of health care services that goes beyond dissemination of evidence-based guidelines (Berwick, 2003; Rogers, 2003; Titler & Everett, 2001). Dissemination activities take many forms, including publications, conferences, consultations, and training programs, but promoting knowledge uptake and changing practitioner behavior requires active interchange with those in direct care (Scott et al., 2008; Titler et al., 2008).This chapter presents an overview of evidence-based practice, and the process of applying evidence in practice to improve patient outcomes.

## OVERVIEW OF EVIDENCE-BASED PRACTICE

The relationships among conduct, dissemination, and use of research are illustrated in Figure 20-1. Conduct of research is the analysis of data collected from subjects who meet study inclusion and exclusion criteria for the purpose of answering research questions or testing hypotheses. Traditionally, the conduct of research has included dissemination of findings via research reports in journals and at scientific conferences.

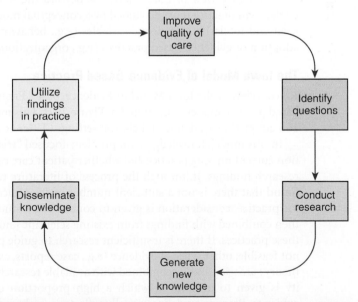

**FIGURE 20-1** The model of the relationship among conduct, dissemination, and use of research. (Redrawn from Weiler, K., Buckwalter, K., Titler, M. (1994). Debate: is nursing research used in practice? In J. McCloskey, & H. Grace (Eds.), *Current issues in nursing* (4th ed.). St Louis, MO: Mosby.)

Evidence-based practice is the conscientious and judicious use of current best evidence in conjunction with clinical expertise and patient values to guide health care decisions (Sackett et al., 2000). When enough research evidence is available, practice should be guided by research evidence in conjunction with clinical expertise and patient values. In some cases, however, a sufficient research base may not be available, and health care decision making is derived principally from nonresearch evidence sources such as expert opinion and scientific principles. As illustrated in Figure 20-1, application of research findings in practice may not only improve quality care but create new and exciting questions to be addressed via conduct of research.

The terms research utilization and evidence-based practice are sometimes used interchangeably. Although these two terms are related, they are not the same. Adopting the definition of evidence-based practice as the conscious and judicious use of the current "best" evidence in the care of patients and delivery of health care services; research utilization is a subset of evidence-based practice that focuses on the application of research findings. Evidence-based practice is a broader term that not only encompasses research utilization but also includes use of case reports and expert opinion in deciding the practices to be used in health care.

## Models of Evidence-Based Practice

Multiple models of evidence-based practice and translation science are available. Common elements of these models are syntheses of evidence, implementation, evaluation of the impact on patient care, and consideration of the context/setting in which the evidence is implemented. For a summary of models, the review by Grol and colleagues (2007) is recommended.

Although review of these models is beyond the scope of this chapter, implementing evidence in practice must be guided by a conceptual model to organize the strategies being used and to clarify extraneous variables (e.g., behaviors, facilitators) that may influence adoption of evidence-based practices (e.g., organizational size, characteristics of users).

## The Iowa Model of Evidence-Based Practice

An overview of the Iowa Model of Evidence-Based Practice as an example of an evidence-based practice model is illustrated in Figure 20-2. This model has been widely disseminated and adopted in academic and clinical settings (Titler et al., 2001).

In this model, knowledge- and problem-focused "triggers" lead staff members to question current nursing practice and whether patient care can be improved through the use of research findings. If, through the process of literature review and critique of studies, it is found that there is not a sufficient number of scientifically sound studies to use as a base for practice, consideration is given to conducting a study. Findings from such studies are then combined with findings from existing scientific knowledge to develop and implement these practices. If there is insufficient research to guide practice, and conducting a study is not feasible, other types of evidence (e.g., case reports, expert opinion, scientific principles, theory) are used and/or combined with available research evidence to guide practice. Priority is given to projects in which a high proportion of practice is guided by research evidence. Practice guidelines usually reflect research and nonresearch evidence and therefore are called evidence-based practice guidelines (see Chapter 11).

Recommendations for practice are developed based on evidence synthesis. The recommended practices, based on evidence, are compared to current practice and a decision is

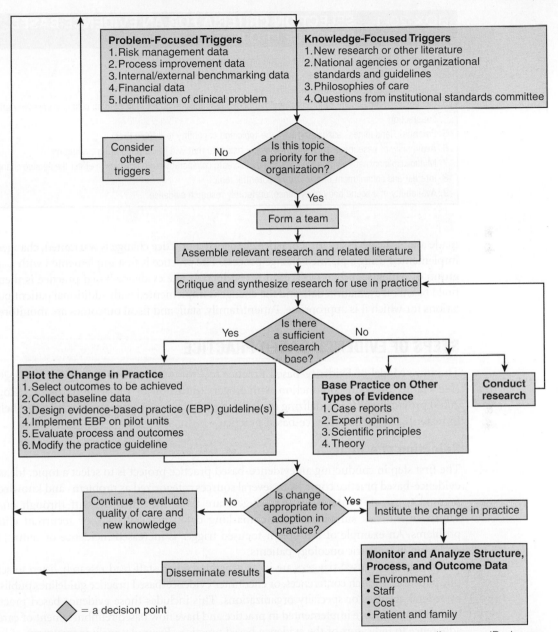

**FIGURE 20-2** The Iowa model of evidence-based practice to promote quality care. (Redrawn from Titler, M., et al. (2001). The Iowa model of evidence-based practice to promote quality care. *Critical Care Nursing Clinics of North America, 13*(4), 497–509.)

**BOX 20-1   SELECTION CRITERIA FOR AN EVIDENCE-BASED PRACTICE PROJECT**

1. Priority of the topic for nursing and for the organization
2. Magnitude of the problem (small, medium, large)
3. Applicability to several or few clinical areas
4. Likelihood of the change to improve quality of care, decrease length of stay, contain costs, or improve patient satisfaction
5. Potential "land mines" associated with the topic and capability to diffuse them
6. Availability of baseline quality improvement or risk data that will be helpful during evaluation
7. Multidisciplinary nature of the topic and ability to create collaborative relationships to effect the needed changes
8. Interest and commitment of staff to the potential topic
9. Availability of a sound body of evidence, preferably research evidence

made about the necessity for a practice change. If a practice change is warranted, changes are implemented using a planned change process. The practice is first implemented with a small group of patients, and an evaluation is conducted. The evidence-based practice is then refined based on evaluation data and the change is implemented with additional patient populations for which it is appropriate. Patient/family, staff, and fiscal outcomes are monitored.

## STEPS OF EVIDENCE-BASED PRACTICE

The Iowa Model of Evidence-Based Practice to Promote Quality Care (Titler et al., 2001) (see Figure 20-2), in conjunction with Rogers' diffusion of innovations model (Rogers, 2003) provide steps for actualizing evidence-based practice. A team approach is most helpful in fostering a specific evidence-based practice.

### Selection of a Topic

The first step in conducting an evidence-based practice project is to select a topic. Ideas for evidence-based practice come from several sources categorized as problem- and knowledge-focused triggers. Problem-focused triggers are those identified by staff through quality improvement, risk surveillance, benchmarking data, financial data, or recurrent clinical problems. An example of a problem-focused trigger is increased incidence of central line occlusion in pediatric oncology patients.

Knowledge-focused triggers are ideas generated when staff read research, listen to scientific papers at research conferences, or encounter evidence-based practice guidelines published by federal agencies or specialty organizations. This includes those evidence-based practices that CMS expects are implemented in practice and have now based reimbursement of care on adherence to indicators of the evidence-based practices. Examples include treatment of heart failure, community-acquired pneumonia, and prevention of nosocomial pressure ulcers. Each of these topics includes a nursing component, such as discharge teaching, instructions for patient self care, or pain management. Sometimes topics arise from a combination of problem- and knowledge-focused triggers, such as the length of bed rest time after femoral artery catheterization. In selecting a topic, it is essential that nurses consider how the topic fits with organization, department, and unit priorities to garner support from leaders within the organization and the necessary resources to successfully complete the project. Criteria to consider when selecting a topic are outlined in Box 20-1.

---

**HELPFUL HINT**

Regardless of which method is used to select an evidence-based practice topic, it is critical that the staff members who will implement the potential practice changes are involved in selecting the topic and view it as contributing significantly to the quality of care.

---

## Forming a Team

A team is responsible for development, implementation, and evaluation of the evidence-based practice. A task force approach also may be used, in which a group is appointed to address a practice issue. The composition of the team is directed by the topic selected and should include interested stakeholders in the delivery of care. For example, a team working on evidence-based pain management should be interdisciplinary and include pharmacists, nurses, physicians, and psychologists. In contrast, a team working on the evidence-based practice of bathing might include a nurse expert in skin care, assistive nursing personnel, and staff nurses.

In addition to forming a team, key stakeholders who can facilitate the evidence-based practice project or put up barriers against successful implementation should be identified. A stakeholder is a key individual or group of individuals who will be directly or indirectly affected by the implementation of the evidence-based practice. Some of these stakeholders are likely to be members of the team. Others may not be team members but are key individuals within the organization or unit who can adversely or positively influence the adoption of the evidence-based practice. Questions to consider in identification of key stakeholders include the following:

- How are decisions made in the practice areas where the evidence-based practice will be implemented?
- What types of system changes will be needed?
- Who is involved in decision making?
- Who is likely to lead and champion implementation of the evidence-based practice?
- Who can influence the decision to proceed with implementation of the practice?
- What type of cooperation is needed from the stakeholders for the project to be successful?

Failure to involve or keep supportive stakeholders informed may place the success of the project at risk because they are unable to anticipate and/or defend the rationale for changing practice, particularly with resistors (nonsupportive stakeholders) who have a great deal of influence among their peer group.

An important early task for the evidence-based practice team is to formulate the PICO question. This helps set boundaries around the project and assists in evidence retrieval. This approach is illustrated in Table 20-1 (see Chapters 1, 2, 3, and 19).

## Evidence Retrieval

Once a topic is selected, relevant research and related literature need to be retrieved, including clinical studies, meta-analyses, and existing evidence-based practice guidelines (see Chapters 3 and 11). AHRQ (www.AHRQ.gov) sponsors the Evidenced-Based Practice Centers and a National Guideline Clearinghouse where abstracts of evidence-based practice guidelines are available. Current best evidence from specific studies of clinical problems can

| TABLE 20-1 | USING PICO TO FORMULATE THE EVIDENCE-BASED PRACTICE QUESTION | | | |
|---|---|---|---|---|
| | PATIENT/ POPULATION/ PROBLEM | INTERVENTION/ TREATMENT | COMPARISON INTERVENTION | OUTCOME(S) |
| Tips for Building the Question | How would we describe a group of patients similar to ours? | Which main intervention are we considering? | What is the main alternative to compare with the intervention? | What can we hope to accomplish? |
| Example 1 | Pain management for elders admitted to a hospital with a hip fracture | Pain assessment—pain tool Patient-controlled analgesia | Standard of care Nurse-administered analgesic | Regular (e.g., q4hr) pain assessment Less pain intensity Earlier mobility Decreased length of stay |
| Example 2 | Pain assessment of cognitively impaired elders | Pain assessment tool designed for assessing pain in cognitively impaired elders in long-term care setting | Not assess pain Yes/no question | Regular pain assessment with treatment of pain Fewer residents in pain |

Modified from University of Illinois at Chicago, P.I.C.O. Model for Clinical Questions, www.uic.edu/depts/lib/lhsp/resources/pico.shtml.

be found in an increasing number of electronic databases such as the Cochrane Library (www.thecochranelibrary.com), the Centers for Health Evidence (www.cche.net), and Best Evidence (www.acponline.org) (see Chapter 3). Once the literature is located, it is helpful to classify the articles as clinical (nonresearch), theory articles, research articles, systematic reviews, and evidence-based practice guidelines. Before reading and critiquing the research, it is useful to read background articles to have a broad view of the topic and related concepts, and to then review existing evidence-based practice guidelines. It is helpful to read articles in the following order:

1. Clinical articles to understand the state of the practice
2. Theory articles to understand the theoretical perspectives and concepts that may be encountered in critiquing studies
3. Systematic reviews and synthesis reports to understand the state of the science
4. Evidence-based practice guidelines and evidence reports
5. Research articles, including meta-analyses

## Schemas for Grading the Evidence

There is no consensus among professional organizations or across health care disciplines regarding the best system to use for denoting the type and quality of evidence, or the grading schemas to denote the strength of the body of evidence (Guyatt et al., 2008a; Institute of Medicine, 2011). See Tables 20-2 and 20-3 for grading and assessing quality of research studies. The important domains and elements to include in grading the strength of the evidence are defined in Table 20-4.

In grading the evidence, two important areas are essential to address: (1) the quality of the individual research; and (2) the strength of the body of evidence. Important domains and elements of any system used to rate quality of individual studies are in Table 20-3 by type of

## TABLE 20-2  EXAMPLES OF EVIDENCE-BASED PRACTICE RATING SYSTEMS

| GRADE WORKING GROUP (GRADE WORKING GROUP, 2004; GUYATT et al., 2008b) | U.S. PREVENTATIVE SERVICES TASK FORCE AFTER MAY 2007 (HARRIS et al., 2001; U.S. PREVENTIVE SERVICES TASK FORCE, 2008) |
|---|---|
| **Strength of Evidence: Quality of the Evidence** | **Levels of Certainty Regarding Net Benefit** |
| High: Further research is very unlikely to change confidence in the estimate of effect. Scientific evidence provided by well-designed, well-conducted, controlled trials (randomized and nonrandomized) with statistically significant results that consistently support the recommendation. | High: Available evidence usually includes consistent results from well-designed, well-conducted studies in representative primary care populations. These studies assess effects of the preventive service on health outcomes. This conclusion is therefore unlikely to be strongly affected by the results of future studies. |
| Moderate: Further research is likely to have an important impact on confidence in the estimate of effect and may change the estimate. | Moderate: The available evidence is sufficient to determine the effects of the preventive service on health outcomes, but confidence in the estimate is constrained by such factors as: |
| Low: Further research is very likely to have an important impact on confidence in the estimate of effect and is likely to change the estimate | The number, size, or quality of individual studies. Inconsistency of findings across individual studies. |
| Very Low: Any estimate of effect is very uncertain. | Limited generalizability of findings to routine primary care practice. |
| Note: The type of evidence is first ranked as follows: Randomized trial = high. Observational study = low. Any other evidence = very low. | Lack of coherence in the chain of evidence. |
| Limitations in study quality, important inconsistency of results, uncertainty about the directness of the evidence, imprecise or sparse data, and high probability of reporting bias can lower the evidence grade. Expert opinion that supports the guideline recommendation because the available scientific evidence did not present consistent results or because controlled trials were lacking. Grade of evidence can be increased if there is (1) strong evidence of association—significant relative risk of $>2.0$ $(< 0.5)$ based on consistent evidence from two or more observational studies, with no plausible confounders (1); (2) very strong evidence of association—significant relative risk of $>5.0$ $(<0.2)$ based on direct evidence with no major threats to validity (2); (3) evidence of a dose response gradient (1); and (4) all plausible confounders would have reduced the effect (1). | As more information becomes available, the magnitude or direction of the observed effect could change, and this change may be large enough to alter the conclusion. |
| | Low: The available evidence is insufficient to assess effects on health outcomes. Evidence is insufficient because of one or more of the following: The limited number or size of studies. Important flaws in study design or methods. Inconsistency of findings across individual studies. Gaps in the chain of evidence. Findings not generalizable to routine primary care practice. Lack of information on important health outcomes. More information may allow estimation of effects on health outcomes. |

*Continued*

## TABLE 20-2 EXAMPLES OF EVIDENCE-BASED PRACTICE RATING SYSTEMS—cont'd

### GRADE WORKING GROUP (GRADE WORKING GROUP, 2004; GUYATT et al., 2008b)

**Strength of Recommendations**

Strong: confident that desirable effects of adherence to a recommendation outweigh undesirable effects.

Weak: desirable effects of adherence to a recommendation probably outweigh the undesirable effects, but developers are less confident.

Note: Strength of recommendation is determined by the balance between desirable and undesirable consequences of alternative management strategies, quality of evidence, variability in values and preferences, and resource use.

### U.S. PREVENTATIVE SERVICES TASK FORCE AFTER MAY 2007 (HARRIS et al., 2001; U.S. PREVENTIVE SERVICES TASK FORCE, 2008)

**Recommendation Grades**

A. USPSTF recommends the service. There is high certainty that the net benefit is substantial. Practice: Offer or provide this service.

B. USPSTF recommends the service. There is high certainty that the net benefit is moderate or there is moderate certainty that the net benefit is moderate to substantial. Practice: Offer or provide this service.

C. USPSTF recommends against routinely providing the service. There may be considerations that support providing the service in an individual patient. There is at least moderate certainty that the net benefit is small. Practice: Offer or provide this service only if other considerations support the offering or providing the service in an individual patient.

D. USPSTF recommends against the service. There is moderate or high certainty that the service has no net benefit or that the harms outweigh the benefits. Practice: Discourage the use of this service.

E. The USPSTF concludes that the current evidence is insufficient to assess the balance of benefits and harms of the service. Evidence is lacking, of poor quality, or conflicting, and the balance of benefits and harms cannot be determined. Practice: Read the clinical considerations section of USPSTF Recommendation Statement. If the service is offered, patients should understand the uncertainty about the balance of benefits and harms.

study. The domains and elements to include in grading the strength of the evidence are defined in Table 20-4. The information posted on the GRADE Web site (www.gradeworkinggroup.org) is also important information to understand the challenges and approaches for assessing the quality of evidence and strength of recommendations. In Chapter 1, Figure 1-1 provides an evidence hierarchy used for grading the evidence that is an adaptation similar to the evidence hierarchies that appear in Table 20-2.

## TABLE 20-3 IMPORTANT DOMAINS AND ELEMENTS FOR SYSTEMS TO RATE QUALITY OF INDIVIDUAL ARTICLES

| SYSTEMATIC REVIEWS | RANDOMIZED CLINICAL TRIALS | OBSERVATIONAL STUDIES | DIAGNOSTIC TEST STUDIES |
|---|---|---|---|
| *Study question* | Study question | Study question | *Study population* |
| *Search strategy* | *Study population* | Study population | *Adequate description of test* |
| *Inclusion and exclusion criteria* | *Randomization* | *Comparability of subjects* | *Appropriate reference standard* |
| Interventions | *Blinding* | *Exposure or intervention* | *Blinded comparison of test and reference* |
| Outcomes | Interventions | Outcome measurement | *Avoidance of verification bias* |
| *Data extraction* | Outcomes | *Statistical analysis* | |
| Study quality and validity | *Statistical analysis* | Results | |
| Data synthesis and analysis | Results | Discussion | |
| Results | Discussion | *Funding or sponsorship* | |
| Discussion | *Funding or sponsorship* | | |
| *Funding or sponsorship* | | | |

Modified from Agency for Healthcare Research and Quality. (2002). *Systems to rate the strength of scientific evidence: evidence report/technology assessment number 47*. Rockville, MD: Agency for Healthcare Research and Quality, U.S. Department of Health and Human Services.
Key domains are in *italics*.

## TABLE 20-4 IMPORTANT DOMAINS AND ELEMENTS FOR SYSTEMS TO GRADE THE STRENGTH OF EVIDENCE

| | |
|---|---|
| Quality | The aggregate of quality ratings for individual studies, predicated on the extent to which bias was minimized. |
| Quantity | Magnitude of effect, numbers of studies, and sample size or power. |
| Consistency | For any given topic, the extent to which similar findings are reported using similar and different study designs. |
| Relevance | Relevance of findings to characteristics of individual groups. |

Modified from IOM (2011).

## Critique and Synthesis of Research

Critique of evidence-based guidelines (see Chapter 11) and studies (see Chapters 8, 9 and 10) should use the same methodology, and the critique process should be a shared responsibility. It is helpful, however, to have one individual provide leadership for the project and design strategies for completing critiques. A group approach to critiques is recommended because it distributes the workload, helps those responsible for implementing the changes to understand the scientific base for the practice change, arms nurses with citations and research-based language to use in advocating for practice changes with peers and those in other disciplines, and provides novices an environment to learn critique and application of research findings. Methods to make the critique process fun and interesting include the following:

- Using a journal club to discuss critiques done by each member of the group
- Pairing a novice and expert to do critiques
- Eliciting assistance from students who may be interested in the topic and want experience doing critiques

- Assigning the critique process to graduate students interested in the topic
- Making a class project of critique and synthesis of research for a given topic
- Critiquing criteria at the end of each chapter and the critiquing criteria summary tables in Chapters 6 and 18

**HELPFUL HINT**

Keep critique processes simple, and encourage participation by staff members who are providing direct patient care.

Once studies are critiqued, a decision is made regarding use of each study in the synthesis of the evidence for application in practice. Factors that should be considered for inclusion of studies in the synthesis of findings are overall scientific merit of the study; type (e.g., age, gender, pathology) of subjects enrolled in the study and the similarity to the patient population to which the findings will be applied; and relevance of the study to the topic of question. For example, if the practice area is prevention of deep venous thrombosis in postoperative patients, a descriptive study using a heterogeneous population of medical patients is not appropriate for inclusion in the synthesis of findings.

To synthesize the findings from research critiques, it is helpful to use a summary table in which critical information from studies can be documented. Essential information to include in such summary is the following:

- Research questions/hypotheses
- The independent and dependent variables studied
- A description of the study sample and setting
- The type of research design
- The methods used to measure each variable and outcome
- The study findings

An example of a summary form is illustrated in Table 20-5.

**HELPFUL HINT**

Use of a summary form helps identify commonalities across several studies with regard to study findings and the types of patients to which study findings can be applied. It also helps in synthesizing the overall strengths and weakness of the studies as a group.

## Setting Forth Evidence-Based Practice Recommendations

Based on the critique of practice guidelines and synthesis of research, recommendations for practice are set forth. The type and strength of evidence used to support the practice needs to be clearly delineated in your evidence table. Box 20-2 is another useful tool to assist with this activity.

## Decision to Change Practice

After studies are critiqued and synthesized the next step is to decide if the findings are appropriate for use in practice. Criteria to consider include the following:

- Relevance of evidence for practice
- Consistency in findings across studies and/or guidelines

| TABLE 20-5 | EXAMPLE OF A SUMMARY TABLE FOR RESEARCH CRITIQUES | | | | | | | | | |
|---|---|---|---|---|---|---|---|---|---|---|
| CITATION | RESEARCH QUESTION | RESEARCH DESIGN | SAMPLE | INDEPENDENT VARIABLES AND MEASURES | DEPENDENT VARIABLES AND MEASURES | RESULTS | GENERAL STRENGTHS | GENERAL WEAKNESSES | OVERALL QUALITY OF STUDY* | SUMMARY STATEMENTS FOR PRACTICE |
|  |  |  |  |  |  |  |  |  |  |  |
|  |  |  |  |  |  |  |  |  |  |  |
|  |  |  |  |  |  |  |  |  |  |  |
|  |  |  |  |  |  |  |  |  |  |  |

*Use a consistent rating system (e.g., good, fair, poor).

| BOX 20-2 | **CONSISTENCY OF EVIDENCE FROM CRITIQUED RESEARCH, APPRAISALS OF EVIDENCE-BASED PRACTICE GUIDELINES, CRITIQUED SYSTEMATIC REVIEWS, AND NONRESEARCH LITERATURE** |
|---|---|

1. Are there replication of studies with consistent results?
2. Are the studies well designed?
3. Are recommendations consistent among systematic reviews, evidence-based practice guidelines, and critiqued research?
4. Are there identified risks to the patient by applying evidence-based practice recommendations?
5. Are there identified benefits to the patient?
6. Have cost analysis studies been conducted on the recommended action, intervention, or treatment?
7. Summary recommendations about assessments, actions, interventions/treatments from the research, systematic reviews, evidence-based guidelines with an assigned evidence grade.

Modified from Titler, M. G. (2002). *Toolkit for promoting evidence-based practice.* Iowa City, IA: Department of Nursing Services and Patient Care, University of Iowa Hospitals and Clinics.

- A significant number of studies and/or evidence-based practice guidelines with sample characteristics similar to those to which the findings will be used
- Consistency among evidence from research and other nonresearch evidence
- Feasibility for use in practice
- The risk/benefit ratio (risk of harm versus the potential benefit for the patient)

Synthesis of study findings and other evidence may result in supporting current practice, making minor practice modifications, undertaking major practice changes, or developing a new area of practice.

## Development of Evidence-Based Practice

The next step is to document the evidence base of the practice using the agreed upon grading schema. When critique results and synthesis of evidence support current practice or suggest a practice change, a written evidence-based practice standard (e.g., policy, procedure, guideline) is warranted. This is necessary so that individuals in the setting know (1) that the practices are based on evidence, and (2) the type of evidence (e.g., randomized controlled trial, expert opinion) used in development of the practice.

It is imperative that once the evidence-based practice standard is written, key stakeholders have an opportunity to review it and provide feedback to the individual(s) responsible for developing it. Use of focus groups is a useful way to provide discussion about the evidence-based practice and to identify key areas that may be potentially troublesome during the implementation phase. Key questions that can be used in the focus groups are in Box 20-3.

| **HELPFUL HINT** |
|---|
| Use a consistent approach to writing evidence-based practice standards and referencing the research and related literature. |

## BOX 20-3 KEY QUESTIONS FOR FOCUS GROUPS

1. What is needed by staff (e.g., nurses, physicians) to use the evidence-based practice with patients in units (specify unit)?
2. In your opinion, how will this standard improve patient care in your unit/practice?
3. What modifications would you suggest in the evidence-based practice standard before using it in your practice?
4. What content in the evidence-based practice standard is unclear? Needs revision?
5. What would you change about the format of the evidence-based practice standard?
6. What part of this evidence-based practice change do you view as most challenging?
7. Any other suggestions?

## Implementing the Practice Change

If a practice change is warranted, the next steps are to make the changes in practice. This goes beyond writing a policy or procedure that is evidence based; it requires interaction among direct care providers to champion and foster evidence adoption, leadership support, and system changes. Rogers's (2003) seminal work on diffusion of innovations is extremely useful in selecting strategies for promoting adoption of evidence-based practices. According to this model, adoption of evidence-based practice innovations is influenced by the nature of the innovation (e.g., the type and strength of evidence, the clinical topic) and the manner in which it is communicated (disseminated) to members (nurses) of a social system (organization, nursing profession). Strategies for promoting adoption of evidence-based practices must address these areas within a context of participative, planned change (Figure 20-3).

### Nature of the Innovation/Evidence-Based Practice

Characteristics of an innovation or evidence-based practice that affect adoption include the relative advantage of the evidence-based practice (e.g., effectiveness, relevance to the task, social prestige); the compatibility with values, norms, work, and perceived

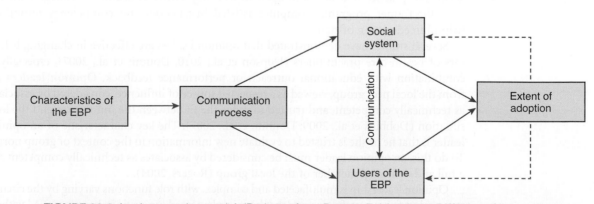

FIGURE 20-3 Implementation model. (Redrawn from Rogers, E. M. (2003). *Diffusion of innovations* (5th ed.). New York, NY: Free Press; Titler, M. G., & Everett, L. Q. (2001). Translating research into practice: considerations for critical care investigators. *Critical Care Nursing Clinics of North America, 13*(4), 587–604.)

needs of users; and complexity of the evidence-based practice topic (Rogers, 2003). For example, evidence-based practice topics that are perceived by users as relatively simple (e.g., influenza vaccines for older adults) are more easily adopted in less time than those that are more complex (e.g., acute pain management for hospitalized older adults).

An important principle to remember when planning implementation of an evidence-based practice is that the attributes of the evidence-based practice topic as perceived by users and stakeholders (e.g., ease of use, valued part of practice) are neither stable features nor sure determinants of their adoption. Rather, it is the interaction among the characteristics of the evidence-based practice topic, the intended users, and a particular context of practice that determines the rate and extent of adoption (Dogherty et al., 2012; Greenhalgh et al., 2005). An example of a quick reference guide is shown in Figure 20-4.

## Methods of Communication

Interpersonnel communication methods and influence among social networks of users affect adoption of evidence-based practices (Rogers, 2003). Use of opinion leaders, change champions, consultation with experts in the field, and education are strategies tested to promote adoption of evidence-based practices. Education is necessary but not sufficient to change practice, and didactic continuing education alone does little to change practice behavior (Farmer et al., 2008; Forsetlund et al., 2009). It is important that staff know the scientific basis and improvements in quality of care anticipated by the changes. Disseminating information to staff needs to be done creatively. A staff in-service may not be the most effective method nor reach the majority of the staff. Although it is unrealistic for all staff to have participated in the critique process or to have read all studies used, it is important that they know the myths and realities of the practice. Staff education must also include ensuring competence in the skills necessary to carry out the new practice.

One method of communicating information to staff is through use of colorful posters that identify myths and realities or describe the essence of the change in practice (Titler et al., 2001). Visibly identifying those who have learned the information and are using the evidence-based practice (e.g., buttons, ribbons, pins) stimulates interest in others who may not have internalized the change. As a result, the "new" learner may begin asking questions about the practice and be more open to learning. Other educational strategies such as train-the-trainer programs, computer-assisted instruction, and competency testing are helpful in education of staff.

Several studies have demonstrated that opinion leaders are effective in changing behaviors of health care practitioners (Dopson et al., 2010; Doumit et al., 2007), especially in combination with educational outreach or performance feedback. **Opinion leaders** are from the local peer group, viewed as a respected source of influence, considered by associates as technically competent, and trusted to judge the fit between the innovation and the local situation (Dobbins et al., 2009; Doumit, et al., 2007). The key characteristic of an opinion leader is that he or she is trusted to evaluate new information in the context of group norms. To do this, an opinion leader must be considered by associates as technically competent and a full and dedicated member of the local group (Rogers, 2003).

Opinion leadership is multifaceted and complex, with role functions varying by the circumstances, but few successful projects that have implemented innovations have managed without the input of identifiable opinion leaders (Greenhalgh et al., 2005). Social interactions such as "hallway chats," one-on-one discussions, and addressing questions are important yet often overlooked components of translation (Jordan et. al., 2009). If the evidence-based practice that

*Use this quick reference guide to help in the assessment of pain:*
- Before patients undergo medical procedures or surgeries that can cause pain
- When patients are experiencing pain from recent surgeries, medical procedures, trauma, or other acute illness

*General principles for assessing pain in older adults:*
- Verify sensory ability (Can the person see you? Hear you?).
- Allow time to respond.
- Repeat questions/instructions as necessary.
- Use printed materials with large type and dark lines.

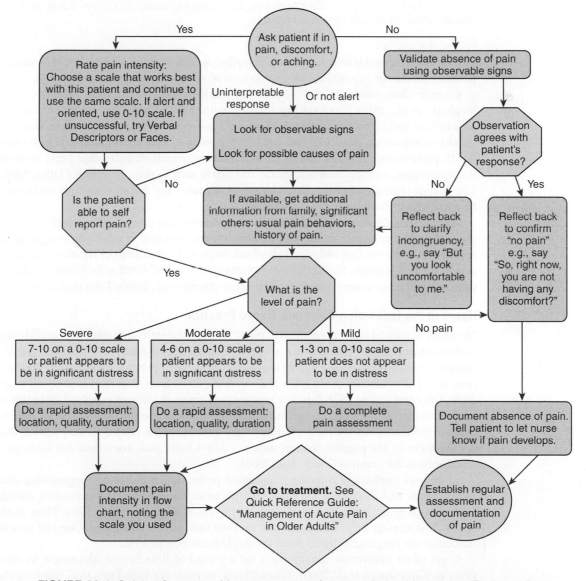

**FIGURE 20-4** Quick reference guide: assessment of acute pain in older adults. (Redrawn from Harris, R. P., et al. (2001). Current methods of the U.S. Preventive Services Task Force: a review of the process, *American Journal of Preventative Medicine*, 20(Suppl 3), 21–35; Herr, K., et al. (2000). *Evidence-based guideline: from book to bedside–acute pain management in the elderly.* Iowa City, IA: University of Iowa.)

| BOX 20-4    **ROLE EXPECTATIONS OF AN OPINION LEADER** |
| --- |
| 1. Be/become an expert in the evidence-based practice. |
| 2. Provide organizational/unit leadership for adopting the evidence-based practice. |
| 3. Implement various strategies to educate peers about the evidence-based practice. |
| 4. Work with peers, other disciplines, and leadership staff to incorporate key information about the evidence-based practice into organizational/unit standards, policies, procedures, and documentation systems. |
| 5. Promote initial and ongoing use of the evidence-based practice by peers. |

From Titler, M. G., et al. (2006). *Book to bedside: promoting and sustaining EBPs in elders.* Iowa City, IA: University of Iowa College of Nursing.

is being implemented is interdisciplinary, discipline-specific opinion leaders should be used to promote the change in practice. Role expectations of an opinion leader are in Box 20-4.

Change champions are also helpful for implementing innovations (Rogers, 2003; Dogherty et al., 2012). They are practitioners within the local group setting (e.g., clinic, patient care unit) who are expert clinicians, are passionate about the innovation, are committed to improving quality of care, and have a positive working relationship with other health professionals (Rogers, 2003). They circulate information, encourage peers to adopt the innovation, arrange demonstrations, and orient staff to the innovation (Titler, 2004). The change champion believes in an idea; will not take "no" for an answer; is undaunted by insults and rebuffs; and above all, persists.

Advanced practice nurses (APNs) can provide one-on-one consultation to staff regarding use of the evidence-based practice with specific patients, assist staff in troubleshooting issues in application of the practice, and provide feedback on provider performance regarding use of the evidence-based practices. Studies have demonstrated that use of APNs as facilitators of change promote adherence to the evidence-based practice (Stetler et al., 2006a; Titler et al., 2008).

## Users of the Innovation/Evidence-Based Practice

Members of a social system (e.g., nurses, physicians, clerical staff) influence how quickly and widely evidence-based practices are adopted (Rogers, 2003). Audit and feedback, performance gap assessment (PGA), and trying the evidence-based practice are strategies that have been tested (Greenhalgh et al., 2005; Hysong et al., 2006; Ivers et al., 2012; Jamtvedt et al., 2010; Titler et al., 2006). PGA (baseline practice performance) informs members at the beginning of change about a practice performance and opportunities for improvement. Specific practice indicators selected for performance gap assessment are related to the practices that are the focus of the practice change, such as every-4-hour pain assessment for acute pain management, for example (Titler et al., 2006).

Audit and feedback is ongoing auditing of performance indicators, aggregating data into reports, and discussing the findings with practitioners during the practice change (Greenhalgh et al., 2005; Ivers et al., 2012; Jamtvedt et al., 2010; Titler, 2004; Titler et al., 2006). This strategy helps staff know and see how their efforts to improve care and patient outcomes are progressing throughout the implementation process.

Users of an innovation usually try it for a period of time before adopting it in their practice (Greenhalgh et al., 2005). When "trying an evidence-based practice" (piloting the change) is incorporated as part of the implementation process, users have an opportunity to use it, provide feedback to those in charge of implementation, and modify the practice if necessary. Piloting the practice as part of implementation has a positive influence on the extent of adoption of the new practice (Greenhalgh et al., 2005; Rogers, 2003; Stetler et al., 2006b).

### Social System

Clearly, the social system or context of care delivery matters when implementing evidence-based practices (Kochevar & Yano, 2006; Rogers, 2003). For example, investigators demonstrated the effectiveness of a prompted voiding intervention for urinary incontinence in nursing homes, but sustaining the intervention in day-to-day practice was limited when the responsibility of carrying out the intervention was shifted to nursing home staff (rather than the investigative team) and required staffing levels in excess of a majority of nursing home settings (Engberg et al., 2004). This illustrates the importance of embedding interventions into ongoing care processes.

As part of the work of implementing evidence-based practices, it is important that the social system (e.g., unit, service line, clinic) ensure that policies, procedures, standards, clinical pathways, and documentation systems support the use of the evidence-based practices (Titler, 2004). Documentation forms or clinical information systems may need revision to support practice changes; documentation systems that fail to readily support the new practice thwart change. For example, if staff members are expected to reassess and document pain intensity within 30 minutes after administration of an analgesic agent, documentation forms must reflect this practice standard. It is the role of leadership to ensure that organizational documents and systems are flexible and supportive of the evidence-based practices.

A learning organizational culture and proactive leadership that promotes knowledge sharing are important components for building an evidence-based practice (Lozano et al., 2004). Components of a receptive context for evidence-based-practice include the following:

- Strong leadership
- Clear strategic vision
- Good managerial relations
- Visionary staff in key positions
- A climate conducive to experimentation and risk taking
- Effective data-capture systems

An organization may be generally amenable to innovations but not ready or willing to assimilate a particular evidence-based practice. Elements of system readiness include the following:

- Tension for change
- Evidence-based practice–system fit
- Assessment of implications
- Support and advocacy for the evidence-based practice
- Dedicated time and resources
- Capacity to evaluate the impact of the evidence-based practice during and following implementation

Leadership support is critical for promoting use of evidence-based practices (Berwick, 2003), and is expressed verbally, and by providing necessary resources, materials, and time to fulfill responsibilities (Stetler et al., 2006b). Senior leadership needs to create an organizational mission, vision, and strategic plan that incorporates evidence-based practice, implements performance expectations for staff that include evidence-based practice work, integrates the work of evidence-based practice into the governance structure of the health care system, demonstrates the value of evidence-based practices through

## BOX 20-5    STEPS OF EVALUATION FOR EVIDENCE-BASED PROJECTS

1. Identify process and outcome variables of interest.
   *Example:* Process variable—Patients > 65 years will have a Braden scale completed on admission.
   Outcome variable—Presence/absence of nosocomial pressure ulcer; if present, determine stage as I, II, III, IV.
2. Determine methods and frequency of data collection.
   *Example:* Process variable—Chart audit of all patients > 65 years, 1 day a month.
   Outcome variable—Patient assessment of all patients > 65 years, 1 day a month.
3. Determine baseline and follow-up sample sizes.
4. Design data collection forms.
   *Example:* Process chart audit abstraction form.
   Outcome variable—pressure ulcer assessment form.
5. Establish content validity of data collection forms.
6. Train data collectors.
7. Assess interrater reliability of data collectors.
8. Collect data at specified intervals.
9. Provide "on-site" feedback to staff regarding the progress in achieving the practice change.
10. Provide feedback of analyzed data to staff.
11. Use data to assist staff in modifying or integrating the evidence-based practice change.

administrative behaviors, and establishes explicit expectations that nurse leaders will create microsystems that value and support clinical inquiry (Titler, 2002).

In summary, making an evidence-based change in practice involves a series of action steps in a complex, nonlinear process. Implementing the change takes time to integrate depending on the nature of the practice change. Merely increasing staff knowledge about an evidence-based practice and passive dissemination strategies are not likely to work, particularly in complex health care settings. Strategies that seem to have a positive effect on promoting use of evidence-based practices include audit and feedback, use of clinical reminders and practice prompts, opinion leaders, change champions, interactive education, mass media, educational outreach/academic detailing, and the context of care delivery (e.g., leadership, learning, questioning). It is important that senior leadership and those leading evidence-based practice improvements are aware of change as a process and continue to encourage and teach peers about the change in practice. The new practice must be continually reinforced and sustained or the practice change will be intermittent and soon fade, allowing more traditional methods of care to return.

## Evaluation

Evaluation provides an opportunity to collect and analyze data with regard to use of a new evidence-based practice and then to modify the practice as necessary. It is important that the evidence-based change is evaluated, both at the pilot testing phase and when the practice is changed in additional patient care areas. The importance of the evaluation cannot be overemphasized; it provides information for performance gap assessment, audit, and feedback, and provides information necessary to determine if the evidence-based practice should be retained, modified, or eliminated.

An outcome achieved in a controlled environment (as when a researcher is implementing a study protocol for a homogeneous group of study patients) may not result in the same outcome when the practice is implemented in the natural clinical setting by several caregivers to a more heterogeneous patient population. Steps of the evaluation process are summarized in Box 20-5.

| TABLE 20-6 | EXAMPLES OF EVALUATION MEASURES | | | | | |
|---|---|---|---|---|---|---|
| | | NURSES' SELF-RATING | | | | |
| **EXAMPLE PROCESS QUESTIONS** | | SD | D | NA/D | A | SA |
| I feel well prepared to use the Braden Scale with older patients. | | 1 | 2 | 3 | 4 | 5 |
| Malnutrition increases patient risk for pressure ulcer development. | | 1 | 2 | 3 | 4 | 5 |
| **EXAMPLE OUTCOME QUESTION** | | | | | | |
| **PATIENT** | | | | | | |
| On a scale of 0 (no pain) to 10 (worst possible pain), how much pain have you experienced over the past 24 hours? | (Pain intensity) | | | | | |

SD, strongly disagree; D, disagree; NA/D, neither agree nor disagree; A, agree; SA, strongly agree.

Evaluation should include both process and outcome measures. The process component focuses on how the practice change is being implemented. It is important to know if staff are using the practice and implementing the practice as noted in the evidence-based practice guideline. Evaluation of the process also should note (1) barriers that staff encounter in carrying out the practice (e.g., lack of information, skills, or necessary equipment), (2) differences in opinions among health care providers, and (3) difficulty in carrying out the steps of the practice as originally designed (e.g., shutting off tube feedings 1 hour before aspirating contents for checking placement of nasointestinal tubes). Process data can be collected from staff and/or patient self-reports, medical record audits, or observation of clinical practice. Examples of process and outcome questions are shown in Table 20-6.

Outcome data are an equally important part of evaluation. The purpose of outcome evaluation is to assess whether the patient, staff, and/or fiscal outcomes expected are achieved. Therefore it is important that baseline data be used for a preintervention/postintervention comparison (Titler et al., 2001). The outcome variables measured should be those that are projected to change as a result of changing practice. For example, research demonstrates that less restricted family visiting practices in critical care units result in improved satisfaction with care. Thus patient and family member satisfaction should be an outcome measure that is evaluated as part of changing visiting practices in adult critical care units. Outcome measures should be measured before the change in practice is implemented, after implementation, and every 6 to 12 months thereafter. Findings must be provided to clinicians to reinforce the impact of the change and to ensure that they are incorporated into quality improvement programs. When collecting process and outcome data for evaluation of a practice change, it is important that the data collection tools are user-friendly, short, concise, easy to complete, and have content validity. Focus must be on collecting the most essential data. Those responsible for collecting evaluative data must be trained on data collection methods and be assessed for interrater reliability (see Chapters 14 and 15). It is our experience that those individuals who have participated in implementing the protocol can be very helpful in evaluation by collecting data, providing timely feedback to staff, and assisting staff to overcome barriers encountered when implementing the changes in practice.

One question that often arises is how much data are needed to evaluate this change. The preferred number of patients (N) is somewhat dependent on the size of the patient population affected by the practice change. For example, if the practice change is for families of critically ill adult patients and the organization has 1,000 adult critical care patients annually, 50 to 100 satisfaction responses preimplementation, and 25 to 50 responses postimplementation, at 3 and 6 months should be adequate to look for trends in satisfaction and possible areas that need to be addressed in continuing this practice (e.g., more bedside chairs in patient rooms). The rule of thumb is to keep the evaluation simple, because data often are collected by busy clinicians who may lose interest if the data collection, analysis, and feedback are too long and tedious. It is also important to check with your institution's guidelines for collecting data related to practice changes as institutional approval may be needed.

The evaluation process includes planned feedback to staff who are making the change. The feedback includes verbal and/or written appreciation for the work and visual demonstration of progress in implementation and improvement in patient outcomes. The key to effective evaluation is to ensure that the evidence-based change in practice is warranted (e.g., will improve quality of care) and that the intervention does not bring harm to patients.

---

### HELPFUL HINT

Include patient outcome measures (e.g., pressure ulcer prevalence) and cost (e.g., cost savings, cost avoidance) in evaluation practice projects.

---

## FUTURE DIRECTIONS

Education must include knowledge and skills in the use of research evidence in practice. Nurses are increasingly being held accountable for practices based on scientific evidence. Thus we must communicate and integrate into our profession the expectation that it is the professional responsibility of all nurses to read and use research in their practice, and to communicate with nurse scientists the many and varied clinical problems for which we do not yet have a scientific base.

## ■ KEY POINTS

- The terms *research utilization* and *evidence-based practice* are sometimes used interchangeably. These terms, though related, are not the same. Research utilization is the process of using research findings to improve practice. Evidence-based practice is a broad term that not only encompasses use of research findings, but also use of other types of evidence, such as case reports and expert opinion in deciding the evidence base for practice.
- There are several models of evidence-based practice. A key feature of all models is the judicious review and synthesis of research and other types of evidence to develop an evidence-based practice standard.
- The steps of evidence-based practice using the Iowa Model of Evidence-Based Practice are as follows: selection of a topic, forming a team, retrieval of the evidence, grading the

evidence, developing an evidence-based practice standard, implementing the evidence-based practice, and evaluating the effect on staff, patient, and fiscal outcomes.

- Adoption of evidence-based practice standards requires education and dissemination to staff as well as the use of change strategies such as opinion leaders, change champions, use of a core group, and consultants.
- It is important to evaluate the change. Evaluation provides data for performance gap assessment, audit, and feedback, and provides information necessary to determine if the practice should be retained.
- Evaluation includes both process and outcome measures.
- It is important for organizations to create a culture of evidence-based practice. To create this culture requires an interactive process. Organizations need to provide access to information, access to individuals who have skills necessary for evidence-based practice, and a written and verbal commitment to evidence-based practice in the organization's operations.

## CRITICAL THINKING CHALLENGES

- Discuss the differences among nursing research, research utilization, and evidence-based practice. Support your discussion with examples.
- Why would it be important to use an evidence-based practice model, such as the Iowa Model of Evidence-Based Practice, to guide a practice project focused on justifying and implementing a change in clinical practice?
- You are a staff nurse working on a cardiac step-down unit. Many of your colleagues do not understand evidence-based practice. How would you help them to understand the relevance of evidence-based practice to providing optimal care to this patient population?
- What barriers do you see to applying evidence-based practice in your clinical setting? Discuss strategies to use in overcoming these barriers.

## REFERENCES

Berwick, D. M. (2003). Disseminating innovations in health care. *Journal of the American Medical Association*, *289*(15), 1969–1975.

Centers for Medicare and Medicaid Services. (2008). Retrieved December 2012 from www.cms.hhs.gov/.

Dobbins, M., Robeson, P., Ciliska, D., et al. (2009). A description of a knowledge broker role implemented as part of a randomized controlled trial evaluating three knowledge translation strategies. *Implementation Science*, *4*, 23.

Dogherty, E. J., Harrison, M. B., Baker, C., & Graham, I. D. (2012). Following a natural experiment of guideline adaptation and early implementation: a mixed methods study of facilitation. *Implementation Science*, *7*, 9.

Dopson, S., FitzGerald, L., Ferlie, E., et al. (2010). No magic targets! Changing clinical practice to become more evidence based. *Health Care Management Review*, *27*(3), 35–47.

Doumit, G., Gattellari, M., Grimshaw, J., & O'Brien, M. A. (2007). Local opinion leaders: effects on professional practice and health care outcomes. *Cochrane Database of Systematic Reviews*, *2007*(1), CD000125.

Engberg, S., Kincade, J., & Thompson, D. (2004). Future directions for incontinence research with frail elders. *Nursing Research*, *53*(Suppl 6), S22-S29.

Farmer AP, Légaré F, Turcot L, et al. (2008). Printed educational materials: effects on professional practice and health care outcomes. *Cochrane Database of Systematic Reviews*, *2008*(3), CD004398.

Forsetlund, L., Bjorndal, A., Rashidian, A., et al. (2009). Continuing education meetings and workshops: effects on professional practice and health care outcomes. *Cochrane Database of Systematic Reviews, 2009*(2), CD003030.

GRADE Working Group. (2004). Grading quality of evidence and strength of recommendations. *British Medical Journal, 328*, 1490–1494.

Greenhalgh, T., Robert, G., Bate, P., et al. (2005). *Diffusion of innovations in health service organizations: a systematic literature review*. Malden, MA: Blackwell.

Grol, R. P., Bosch, M. C., Hulscher, M. E., et al. (2007). Planning and studying improvement in patient care: the use of theoretical perspectives. *Milbank Quarterly, 85*(1), 93–138.

Guyatt, G. H., Oxman, A. D., Kunz, R., et al. (2008a). Rating quality of evidence and strength of recommendations: what is "quality of evidence" and why is it important to clinicians? *British Medical Journal, 336*(7651), 995–998.

Guyatt, G. H., Oxman, A. D., Vist, G., et al. (2008b). Rating quality of evidence and strength of recommendations GRADE: an emerging consensus on rating quality of evidence and strength of recommendations. *British Medical Journal, 336*, 924–926.

Hysong, S. J., Best, R. G., & Pugh, J. A. (2006). Audit and feedback and clinical practice guideline adherence: making feedback actionable. *Implementation Science, 1*, 9.

Harris, RP, Helfan,M., Woolf, SH et al. (2001). Currents methods of the US Preventive Services Task force: a review of the process, *Am J. Prev. Med*, 20(3S): 21-35.

Institute of Medicine. (2001). *Crossing the quality chasm: a new health system for the 21st century*. Washington, DC: National Academies Press.

Institute of Medicine. (2011). *Clinical practice guidelines we can trust*. Washington, DC: The National Academy Press.

Ivers, N., Jamtvedt, G., Flottorp, S., et al. (2012). Audit and feedback: effects on professional practice and healthcare outcomes. *Cochrane Database of Systematic Reviews, 2012*(6), CD000259. doi: 10.1002/14651858.CD000259.pub3.

Jamtvedt, G., Young, J. M., Kristoffersen, D. T., et al. (2010). Audit and feedback: effects on professional practice and health care outcomes (Review). *Cochrane Database of Systematic Reviews, 2007*(7), CD000259.

Jordan, M. E., Lanham, H. J., Crabtree, B. F., et al. (2009). The role of conversation in health care interventions: enabling sensemaking and learning. *Implementation Science, 4*, 15.

Kochevar, L. K., & Yano, E. M. (2006). Understanding health care organization needs and context: beyond performance gaps. *Journal of General Internal Medicine, 21*, S25–S29.

Leape, L. L. (2005). *Advances in patient safety: from research to implementation* (Vol. 3).Rockville, MD: Agency for Healthcare Research and Quality.

Lozano, P. Finkelstein, JA, Carey, VJ et al., (2004). A multisite randomized trial of the effects of physician education and organizational change in chronic-asthma care. *Arch. Pediatric Adolesc. Medicine*, 158: 875-883.

Rogers, E. M. (2003). *Diffusion of innovations* (5th ed.). New York, NY: Free Press.

Sackett, D. L., Straus, S. E., Richardson, W. S., et al. (2000). *Evidence-based medicine: how to practice and teach EBM*. London, UK: Churchill Livingstone.

Scott, S. D., Plotnikoff, R. C., Karunamuni, N., et al. (2008). Factors influencing the adoption of an innovation: an examination of the uptake of the Canadian Heart Health Kit (HHK). *Implementation Science, 3*, 41.

Stetler, C. B., Legro, M. W., Rycroft-Malone, J., et al. (2006a). Role of "external facilitation" in implementation of research findings: a qualitative evaluation of facilitation experiences in the Veterans Health Administration. *Implementation Science, 1*, 23.

Stetler, C. B., Legro, M. W., Wallace, C. M., et al. (2006b). The role of formative evaluation in implementation research and the QUERI experience. *Journal of General Internal Medicine, 21*, S1–S8.

Titler, M. G. (2002). *Toolkit for promoting evidence-based practice*. Iowa City, IA: Department of Nursing Services and Patient Care, University of Iowa Hospitals and Clinics.

Titler, M. G. (2004). Methods in translation science. *Worldviews on Evidence-Based Nursing, 1*, 38–48.

Titler, M. G. (2008). The evidence for evidence-based practice implementation. In R. Hughes (Ed.), *Patient safety and quality—an evidence-based handbook for nurses* (pp. 1–49). Rockville, MD: Agency for Healthcare Research and Quality.

Titler, M. G., et al. (2006). *Book to bedside: promoting and sustaining EBPs in elders.* Iowa City, IA: University of Iowa College of Nursing.

Titler, M. G., & Everett, L. Q. (2001). Translating research into practice: considerations for critical care investigators. *Critical Care Nursing Clinics of North America, 13*(4), 587–604.

Titler, M. G., Herr, K., Brooks, J. M., et al. (2008). A translating research into practice intervention improves management of acute pain in older hip fracture patients. *Health Services Research.* Retrieved from www3.interscience.wiley.com/journal/120120473/issue.

Titler, M. G., Kleiber, C., Steelman, V. J., et al. (2001). The Iowa model of evidence-based practice to promote quality care. *Critical Care Nursing Clinics of North America, 13*(4):497–509.

US Preventive Services Task Force (2008). *US Preventive Services Task Force grade definitions, 2008.* Retrieved from www.ahrq.gov/clinic/uspstf/grades.htm

## evolve WEBSITE

*Go to Evolve at http://evolve.elsevier.com/LoBiondo/ for review questions, critiquing exercises, and additional research articles for practice in reviewing and critiquing.*

# CHAPTER

# 21

# Quality Improvement

*Maja Djukic and Mattia J. Gilmartin*

## Evolve WEBSITE

*Go to Evolve at http://evolve.elsevier.com/LoBiondo/ for review questions, critiquing exercises, and additional research articles for practice in reviewing and critiquing.*

## LEARNING OUTCOMES

- Discuss the characteristics of quality health care defined by the Institute of Medicine.
- Compare the characteristics of the major quality improvement (QI) models used in health care.
- Identify two databases used to report health care organization's performance to promote consumer choice and guide clinical QI activities.
- Describe the relationship between nursing-sensitive quality indicators and patient outcomes.

- Describe the steps in the improvement process and determine appropriate QI tools to use in each phase of the improvement process.
- List four themes for improvement to apply to the unit where you work.
- Describe ways that nurses can lead QI projects in clinical settings.
- Use the SQUIRE Guidelines to critique a journal article reporting the results of a QI project.

## KEY TERMS

accreditation
benchmarking
Clinical Microsystems
common cause and
    special cause
    variation
control chart
flowchart

Lean
nursing-sensitive
    quality indicators
performance
    measurement
Plan-Do-Study-Act
    Improvement
    Cycles

public reporting
quality health care
quality improvement
root cause analysis
run chart
Six Sigma
SQUIRE Guidelines

Total Quality
    Management/
    Continuous Quality
    Improvement

---

**BOX 21-1 SIX DIMENSIONS AND DEFINITIONS OF HEALTH CARE QUALITY**

1. **Safe:** avoiding injuries to patients from the care that is intended to help them.
2. **Effective:** providing services based on scientific knowledge to all who could benefit, and refraining from providing services to those not likely to benefit.
3. **Patient-centered:** providing care that is respectful of and responsive to individual patient preferences, needs, and values, and ensuring that patient values guide all clinical decisions.
4. **Timely:** reducing waits and sometimes harmful delays for both those who receive and those who give care.
5. **Efficient:** avoiding waste, including waste of equipment, supplies, ideas, and energy.
6. **Equitable:** providing care that does not vary in quality because of personal characteristics such as gender, ethnicity, geographic location, and socioeconomic status.

From Institute of Medicine. (2001). Crossing the quality chasm: A new health system for the 21st century. Executive summary. Washington, DC: The National Academies Press.

---

The Institute of Medicine (IOM, 2001) defines quality health care as care that is safe, effective, patient-centered, timely, efficient, and equitable (Box 21-1). The quality of the health care system was brought to the forefront of national attention in several important reports (IOM, 1999; 2001), including *Crossing the Quality Chasm,* which concluded that "between the health care we have and the care we could have lies not just a gap, but a chasm" (IOM, 2001, p. 1). The report notes that "the performance of the health care system varies considerably. It may be exemplary, but often is not, and millions of Americans fail to receive effective care" (IOM, 2001, p. 3). The first national report card on U.S. health care quality (McGlynn et al., 2003) identified that adults, regardless of their race, gender, or financial status, receive only about half of the recommended care for leading causes of death and disability such as pneumonia, diabetes, asthma, and coronary artery disease.

Quality of care has improved for some conditions (Chassin et al., 2010). For example, prophylactic antibiotic administration within 1 hour of starting a surgical incision is now a recommended practice. In 2002, only about 10% of hospitals were in compliance with this practice, but in 2009 about 90% of hospitals reported being in compliance. Still, much room for improvement of quality remains, as evident from the latest report of the Agency for Healthcare Research and Quality (AHRQ, 2012). The report concluded that health care effectiveness, patient safety, timeliness, patient centeredness, care coordination, efficiency, health system infrastructure, and access are suboptimal, especially for minority and low-income groups. For example, fewer than 25% of adults age 40 years and older with diabetes receive all four recommended interventions (Hemoglobin A1c tests, foot exam, dilated eye exam, and flu shot) (AHRQ, 2012). Also, almost 20% of adults report sometimes or never receiving care as soon as they want it, even if they need care right away for an illness, injury, or condition (AHRQ, 2012). Despite these quality issues, the U.S. spends twice as much on health care per capita per year at $7,290, compared with other developed nations, while ranking last in health care quality (Davis et al., 2010).

The purpose of this chapter is to introduce you to the principles of quality improvement (QI) and provide examples of how to apply these principles in your practice so you can effectively contribute to needed health care improvements. QI "uses data to monitor the outcomes of care processes and improvement methods to design and test changes to continuously improve the quality and safety of health care systems" (Cronenwett et al., 2007, p. 127).

## BOX 21-2    NATIONAL QUALITY AIMS AND PRIORITIES

| NATIONAL QUALITY AIMS | NATIONAL QUALITY PRIORITIES FOR ACHIEVING THE AIMS |
|---|---|
| • **Better Care:** Improve the overall quality of care, by making health care more patient-centered, reliable, accessible, and safe.<br>• **Healthy People/Healthy Communities:** Improve the health of the U.S. population by supporting proven interventions to address behavioral, social, and environmental determinants of health in addition to delivering higher-quality care.<br>• **Affordable Care:** Reduce the cost of quality health care for individuals, families, employers, and government. | • Make care safer by reducing harm caused in the delivery of care.<br>• Ensure each person and family are engaged as partners in their care.<br>• Promote effective communication and care coordination.<br>• Promote the most effective prevention and treatment practices for the leading causes of mortality, starting with cardiovascular disease.<br>• Work with communities to promote wide use of best practices to enable healthy living.<br>• Make quality care more affordable for individuals, families, employers, and governments by developing and spreading new health care delivery models. |

From the U.S. Department of Health and Human Services. (2012a). *National strategy for quality improvement in health care.* www.ahrq.gov/workingforquality/nqs/nqs2012annlrpt.pdf

## NURSES' ROLE IN HEALTH CARE QI

Florence Nightingale championed QI by systematically documenting high rates of morbidity and mortality resulting from poor sanitary conditions among soldiers serving in the Crimean War of 1854 (Henry et al., 1992). She used statistics to document changes in soldiers' health, including reductions in mortality resulting from a number of nursing interventions such as hand hygiene, instrument sterilization, changing of bed linens, ward sanitation, ventilation, and proper nutrition (Henry et al., 1992). Today, nurses continue to be vital to health system improvement efforts (IOM, 2011). One main initiative developed to bolster nurses' education in health system improvements is *Quality and Safety Education for Nurses* (QSEN) (Cronenwett et al., 2007). The overall goal of this project is to help build nurses' competence in the areas of QI, patient-centered care, teamwork and collaboration, patient safety, informatics, and evidence-based practice (EBP). Other initiatives, including *Transforming Care at the Bedside* (TCAB), *Integrated Nurse Leadership Program*, and the *Clinical Scene Investigator Academy* have been developed to increase nurses' engagement in QI (Kliger et al., 2010). To effectively influence improvements in the work setting and ensure that all patients consistently receive excellent care, it is important to

• Align national, organizational, and unit level goals for QI
• Recognize external drivers of quality, such as accreditation, payment, and performance measurement
• Develop skills to apply QI models and tools

## NATIONAL GOALS AND STRATEGIES FOR HEALTH CARE QI

The first National Quality Strategy (U.S. Department of Health and Human Services [HHS], 2012a) established aims and priorities for QI (Box 21-2). Achieving these national quality targets requires major redesign of the health care system. One way you can contribute to this redesign is to familiarize yourself with the national priorities, improvement targets, and corresponding national initiatives (described in Table 21-1) and use them to guide improvements in your work setting.

| TABLE 21-1 | NATIONAL QUALITY STRATEGY PRIORITIES, IMPROVEMENT TARGETS, AND RELATED INITIATIVES | | | |
|---|---|---|---|---|
| **NATIONAL QUALITY STRATEGY PRIORITY** | **MEASURE FOCUS** | **MEASURE NAME/DESCRIPTION** | **ASPIRATIONAL TARGET** | **RELATED NATIONAL INITIATIVES** |
| Making care safer by reducing the harm caused in care delivery. | Hospital-Acquired Conditions (HACs) | Incidence of measurable HAC | Reduce preventable HACs by 40% by end of 2013. | **Partnership for Patients:** national patient safety and QI initiative with goals for reducing preventable HACs by 40%, and reducing 30-day hospital readmissions by 20% by end of 2013. www.healthcare.gov/compare/partnership-for-patients/index.html |
| | Hospital Readmissions | All-payer 30-day readmission rate | Reduce all readmissions by 20% by end of 2013. | |
| Ensuring each person and family is engaged in their care. | Timely Care | Adults who needed care right away for an illness, injury, or condition in the last 12 months or who sometimes or never acquired care as wanted | Not available. | **Linking Patient Experiences to Provider Payment:** part of Medicare payments for services. Surveys measuring patient-provider communications and patient satisfaction known as Consumer Assessment of Health Care Providers and Systems (HCAHPS) surveys, allows Medicare to learn which providers and hospitals are successfully engaging patients in their care. www.cms.gov/aco; www.cms.gov/Hospital-Value-Based-Purchasing |
| | Decision Making | People with a usual source of care whose health care providers sometimes or never discuss decisions with them | Not available. | |
| Promoting effective communication and care coordination. | Patient-Centered Medical Home (PCMH) | Percentage of children needing care coordination who receive effective care coordination | Not available. | **Multi-State Initiative: The Multi-Payer Advanced Primary Care Practice Demonstration:** Centers for Medicare and Medicaid Services (CMS) is partnering with State Medicaid programs, private insurers, and employers to support primary care practices emphasizing prevention, health information technology, care coordination, and shared decision making between patients and providers. www.cms.gov/Medicare/Demonstration-Projects/DemoProjectsEvalRpts/Medicare-Demonstrations-Items/CMS1230016.html |
| | 3-Item Care Transition Measure | • Patients are asked if staff took patient and family's preferences into account in deciding what health care needs would be when discharged<br>• When discharged, was there a good understanding of what patient and family were responsible for in managing their health<br>• When discharged patient clearly understood purpose for taking medications | Not available. | |

*Continued*

| TABLE 21-1 | NATIONAL QUALITY STRATEGY PRIORITIES, IMPROVEMENT TARGETS, AND RELATED INITIATIVES—cont'd | | | |
|---|---|---|---|---|
| **NATIONAL QUALITY STRATEGY PRIORITY** | **MEASURE FOCUS** | **MEASURE NAME/DESCRIPTION** | **ASPIRATIONAL TARGET** | **RELATED NATIONAL INITIATIVES** |
| Promoting the most effective prevention and treatment practices for the leading causes of mortality, starting with cardiovascular disease. | Aspirin Use | Those at increased risk of cardiovascular disease are taking aspirin | 65% by 2017 | **The Million Hearts Campaign** is a public-private sector initiative led by the Department of Health and Human Services (DHHS) to prevent 1 million heart attacks and strokes over the next 5 years. millionhearts.hhs.gov/index.html |
| | Blood Pressure Control | Those with hypertension have adequately controlled blood pressure | 65% by 2017 | |
| | Cholesterol Management | Those with high cholesterol have adequately managed hyperlipidemia | 65% by 2017 | |
| | Smoking Cessation | People trying to quit smoking who get help | 65% by 2017 | |
| Working with communities to promote best practices for healthy living. | Depression | Percentage of adults who reported symptoms of a major depressive episode (MDE) in the last 12 months who received treatment in the last 12 months | Not available. | **The Community Transformation Grants** program supports community level efforts to reduce chronic diseases such as heart disease, cancer, stroke, and diabetes. For example, making healthy meals possible in school vending machines. www.cdc.gov/communitytransformation/ |
| | Obesity | Proportion of adults who are obese | Not available. | |
| Making quality care more affordable by developing and spreading new health care delivery models. | Out of Pocket Expenses | Percentage of people under 65 years of age with out-of-pocket medical and premium expenses greater than 10% of income | Not available. | **The CMS Innovation Center** as a new engine for testing innovative care delivery and payment models that have potential to deliver better health care at lower cost for Medicare, Medicaid and Children's Health Insurance Program (CHIP) beneficiaries. www.innovations.cms.gov |
| | Health Spending per Capita | Annual all payer health care spending per person | | |

From the U.S. Department of Health and Human Services. (2012a). National strategy for *quality improvement in health care.* Retrieved from www.ahrq.gov/workingforquality/nqs/nqs2012annlrpt.pdf

## EXTERNAL DRIVERS OF QUALITY

QI relies on aligning institutional priorities with external incentives that drive QI, including accreditation, financial incentives, performance measurement, and public reporting (Ferlie & Shortell, 2001).

## BOX 21-3 QI ACCREDITING ORGANIZATIONS

- **Joint Commission:** responsible for ensuring a minimum standard of structures, processes and outcomes for patient care. Accreditation by the Joint Commission is voluntary, but it is required to receive reimbursement for patient care services. For more information: www.jointcommission.org/
- **National Committee for Quality Assurance Accreditation for Health Plans (NCQA):** a private not-for-profit organization dedicated to improving health care quality. The NCQA is responsible for accrediting health insurance programs. Accredited health insurance programs are exempt from many or all elements associated with annual state audits. The NCQA developed and maintains **The Healthcare Effectiveness Data and Information Set (HEDIS):** a tool used by the majority of America's health plans to measure performance on important dimensions of care and service. HEDIS allows for comparison of performance across health plans. For more information: www.ncqa.org/Programs/Accreditation/HealthPlanHP.aspx
- **American Nurses' Credentialing Center Magnet Recognition Program** recognizes health care organizations that provide the very best in nursing care and uphold the tradition of professional nursing practice. For more information: www.nursecredentialing.org/Magnet.aspx

## Accreditation

Accreditation is a process in which an organization demonstrates attainment of predetermined standards set by an external nongovernmental organization responsible for setting and monitoring compliance in a particular industry sector (Scrivens, 1997). Several accrediting bodies are listed in Box 21-3.

## Financial Incentives

Financial incentives seek to align providers' behaviors with improvements in the quality, efficiency, and effectiveness of health care services by paying a bonus to individuals and organizations that deliver care within a set budget or meet preestablished performance targets (Rosenthal & Frank, 2006). Box 21-4 on p. 448 shows examples of financial incentives.

## Performance Measurement

Performance measurement is a tool that tracks an organization's performance using standardized measures to document and manage quality. National health care performance standards are developed using a consensus process in which stakeholder groups, representing the interests of the public, health professionals, payers, employers, and government identify priorities, measures, and reporting requirements to document and manage the quality of care (National Quality Forum [NQF], 2004). See Box 21-5 on p. 449 for examples of groups responsible for developing measurement standards.

## Public Reporting

Public reporting provides objective information to promote consumer choice, guide QI efforts, and promote accountability for performance among providers and delivery organizations. It also allows organizations to compare their performance across standard measures against their peer organizations locally and nationally (Giordano et al., 2010). Several major public reporting systems are described in Box 21-6 on p. 449.

> ## BOX 21-4 FINANCIAL INCENTIVES TO PROMOTE QUALITY IN THE HEALTH CARE SECTOR
>
> [1]**Capitation:** a payment arrangement for health care services. Pays a provider (physician or nurse practitioner) or provider group a set amount for each enrolled person assigned to them, per period of time, whether or not that person seeks care. These providers generally are contracted with a type of health maintenance organization (HMO). Payment levels are based on average expected health care use of a particular patient, with greater payment for patients with significant medical history.
>
> [2]**Bundled Payments Initiative:** links payments for multiple services that patients receive during an episode of care. Payments seek to align incentives for hospitals, post acute care providers, doctors, and other practitioners to improve the patient's care experience during a hospital stay in an acute care hospital through post-discharge recovery.
>
> [3]**Pay for Performance:** an emerging movement in health insurance where providers are rewarded for meeting preestablished targets for health care delivery services. This model rewards physicians, hospitals, medical groups, and other health care providers for meeting certain performance measures for quality and efficiency.
>
> [4]**Value-Based Health Care Purchasing:** a project of participating health plans, including the CMS, where buyers hold providers of health care accountable for both cost and quality of care. Value-based purchasing brings together information on health care quality, patient outcomes and health status, with data on the dollar outlays going towards health. The focus is on managing health care system use to reduce inappropriate care and to identify and reward the best-performing providers.
>
> [5]**Accountable Care Organization (ACO):** a payment and care delivery model that seeks to tie provider reimbursements to quality metrics and reductions in the total cost of care for an assigned population of patients. A group of coordinated health care providers form an ACO, which then provides care to a group of patients. The ACO may use a range of payment models (e.g., capitation, fee-for-service). The ACO is accountable to the patients and the third-party payer for the quality, appropriateness, and efficiency of the health care provided.

1. American Medical Association. (2012). *Capitation.* Retrieved from www.ama-assn.org/ama/pub/physician-resources/practice-management-center/claims-revenue-cycle/managed-care-contracting/evaluating-payment-options/capitation.page
2. Centers for Medicare and Medicaid Services. (2012). *Bundled payments for care improvement.* Retrieved from www.innovations.cms.gov/initiatives/bundled-payments/index.html
3. Integrated Healthcare Association. (2012). *National pay for performance overview.* Retrieved from www.iha.org/p4p_national.html
4. Agency for Healthcare Research and Quality. (1998). *Theory and reality of value-based purchasing: Lessons from the pioneers* (AHRQ Publication No. 98-0004). Retrieved from www.ahrq.gov/qual/meyerrpt.htm
5. American Hospital Association. (2010). *Accountable care organizations: AHA research synthesis report.* Retrieved from www.aha.org/research/cor/accountable/index.shtml

## Measuring Nursing Care Quality

Nurses deliver the majority of health care and therefore have a substantial influence on its overall quality (IOM, 2011). However, nursing's contribution to the overall quality of health care has been difficult to quantify, owing in part to insufficient standardized measurement systems capable of capturing nursing care contribution to patient outcomes. The Robert Wood Johnson Foundation has funded the NQF to recommend nursing-sensitive consensus standards to be used to set standards for public accountability and QI. The work of the NQF (2004) resulted in endorsement of **15 nursing-sensitive quality indicators** (Table 21-2 on p. 450). Since the endorsement of "NQF 15," several data reporting mechanisms have been established for performance sharing internally among providers to identify areas in need of improvement, externally for purposes of accreditation and payment, and with health care

## BOX 21-5 PERFORMANCE MEASUREMENT STANDARD SETTING GROUPS

[1]**National Quality Forum (NQF)** is a nonprofit organization that operates under a three-part mission to improve the quality of health care in the United States. NQF builds consensus on national priorities for performance improvement, endorses national consensus standards for measuring and publically reporting on performance, and promotes the attainment of national performance goals through education and outreach.

[2]**Hospital Quality Alliance (HQA)** is a multi-stakeholder organization comprised of more than 350 organizations representing consumers, purchasers, health professionals, providers, health systems, insurers and state government and federal agencies. It is responsible for developing and managing the *Hospital Compare* database of the nation's 4,000 Medicare-certified hospitals.

[3]**Ambulatory Quality Alliance (AQA)** consists of a large body of stakeholders that represents clinicians, consumers, purchasers, health plans and others. Creates and maintains performance data at the physician and other clinical level in the ambulatory and primary care sectors. Develops and maintains the *Physician Quality Reporting Initiative*.

1. National Quality Forum. (2012). *About NQF*. Retrieved from www.qualityforum.org/About_NQF/About_NQF.aspx
2. Hospital Quality Alliance. (n.d.). *About us*. Retrieved from www.hospitalqualityalliance.org/hospital-qualityalliance/aboutus/aboutus.html
3. Ambulatory Quality Alliance. (2012). *Homepage*. Retrieved from www.aqaalliance.org/default.htm

## BOX 21-6 PUBLIC REPORTING SYSTEMS

- **Hospital Compare** allows consumers to compare information on hospitals. The database includes performance measures on: timely and efficient care; readmissions; complications and deaths; use of medical imaging; survey of patient's experiences;' number of Medicare patients; and Medicare payment. For more information, visit www.hospitalcompare.hhs.gov/
- **Nursing Home Compare** allows consumers to compare information about nursing homes. It contains quality of care information on every Medicare and Medicaid-certified nursing home in the country. The database includes performance measures on health inspections, staffing, and clinical quality. For more information, visit www.medicare.gov/NursingHomeCompare/
- **Home Health Compare** has information about the quality of care provided by Medicare-certified home health agencies that meet Federal health and safety requirements throughout the nation. For more information, visit www.medicare.gov/homehealthcompare
- **Hospital Consumer Assessment of Healthcare Providers and Systems (HCAHPS)** Developed by the Agency for Healthcare Research and Quality, the HCAHPS is a standardized survey and data collection method for measuring patients' perspectives on hospital care. The HCAHPS survey contains 18 patient perspectives on care for eight key topics: communication with doctors, communication with nurses, responsiveness of hospital staff, pain management, communication about medicines, discharge information, cleanliness of the hospital environment, and quietness of the hospital environment. HCAHPS performance is used to calculate incentive payments in the Hospital Value-Based Purchasing program for hospital discharges beginning in October 2012. For more information, visit www.hcahpsonline.org
- **Physician Quality Reporting Initiative** is a program administered by the CMS that collects performance data at the physician/provider clinical level in the ambulatory and primary care sectors. For more information, visit www.cms.gov/Medicare/Quality-Initiatives-Patient-Assessment-Instruments/PQRS/index.html
- **The Leapfrog Group** is an initiative of organizations that buy health care who are working to improve the safety, quality and affordability of health care for Americans. The Leapfrog Group conducts a survey for comparing hospitals' performance on the national standards of safety, quality, and efficiency that are most relevant to consumers and purchasers of care. For more information, visit www.leapfroggroup.org/

| TABLE 21-2 | NATIONAL VOLUNTARY STANDARDS FOR NURSING-SENSITIVE CARE | |
|---|---|---|
| **FRAMEWORK CATEGORY** | **MEASURE** | **DESCRIPTION** |
| Patient-centered outcome measures | Death among surgical inpatients with treatable serious complications (failure to rescue) | Percent of major surgical inpatients who experience a hospital-acquired complication (e.g., sepsis, pneumonia, gastrointestinal bleeding, shock/cardiac arrest, deep vein thrombosis/pulmonary embolism) that results in death. |
| | Pressure ulcer prevalence* | Percent of inpatients who have hospital-acquired pressure ulcer (Stage 2 or greater). |
| | Falls prevalence* | Number of inpatient falls per inpatient days. |
| | Falls with injury | Number of inpatient falls with injuries per inpatient days. |
| | Restraint prevalence (vest and limb only) | Percent of patients who have a vest or limb restraint. |
| | Urinary catheter-associated urinary tract infection (UTI) for intensive care unit (ICU) patients* | Rate of UTI associated with use of urinary catheters for ICU patients. |
| | Central line catheter-associated blood stream infection rate for ICU and high-risk nursery (HRN) patients* | Rate of blood stream infections associated with use of central line catheters for ICU or HRN patients. |
| | Ventilator-associated pneumonia for ICU and HRN patients* | Rate of pneumonia associated with use of ventilators for ICU and HRN patients. |
| Nursing-centered intervention measures | Smoking cessation counseling for acute myocardial infarction (AMI)* | Percent of AMI inpatients with smoking history in the past year who received smoking cessation advice or counseling during hospitalization. |
| | Smoking cessation counseling for heart failure (HF)* | Percent of HF inpatients with smoking history within the past year who received smoking cessation advice or counseling during hospitalization. |
| | Smoking cessation counseling for pneumonia* | Percent of pneumonia inpatients with smoking history within the past year who received smoking cessation advice or counseling during hospitalization. |
| System-centered measures | Skill mix (Registered Nurse [RN], Licensed Vocational/Practical Nurse [LVN/LPN], unlicensed assistive personnel [UAP] and contract) | • Percent of RN care hours to total nursing care hours.<br>• Percent of LVN/LPN care hours to total nursing care hours.<br>• Percent of UAP care hours to total nursing care hours<br>• Percent of contract hours (RN, LVN/LPN, and UAP) to total nursing care hours. |
| | Nursing care hours per inpatient day (RN, LVN/LPN, and UAP) | • Number of RN care hours per patient day.<br>• Number of nursing staff hours (RN, LVN, LPN, UAP). |
| | Practice Environment Scale-Nursing Work Index (PES-NWI) (composite and five subscales) | Composite score and mean presence scores for each of the following subscales derived from PES-NWI:<br>• Nurse participation in hospital affairs.<br>• Nursing foundations for quality of care.<br>• Nurse manager ability, leadership, and support of nurses.<br>• Staffing and resource adequacy.<br>• Collegial nurse-physician relations. |
| | Voluntary turnover | Number of voluntary uncontrolled separations during the month for RNs and advanced practice nurses, LVN/LPNs, and nurse assistant/aides. |

Reproduced with permission from National Quality Forum. (2012). *Measuring performance.* Retrieved from www.qualityforum.org/Measuring_Performance/ABCs_of_Measurement.aspx
*Note.*(*) indicates NQF-endorsed national voluntary consensus standard for hospital care.

consumers so that they can choose providers based on the quality of services provided. Examples include *Hospital Compare* (USDHHS, 2012b) and the nursing-specific databases described by Alexander (2007):

- **The National Database of Nursing Quality Indicators®** is a proprietary database of the American Nurses Association. The database collects and evaluates unit-specific nurse-sensitive data from hospitals in the U.S. Participating facilities receive unit-level comparative data reports to use for QI purposes.
- **California Nursing Outcomes Coalition (CalNOC)** is a data repository of hospital-generated, unit-level, acute nurse staffing and workforce characteristics and processes of care, as well as key NQF-endorsed, nursing-sensitive outcome measures, submitted electronically via the web.
- **Veterans Affairs Nursing Outcomes Database** was originally modeled after CalNOC. Data are collected at the unit and hospital levels to facilitate evaluation of quality and enable benchmarking within and among Veterans Affairs facilities.

> **HELPFUL HINT**
>
> To find out how your hospital compares in nursing-sensitive quality indicators such as pressure ulcers, infections, and falls with another hospital in your area, go to www.hospitalcompare.hhs.org. Identify high performing organizations in your area from which you can learn.

## Benchmarking

Measurement of quality indicators must be done methodically using standardized tools. Standardized measurement allows for benchmarking, which is "a systematic approach for gathering information about process or product performance and then analyzing why and how performance differs between business units" (Massoud et al., 2001, p. 74). Benchmarking is critical for QI because it helps identify when performance is below an agreed-upon standard, and it signals the need for improvement. For example, when you record assessment of your patient's skin status using a standardized assessment tool such as the *Braden Scale for Predicting Pressure Score Risk* (Stotts & Gunningberg, 2007), it allows for comparison of your assessment to those of providers in other organizations who provide care to a similar patient population and who use the same tool to document assessments. Tracking changes in the overall Braden Scale score over time allows you to intervene, if the score falls below a set standard, indicating high risk for pressure ulcer development. Equally, after you implement needed interventions such as changes in feeding or mobility, you can track changes in the Braden Scale score to determine whether the interventions were effective in reducing risk for pressure ulcer development. Therefore, standardized measurement can tell you when changes in care are needed and whether implemented interventions have resulted in actual improvement of patient outcomes.

When all clinical units document care in the same way, it is possible to document pressure ulcer care across units. These performance data are useful for benchmarking efforts where clinical teams learn from each other how to apply best practices from high-performing units to the care processes of lower-performing units. Benchmarking (Massoud et al., 2001, p. 75) can be used to

- Develop plans to address improvement needs
- Borrow and adapt successful ideas from others
- Understand what has already been tried

# COMMON QI PERSPECTIVES AND MODELS

QI as a management model is both a philosophy of organizational functioning and a set of statistical analysis tools and change techniques used to reduce variations in the quality of goods or services that an organization produces (Nelson et al., 2007). The QI model emphasizes customer satisfaction, teams and teamwork, and the continuous improvement of work processes. Other defining features of QI include the use of transformational leadership by leaders at all levels to set performance goals and expectations, use of data to make decisions, and standardization of work processes to reduce variation across providers and service encounters (Nelson et al., 2007). The key principles associated with QI are shown in Table 21-3.

Although QI has its roots in the manufacturing sector, many of the ideas, tools, and techniques used to measure and manage quality have been applied in health care organizations to improve clinical outcomes and reduce waste (DelliFraine et al., 2010; Seidl & Newhouse, 2012). The major QI models used in health care include

- Total Quality Management/Continuous Quality Improvement (TQM/CQI)
- Six Sigma
- Lean
- Clinical Microsystems

The key characteristics of each of these models are described in Table 21-4 on p. 454. Because QI uses a holistic approach, leaders often select one quality model that is used to guide the organization's overarching improvement agenda.

It is important to note that health care organizations have adopted principles and practices associated with the industrial QI approach relatively recently. Historically, the quality of health care was assessed retrospectively using the quality assurance (QA) model. The QA model uses chart audits to compare care against a predetermined standard. Corrective actions associated with QA focus on assigning individual blame and correcting deficiencies in operations. Another model commonly associated with health care QI is the *Structure-Process-Outcome Framework* (Donabedian, 1966). This framework is used to examine the resources that make up health care delivery services, clinicians' work practices, and the outcomes associated with the structure and processes. The evolution of the key perspectives, used to understand and manage QI in health care organizations, is summarized in Table 21-5 on p. 455.

# QI STEPS AND TOOLS

Similar to the nursing process, which you use to guide your assessment, diagnoses, and treatment of patient problems, you can use the QI process steps (Massoud et al., 2001) for the following:

1. Assessing health system performance by collecting and monitoring data
2. Analyzing data to identify a problem in need of improvement
3. Developing a plan to treat the identified problem
4. Testing and implementing the improvement plan

Several tools facilitate each step of the QI process (Table 21-6 on p. 456). You can use these tools to assist with collecting and analyzing data and to identify and test improvement ideas. A case example, *Nurse Response Time to Patient Call Light Requests* (Box 21-7 on p. 456), is presented to introduce the steps of the improvement process and apply several basic QI tools used to measure and manage system performance.

## TABLE 21-3 PRINCIPLES OF QUALITY IMPROVEMENT

| IMPROVEMENT PRINCIPLE | KEY BENEFITS |
|---|---|
| **Principle 1 – Customer focus/Patient focus**<br>Health care organizations rely on patients and therefore should understand current and future patient needs, should meet patient requirements and strive to exceed patient expectations. | • Increased revenue and market share obtained through flexible and fast responses to market opportunities<br>• Increased effectiveness in the organization's resources use to enhance patient satisfaction<br>• Improved patient loyalty leading to repeat business |
| **Principle 2 – Leadership**<br>Leaders establish unity of purpose and the organization's direction should create and maintain an internal environment in which people can become fully involved in organization's objectives achievement. | • People understand and are motivated towards the organization's goals and objectives<br>• Activities are evaluated, aligned and implemented in a unified way<br>• Miscommunication between organization levels are minimized |
| **Principle 3 – Involvement of people**<br>People at all levels are the essence of an organization and their full involvement enables their abilities to be used for the organization's benefit. | • Motivated, committed and involved people within the organization<br>• Innovation and creativity further the organization's objectives<br>• People are accountable for own performance<br>• People are eager to participate in and contribute to continual improvement |
| **Principle 4 – Process approach**<br>A desired result is achieved more efficiently when activities and related resources are managed as a process. | • Lower costs and shorter cycle times through effective use of resources<br>• Improved, consistent and predictable results<br>• Focused and prioritized Improvement opportunities |
| **Principle 5 – System approach to management**<br>Identifying, understanding and managing interrelated processes as a system contributes to the organization's effectiveness and efficiency in achieving its objectives. | • Integration and alignment of processes that will best achieve desired results<br>• Ability to focus effort on the key processes<br>• Improve confidence among key stakeholders as to the organization's consistency, effectiveness and efficiency |
| **Principle 6 – Continual improvement**<br>Continual improvement of the organization's overall performance should be a permanent objective of the organization. | • Performance advantage through improved organizational capabilities<br>• Alignment of improvement activities at all levels to an organization's strategic intent<br>• Flexibility to react quickly to opportunities |
| **Principle 7 – Factual approach to decision making**<br>Effective decisions are based on the analysis of data and information. | • Informed decisions<br>• Increased ability to demonstrate past decisions effectiveness through reference to factual records<br>• Increased ability to review, challenge and change opinions and decisions |
| **Principle 8 – Mutually beneficial supplier relationships**<br>An organization and its suppliers are interdependent and a mutually beneficial relationship enhances ability of both to create value. | • Increased ability to create value for both parties<br>• Flexibility and speed of joint responses to changing market or customer needs and expectations<br>• Optimization of costs and resources |

Adapted with permission from International Organization for Standardization. (2012). *ISO 9000 series quality management principles.* Retrieved from www.iso.org/iso/qmp_2012.pdf

| TABLE 21-4 | OVERVIEW OF QUALITY IMPROVEMENT MODELS USED IN HEALTH CARE | |
|---|---|---|
| **MODEL** | **MAIN CHARACTERISTICS** | **RELATED RESOURCES** |
| TQM/CQI (Langley et al., 2009) | • A holistic management approach used to improve organizational performance<br>• Seeks to understand and manage variation in service delivery<br>• Emphasizes customer satisfaction as an important performance measure<br>• Relies on team work and collaboration among workers to deliver technically excellent and customer/patient-centered services<br>• Quality management science uses tools and techniques from statistics, engineering, operations research, management, market research and psychology<br>• TQM/CQI tools and techniques are applied to specific performance problems in the form of improvement projects<br>• The extent to which unit-level QI projects align with larger organizational quality goals, is related to their success and sustainability | United States Agency for International Development (USAID) Healthcare Improvement Project: www.hciproject.org/improvement_tools/improvement_methods/approaches/quality<br>Institute for Healthcare Improvement: www.ihi.org/Pages/default.aspx |
| Six Sigma (DelliFraine et al., 2010) | • Developed at Motorola in the 1980s<br>• Six Sigma takes its name from the statistical notation of sigma ($\sigma$) used to measure variation from the mean<br>• Emphasizes meeting customer requirements and eliminating errors or rework with the goal of reducing process variation<br>• Focuses on tightly controlling variations in production processes with the goal of reducing the number of defects to 3.4 units per 1 million units produced<br>• Process control achieved by applying DMAIC improvement model<br>• DMAIC includes: defining, measuring, analyzing, improving, and controlling<br>• Practitioners achieve mastery levels using statistical tools to measure and manage process variation (e.g., yellow-belt, green-belt, black-belt) | AHRQ Innovations Exchange: www.innovations.ahrq.gov/innovations_qualitytools.aspx |
| Lean (DelliFraine et al., 2010) | • Sometimes referred to as the Toyota Quality Model<br>• Focus: Eliminating waste from the production system by designing the most efficient and effective system<br>• Production controlled through standardization and placing the right person and materials at each step of the process<br>• Uses the PDSA improvement cycle<br>• Statistical tools include value stream mapping and Kanban, or a visual cue, used to warn clinicians that there is a process problem<br>• Performance measures vary from project to project and may inform the creation of new performance measures<br>• Uses a master teacher ("Sensei") to spread the practices of Lean though the organizational culture | Institute for Healthcare Improvement: www.ihi.org/knowledge/Pages/IHIWhitePapers/GoingLeaninHealthCare.aspx |
| Clinical Microsystems (Nelson et al., 2007) | • Model of service excellence developed specifically for health care<br>• Clinical microsystem is considered the building block of any health care system and is the smallest replicable unit in an organization<br>• Members of a clinical microsystem are interdependent and work together toward a common aim | Clinical Microsystems: www.clinicalmicrosystem.org/ |

| TABLE 21-5 | EVOLUTION OF QUALITY IMPROVEMENT PERSPECTIVES IN HEALTH CARE | | |
|---|---|---|---|
| **MODEL** | **KEY FEATURES** | **QUALITY MONITORING MECHANISMS** | **REPRESENTATIVE RESEARCH QUESTIONS** |
| 1920s-1980s<br>QA<br>Used to correct differences between what should be and what actually is (Asubonteng et al., 1996) | • Uses external standards to guide quality<br>• Quality assessed after the fact<br>• Corrective action is punitive<br>• The focus is on symptoms, individual failures, and compliance with standards | • Accreditation<br>• Chart audit<br>• Morbidity & Mortality Rounds | What factors affect the adoption of innovative QA techniques in hospital settings?<br>Adapted from Storey (2013). |
| 1960s-2010s<br>Structure-Process-Outcome Framework examines system components that lead to health care quality (Donabedian, 1966) | • Stresses professional responsibility for evaluating care quality<br>• *Structure* focuses on provider and organizational characteristics *Process* focuses on how care is delivered<br>• *Outcome* focuses on the end results of medical care | • Accreditation<br>• Work redesign<br>• Benchmarking<br>• Professional education and credentialing | What is the relationship between processes, outcomes, and satisfaction with care expected of acute care nurse practitioners (ACNPs)?<br>Adapted from Sidani & Doran (2010). |
| 1990s-2010s TQM/CQI<br>Model used to continually improve services and organizational performance (Bigelow & Arndt, 1995) | • Systems approach to improve efficiency<br>• Incorporates clinical, financial, administrative and patient satisfaction perspectives<br>• Focuses on meeting actual and unanticipated patient needs<br>• Uses statistical analysis to reduce variation in service processes<br>• Relies on team work and data-based decisions | • Accreditation<br>• Benchmarking (HCAHPS)<br>• Clinical practice guidelines<br>• PDSA cycles<br>• Process redesign<br>• Lean<br>• Six Sigma | Do P-D-S-A cycles of change eliminate elective birth inductions for neonates less than 39 weeks to align unit practice with national recommendations?<br>Adapted from Doyle et al. (2012). |
| 2000s-2010s<br>Patient Safety Systems approach to reduce harm to patients (Chassin & Loeb, 2011) | • Applies safety science methods to design health care delivery systems.<br>• Focuses on reducing or avoiding adverse events<br>• Domains include patients; providers; care routines; system design | • Accreditation<br>• Sentinel event reporting;<br>• National Patient Safety Goals<br>• High reliability organization model<br>• Root cause analysis | Does learning climate moderate the relationship between work dynamics and nurse mix and medication errors? Adapted from Chang & Mark (2011). |

## Forming a Lead QI Team

QI is inherently a team process and requires involvement of multiple professionals from various perspectives to assess the potential causes of system malfunction and improvement ideas (Nelson et al., 2007). A lead QI team should be composed of representatives from multiple professions involved in patient care, support staff, patients, and families. While all professional staff, support staff, and patients should be involved throughout the improvement process, members of the lead team are responsible for

## TABLE 21-6    QI TOOLS AND ACTIVITIES

| BASIC TOOLS AND ACTIVITIES | STEP 1 ASSESS | STEP 2 ANALYZE | STEP 3 PLAN & IMPLEMENT | STEP 4 TEST AND EVALUATE |
|---|---|---|---|---|
| Data collection | X | X | X | X |
| Flowcharts | X | X | X | X |
| Cause-and-effect analysis | | X | | |
| Bar and pie charts | X | X | | X |
| Run charts | X | X | | X |
| Control charts | X | X | | X |
| Histograms | X | X | | X |
| Pareto charts | X | X | | X |
| Benchmarking | X | | | X |
| Gantt charts | | X | | X |

From Massoud et al. (2001). A modern paradigm for improving healthcare quality. *QA Monograph Series* 1(1). Bethseda, MD: Published for the U.S. Agency for International Development by the Quality Assurance Project.

## BOX 21-7    APPLYING THE QI STEPS TO A CLINICAL PERFORMANCE PROBLEM

### A Case Study of a Call Bell Response Time Improvement Project

**Case Study Background**

After reviewing a year of HCAHPS patient satisfaction data, the QI team on the 6 East orthopedic unit noticed that the unit consistently scored below the hospital average on the call bell response time. In addition to the somewhat mediocre patient satisfaction scores, the nurses were also frustrated with the way that the staff responded to patient calls on the unit. Using the patient and staff satisfaction data as a starting point, the QI team selected call bell response time as an opportunity for improvement.

**Improvement Step 1: Assessment**

The goal of the 6 East QI project was to understand and manage system variation associated with patient's satisfaction with call bell response time. The QI team began the improvement project by asking the broad questions:

- What time of day is associated with a higher frequency of call bell use?
- What is the average time that it takes a staff member to answer a call bell?
- Are there variations in call bell response time based on the location of the patient's room in relation to the central nursing station?

The QI team designed a **check sheet** to collect data on the number of call bell requests each hour by patient's room number. The charge nurse and unit clerk took turns recording call bell requests during a 24-hour period. The QI team downloaded data from the call bell system to gain information on the average response time as well as information about unit staffing patterns and patient's admitting diagnoses.

**Improvement Step 2: Analysis**

To begin, the QI team tallied the call response time with a histogram using 5-minute intervals. In graphing the data, a clear pattern emerged. The patient wait times fell into three groups:

- One group waited an average of 8 minutes,
- The second group waited an average of 12 minutes, and
- A third group waited an average of 20 minutes for a member of staff to respond to the call bell request.

Upon further analysis of the data, the QI team discovered that the patients with the longest waiting times were in rooms that are the furthest from the central nursing station. The QI team constructed a **pareto diagram** to understand the nature and frequency of the patients' requests. This analysis revealed that the three most frequently occurring patient requests were:

- Pain medication,
- Assistance with repositioning,
- Assistance with opening and positioning food on the tray table at meal time.

## BOX 21-7 APPLYING THE QI STEPS TO A CLINICAL PERFORMANCE PROBLEM—cont'd

Finally, the team constructed a *fishbone diagram* to identify the factors associated with the twenty-minute response delays. Using these data, the QI team was able to identify the likely cause of the problem and its symptoms.

### Improvement Step 3: Develop a Plan for Improvement

The QI team worked with the hospital librarian to identify relevant studies to develop their improvement project plan. The QI team reviewed a number of research studies about patient requests and response rates from both the patient and nurse perspectives. The team also reviewed studies about work redesign to involve the food service team more directly into the unit's work flow. Based on a critical appraisal of the evidence, the QI team decided to try two interventions for the improvement project:

1) Hourly nurse rounding to improve responsiveness for patient's pain medication requests, and
2) Role redesign for the dietary staff to reduce request for meal assistance.

The QI team agreed on the *specific aim statements* to guide the project:
1. In 30 days, we aim to reduce the number of call bell requests for pain medication from 15 per hour to 3 per 8-hour shift.
2. In 30 days, we aim to decrease average wait time for pain medication from 12 minutes to 5 minutes.

### Improvement Step 4: Test and Implement the Improvement Plan

**Case Study Continues:** The QI team tested the two change ideas using *PDSA cycles* during two successive weeks. Hourly nurse rounding was tested using three nurses on the day and evening shift with patients admitted to three randomly assigned rooms for a 3-day period. During the hourly rounds the nurses conducted pain assessments and administered medication and other pain management interventions. The nurses recorded their interventions on a data collection sheet in each patient's bedside chart. The unit clerk collected the call bell frequency and response time from the central system for the patients in the randomly assigned rooms during the PDSA testing period. During the testing period, the improvement team reviewed the data at the end of each shift to assess changes in performance.

During the next week, the improvement team piloted the change in the dietary aid's work responsibilities to include opening the food trays at the bedside, positioning patients to eat and filling the water pitchers at the time the meals were served. The change in the dietary aid job responsibilities required training in infection control, body mechanics, and the creating of a new sign system to alert the dietary staff about the patients' dietary restrictions. This *change idea* was piloted using the same number of staff members, duration, patient rooms, and unit clerk documentation responsibilities as the PDSA cycle for the hourly nurse rounds. Staff feedback about the strengths and drawbacks of the hourly rounding and expanded food preparation responsibilities for the dietary aids, including suggestions for improving the practice changes, were collected.

Finally, to evaluate the effectiveness of the change ideas, the QI team used a *run chart* to track performance for the unit's call bell response time. The run chart was annotated to include the days that the team implemented the PDSA cycles to refine the process used for hourly nurse rounding and the change in the dietary aid's responsibilities to set-up patients' meal trays. At the end of a month of experimentation, the QI team was able to reduce the number of call bell requests for pain medication from a high of 15 per hour at the beginning of the project, to three per shift. Similarly, the average time that patients waited for their pain medication dropped from 12 minutes to 5 minutes. The team was able to achieve similar reductions in the call bell requests at meal time by expanding the role of the dietary aid to include meal set-up. Based on the performance data, the QI team recommended that hourly nurse rounding and meal set-up by the dietary aids become the standard of practice for the unit.

To embed the new practices into the unit's routines, the QI team supervised PDSA cycles until the entire unit reached the performance goal in the specific aim statement. The run chart data suggested that the call bell response process was mostly stable with some variation attributed to new staff hired for the weekend day shift that were not fully oriented to the unit's new routines for hourly nurse rounding and the dietary aid's responsibilities for setting up meal trays for the patients.

planning, coordinating, implementing, and evaluating improvement efforts. To maintain a productive lead team, it is important to set a meeting schedule and use effective meeting tools such as the following (Nelson et al., 2007):
- Meeting agenda
- Meeting roles
- Ground rules

- Brainstorming
- Multi-voting

Other tools that can help with project management to keep team and activities organized and focused include action plans and Gantt charts (Nelson et al., 2007). To download templates of meeting agendas, meeting role cards, action plans, and Gantt charts, go to the Clinical Microsystems website at www.clinicalmicrosystem.org/ and select the Materials/Worksheets tabs. After the lead team is assembled and team processes established, the team can begin assessment of the health system.

---

**HELPFUL HINT**

To keep the QI lead team engaged and on schedule, hold team meetings at least weekly and display a timeline of QI activities such as data collection, analysis, and results of PDSA cycles with completion progress for each activity where all team members can see it.

---

## Improvement Process Step 1: Assessment

In the assessment phase, the first step is to complete a structured assessment to understand more about performance patterns. The improvement team typically begins with a series of broad questions that are used to guide data collection. Common methods used to collect system performance data include *check sheets* and *data sheets* to understand performance patterns and *surveys, focus groups, and interviews* to gather information about patient and staff perceptions of system performance. Commonly collected data elements include information about the following (Nelson et al., 2007):

- Patients: What are the average age, gender, top diagnoses, and satisfaction scores?
- Professionals: What is the level of staff satisfaction? What is their skill set?
- Processes and patterns: What are the processes for admitting and discharging patients?
- Common performance metrics: What are the rates of pressure ulcers and falls with injury? For useful data collection templates, select the Tools tab at www.clinicalmicrosystem.org/.

---

**HELPFUL HINT**

To reduce data collection burden related to QI projects, when starting the assessment phase of the QI process first identify what performance data already exist in your organization. For example, find out if your organization is participating in the National Database of Nursing Care Quality Indicators program, which collects quarterly data on pressure ulcers, infections, falls, staff satisfaction, and other quality indicators.

---

## Improvement Step 2: Analysis

The next phase of the improvement process focuses on data analysis. Because QI uses a team problem-solving approach, data are displayed in graphic form so all team members can see how the system is performing and generate ideas for what to improve. Several tools exist to help display and analyze performance data.

### Trending Variation in System Performance with Run and Control Charts

If quality health care means that the right care is delivered to the right people, in the right way, at the right time, for every person, during each clinical encounter, it is important to learn when criteria are not met and why (IOM, 2001). One method is to track performance

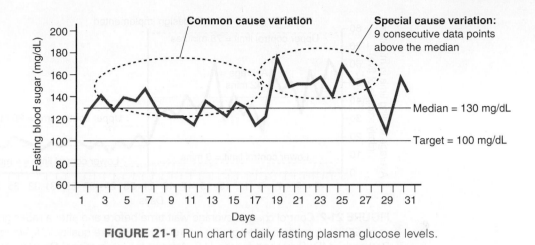

**FIGURE 21-1** Run chart of daily fasting plasma glucose levels.

over time and understand sources of variation in system performance, which can guide improvement activities to design a better-functioning health system. Minimizing performance variation is one of the main QI goals. There are two main types of system variation (Nelson et al., 2007, p. 346):

- Common cause variation occurs at random and is considered a characteristic of the system. For example, you might never leave your house in time for prompt arrival to class. In this case, you must work on better managing multiple random causes of tardiness, such as getting up late or taking too long to shower, dress, and eat to improve your overall punctuality record.

- Special cause variation arises from a special situation that disrupts the causal system beyond what can be accounted for by random variation. An example might be that you usually leave your house on time for a prompt arrival to class, but special circumstances such as road construction or a broken elevator delay your arrival to class. Once these special causes of tardiness are resolved, you will arrive to class on time.

Variations in system performance over time are commonly displayed with run charts and control charts. A **run chart** is a graphical data display that shows trends in a measure of interest; trends reveal what is occurring over time (Nelson et al., 2007). The vertical axis of the run chart depicts the value of measure of interest and the horizontal axis depicts the value of each measure running over time. A run chart shows whether the outcome of interest is running in a targeted area of performance and how much variation there is from point to point and over time. For example, a patient newly diagnosed as having diabetes can record her blood glucose levels over a month using a run chart. By regularly charting blood glucose levels, the patient is able to reveal when blood glucose runs higher or lower than the target level of less than 100 mg/dl for fasting plasma glucose (FPG) test. The run chart in Figure 21-1 shows that FPG levels are consistently higher than the target, with a median FPG of 130 mg/dl; the trend of FPG readings in the first 19 days of the month is indicative of common cause variation. These random variations in FPG readings are likely caused by confluence of several factors such as diet, exercise, and medication adherence. To correct the undesirable variation, the patient can assess what factors might be influencing the higher FPG values and then work with her primary care provider to develop necessary interventions to better control her blood glucose by better managing multiple causal

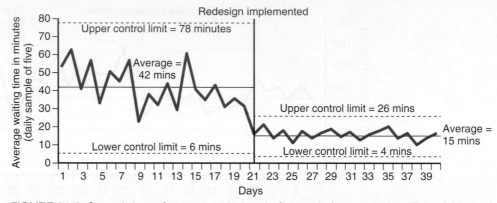

**FIGURE 21-2** Control chart of average wait time before and after a redesign. (From Massoud et al. (2001). A modern paradigm for improving healthcare quality. *QA Monograph Series* 1(1). Bethseda, MD: Published for the U.S. Agency for International Development by the Quality Assurance Project.)

factors. To determine whether interventions were successful, the patient and her provider should continue to document blood glucose levels and then compare the median FPG values before and after interventions are implemented.

In addition, special cause variation in FPG is evident on days 19 to 28, where nine consecutive FPG readings are above the median line. It turns out that on these days, the patient had run out of her glucose-lowering medication; this special circumstance caused increased FPG. Although various rules exist for accurately determining the presence of special cause variation, generally special cause variation is present if the following are true (Nelson et al., 2007, p. 349):

• Eight data points in a row are above or below the median or mean
• Six data points in a row are going up
• Six data points in a row are going down

Determining common and special causes of variation is important because treatment strategies for eliminating each type of variation will vary.

A **control chart** (Figure 21-2) is also used to track system performance over time, but it is a more sophisticated data tool than a run chart (Nelson et al., 2007). A control chart includes information on the average performance level for the system depicted by a center line displaying the system's average performance (the mean value), and the upper and lower limits depicting one to three standard deviations from average performance level. The rules to detect special cause variation are the same for run and control charts, except that for control charts the upper and lower limits are additional tools used to detect special cause variation. Any point that falls outside the control limit is considered an outlier that merits further examination.

**HELPFUL HINT**

Use a run chart in step two of the QI process to analyze causes of variation in fasting plasma glucose (FPG) levels from the target level of 100mg/dl and in step four of the QI process to evaluate if changes in diet, exercise, and medication adherence helped the patient achieve the targeted FPG.

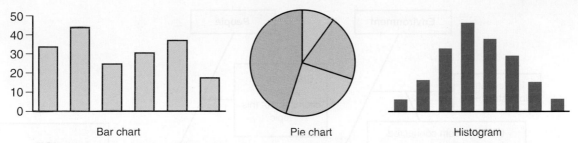

**FIGURE 21-3** Examples of bar chart, pie chart, and histogram. (From Massoud et al. (2001). A modern paradigm for improving healthcare quality. *QA Monograph Series* 1(1). Bethseda, MD: Published for the U.S. Agency for International Development by the Quality Assurance Project.)

## Graphs

Graphs commonly used to understand system performance, displayed in Figure 21-3, include **pie charts**, **bar charts**, and **histograms.** Selecting the appropriate chart depends on the type of data collected and the performance pattern the improvement team is trying to understand. A bar chart is used to display categorical-level data. A pareto diagram is a special type of bar chart used to understand the frequency of factors that contribute to a common effect. It is used to display the Pareto Principle, sometimes referred to as the **80-20 Rule**, or the Law of the Few (Massoud et al., 2001), which states that 80% of variation in a problem originates with 20% of cases. In a pareto diagram, the bars are displayed in descending order of frequency. A histogram is another type of bar chart used for continuous-level data to show the distribution of the data around the mean, commonly called the *bell curve* (Massoud et al., 2001).

## Cause and Effect Diagrams

More sophisticated visual data displays include **cause and effect diagrams** used to identify and treat the causes of performance problems. Two common tools in this category are a fishbone or Ishikawa diagram and a tree diagram (Massoud et al., 2001). The **fishbone diagram** facilitates brainstorming about potential causes of a problem by grouping potential causes into the categories of environment, people, materials, and process (Figure 21-4 on p. 462). Fishbone diagrams can be used proactively to prevent quality defects, including errors, and retrospectively to identify factors that potentially contributed to quality defect or an error that has already occurred. An example of when fishbone diagram is used retrospectively is during root cause analyses (RCAs) to identify system design failures that caused errors.

An RCA is a structured method used to understand sources of system variation that lead to errors or mistakes, including sentinel events, with the goal of learning from mistakes and mitigating hazards that arise as a characteristic of the system design (Percarpio et al., 2008). An RCA is conducted by a team that includes representatives from nursing, medicine, management, QI, or risk management, and the individual(s) involved in the incident (sometimes including the patient or family members in the discovery process), and it emphasizes system failures while avoiding individual blame (Percarpio et al., 2008). An RCA seeks to answer three questions to learn from mistakes:

- What happened?
- Why did it happen?
- What can be done to prevent it from happening again?

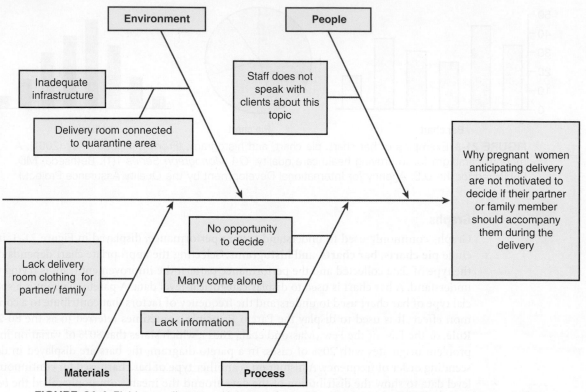

**FIGURE 21-4** Fishbone diagram. (Adapted from Massoud et al. (2001). A modern paradigm for improving healthcare quality. *QA Monograph Series* 1(1). Bethseda, MD: Published for the U.S. Agency for International Development by the Quality Assurance Project.)

Because the RCA is viewed as an opportunity for organizational learning and improvement, the most effective RCAs include a change in practice or work system design to lessen the chances of similar errors occurring in the future.

A **tree diagram** is particularly useful for identifying the chain of causes with the goal of identifying the root cause of a problem. For example, consider medication errors. The improvement team could use the **Five Why's** method to establish the chain of causes leading to the medication error:

- Question 1: Why did the patient get the incorrect medicine?
  Answer 1: Because the prescription was wrong.
- Question 2: Why was the prescription wrong?
  Answer 2: Because the doctor made the wrong decision.
- Question 3: Why did the doctor make the wrong decision?
  Answer 3: Because he did not have complete information in the patient's chart.
- Question 4: Why wasn't the patient's chart complete?
  Answer 4: Because the doctor's assistant had not entered the latest laboratory report.
- Question 5: Why hadn't the doctor's assistant charted the latest laboratory report?
  Answer 5: Because the lab technician telephoned the results to the receptionist, who forgot to tell the assistant.

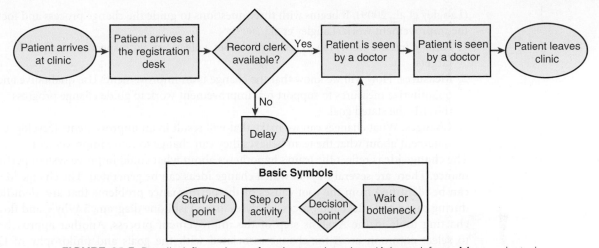

**FIGURE 21-5** Detailed flow chart of patient registration. (Adapted from Massoud et al. (2001). A modern paradigm for improving healthcare quality. *QA Monograph Series* 1(1). Bethseda, MD: Published for the U.S. Agency for International Development by the Quality Assurance Project.)

In this case, using Five Why's technique suggests that a potential solution for avoiding wrong prescriptions in the future might be to develop a system for tracking lab reports (Massoud et al., 2001).

### Flowcharting

A flowchart depicts how a process works, detailing the sequence of steps from the beginning to the end of a process (Massoud et al., 2001). Several types of flowcharts exist, including the most simple (*high level*), a detailed version (*detailed*), and one that also indicates the people involved in the steps (*deployment or matrix*). Figure 21-5 shows an example of a detailed flowchart. Massoud and colleagues (2001, p. 59) suggest using flowcharts to

- Understand processes
- Consider ways to simplify processes
- Recognize unnecessary steps in a process
- Determine areas for monitoring or data collection
- Identify who will be involved in or affected by the improvement process
- Formulate questions for further research

When flowcharting, it is important to identify a start and an end point of a process, then make a record of the actual, not the ideal, process. To obtain an accurate picture of the process, perform direct observation of the process steps and communicate with people who are directly part of the process to clarify all the steps.

### Improvement Step 3: Develop a Plan for Improvement

By identifying potential sources of variation, the improvement team can pinpoint the problem areas in need of improvement. The next phase is to treat the performance problem. This phase involves developing and testing a plan for improvement. A simple yet powerful model for developing and testing improvements is **The Model for Improvement**

(Langley et al., 2009). It begins with three questions to guide the change process and focus the improvement work (Langley et al., 2009):

1. **Aim.** What are we trying to accomplish? Set a clear aim with specific measurable targets.
2. **Measures.** How will we know that the change is an improvement? Use qualitative and quantitative measures to support real improvement work to guide change progress towards the stated goal.
3. **Changes.** What changes can we make that will result in an improvement? Develop a statement about what the team believes they can change to cause improvement.

The **change ideas** reflect the team's hypotheses about what could improve system performance. There are several ways in which change ideas can be generated. The change ideas can be identified from the root causes of the performance problems that are identified during cause and effect and process analyses using Fishbone diagram, 5 Why's, and flowcharting tools in the Analysis step of the improvement process. Another approach is to select common areas for change associated with the goals and philosophy of QI. Common **change topics**, also referred to as **themes for improvement**, include (Langley et al., 2009, p. 359):

- eliminating waste
- improving work flow
- optimizing inventory
- changing the work environment
- managing time more effectively
- managing variation
- designing systems to avoid mistakes
- focusing on products or services

Change ideas can also come from the evidence provided by your review of the available literature. This is where your EBP skills will be most helpful. You will need to critically appraise both research studies and QI studies of interventions that can be applied to remedy the identified problem. To help you decide whether a journal article is a research study or a QI study, see the *critical decision tree* in Figure 21-6 on p. 465. Because QI studies capture the experiences of a particular organization or unit, the results of these studies are usually not generalizable. In an effort to promote knowledge transfer and learning from other's improvement experiences, the *Standards for Quality Improvement Reporting Excellence,* or the SQUIRE Guidelines (Davidoff et al., 2008), were developed to promote the publication and interpretation of this type of applied research. The SQUIRE Guidelines are presented in Table 21-7 on p. 466; you should use them to evaluate QI studies.

## Improvement Step 4: Test and Implement the Improvement Plan

The improvement changes that are identified in the planning phase are tested using the **Plan-Do-Study-Act (PDSA) Improvement cycle,** which is the last step of The Improvement Model (Langley et al., 2009; Massoud et al., 2001) depicted in Figure 21-7 on p. 468. The focus of PDSA is experimentation using small and rapid tests of change. Actions involved in each phase of the PDSA cycle are detailed in Figure 21-7. In this step, you evaluate the success of the intervention in bringing about improvement. It is important for the team to monitor the intended and unintended changes in system performance, the patient and staff perceptions of the change, and, ideally, the costs of the change. Also, in this phase of the improvement process, it is useful to track the stability and sustainability of the new

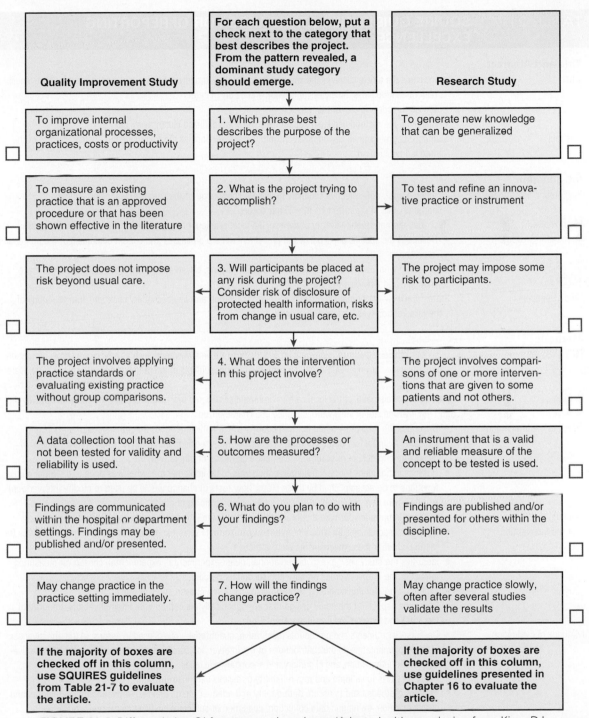

**FIGURE 21-6** Differentiating QI from research projects. (Adapted with permission from King, D.L. (2008). Research and quality improvement: Different processes, different evidence. *Medsurg Nursing, 17*(3), 167.)

| TABLE 21-7 | SQUIRE GUIDELINES STANDARDS FOR QI REPORTING EXCELLENCE |
|---|---|

**Title and Abstract**

| | |
|---|---|
| Title | • Indicates the article concerns the improvement of quality (broadly defined to include the safety, effectiveness, patient-centeredness, timeliness, efficiency, and equity of care)<br>• States the specific aim of the intervention<br>• Specifies the method used (e.g., qualitative study, randomized cluster trial, etc.) |
| Abstract | Summarizes precisely all key information from various sections of the text using the abstract format of the intended publication |

**Introduction**

| | |
|---|---|
| Background and Knowledge | Provides a brief, non-selective summary of current knowledge of the care problem being addressed, and characteristics of organizations in which it occurs |
| Local Problem | Describes the nature and severity of the specific local problem or system dysfunction that was addressed |
| Intended Improvement | • Describes the specific aim (changes/improvement in care processes and patient outcomes) of the proposed intervention<br>• Specified who (champions, supporters) and what (events, observations) triggered the decision to make changes, and why now (timing) |
| Study Question | States precisely the primary improvement-related question and any secondary questions that the study of the intervention was designed to answer |

**Methods**

| | |
|---|---|
| Ethical Issues | Describes ethical aspects of implementing and studying the improvement, such as privacy concerns, protection of participants' physical well-being, and potential author conflicts of interest, and how ethical concerns were addressed |
| Setting | Specifies how elements of the local care environment considered most likely to influence change/improvement in the involved site or sites were identified and characterized |
| Planning the Intervention | • Describes the intervention and its component parts in sufficient detail that others could reproduce it<br>• Indicates main factors that contribute to choice of the specific intervention (e.g., analysis of causes of dysfunction; matching relevant improvement experience of others with the local situation)<br>• Outlines initial plans for how the intervention was to be implemented: what was done (e.g., initial steps; functions to be accomplished by those steps; how tests of change would be used to modify intervention). and by whom (e.g., intended roles, qualifications and training of staff) |
| Planning the Study of the Intervention | • Outlines initial plans for how the intervention was implemented (e.g., dose and intensity of exposure)<br>• Describes mechanisms by which intervention components were expected to cause changes, and plans for testing whether those mechanisms were effective<br>• Identifies the study design (e.g., observational, quasi-experimental, experimental) chosen for measuring impact of the intervention on primary and secondary outcomes<br>• Explains plans for implementing essential aspects of the chosen study design<br>• Describes aspects of the study design that are specifically concerned with internal validity (integrity of the data) and external validity (generalizability) |
| Methods of Evaluation | • Describes instruments and procedures (qualitative, quantitative, mixed) used to assess: a) the effectiveness of the implementation, b) the contributions of the intervention components and context factors to effectiveness of the intervention, and c) primary and secondary outcomes<br>• Reports efforts to validate and test reliability of assessment instruments<br>• Explains methods used to assure data quality and adequacy (e.g., blinding; repeating measurements and data extraction; training in data collection; collection of sufficient baseline measurements) |
| Analysis | • Provides details of qualitative and quantitative (statistical) methods used to draw inferences from the data<br>• Aligns unit of analysis with level at which the intervention was implemented<br>• Specifies degree of variability expected in implementation, change expected in primary outcomes (effect size), and ability of study design (including size) to detect such effects |

| TABLE 21-7 | SQUIRE GUIDELINES STANDARDS FOR QI REPORTING EXCELLENCE—cont'd |
|---|---|

**Results**

Outcomes

Nature of setting and improvement intervention
- Characterizes relevant elements of setting or settings (e.g., geography, physical resources, organizational culture, history of change efforts) and structures and patterns of care (e.g., staffing, leadership) that provided context for intervention
- Explains the actual course of the intervention (e.g., sequence of steps, events or phases; types and numbers of participants at key points), preferably using a time-line or flow diagram
- Documents degree of success in implementing intervention components
- Describes how and why the initial plan evolved, and the most important lessons learned from that evolution, particularly the effects of internal feedback from tests of change

Changes in process of care and patient outcomes associated with the intervention
- Presents data on changes observed in the care delivery process
- Presents data on changes observed in measures of patient outcomes (e.g., morbidity, mortality, function, patient/staff satisfaction, service use, cost, care disparities)
- Considers benefits, harms, unexpected results, problems, failures
- Presents evidence regarding the strength of association between observed changes/improvements and intervention components/context factors
- Includes summary of missing data for intervention and outcomes

**Discussion**

Summary
- Summarizes the most important successes and difficulties in implementing intervention components, and main changes observed in care delivery and clinical outcomes
- Highlights the study's particular strengths

Relation to other evidence

Compares and contrasts study results with relevant findings of others, drawing on broad review of the literature; use of a summary table may be helpful in building on existing evidence

Limitations
- Considers possible sources of confounding, bias, or imprecision in design, measurement, and analysis that may have affected study outcomes (internal validity)
- Explores factors that could affect generalizability (external validity). For example: representativeness of participants; effectiveness of implementation; dose-response effects; features of local care setting
- Addresses likelihood that observed gains may weaken over time, and describes plans, if any, for monitoring and maintaining improvement, explicitly states if such planning was not done
- Reviews efforts made to minimize and adjust for study limitations
- Assesses the effect of study limitations on interpretation and application of results

Interpretation
- Explores possible reasons for differences between observed and expected outcomes
- Draws inferences consistent with the strength of data about causal mechanism and size of observed changes, paying particular attention to components of the intervention and context factors that helped determine the intervention's effectiveness (of lack thereof), and types of settings in which this intervention is most likely to be effective
- Suggests steps that might be modified to improve future performance
- Reviews issues of opportunity costs and actual financial cost of the intervention

Conclusions
- Considers overall practical usefulness of the intervention
- Suggests implications of this report for further studies of improvement interventions

**Other Information**

Funding

Describes funding sources, if any, and role of funding organization in design, implementation, interpretation and publication of study

Reproduced with permission from Davidoff et al. (2008). Publication guidelines for improvement studies in health care: evolution of the SQUIRE project. *Annals of Internal Medicine, 149*(9), 670–676.
*Note:* See www.squire-statement.org/ for more information on publishing QI studies.

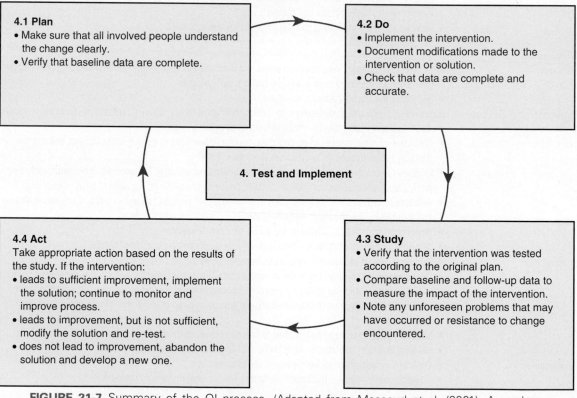

| **1. Assess** | **Activities**<br>• Define a specific goal for improvement<br>• Decide who needs to be on the problem-solving team<br>• Achieve group consensus on improvement goals |
|---|---|

| **2. Analyze** | **Activities**<br>• Analyze available and readily accessible data and information<br>• Identify indicators (measures of improvement)<br>• Collect data prior to the intervention if necessary |
|---|---|

| **3. Develop** | **Activities**<br>• Generate possible interventions<br>• Rank interventions according to priority and feasibility<br>• If possible, test interventions sequentially(one at a time) |
|---|---|

**4.1 Plan**
• Make sure that all involved people understand the change clearly.
• Verify that baseline data are complete.

**4.2 Do**
• Implement the intervention.
• Document modifications made to the intervention or solution.
• Check that data are complete and accurate.

**4. Test and Implement**

**4.4 Act**
Take appropriate action based on the results of the study. If the intervention:
• leads to sufficient improvement, implement the solution; continue to monitor and improve process.
• leads to improvement, but is not sufficient, modify the solution and re-test.
• does not lead to improvement, abandon the solution and develop a new one.

**4.3 Study**
• Verify that the intervention was tested according to the original plan.
• Compare baseline and follow-up data to measure the impact of the intervention.
• Note any unforeseen problems that may have occurred or resistance to change encountered.

**FIGURE 21-7** Summary of the QI process. (Adapted from Massoud et al. (2001). A modern paradigm for improving healthcare quality. *QA Monograph Series* 1(1). Bethseda, MD: Published for the U.S. Agency for International Development by the Quality Assurance Project.)

work process by monitoring system performance over time. Results data should be presented in graphic data displays (explained earlier in the chapter) and compared to the baseline performance.

## TAKING ON THE QI CHALLENGE AND LEADING THE WAY

Hospital leaders and other key stakeholders agree that enabling nurses to lead and participate in QI is vital for strengthening our health system's capacity to provide high-quality patient care (Draper et al., 2008; IOM, 2011). Nurses are on the front lines of delivering care and they offer unique perspectives on the root causes of dysfunctional care, as well as what interventions might work reliably and sustainably in everyday clinical practice to achieve best care. However, multiple barriers to nurses' participation in QI exist, including insufficient staffing, lack of leadership support and resources for nurses' participation in QI, and not enough educational preparation for knowledgeable and meaningful QI involvement (Draper et al., 2008). For nurses to contribute their knowledge and expertise to patient care delivery and the organization's quality enterprise, nursing leadership must engage in (Berwick, 2011, p. 326)

- Setting aims and building the will to improve
- Measurement and transparency
- Finding better systems
- Supporting PDSA activities, risk, and change
- Providing resources

Several common elements that make improvement work doable are captured in two bodies of knowledge (Berwick, 2011). One is **professional knowledge** that includes knowledge of one's discipline, subject matter, and values of the discipline. The other is **knowledge of improvement**, which includes knowledge of complex systems functioning through dynamic interplay among various technical and human elements; knowledge of how to detect and manage variation in system performance; knowledge of managing group processes through effective conflict resolution and communication; and knowledge of how to gain further knowledge by continual experimentation in local settings through rapid tests of change. Linking these two knowledge systems promotes continuous improvement in health care. This chapter provides a starting point for you to develop basic knowledge and skills for the improvement work, so you can better meet the challenges of expectation of contemporary nursing practice.

## KEY POINTS

- There is much room for improving the quality of care in the U.S.
- The quality of health care is evaluated in terms of its effectiveness, efficiency, access, safety, timeliness, and patient centeredness.
- As the largest group of health professionals, nurses play a key role in leading QI efforts in clinical settings.
- Accreditation, payment, and performance measurement are external incentives used to improve the quality of care delivered by hospitals and health professionals. One example of such is the Joint Commission accreditation for health care delivery organizations.
- The National Quality Forum "15" (NQF 15) is a set of 15 nursing-sensitive measures to assess and improve the quality of nursing care delivered in the U.S.
- Standardized measures such as patient fall rates are used to compare performance across nursing units and organizations.

- Health care payers use quality performance measures such as 30-day readmission rates as a basis for paying hospitals and providers.
- QI is both a philosophy of organizational functioning and a set of statistical analysis tools and change techniques used to reduce variation.
- The major approaches used to manage quality in health care are Total Quality Management/Continuous Quality Improvement; Lean; Six Sigma; and the Clinical Microsystems model.
- The defining characteristics of QI are focus on patients/customers; teams and teamwork to improve work processes; and use of data and statistical analysis tools to understand system variation.
- QI uses benchmarking to compare organizational performance and learn from high-performing organizations.
- QI tools, techniques, and principles are applied to clinical performance problems in the form of improvement projects, such as using a presurgical checklist to prevent wrong-side surgeries, a national patient safety goal.
- Unit-level improvement projects should align with organizational-level improvement priorities to promote the sustainability of the unit-level projects.
- There are four major steps in the QI process: assessment, analysis, improvement, and evaluation.
- Patient safety focuses on designing systems to remove factors known to cause errors or adverse events.
- Barriers exist that impede nurses' participation in QI, including insufficient staffing, lack of leadership support, and nurses' unfamiliarity with QI principles and practices.

## CRITICAL THINKING CHALLENGES

- Discuss the similarities and differences among total quality improvement, Lean, Six Sigma, and the Clinical Microsystems models.
- Consider your unit's performance on the HCAHPS (*Hospital Consumer Assessment of Healthcare Providers and Systems*) Survey. What suggestions do you have for applying QI principles to improve your unit's score on these key performance indicators?
- Why is it important to document nurse-sensitive care outcomes using standardized performance measurement systems? How does performance measurement relate to QI activities?
- What barriers do you see for participating in unit-level quality improvement initiatives? What suggestions do you have for overcoming these barriers?
- In what ways do QI studies differ from research studies? How would you use the results of a QI study to inform a change in practice on your unit?

## REFERENCES

Agency for Healthcare Research and Quality. (2012). *National healthcare quality report (AHRQ Publication No.* 12-0005). Retrieved from http://www.ahrq.gov/qual/nhqr11/nhqr11.pdf

Alexander, G. R. (2007). Nursing sensitivity databases: their existence, challenges, and importance. *Medical Care Research and Review, 64*(2), 44S–63S. doi: 10.1177/558707299244.

Asubonteng, P., McCleary, K. J., & Munchus, G. (1996). The evolution of quality in the US health care industry: an old wine in a new bottle. *International Journal of Health Care Quality Assurance, 9*(3), 11–19. doi: 10.1108/09526869610117739.

Berwick, D. M. (2011). Preparing nurses for participation in and leadership of continual improvement. *Journal of Nursing Education, 50*(6), 322–327.

Bigelow, B., & Arndt, M. (1995). Total quality management: field of dreams? *Health Care Management Review, 20*(4), 15–25.

Chang, Y., & Mark, B. (2011). Effects of learning climate and registered nurse staffing on medication errors. *Nursing Research, 60*(1), 32–39. doi: 10.1097/NNR.0b013e3181ff73cc.

Chassin, M. R., & Loeb, J. M. (2011). The ongoing quality improvement journey: next stop, high reliability. *Health Affairs, 30*(4), 559–568. doi: 10.1377/hlthaff.2011.0076.

Chassin, M. R., Loeb, J. M., Schmaltz, S. P., Wachter, R. M. (2010). Accountability measures: using measurement to promote quality improvement. *The New England Journal of Medicine, 363*(7), 683–688. doi.10.1056/NEJMsb1002320.

Cronenwett, L., Sherwood, G., Barnsteiner, J., et al. (2007). Quality and safety education for nurses. *Nursing Outlook, 55*(3), 122–131. doi:10.1016/j.outlook.2007.02.006.

Davidoff, F., Batalden, P., Stevens, D., et al. (2008). Publication guidelines for improvement studies in health care: evolution of the SQUIRE project. *Annals of Internal Medicine, 149*(9), 670–676.

Davis, K., Schoen, C., & Stremikis, K. (2010). *How the performance of the U.S. health care system compares internationally*. Retrieved from http://www.commonwealthfund.org/~/media/Files/Publications/Fund%20Report/2010/Jun/1400_Davis_Mirror_Mirror_on_the_wall_2010.pdf

DelliFraine, J. L., Langabeer, J. R. II, Nembhard, I. M. (2010). Assessing the evidence of Six Sigma and Lean in the health care industry. *Quality Management in Health Care, 19*(3), 211–225. doi: 10.1097/QMH.0b013e3181eb140e.

Donabedian, A. (1966). Evaluating the quality of medical care. *The Milbank Memorial Fund Quarterly, 44*(3), 166–206.

Doyle, J. L., Kenny, T. H., von Grueigen, et al. (2012). Implementing an induction scheduling procedure and consent form to improve quality of care. *Journal of Obstetric, Gynecologic & Neonatal Nursing, 41*(4), 462–473.

Draper, D. A., Felland, L. E., Liebhaber, A., & Melichar, L. (2008). *The role of nurses in hospital quality improvement (CSHSC Report no. 3)*. Retrieved from http://www.hschange.org/CONTENT/972/

Ferlie, E. B., & Shortell, S. M. (2001). Improving the quality of health care in the United Kingdom and the United States: A framework for change. *Milbank Quarterly, 79*(2), 281–315. doi: 10.1111/1468-0009.00206.

Giordano, L. A., Elliott, M. N., Goldstein, E., et al. (2010). Development, implementation, and public reporting of the HCAHPS survey. *Medical Care Research and Review, 67*(1), 23–37. doi: 10.1177/1077558709341065.

Henry, B., Wood, S., Nagelkerk, J. (1992). Nightingale's perspective of nursing administration. *Sogo Kango: Comprehensive Nursing Quarterly, 27*, 16–26.

Institute of Medicine. (1999). *To err is human: building a safer health system: executive summary*. Washington, DC: The National Academies Press. Retrieved from http://books.nap.edu/openbook.php?record_id=9728

Institute of Medicine. (2001). *Crossing the quality chasm: a new health system for the 21st century: executive summary*. Washington, DC: The National Academies Press. Retrieved from http://books.nap.edu/catalog/10027.html

Institute of Medicine. (2011). *The future of nursing: leading change, advancing health*. Washington, DC: The National Academies Press.

Kliger, J., Lacey, S. R., Olney, A., et al. (2010). Nurse driven programs to improve patient outcomes. *Journal of Nursing Administration, 40*(3), 109–114. doi: 10.1097/NNA.0b013e3181d042ac.

Langley, G. J., Moen, R. D., Nolan, K. M., et al. (2009). *The improvement guide: a practical approach to enhancing organizational performance* (2nd ed.). San Francisco, CA: Jossey-Bass.

Massoud, R., Askov, K., Reinke, J., et al. (2001). A modern paradigm for improving healthcare quality. *QA Monograph Series 1*(1). Bethseda, MD: the Quality Assurance Project.

McGlynn, E. A., Asch, S. M., Adams, J., et al. (2003). The quality of health care delivered to adults in the United States. *New England Journal of Medicine, 348*(26), 2635–2645. doi: 10.1056/NEJMsa022615.

National Quality Forum. (2004). *National voluntary consensus standard for nursing-sensitive care: an initial performance measure set*. Retrieved from http://www.qualityforum.org/Publications/2004/10/National_Voluntary_Consensus_Standards_for_Nursing-Sensitive_Care__An_Initial_Performance_Measure_Set.aspx

Nelson, E. C., Batalden, P. B., & Godfrey, M. M. (2007). *Quality by design: a clinical microsystems approach*. San Francisco, CA: Jossey-Bass.

Percarpio, K. B., Watts, V., & Weeks, W. B. (2008). The effectiveness of root cause analyses: what does the literature tell us? *Joint Commission Journal of Quality and Patient Safety, 34*(7), 391–398.

Rosenthal, M. B., & Frank, R. G. (2006). What is the empirical basis for paying for quality in health care? *Medical Care Research and Review, 63*(2), 135–157. doi: 10.1177/1077558705285291.

Scrivens, E. (1997). Putting continuous quality improvement into accreditation: improving approaches to quality assessment. *Quality in Health Care, 6*(4), 212–218. doi: 10.1136/qshc.6.4.212.

Seidl, K. L., & Newhouse, R. P. (2012). The intersection of evidence-based practice with five quality improvement methodologies. *Journal of Nursing Administration, 42*(6), 299–304. doi: 10.1097/NNA.0b013e31824ccdc9

Sidani, S., & Doran, D. (2010). Relationship between processes and outcomes of nurse practitioners in acute care: an exploration. *Journal of Nursing Care Quality, 25*(1), 31–35.

Storey, J. (2013). Factors affecting the adoption of quality assurance technologies in healthcare. *Journal of Health Organization and Management*, in press. Retrieved from oro.open.ac.uk/34536/

Stotts, N. A., & Gunningberg, L. (2007). Predicting pressure ulcer risk. *American Journal of Nursing, 107*(1), 41–48.

U. S. Department of Health and Human Services. (2012a). *National strategy for quality improvement in health care*. Retrieved from http://www.ahrq.gov/workingforquality/nqs/nqs2012annlrpt.pdf

U. S. Department of Health and Human Services. (2012b). *Hospital Compare*. Retrieved from http://www.hospitalcompare.hhs.gov/

# ℮volve WEBSITE

*Go to Evolve at http://evolve.elsevier.com/LoBiondo/ for review questions, critiquing exercises, and additional research articles for practice in reviewing and critiquing.*

# A Randomized, Clinical Trial of Education or Motivational-Interviewing–Based Coaching Compared to Usual Care to Improve Cancer Pain Management

*Mary Laudon Thomas, RN, MS, AOCN®, Janette E. Elliott, RN-BC, MS, AOCN®, Stephen M. Rao, PhD, Kathleen F. Fahey, RN, MS, CNS, Steven M. Paul, PhD, and Christine Miaskowski, RN, PhD, FAAN*

**Purpose/Objectives:** To test the effectiveness of two interventions compared to usual care in decreasing attitudinal barriers to cancer pain management, decreasing pain intensity, and improving functional status and quality of life (QOL).

**Design:** Randomized clinical trial.

**Setting:** Six outpatient oncology clinics (three Veterans Affairs [VA] facilities, one county hospital, and one community-based practice in California, and one VA clinic in New Jersey)

**Sample:** 318 adults with various types of cancer-related pain.

**Methods:** Patients were randomly assigned to one of three groups: control, standardized education, or coaching. Patients in the education and coaching groups viewed a video and received a pamphlet on managing cancer pain. In addition, patients in the coaching group participated in four telephone sessions with an advanced practice nurse interventionist using motivational interviewing techniques to decrease attitudinal barriers to cancer pain management. Questionnaires were completed at baseline and six weeks after the final telephone calls. Analysis of covariance was used to evaluate for differences in study outcomes among the three groups.

**Main Research Variables:** Pain intensity, pain relief, pain interference, attitudinal barriers, functional status, and QOL.

**Findings:** Attitudinal barrier scores did not change over time among groups. Patients randomized to the coaching group reported significant improvement in their ratings of pain-related interference with function, as well as general health, vitality, and mental health.

**Conclusions:** Although additional evaluation is needed, coaching may be a useful strategy to help patients decrease attitudinal barriers toward cancer pain management and to better manage their cancer pain.

**Implications for Nursing:** By using motivational interviewing techniques, advanced practice oncology nurses can help patients develop an appropriate plan of care to decrease pain and other symptoms.

Despite important advances in its management, cancer pain remains a significant clinical problem (Apolone et al., 2009; McGuire, 2004; van den Beuken-van Everdingen et al., 2007). In a meta-analysis, cancer pain was found in 64% of patients with metastatic disease, 59% of patients receiving antineoplastic therapy, and 33% of patients who had received curative cancer treatment (van den Beuken-van Everdingen et al., 2007). Cancer pain also has a negative effect on patients' functional status (Ferreira et al., 2008; Holen, Lydersen, Klepstad, Loge, & Kassa, 2008; Vallerand, Templin, Sasenau, & Riley-Doucet, 2007) and is associated with psychological distress (Cohen et al., 2003; Vallerand, Hasenau, Templin, & Collins-Bohler, 2005). The effect of cancer pain on an individual's quality of life (QOL) can be significant and extend beyond disturbances in mood and physical function (Burckhardt & Jones, 2005; Dahl, 2004; Fortner et al., 2003).

Although advances in pain management can reduce cancer pain for a significant number of patients, numerous clinician, healthcare system, and **societal barriers (e.g., knowledge deficits, reimbursement** and regulatory constraints, religious or cultural views) contribute to ineffective pain management (Brockopp et al., 1998; Dahl, 2004; Hill, 1993; Sun et al., 2007). Attitudinal barriers held by patients can be a substantive factor in the inadequate treatment of cancer pain (Anderson et al., 2002; Ward et al., 2008). Those attitudinal barriers need to be addressed if cancer pain management is to be improved (Fahey et al., 2008).

In a meta-analysis of the benefits of patient-based psychoeducational interventions for cancer pain management, Bennett, Bagnall, and Closs (2009) concluded that, compared to usual care, educational interventions improved knowledge and attitudes and reduced average and worst pain intensity scores. However, those interventions had no effect on medication adherence or in reducing pain's level of interference with daily activities. Bennett et al. (2009) suggested that additional trials are warranted to test different approaches to cancer pain education and to clarify the exact relationships between education and improved patient outcomes.

Many psychoeducational intervention studies were conducted in the hospital setting (Chang, Chang, Chiou, Tsou, & Lin, 2002; de Wit et al., 2001; Jahn et al., 2010) or in patients' homes (Given et al., 2002; Miaskowski et al., 2004), which limited the generalizability of the findings to the outpatient clinic setting. In addition, although they achieved a positive outcome, many of the studies were labor-intensive, which also limited their ability to be implemented in a busy oncology clinic (Given et al., 2002; Miaskowski et al., 2004). Unfortunately, studies using less labor-intensive interventions were not as successful in decreasing cancer pain (Anderson et al., 2002; Oliver, Kravitz, Kaplan, & Meyers, 2001; Syrjala et al., 2008).

Coaching is a useful strategy to improve cancer pain management (Kalauokalani, Franks, Oliver, Meyers, & Kravitz, 2007; Miaskowski et al., 2004). Incorporating principles of motivational interviewing into a coaching intervention affords a unique method of exploring personal attitudes, behaviors, and beliefs that can interfere with effective cancer pain management (Fahey et al., 2008; Prochaska & DiClemente, 1984).

Change theory, specifically the Transtheoretical Model (Prochaska & DiClemente, 1984), is a useful conceptual framework for coaching. In this model, behavioral change is a function of a person's state of readiness or motivation to modify a particular behavior. Motivational interviewing is a nonauthoritarian counseling technique that can assist patients in recognizing and resolving ambivalence about making constructive behavioral changes. It matches the patients' readiness to change and can motivate the patient to move through the stages of the Transtheoretical Model: precontemplation (unaware of need for change), contemplation (thinking about change), preparation (actively considering change), action (engaging in changing behavior), and maintenance (maintaining a changed behavior) (Fahey et al., 2008; Prochaska & DiClemente, 1984).

Given the limitations of previous intervention studies, additional research is warranted using approaches that can be implemented in the outpatient setting. Therefore, the purposes of this randomized clinical trial were to test the effectiveness of two interventions compared to usual care in decreasing attitudinal barriers to cancer pain management, decreasing pain intensity, and improving pain relief, functional status, and QOL. The authors hypothesized that the motivational-interviewing–based coaching group would demonstrate greater benefit (i.e., decreasing attitudinal barriers; decreasing pain intensity; and improving pain relief, functional status, and QOL) than either the conventional education or usual care groups.

## METHODS

### Sample and Settings

A convenience sample was obtained by recruiting patients from six outpatient oncology clinics (three Veterans Affairs [VA] facilities, one county hospital, and one community-based practice in California, and one VA clinic in New Jersey). Patients were eligible to participate if they were able to read and understand the English language, had access to a telephone, had a life expectancy longer than six months, and had an average pain intensity score of 2 or higher as measured on a 0–10 scale, with higher scores indicating more pain. Patients were excluded if they had a concurrent cognitive or psychiatric condition or substance abuse problem that would prevent adherence to the protocol, had severe pain unrelated to their cancer, or resided in a setting where the patient could not self-administer pain medication (e.g., nursing home, board and care facility). The study was approved by the institutional review board and research committee at each of the sites. To test the interaction of time (change in scores from pre- to post-study) by assignment to the three treatment groups (i.e., control, education, or coaching), a sample size of 240 was needed to detect a medium effect ($f = 0.25$; $h_2 = 6\%$ of explained variance). As shown in Figure 1, of the 1,911 patients who were screened, 406 were eligible to participate, 322 provided written informed consent, and 289 completed baseline assessments after being randomized to one of three groups.

### Procedures

Prior to beginning participant recruitment, all research team members were trained extensively so that the procedures for enrollment, data collection, and interventions were standardized across all clinic sites. Research associates (RNs or psychology interns) were trained in procedures for evaluating potential participants, approaching them, obtaining consent to participate, and administering the instruments and videotapes. Importantly, the research associates were trained in providing attention-control telephone calls. The nurse interventionist was trained extensively in motivational interviewing and change theory by

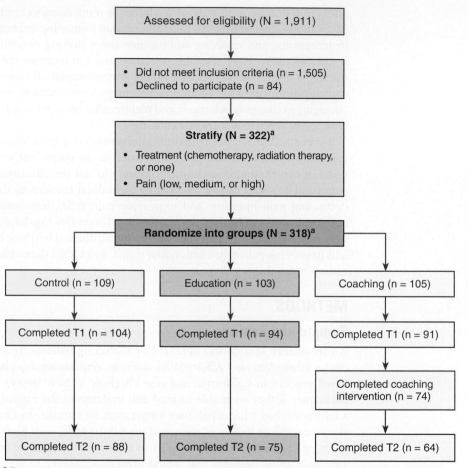

Assessed for eligibility (N = 1,911)

- Did not meet inclusion criteria (n = 1,505)
- Declined to participate (n = 84)

**Stratify (N = 322)**[a]
- Treatment (chemotherapy, radiation therapy, or none)
- Pain (low, medium, or high)

**Randomize into groups (N = 318)**[a]

| Control (n = 109) | Education (n = 103) | Coaching (n = 105) |

| Completed T1 (n = 104) | Completed T1 (n = 94) | Completed T1 (n = 91) |

Completed coaching intervention (n = 74)

| Completed T2 (n = 88) | Completed T2 (n = 75) | Completed T2 (n = 64) |

[a] Four patients withdrew before randomization, and one was lost to follow-up before completing T1.
*Note.* Reasons for lack of completion included being too ill, withdrawing, fatigue, being lost to follow-up, death, ineligibility, prolonged hospitalization, protocol violation, or other.

**FIGURE 1** Trial Participation at Baseline (T1) and Six Months (T2)

a cognitive behavioral psychologist and then in procedures related to the specific coaching protocol. Details of this training are described in Fahey et al. (2008). Monthly team meetings were held throughout the study to ensure procedural fidelity was maintained.

Patients were identified by clinic staff and screened for eligibility by the research associate, who then approached eligible patients, explained the study, and obtained written informed consent. Patients were stratified based on pain intensity (i.e., low, medium, or high) and cancer treatment (i.e., chemotherapy or radiation therapy) to control for the confounding variables of pain intensity and the effects of cancer treatment. Stratifying by pain intensity accounts for the curvilinear relationship between pain severity and functional status (e.g., changes in pain intensity at the upper levels of the scale have a different effect on functional status compared to changes at the lower levels of the scale). Stratification by cancer therapy was used to control for the effect of treatment in either decreasing pain from shrinking the tumor or increasing pain because of toxicity of treatment. Patients at each clinic site then were randomized based on the stratification criteria using permuted blocks with variable sizes into one of three groups: usual care (control), education, or coaching. This method of randomization was used to ensure balance across the treatment groups within each stratification cell.

Patients and clinicians at the study sites were blinded to the patient's group assignment. At the time of enrollment, patients completed a demographic questionnaire, the Karnofsky Performance Status (KPS) scale (Karnofsky & Burchenal, 1949), the Brief Pain Inventory (Daut, Cleeland, & Flanery, 1983), the Barriers Questionnaire (BQ) (Ward et al., 1993), the 36-Item Short Form Health Survey (SF-36®) (Ware & Sherbourne, 1992), and the Functional Assessment of Cancer Therapy–General (FACT-G) (Cella et al., 1993). The patients' medical records were reviewed for disease and treatment information.

Patients in the usual care group viewed a video on cancer (American Cancer Society, 1994). Patients assigned to the education group viewed a video on managing cancer pain that focused on overcoming attitudinal barriers (Syrjala, Abrams, Du Pen, Niles, & Rupert, 1995) and received the Agency for Health Care Policy and Research (1994) pamphlet entitled, *Managing Cancer Pain, Consumer Version, Clinical Practice Guideline Number 9*. To simulate the time constraints in many oncology outpatient clinics, no reinforcement of the material was provided unless the patient sought additional information or asked questions of the clinic staff. Patients assigned to the coaching group received the same intervention as those assigned to the education group. In addition, they participated in four 30-minute telephone sessions that explored beliefs about pain, use of analgesics and nonpharmacologic pain management strategies, and communication about pain management. Those four calls were conducted about every other week over a six-week time period by the nurse interventionist, a clinical nurse specialist trained in motivational interviewing techniques. For a detailed description of the coaching intervention, see Fahey et al. (2008). Patients assigned to the usual care and education groups also received four telephone calls (about every other week over a six-week time period) from the research assistant for attention-control purposes. Six weeks after the final telephone call (i.e., 12 weeks postrandomization), all patients completed the same questionnaires that were done at enrollment. Participants received a $25 gift certificate after completing each set of questionnaires.

## Instruments

Attitudinal barriers were assessed with the **BQ** (Ward et al., 1993; Ward & Gatwood, 1994), a 27-item instrument that measures eight barriers to cancer pain management (concern about side effects, concern about tolerance, fear of addiction, fatalism, fear of disease progression, desire to be a good patient, fear of injections, and concern about distracting the physician from curing disease). Each item is rated on a scale from 0 (not at all agree) to 5 (agree very much). Mean subscale and total scores were calculated for the BQ, with higher scores reflecting stronger barriers. The BQ has demonstrated adequate validity and reliability (Ward et al., 1993; Ward & Gatwood, 1994).

Pain was assessed with the **Brief Pain Inventory**, a self-report instrument designed to assess the intensity and quality of pain, the extent to which pain relief was obtained, and the extent to which pain interferes with function (Daut et al., 1983). Severity and interference are rated on a numeric score from 0 (does not interfere) to 10 (completely interferes). A mean interference score was calculated (Serlin, Mendoza, Nakamura, & Cleeland, 1995), with higher scores reflecting greater pain intensity and greater interference with function.

Functional status was measured with the **SF-36** (Ware & Sherbourne, 1992). Eight health concepts were assessed (physical functioning, role limitations because of physical health problems, bodily pain, social functioning, role limitations because of emotional health problems, general mental health, vitality, and perception of general health). In addition, physical and mental component summary scores are obtained by combining scores related to physical and mental functioning, respectively. For each scale, scores are reversed (as needed so that higher scores reflect better health states), summed, and linearly transformed on a 0–100 scale, with higher scores reflecting higher functioning. The SF-36 has been used extensively and has well-established validity and reliability (Given, Given, Azzouz, Stommel, & Kozachick, 2000; McHorney, Ware, & Raczek, 1993; Miaskowski et al., 2007; Thong, Mols, Coebergh, Roukema, & van de Poll-Franse, 2009).

QOL was measured with the **FACT-G** (Cella et al., 1993). Four QOL domains (physical, social, emotional, and functional well-being) are measured. Patients were asked to rate the extent to which they agreed with each item using a five-point Likert-type scale that ranged from 0 (not at all) to 4 (very much). Scores for items within each subscale are summed to obtain a subscale score, and all of the individual items are summed to obtain a total score, which can range from 0–112. The FACT-G has been used in numerous studies of patients with cancer (Elting et al., 2008; Wittmann, Vollmer, Schweiger, & Hiddemann, 2006; Zimmerman et al., 2010) and specifically in studies of patients with cancer-related pain (Chang, Hwang, & Kasimis, 2002; Harris et al., 2009). The FACT-G has well-established validity and reliability (Cella et al., 1993).

## Data Analysis

Differences in demographic and clinical characteristics among the three groups were evaluated using analyses of variance and chi-square tests. Analyses of covariance were performed to evaluate for differences in scores on average and worst pain intensity, pain relief, mean pain interference, the BQ, the SF-36, and the FACT-G among the three patient groups. That procedure allows for the evaluation of the end-of-study outcomes while controlling for those same outcomes at baseline. The examination of differences among groups in end-of-study outcomes, with baseline measurements of those outcomes covaried out, often is a preferred method for examining changes in outcome measures from the beginning to the end of a study (Cohen, 1988). All calculations used actual values. Adjustments were not made for missing data; therefore, the cohort for each analysis was dependent on the largest set of data across groups. If the overall analysis of covariance for a particular outcome indicated differences among the three groups, pairwise contrasts were conducted to determine the location of the difference. The Bonferroni procedure was used to distribute a family alpha of 0.05 across the three pairwise contrasts. All p values have been adjusted so that values lower than 0.05 are considered statistically significant.

## RESULTS

### Sample

Of the 289 patients who enrolled, 227 completed the end-of-study evaluation. The length of time from cancer diagnosis to study enrollment averaged 30–38 months. The most common cancer types were lung, prostate, and head and neck. Most patients were men and middle-aged, and about half of the sample was married or partnered. No differences were found among the three groups on any demographic or clinical characteristic except KPS score. Patients in the education group reported significantly lower KPS scores than patients in the coaching group (p = 0.03) (see Table 1).

## TABLE 1    DEMOGRAPHIC AND CLINICAL CHARACTERISTICS BY STUDY GROUP

| CHARACTERISTIC | CONTROL (N = 88)[a] | | EDUCATION (N = 75)[b] | | COACHING (N = 64) | | STATISTICS |
|---|---|---|---|---|---|---|---|
| | $\overline{X}$ | SD | $\overline{X}$ | SD | $\overline{X}$ | SD | |
| Age (years) | 58.7 | 11.5 | 62.5 | 11.2 | 61.8 | 11.3 | $F_{(2, 223)} = 2.54$, $p = 0.08$ |
| Education (years) | 13.8 | 2.7 | 12.8 | 2.6 | 13.1 | 3.2 | $F_{(2, 222)} = 2.57$, $p = 0.08$ |
| Time since diagnosis (months) | 31.9 | 52.7 | 37.5 | 45 | 30 | 42.5 | $F_{(2, 222)} = 0.48$, $p = 0.62$ |
| Karnofsky Performance Status score[c] | 76.6 | 12.5 | 72.3 | 12.7 | 77.6 | 13.2 | $F_{(2, 222)} = 3.53$, $p = 0.03$* |

| CHARACTERISTIC | N | % | N | % | N | % | STATISTICS |
|---|---|---|---|---|---|---|---|
| **Gender** | | | | | | | $\chi^2 = 4$; $p = 0.13$ |
| Male | 79 | 90 | 71 | 95 | 54 | 84 | |
| Female | 9 | 10 | 4 | 5 | 10 | 16 | |
| **Ethnicity** | | | | | | | $\chi^2 = 13.4$, $p = 0.65$ |
| African American | 21 | 24 | 15 | 20 | 7 | 11 | |
| Caucasian | 48 | 56 | 44 | 60 | 44 | 69 | |
| Latino | 6 | 7 | 8 | 11 | 7 | 11 | |
| Other | 11 | 13 | 7 | 10 | 6 | 9 | |
| **Marital status** | | | | | | | $\chi^2 = 8.3$, $p = 0.61$ |
| Married or partnered | 40 | 46 | 37 | 50 | 33 | 52 | |
| Widowed, divorced, or separated | 33 | 38 | 23 | 31 | 27 | 42 | |
| Never married | 15 | 17 | 14 | 19 | 4 | 6 | |
| **Living arrangements** | | | | | | | $\chi^2 = 6.4$, $p = 0.38$ |
| Alone | 23 | 26 | 12 | 16 | 15 | 23 | |
| With family or friends | 55 | 63 | 57 | 76 | 47 | 73 | |
| Other | 10 | 11 | 6 | 8 | 2 | 3 | |
| **Employment** | | | | | | | $\chi^2 = 10.1$, $p = 0.61$ |
| Full- or part-time | 10 | 12 | 4 | 5 | 5 | 8 | |
| Disability, leave of absence, or retired | 54 | 63 | 57 | 77 | 48 | 75 | |
| Unemployed | 18 | 21 | 11 | 15 | 10 | 16 | |
| Other | 4 | 5 | 2 | 3 | 1 | 2 | |
| **Cancer diagnosis** | | | | | | | $\chi^2 = 45.7$, $p = 0.72$ |
| Breast | 5 | 6 | 3 | 4 | 8 | 13 | |
| Colon | 6 | 7 | 2 | 3 | 4 | 6 | |
| Head and neck | 12 | 14 | 7 | 9 | 6 | 9 | |
| Lung | 21 | 24 | 14 | 19 | 9 | 14 | |
| Myeloma | 6 | 7 | 5 | 7 | 6 | 9 | |
| Prostate | 12 | 14 | 16 | 21 | 11 | 17 | |
| Other (mixed types) | 26 | 30 | 28 | 37 | 20 | 31 | |

*Education < coaching, $p < 0.05$
[a]Because patients could refuse to complete items, N = 86 for ethnicity and employment.
[b]Because patients could refuse to complete items, N = 74 for ethnicity, marital status, and employment.
[c]Scores indicate functional status on a 0–100 scale, with higher scores reflecting higher function.
*Note.* Because of rounding, not all percentages total 100.

## Instrument Scores

**Barrier Questionnaire:** Barrier subscale scores were modest in all three groups, with concerns about addiction and disease progression rated higher than those related to fatalism or the need to be a "good patient" (data not shown). However, after controlling for each of the BQ scores at baseline, no differences were found among the three groups in any of the subscale or total BQ scores.

**Pain intensity, interference, and relief:** After controlling for average pain at baseline, no differences were found among the three groups in average pain intensity scores at the end of the study (p = 0.08) (see Figure 2). Similarly, nonsignificant scores were found among the three groups in worst pain intensity scores (data not shown). However, significant differences were found among the three groups in mean pain interference scores at the end of the study (p = 0.01) (see Figure 3). Post-hoc contrasts demonstrated that the coaching group had lower mean pain interference scores at the end of the study compared to the education and control groups (p = 0.03 and 0.02, respectively). After controlling for baseline pain relief scores, no significant differences were found among the three groups in the percentage of pain relief (p = 0.07) at the end of the study.

**Short-Form Health Survey:** Table 2 lists the pre- and post-study SF-36 subscale and component scores for the three groups. After controlling for each of the baseline SF-36 subscale and component scores, no significant differences were found among the groups in social functioning, physical or emotional role functioning, bodily pain, or physical component scores. However, after controlling for each of the subscale scores at baseline, significant differences were found among the groups in general health, vitality, mental health, and the mental component summary score. Post-hoc contrasts demonstrated that the coaching group had higher mental health component scores compared to the control group. All other post-hoc comparisons were not significant.

**Functional Assessment of Cancer Therapy–General:** Table 3 lists the pre- and post-study subscale and total QOL scores for the three groups. Scores for all four subscales remained stable over time. After controlling for each of the FACT-G scores at baseline, no significant differences were found among the groups on any of the subscale or total scores.

## DISCUSSION

Educational interventions have demonstrated positive outcomes in decreasing cancer pain (Clotfelter, 1999; Dalton, Keefe, Carlson, & Youngblood, 2004; de Wit et al., 2001; Syrjala et al., 2008; Ward et al., 2008; Yates et al., 2004). Coaching has been tested less

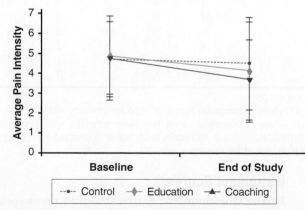

*Note.* F = 2.58; p = 0.08

**FIGURE 2** Changes Over Time in Average Pain Intensity Scores by Patient Group

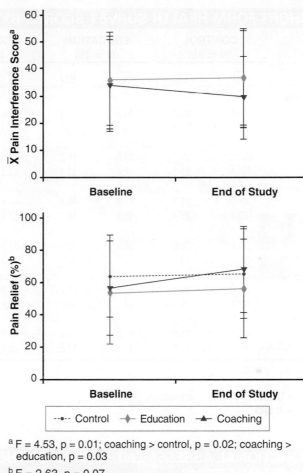

<sup>a</sup> F = 4.53, p = 0.01; coaching > control, p = 0.02; coaching > education, p = 0.03

<sup>b</sup> F = 2.63, p = 0.07

*Note.* All values are plotted as means and standard deviations of the mean.

**FIGURE 3** Changes Over Time in Mean Pain Interference and Pain Relief Scores by Group

frequently as a pain management intervention, but it resulted in positive outcomes in three studies (Kalauokalani et al., 2007; Miaskowski et al., 2004; Oliver et al., 2001). Although successful, the labor-intensive nature of those interventions may limit their use in clinical practice.

The current study tested the effects of two interventions (standardized education and coaching) that were feasible for implementation in an outpatient oncology clinic setting. The coaching intervention was designed to afford flexibility for both the patient and the nurse interventionist to enhance its utility in clinical practice. Patients assigned to the coaching group reported a statistically significant decrease in pain's interference with function and improved ratings of vitality, mental health, and general health. Compared to standardized education, coaching also was associated with clinical improvements in cancer pain management (i.e., decreased cancer pain intensity and improvement or stability in functional status and quality of life). However, most of the improvements were not statistically significant.

## TABLE 2    SHORT-FORM HEALTH SURVEY SCORES BY STUDY GROUP

| SUBSCALE | CONTROL (N = 88) | | EDUCATION (N = 75) | | COACHING (N = 64) | | STATISTICS |
|---|---|---|---|---|---|---|---|
| | $\overline{X}$ | SD | $\overline{X}$ | SD | $\overline{X}$ | SD | |
| **Physical functioning** | | | | | | | $F = 1.179, p = 0.309$ |
| Prestudy | 42.4 | 25.4 | 40.3 | 27.4 | 43.5 | 27.9 | |
| Post-study | 37.3 | 23.7 | 35 | 25.3 | 42.2 | 29.2 | |
| **Body pain** | | | | | | | $F = 2.817, p = 0.062$ |
| Prestudy | 36.9 | 19 | 32.5 | 16.2 | 33.9 | 20.6 | |
| Post-study | 37.4 | 21.3 | 38.4 | 23.4 | 43.2 | 21.8 | |
| **General health** | | | | | | | $F = 4.249, p = 0.015$[a] |
| Prestudy | 41.7 | 21.5 | 41.4 | 19.3 | 47.8 | 23.6 | |
| Post-study | 40.4 | 22.9 | 35.3 | 18.2 | 47.4 | 24.3 | |
| **Vitality** | | | | | | | $F = 3.963, p = 0.02$[b] |
| Prestudy | 34.7 | 18.9 | 35.5 | 20.8 | 37.1 | 21.2 | |
| Post-study | 32 | 19.7 | 30 | 19.5 | 39.3 | 22.7 | |
| **Mental health** | | | | | | | $F = 3.207, p = 0.042$[c] |
| Prestudy | 64 | 20.6 | 62.3 | 21.2 | 66.3 | 19.4 | |
| Post-study | 63.6 | 19.3 | 62 | 22 | 70.8 | 20.4 | |
| **Mental component** | | | | | | | $F = 3.397, p = 0.035$[d] |
| Prestudy | 42.5 | 11.9 | 41.6 | 12.6 | 43.3 | 11.8 | |
| Post-study | 41 | 12.1 | 41.1 | 12.5 | 45.7 | 12.1 | |

[a]Coaching > education, p = 0.016
[b]Coaching > education, p = 0.02
[c]Coaching > control, p = 0.089; coaching > education, p = 0.07
[d]Coaching > control, p = 0.043

## TABLE 3    FUNCTIONAL ASSESSMENT OF CANCER THERAPY–GENERAL SCORES BY STUDY GROUP

| SUBSCALE | CONTROL (N = 88) | | EDUCATION (N = 75) | | COACHING (N = 64) | | STATISTICS |
|---|---|---|---|---|---|---|---|
| | $\overline{X}$ | SD | $\overline{X}$ | SD | $\overline{X}$ | SD | |
| **Physical well-being** | | | | | | | $F = 1.373, p = 0.26$ |
| Prestudy | 15.5 | 6.1 | 15.2 | 5.8 | 16.9 | 5.5 | |
| Post-study | 15.7 | 5.7 | 15.5 | 6.1 | 17.6 | 6.2 | |
| **Social well-being** | | | | | | | $F = 0.465, p = 0.63$ |
| Prestudy | 19 | 6.3 | 20.2 | 6.1 | 21.1 | 5.4 | |
| Post-study | 19 | 6.4 | 19.3 | 6.3 | 20.5 | 6.1 | |
| **Emotional well-being** | | | | | | | $F = 2.41, p = 0.09$ |
| Prestudy | 16.7 | 5.3 | 16.7 | 4.7 | 16.5 | 5.6 | |
| Post-study | 16.8 | 4.9 | 16.2 | 5.3 | 17.6 | 5.3 | |
| **Functional well-being** | | | | | | | $F = 1.382, p = 0.25$ |
| Prestudy | 12.4 | 5.3 | 12.9 | 5.7 | 14.1 | 6.1 | |
| Post-study | 12.8 | 5.7 | 12.3 | 5.8 | 14.4 | 6.4 | |
| **Total score** | | | | | | | $F = 2.164, p = 0.12$ |
| Prestudy | 63.6 | 15.6 | 65.1 | 16.9 | 68.8 | 15.9 | |
| Post-study | 64.4 | 16.3 | 63.3 | 17.5 | 70.5 | 17.3 | |

Several possible explanations exist for the lack of statistical significance for most of the outcome measures.

The current study was unique in that the coaching intervention used principles of motivational interviewing and was based on the Transtheoretical Model of change theory. Those basic principles involve addressing issues of greatest importance from the patient's perspective and assessing the individual's readiness to change a particular behavior. Some patients in the coaching group exhibited persistent reluctance to consider changing a given attitude or behavior that might result in improving their cancer pain management. More commonly, the issue of priorities had a significant effect on the nurse interventionist's ability to address attitudinal barriers that might affect cancer pain management. Cancer pain does not exist in a vacuum. Other issues, related—or not—to cancer and its treatment, often were more pressing from the patient's perspective. True to the theoretical underpinnings of the intervention, the nurse interventionist, in turn, focused on those more pressing issues. That adaptation posed challenges in adhering to the attitudinal content within the coaching protocol, but addressed the unique needs presented by the patient. Although the variation was viewed very positively by patients in their study exit interview, its effect on decreasing cancer pain likely was reduced.

Similarly, the researchers had difficulty maintaining the attention-control telephone calls for their intended purpose (i.e., to control for the attention received by those in the coaching group). A substantial number of patients (assigned to either the education or control groups) voiced significant problems or concerns to the research associate during those calls, which required the research associate to notify the patients' clinicians. Although such notification was important from a clinical and ethical standpoint, the patients did not seek intervention on their own, but rather waited for support and assistance from the research associate beyond that offered from the attention control design, which may have blunted the effects of the coaching intervention.

Another possible explanation for the current findings is that the coaching intervention yielded a positive benefit, but the benefit was not sustainable. The study design was modified at the request of the peer reviewers to delay the post-test to six weeks after the coaching intervention was completed. In hindsight, another measurement should have been made immediately after the coaching intervention was completed (six weeks after baseline), with a third measurement at 12 weeks after baseline. The additional measurement would have allowed for an assessment of the immediate effects of the intervention, particularly with patients who were able to complete the intervention, but died or were too ill to complete the questionnaires at 12 weeks. If a more significant effect was seen immediately after completing the intervention, but was not sustained, an argument could then be made for providing some brief ongoing sessions to reinforce the coaching intervention.

In isolation, a behavioral intervention to decrease cancer pain likely will demonstrate a small effect size. Therefore, the lack of statistical significance may simply be a reflection of inadequate sample size. The sample size also was affected by a high attrition rate (30% of those who enrolled to participate), often because of death or disease progression, which could have contributed to the lack of statistical significance in many of the outcome measures. In addition, more patients assigned to the coaching group were unable to complete the end-of-study measures.

Another possible explanation for the lack of statistical significance on many of the outcome measures is that the instruments used were not sensitive enough to detect change. As a group, the sample scored low on each barrier subscale and total score; the scores were similar to those reported in other studies (Ward et al., 2008). Although participants in the coaching group achieved an improvement in each subscale (except fear of injections) that was greater than the improvement in the other two groups, the differences were not significant. Given the low baseline scores and smaller number of patients assigned to the coaching group, the ability to improve those scores would be extremely difficult. More importantly, during the coaching telephone calls, unique barriers were identified by the patients and discussed that were not always reflected in the scores on the BQ (Fahey et al., 2008). The strength of such beliefs or barriers may be so great that four coaching calls may have been inadequate to overcome that enduring attitude. In addition, motivational interviewing is based on change theory, in which an individual's readiness to change behavior is crucial to the success of a behavioral intervention (Prochaska & DiClemente, 1984). The current study did not assess, nor stratify for, an individual's readiness to change a priori, which also could be a contributing factor to those findings.

At baseline, the FACT-G subscale and total scores in the current study were markedly lower than in the general population, particularly the physical and functional well-being subscale scores (Holzner et al., 2004). Similarly, functional well-being scores were lower than those previously reported by patients with cancer (Burckhardt & Jones, 2005; Sherman, Simonton, Latif, Plante, & Anaissie, 2009). However, baseline scores for all FACT-G subscales were similar to those obtained in another study of U.S. Veterans with cancer pain (Chang et al., 2002). QOL scores did not change substantially over time in any group, which suggests that cancer pain was not a significant factor in the QOL of those patients. An alternative explanation is that the stability of scores may reflect the inability of the FACT-G to detect subtle changes in QOL. Niv and Kreitler (2001) acknowledge that pain can be an important factor in one's QOL, but also suggested that it may not always be the most important. Therefore, focusing solely on managing pain may not necessarily have a significant effect on QOL. This view was substantiated in the coaching group, in which other issues that affected the patient's QOL often took precedence over cancer pain (e.g., those related to cancer treatment, family, or economic hardship).

The SF-36 scores reported by patients in the current study were lower than those reported by the general U.S. population (Miaskowski et al., 2007; Wensing, Vingerhoets, & Grol, 2001) and other samples of patients with cancer (Boini, Briançon, Guillemin, Galan, & Hercberg, 2004; Miaskowski et al., 2007; Mols, Coebergh, & van de Poll-Franse, 2007; Wensing et al., 2001). Perhaps reflective of the supportive and alliance-building nature of the intervention, scores related to mental health, mental component summary score, and even vitality and social function improved from baseline in the coaching group. In contrast, those scores declined in the other two groups. As expected, physical functioning and general health declined over time in the control and education groups, yet surprisingly remained stable in the coaching group. Although bodily pain scores improved in the coaching group (p = 0.06), attempts to improve cancer pain management are unlikely to fully explain all of those differences. However, the improvement may better reflect the nurse interventionist's willingness to adapt to more pressing issues facing the patient during the coaching telephone calls. That action is consistent with motivational interviewing, but not captured by standardized instruments.

Finally, the current study was not designed to alter the amount and types of analgesics prescribed. The types and amount of opioids prescribed and taken varied widely among referral sites (Thomas, Annis, & Hwang, 2004). Interestingly, in this subanalysis, the amount of opioids prescribed or taken did not appear to affect pain intensity ratings, pain relief, or satisfaction with pain management. Although interventions that focus on medication use alone also have not been consistently effective in controlling cancer pain, integrating pharmacologic interventions with cognitive-behavioral interventions might produce results that are more significant.

This study highlights the challenges of testing interventions that focus on clinical processes regarding provider advice, communication, and education in a severely ill patient population. Those clinical processes often are complex, and several interacting components may account for the outcomes. As a result, the authors encourage the use of design methodologies and outcome measures that address the complexities of clinical translational studies and use of nonpharmacologic interventions. Future studies should compare a coaching intervention with different types of controls to ensure that the specific effect of the intervention can be better distinguished from those of other controlled factors, such as time, attention, motivation, expectations, and experience (Bennett, 2010; Bennett et al., 2009).

## Conclusions and Implications for Nursing Practice

Findings from the current study did not support the use of mass-produced educational materials as an effective means of managing cancer pain. However, in the busy clinic setting, too often this approach is all a patient with cancer in pain may receive. Symptoms including cancer pain may not be carefully assessed, nor interventions carefully selected, implemented, and discussed. Advanced practice nurses (APNs) provide comprehensive assessments of symptoms and problems faced by patients with cancer. Using motivational interviewing, APNs and patients can jointly develop an appropriate plan of care to decrease those symptoms. Motivational interviewing is a skill that can be mastered by an APN with sufficient training. In working with patients over time, the use of motivational interviewing can yield positive outcomes that extend beyond traditional cancer pain management. Indeed, the use of motivational interviewing is becoming more popular as a mechanism to increase patient adherence with medical treatment. Cancer pain management needs to be addressed from an integrated biopsychosocial approach (e.g., pharmacologic, cognitive, behavioral, motivational, educational) for its effectiveness to be achieved fully.

Mary Laudon Thomas, RN, MS, AOCN®, is a hematology clinical nurse specialist and Janette E. Elliott, RN-BC, MS, AOCN®, is a pain management clinical nurse specialist, both at the Veterans Administration Palo Alto Healthcare System in California; Stephen M. Rao, PhD, is the health behavior coordinator and director of the Training Psychology Postdoctoral Fellowship Program at the San Francisco Veterans Administration Healthcare System in California; Kathleen F. Fahey, RN, MS, CNS, is the palliative care coordinator at El Camino Hospital in Mountain View, CA; and Steven M. Paul, PhD, is the principal statistician and Christine Miaskowski, RN, PhD, FAAN, is a professor and associate dean for Academic Affairs, both in the Department of Nursing at the University of California, San Francisco. This research was supported by the Department of Veterans Affairs, Veterans Health Administration, Health Services Research and Development Service (Project Number NRI-97026).

The authors gratefully acknowledge Marilyn (Marty) Douglas, DNSc, RN, FAAN, who was coprincipal investigator of this study. They also gratefully acknowledge the time and commitment on the part of the patients who participated in this study.

The views expressed in this article are those of the authors and do not necessarily represent the views of the Department of Veterans Affairs. Thomas can be reached at mary.thomas4@va.gov, with copy to editor at ONFEditor@ons.org. (Submitted July 2010. Accepted for publication May 17, 2011.)

Digital Object Identifier: 10.1188/12.ONF.39-49

## REFERENCES

Agency for Health Care Policy and Research. (1994). *Managing cancer pain, consumer version, clinical practice guideline number 9.* Rockville, MD: U.S. Department of Health and Human Services.

American Cancer Society. (1994). *The cancer experience: living with treatment* [Videotape]. Atlanta, GA: American Cancer Society.

Anderson, K. O., Richman, S. P., Hurley, J., et al. (2002). Cancer pain management among underserved minority outpatients: Perceived needs and barriers to optimal control. *Cancer, 94,* 2295–2304. doi:10.1002/cncr.10414.

Apolone, G., Corli, O., Caraceni, A., et al. (2009). Pattern and quality of care of cancer pain management: results from the Cancer Pain Outcome Research Study Group. *British Journal of Cancer, 100,* 1566–1574. doi:10.1038/sj.bjc.6605053.

Bennett, M. I. (2010). Methodological issues in cancer pain: non-pharmacological trials. In J. A. Paice, R. F. Bell, E. A. Kalso, & O. A. Soyannwo (Eds.), *Cancer pain: from molecules to suffering* (pp. 207–218). Seattle, WA: IASP Press.

Bennett, M. I., Bagnall, A., & Closs, S. J. (2009). How effective are patient-based educational interventions in the management of cancer pain? Systematic review and meta-analysis. *Pain, 143,* 192–199. doi:10.1016/j.pain.2009.01.016.

Boini, S., Briançon, S., Guillemin, F., Galan, P., & Hercberg, S. (2004). Impact of cancer occurrence on health-related quality of life: a longitudinal pre-post assessment. *Health and Quality of Life Outcomes, 2,* 4. doi:10.1186/1477-7525-2-4.

Brockopp, D. Y., Brockopp, G., Warden, S., Wilson, J., Carpenter, J. S., & Vandeveer, B. (1998). Barriers to change: a pain management project. *International Journal of Nursing Studies, 35,* 226–232. doi:10.1016/S0020-7489(98)00035-2.

Burckhardt, C. S., & Jones, K. D. (2005). Effects of chronic widespread pain on the health status and quality of life of women after breast cancer surgery. *Health and Quality of Life Outcomes, 3,* 30. doi:10.1186/1477-7525-3-30.

Cella, D., Tulsky, D. S., Gray, G., et al. (1993). The Functional Assessment of Cancer Therapy Scale: development and validation of the general measure. *Journal of Clinical Oncology, 11,* 570–579.

Chang, M. C., Chang, Y. C., Chiou, J.F., Tsou, T. S., & Lin, C. C. (2002). Overcoming patient-related barriers to cancer pain management for home care patients: a pilot study. *Cancer Nursing, 25,* 470–476. doi:10.1097/00002820-200212000-00012.

Chang, V., Hwang, S., & Kasimis, B. (2002). Longitudinal documentation of cancer pain management outcomes: a pilot study at a VA medical center. *Journal of Pain and Symptom Management, 24,* 494–505.

Clotfelter, C. E. (1999). The effect of an educational intervention on decreasing pain intensity in elderly people with cancer. *Oncology Nursing Forum, 26,* 27–33.

Cohen, J. (1988). *Statistical power analysis for the behavioral sciences* (2nd ed.). Hillsdale, NJ: Lawrence Erlbaum Associates.

Cohen, M. Z., Easley, M. K., Ellis, C., et al. (2003). Cancer pain management and the JCAHO's pain standards: an institutional challenge. *Journal of Pain and Symptom Management, 25,* 519–527. doi:10.1016/S0885-3924(03)00068-X.

Dahl, J. L. (2004). Pain: impediments and suggestions for solutions. *Journal of the National Cancer Institute Monographs, 32,* 124–127. doi:10.1093/jncimonographs/lgh022.

Dalton, J., Keefe, F. J., Carlson, J., & Youngblood, R. (2004). Tailoring cognitive-behavioral treatment for cancer pain. *Pain Management Nursing, 5,* 3–18. doi:10.1016/S1524-9042(03)00027-4.

Daut, R. L., Cleeland, C. S., & Flanery, R. (1983). Development of the Wisconsin Brief Pain Questionnaire to assess pain in cancer and other diseases. *Pain, 17,* 197–210.

de Wit, R., van Dam, F., Loonstra, S., et al. (2001). Improving the quality of pain treatment by a tailored pain education programme for cancer patients in chronic pain. *European Journal of Pain, 5,* 241–256.

Elting, E .S., Keefe, D. M., Sonis, S. T., et al. (2008). Patient-reported measurements of oral mucositis in head and neck cancer patients treated with radiotherapy with or without chemotherapy: demonstration of increased frequency, severity, resistance to palliation, and impact on quality of life. *Cancer, 113,* 2704–2713. doi:10.1002/cncr.23898.

Fahey, K. F., Rao, S. M., Douglas, M. K., Thomas, M. L., Elliott, J. E., & Miaskowski, C. (2008). Nurse coaching to explore and modify patient attitudinal barriers interfering with effective cancer pain management. *Oncology Nursing Forum, 35,* 233–240. doi:10.1188/08.ONF.233-240.

Ferreira, K. A., Kimura, M., Teixeira, M. J., Mendoza, T. R., da Nobrega, J. C., Graziani, S. R., & Takagaki, T. Y. (2008). Impact of cancer-related symptom synergisms on health-related quality of life and performance status. *Journal of Pain and Symptom Management, 35,* 604–616. doi:10.1016/j.jpainsymman.2007.07.010.

Fortner, B. V., Demarco, G., Irving, G., Ashley, J., Keppler, G., Chavez, J., & Munk, J. (2003). Description and predictors of direct and indirect costs of pain reported by cancer patients. *Journal of Pain and Symptom Management, 25,* 9–18.

Given, B., Given, C. W., McCorkle, R., Kozachick, S., Cimprich, B., Rahbar, M. H., & Wojcik, C. (2002). Pain and fatigue management: results of a nursing randomized clinical trial. *Oncology Nursing Forum, 29,* 949–955.

Given, C. W., Given, B., Azzouz, F., Stommel, M., & Kozachick, S. (2000). Comparison of changes in physical functioning of elderly patients with new diagnoses of cancer. *Medical Care, 38,* 482–493.

Harris, K., Chow, E., Zhang, L., et al. (2009). Patients' and healthcare professionals' evaluations of health-related quality-of-life issues in bone metastases. *European Journal of Cancer, 45,* 2510–2518. doi:10.1016/j.ejca.2009.05.024.

Hill, C. S., Jr. (1993). The barriers to adequate pain management with opioid analgesics. *Seminars in Oncology, 20*(2, Suppl. 1), 1–5.

Holen, J. C., Lydersen, S., Klepstad, P., Loge, J. H., & Kassa, S. (2008). The Brief Pain Inventory: pain's interference with functions is different in cancer pain compared with noncancer chronic pain. *Clinical Journal of Pain, 24,* 219–225. doi:10.1097/AJP.0b013e31815ec22a.

Holzner, B., Kemmler, G., Cella, D., et al. (2004). Normative data for functional assessment of cancer therapy. *Acta Oncologica, 43,* 153–160. doi:10.1080/02841860310023453.

Jahn, P., Kitzmantel, J.P., Renz, P., et al. (2010). Improvement of pain-related self-management for oncologic patients through a transinstitutional modular nursing intervention: protocol of a cluster randomized multicenter trial. *Trials, 11,* 29. doi:10.1186/1745-6215-11-29.

Kalauokalani, D., Franks, P., Oliver, J. W., Meyers, F. J., & Kravitz, R. L. (2007). Can patient coaching reduce racial/ethnic disparities in cancer pain control? Secondary analysis of a randomized controlled trial. *Pain Medicine, 8,* 17–24. doi:10.1111/j.1526-4637.2007.00170.x.

Karnofsky, D. A., & Burchenal, J. H. (1949). The clinical evaluation of chemotherapeutic agents in cancer. In C. M. Macleod (Ed.), *Evaluation of chemotherapeutic agents* (pp. 191–205). New York, NY: Columbia University Press.

McGuire, D. B. (2004). Occurrence of cancer pain. *Journal of the National Cancer Institute Monographs, 32,* 51–56. doi:10.1093/jncimonographs/lgh015.

McHorney, C. A., Ware, J. E., & Raczek, A. E. (1993). The MOS 36-Item Short Form Health Survey (SF-36): II: psychometric and clinical tests of validity in measuring physical and mental health constructs. *Medical Care, 31,* 247–263.

Miaskowski, C., Dodd, M. J., West, C., Paul, S. M., Schumacher, K. L., Tripathy, D., & Koo, P. (2007). The use of a responder analysis to identify differences in patient outcomes following a self-care intervention to improve cancer pain management. *Pain, 129,* 55–63. doi:10.1016/j.pain.09.031.

Miaskowski, C., Dodd, M. J., West, C., Schumacher, K. L., Paul, S. M., Tripathy, D., & Koo, P. (2004). Randomized clinical trial of the effectiveness of a self-care intervention to improve cancer pain management. *Journal of Clinical Oncology, 22,* 1713–1720. doi:10.1200/JCO.2004.06.140.

Mols, F., Coebergh, J., & van de Poll-Franse, L. V. (2007). Health-related quality of life and healthcare utilisation among older long-term cancer survivors: a population-based study. *European Journal of Cancer, 43,* 2211–2221. doi:10.1016/j.ejca.2007.06.022.

Niv, D., & Kreitler, S. (2001). Pain and quality of life. *Pain Practice, 1,* 150–161.

Oliver, J. W., Kravitz, R. L., Kaplan, S. H., & Meyers, F. J. (2001). Individualized patient education and coaching to improve pain control among cancer outpatients. *Journal of Clinical Oncology, 19,* 2206–2212.

Prochaska, J. O., & DiClemente, C. C. (1984). *The transtheoretical approach: crossing traditional boundaries of therapy.* Homewood, IL: Dow Jones-Irwin.

Serlin, R. C., Mendoza, T. R., Nakamura, Y., & Cleeland, C. S. (1995). When is cancer pain mild, moderate, or severe? Grading pain severity by its interference with function. *Pain, 61,* 277–284.

Sherman, A. C., Simonton, S., Latif, U., Plante, T. G., & Anaissie, E. J. (2009). Changes in quality-of-life and psychosocial adjustment among multiple myeloma patients treated with high-dose melphalan and autologous stem cell transplantation. *Biology of Blood and Marrow Transplantation, 15,* 12–20. doi:10.1016/j.bbmt.2008.09.023.

Sun, V. C. Y., Borneman, T., Ferrell, B., Piper, B., Koczywas, K., & Choi, K. (2007). Overcoming barriers to cancer pain management: An institutional change model. *Journal of Pain and Symptom Management, 34,* 359–369. doi:10.1016/j.jpainsymman.2006.12.011.

Syrjala, K., Abrams, J. R., Du Pen, A. R., Niles, R., & Rupert, J. (1995). *Relieving cancer pain* [Videotape]. Seattle, WA: Synaptic Medical Productions.

Syrjala, K., Abrams, J. R., Polissar, N., et al. (2008). Patient training in cancer pain management using integrated print and video materials: a multisite randomized controlled trial. *Pain, 135,* 175–186. doi:10.1016/j.pain.2007.10.026

Thomas, M. L., Annis, D., & Hwang, S. (2004, April). *Examining the effectiveness of opiate use in cancer pain management: variation across outpatient oncology clinic settings.* Presented at the Oncology Nursing Society 29th Annual Congress in Anaheim, CA.

Thong, M., Mols, F., Coebergh, J., Roukema, J., & van de Poll-Franse, L. V. (2009). The impact of disease progression on perceived health status and quality of life of long-term cancer survivors. *Journal of Cancer Survivorship: Research and Practice, 3,* 164–173.

Vallerand, A. H., Hasenau, S., Templin, T., & Collins-Bohler, D. (2005). Disparities between black and white patients with cancer pain: the effect of perception of control over pain. *Pain Medicine, 6,* 242–250. doi:10.1111/j.1526-4637.2005.05038.x.

Vallerand, A. H., Templin, T., Sasenau, S. M., & Riley-Doucet, C. (2007). Factors that affect functional status in patients with cancer-related pain. *Pain, 132,* 82–90. doi:10.1016/j.pain.2007.01.029.

van den Beuken-van Everdingen, M. H., de Rijke, J. M., Kessels, A. G., Schouten, H. C., van Kleef, M., & Patijn, J. (2007). Prevalence of pain in patients with cancer: a systematic review of the past 40 years. *Annals of Oncology, 18,* 1437–1449. doi:10.1093/annonc/mdm056.

Ward, S., Donovan, H., Gunnarsdottir, S., Serlin, R. C., Shapiro, G. R., & Hughes, S. (2008). A randomized trial of a representational intervention to decrease cancer pain (RIDcancerPain). *Health Psychology, 27,* 59–67. doi:10.1037/0278-6133.27.1.59.

Ward, S., & Gatwood, J. (1994). Concerns about reporting pain and using analgesics: a comparison of persons with and without cancer. *Cancer Nursing, 17,* 200–206.

Ward, S., Goldberg, N., Miller-McCauley, V., et al. (1993). Patient-related barriers to management of cancer pain. *Pain, 52,* 319–324.

Ware, J. E., & Sherbourne, C. D. (1992). The MOS 36-item Short-Form Health Survey (SF-36) I: conceptual framework and item selection. *Medical Care, 30,* 473–483.

Wensing, M., Vingerhoets, E., & Grol, R. (2001). Functional status, health problems, age, and comorbidity in primary care patients. *Quality of Life Research, 10*, 141–148.

Wittmann, M., Vollmer, T., Schweiger, C., & Hiddemann, W. (2006). The relation between the experience of time and psychological distress in patients with hematological malignancies. *Palliative and Supportive Care, 4*, 357–363. doi:10.1017/S1478951506060469.

Yates, P., Edward, H., Nash, R., et al. (2004). A randomized controlled trial of a nurse-administered educational intervention for improving cancer pain management in ambulatory settings. *Patient Education and Counseling, 53*, 227–237. doi:10.1016/S0738-3991(03)00165-4.

Zimmerman, C., Burman, D., Swami, N., et al. (2010). Determinants of quality of life in patients with advanced cancer. *Supportive Care in Cancer, 19*, 621–629. doi:10.1007/s00520-010-0866-1.

# The Influence of Maternal–Fetal Attachment and Health Practices on Neonatal Outcomes in Low-Income, Urban Women

*Jeanne L. Alhusen,[1]\* Deborah Gross,[1]\*\* Matthew J. Hayat,[2]†
Anne B. (Nancy) Woods,[3]‡ Phyllis W. Sharps[1]\*\**

## ABSTRACT

Maternal–fetal attachment (MFA) has been associated with health practices during pregnancy, but less is known about this relationship in low-income women, and no identified studies have examined this relationship to neonatal outcomes. This longitudinal descriptive study was conducted to examine the relationships among MFA, health practices during pregnancy, and neonatal outcomes in a sample of low-income, predominantly African-American women and their neonates. MFA was associated with health practices during pregnancy and adverse neonatal outcomes. Health practices during pregnancy mediated the relationships of MFA and adverse neonatal outcomes. The results support the importance of examining MFA in our efforts to better understand the etiology of health disparities in neonatal outcomes.

Keywords: maternal–fetal attachment; health-promoting behaviors; health disparities; African American; birth outcomes

[1]Johns Hopkins University School of Nursing, 511 N. Washington Street, Balitmore, MD 21205
[2]College of Nursing, Rutgers University, Newark, NJ
[3]Messiah College, Grantham, PA Accepted 28 December 2011
Accepted 28 December 2011
This study was supported by funding from the National Institutes of Health (T32MH20014-08), the National Institute of Nursing Research (F31NR010957-01A), and the National Center for Research Resources (5KL2RR025006), a component of the National Institutes of Health and the NIH Roadmap for Medical Research.
Correspondence to Jeanne L. Alhusen.
\*Morton and Jane Blaustein Post-doctoral Fellow in Mental Health and Psychiatric Nursing.
\*\*Professor.
†Assistant Professor.
‡Associate Professor.
Published online 19 January 2012 in Wiley Online Library (wileyonlinelibrary.com). doi:10.1002/nur.21464
©2012 Wiley Periodicals, Inc. Res Nurs Health 35:112–120, 2012.

Disparities in neonatal outcomes between African-Americans and non-Latino White Americans are one of the most concerning and chronic health disparities affecting our nation (Alexander, Wingate, Bader, & Kogan, 2008). Many of the health disparities in pre-term birth, low birth weight (LBW) and other adverse pregnancy outcomes are more prevalent in ethnic minority and low-income populations (Patrick & Bryan, 2005). Poor and African-American women have twice the rates of preterm births and higher rates of growth restricted neonates than most other women (Mathews, Minino, Osterman, Strobino, & Guyer, 2011). LBW is a major determinant of infant mortality, and LBW neonates die at rates up to 40 times higher than normal birth weight neonates (Goldenberg & Culhane, 2007). Furthermore, LBW neonates are significantly more likely to have short-and long-term morbidities including delays in cognitive development and growth, and heightened risk of cardiovascular and respiratory disease (Goldenberg & Culhane, 2007). A significant body of research has been devoted to better understanding the reasons for persisting racial disparities in neonatal outcomes, yet the causes remain largely unknown.

One factor known to influence neonatal outcomes is the health practices that a mother engages in during pregnancy. Positive health practices include abstaining from tobacco, alcohol, and other illegal substances; obtaining regular prenatal care; maintaining a nutritionally sound diet (Widen & Siega-Riz, 2010); obtaining adequate rest and sleep; engaging in regular exercise (Stutzman et al., 2010); and learning about pregnancy and childbirth (Feinberg, Jones, Kan, & Goslin, 2010). Several variables that correlate with improved health practices during pregnancy include higher socioeconomic status, higher levels of education (Rubio, Kraemer, Farrell, & Day, 2008; Webb, Siega-Riz, & Dole, 2009), and increased social support (Savage, Anthony, Lee, Kappesser, & Rose, 2007). Conversely, negative health practices during pregnancy, such as tobacco and substance use, are higher among young, unmarried, low-income women (Phares et al., 2004). Cigarette smoking is one of the most preventable risk factors associated with adverse perinatal outcomes (Andres & Day, 2000).

Another factor thought to influence health practices during pregnancy is maternal–fetal attachment (MFA). Cranley (1981) created the theoretical construct of MFA and defined it as "the extent to which women engage in behaviours that represent an affiliation and interaction with their unborn child" (Cranley, 1981, p. 281). Higher levels of MFA correlate with the aforementioned high-quality health practices (Lindgren, 2001, 2003). However, studies of the associations between MFA and health practices during pregnancy have largely excluded low-income, ethnic minorities (Alhusen, 2008). Furthermore, no longitudinal studies were found that examined these variables in relation to neonatal outcomes.

An enhanced understanding of the role that MFA plays in neonatal outcomes of those subject to disparities, by virtue of race or socioeconomic status, is necessary to improve understanding of the relationship between health practices and adverse neonatal outcomes. Extant literature supports the influence of maternal health practices on neonatal outcomes, but less is known about factors that contribute to a woman's ability to engage in those positive health practices.

This study was designed to examine the associations between MFA, health practices during pregnancy, and neonatal outcomes in a highly vulnerable sample of predominantly African-American pregnant women reporting low educational attainment and low socioeconomic status. Pre-term birth and LBW are key predictors of neonatal complications and mortality (Halfon & Lu, 2010; Lu et al., 2010; Oken, Kleinman, Rich-Edwards, & Gillman, 2003). Thus, in this study neonatal measures of birth weight and gestational age were collected. This longitudinal study addressed a significant gap in the current literature by examining the following hypotheses:

After controlling for income, pregnancy wantedness, pre-eclampsia, and gestational diabetes:

1 Higher MFA will be negatively related to adverse neonatal outcomes.
2 Higher MFA will be positively related to improved health practices during pregnancy.
3 Improved health practices during pregnancy will be negatively related to adverse neonatal outcomes.
4 Health practices during pregnancy will mediate the relationship between MFA and adverse neonatal outcomes.

## Theoretical Model

The transition to motherhood is a major developmental life event. This transition requires restructuring goals, behaviors, and responsibilities. This study of factors that facilitated or inhibited this transition drew from Rubin's (1967) theory of maternal role attainment (MRA) as well as Mercer's expansion on this theory, which she termed "Becoming a Mother (BAM)" (Mercer, 2004). Although both theories largely focus on processes necessary for the establishment of maternal identity that occur once the child is born, Mercer's first stage, which entails a commitment and attachment to the unborn baby, recognizes the long-term implications of poor attachment (Mercer & Walker, 2006). A woman's active involvement in this stage has been consistently linked to engaging in healthier behaviors that benefit both the woman and her unborn child (Lindgren, 2001, 2003). Women demonstrating higher levels of MFA are presumed to be more vested in taking care of themselves during pregnancy in an effort to improve both the health of their fetus and pregnancy outcomes. Furthermore, researchers have suggested that prenatal attachment facilitates adaptation to the role of motherhood and may even act as a protective factor against perinatal depression (Brandon, Pitts, Denton, Stringer, & Evans, 2009).

The successful attainment of a maternal identity includes the development of an emotional tie between the mother and unborn child as well as an innate desire to protect the unborn child, later described as MFA (Cranley, 1981). This developmental and interactional process occurs over time (Rubin, 1984). MRA and subsequently BAM acknowledge barriers and facilitators to this process, and were therefore ideal theories to direct this study of MFA in a high-risk population where health disparities persist.

## METHODS

### Sample

A convenience sample of pregnant women from three urban obstetrical clinics in the Mid Atlantic region were recruited for the study. The three clinics were all affiliated with a major university health system and all served predominantly poor (>95% receiving Medicaid), African-American (>95%) inner-city populations. To be eligible for inclusion in the study, participants had to be 16 years or older, between 24 and 28 weeks gestation with singleton pregnancies, and able to speak English. This gestational time frame was chosen as research on MFA has demonstrated MFA increases as a pregnancy progresses, and this time period marks the beginning of fetal viability thereby allowing for accurate assessment of neonatal outcomes (Ramsay & Santella, 2010; Seri & Evans, 2008). Participants who met these initial criteria were excluded if prior to data collection they had been

| | n | % |
|---|---|---|
| **Race** | | |
| African-American | 155 | 93 |
| White non-Hispanic | 9 | 5 |
| Other | 2 | 2 |
| **Education** | | |
| Less than High School | 110 | 67 |
| High School Graduate/GED | 45 | 27 |
| Some College/Trade School | 5 | 3 |
| College/Trade School Graduate | 6 | 3 |
| **Marital status** | | |
| Single | 90 | 54 |
| Partnered/not married | 56 | 34 |
| Married | 17 | 10 |
| Other | 3 | 2 |
| **Employment status** | | |
| Unemployed | 127 | 77 |
| Employed full time | 25 | 15 |
| Employed part time | 14 | 8 |
| **Household income** | | |
| Under $10,000 | 76 | 46 |
| $10,001–$20,000 | 66 | 40 |
| $20,001–$30,000 | 12 | 7 |
| $30,001–$40,000 | 8 | 5 |
| >$40,000 | 4 | 2 |
| **Gravidity** | | |
| Primigravida | 54 | 32 |

**TABLE 1  DEMOGRAPHIC CHARACTERISTICS OF THE STUDY SAMPLE ($n = 166$)**

treated with tocolytic therapy, diagnosed with pre-eclampsia or gestational diabetes, diagnosed with a chronic medical condition (e.g., chronic hypertension, diabetes mellitus), or had an abnormal diagnostic result (e.g., known fetal anomaly, abnormal results on first or second trimester screening tests) during the current pregnancy. Additionally, women reporting a history of fetal (spontaneous abortion after 24 weeks gestation) or infant death were excluded. These exclusion criteria were selected given their known contribution to adverse neonatal outcomes (Institute of Medicine, 1988; Mathews et al., 2011).

Of the 174 eligible pregnant women approached to participate, 167 (96%) completed the study instruments. One participant delivered at an outside hospital, which precluded our ability to obtain accurate birth outcomes. Therefore, the final sample consisted of 166 low-income women (93% African-American) receiving prenatal care from one of the three participating clinics and their neonates, resulting in a 95.4% participation rate. Of note, 84% of the sample initiated prenatal care by 14 weeks gestation, 96% by 18 weeks gestation, and 100% by 24 weeks gestation. As seen in Table 1, the sample consisted of predominantly poor, unmarried, African-American younger women.

## Data Collection Procedures

Institutional Review Board approval was obtained prior to participant recruitment. Eligible participants were approached about enrollment in the study during their prenatal care visits. If a woman expressed an interest in participating, but had not reached 24 weeks gestation, her contact information was obtained. The first author re-contacted her and met with her to complete study instruments prior to a scheduled appointment that occurred between 24 and 28 weeks gestation.

After a complete description of the study, informed consent was obtained from those women who agreed to participate. Participants were interviewed in a private space at each of the three study clinic sites. Interviews lasted approximately 30 minutes. The interviews were conducted by the first author or one of two undergraduate nursing students who received research compliance and study procedures training. Participants were compensated $15 for their participation. Measures related to neonatal outcomes (i.e., birth weight and gestational age) were extracted from electronic chart review within 48 hours after delivery. Measures specific to maternal physical health risk factors (i.e., pre-eclampsia and gestational diabetes) were also extracted from electronic chart review during the same time period, in the event these risk factors developed after the initial data collection (Bodnar, Ness, Markovic, & Roberts, 2005; Catalano, Kirwan, Haugel-de Mouzon, & King, 2003).

## Measures

**Maternal–fetal attachment.** MFA was measured with the Maternal–Fetal Attachment Scale (MFAS; Cranley, 1981). The MFAS is a 24-item measure that asks women to respond to questions or thoughts indicative of MFA. The scale contains 5-point Likert-type items with response options ranging from 1 (definitely no) to 5 (definitely yes). Examples of MFAS items include "I talk to my unborn baby" and "I do things to try to stay healthy that I would not do if I were not pregnant." The total score ranges from 24 to 120 with higher scores indicative of higher levels of MFA. This instrument is one of the most frequently used measures of MFA in prenatal studies and has been used in diverse populations including samples of culturally diverse and low SES adolescents (Ahern & Ruland, 2003; Hart & McMahon, 2006; Lindgren, 2003). Content validity was assessed by an expert panel review. In a study of MFA in ethnic minorities a content validity index of 0.91 was found (Ahern & Ruland, 2003). The Cronbach's alpha coefficient reported by Cranley (1981) was 0.85 and for the current study was 0.88.

**Health practices.** The Health Practices in Pregnancy Questionnaire-II (HPQ-II; Lindgren, 2005) is a 34-item measure designed to address adequacy of health practices in six areas: balance of rest and exercise, safety measures, nutrition, avoiding use of harmful substances, obtaining health care, and obtaining information. In addition, 1 item addresses overall pregnancy health practices. Responses range from 1 (never) to 5 (always or daily) or a word or phrase that indicates the woman's level of engagement in a specific activity (e.g., 1— No alcoholic drinks while pregnant to 5— More than 3 alcoholic drinks at one sitting). Negatively worded items were reverse coded. Examples of HPQ-II items include "Since becoming pregnant I drink more than two caffeinated beverages in a day" and "Since becoming pregnant I have smoked cigarettes." The total score ranges from 34 to 170 with a high score indicating a higher quality of health practices. Content validity was established by clinical experts and pregnant women (Lindgren, 2001, 2005). The Cronbach's alpha coefficient reported by Lindgren (2003) was 0.81 and for the current study was 0.90.

**Neonatal outcomes.** Neonatal outcomes were collected from electronic chart review by the first author. Two undergraduate nursing students collected neonatal data on a random 25% sub-sample to assess inter-rater reliability. A kappa statistic of 1.0 was noted indicating excellent agreement (Landis & Koch, 1977). Neonatal outcomes collected included the neonate's gestational age and birth weight. Small for gestational age (SGA) was calculated using comprehensive reference values of birth weight at 22–44 completed weeks of gestation that were established by Oken et al. (2003) based on a national sample of over 6 million infants. The presence of LBW ($<$2,500 g), pre-term birth ($<$37 completed weeks gestation), or SGA ($<$10th percentile weight adjusted for gestational age) was coded as an adverse neonatal outcome during data collection.

**Demographic and pregnancy background.** A measure of demographic and obstetrical data was developed for use in this study. Demographic data included age, race, marital status, insurance status, employment status, educational history, and income status. Pregnancy history included an assessment of current and previous pregnancies (e.g., was this a planned pregnancy; is this pregnancy wanted, unwanted, or ambivalent; number of previous pregnancies, term births, number of therapeutic and/or spontaneous abortions, and number of live children).

## Data Analysis

Data were analyzed using PASW Statistics 18, Release Version 18.0.0 (IBM SPSS Statistics, Chicago, IL). Data analysis began with descriptive and exploratory statistical analyses. Study variables were examined to assess distributions, to identify outlying or extreme observations, and to determine the need for transformation. There were no missing data. The sample size was based on an a priori power analysis with a specified power of 80% to detect a meaningful difference in MFA between participants delivering LBW neonates and participants delivering neonates $>$2,500 g. Pearson correlation and point biserial correlation coefficients were calculated to address hypotheses 1–3. Mediation of the relationship between MFA and adverse neonatal outcomes by health practices during pregnancy was tested with an analytic approach specific to dichotomous outcomes, using the bootstrap with biased-corrected confidence intervals (MacKinnon, Fairchild, & Fritz, 2007). Separate logistic regression equations were conducted sequentially to first examine the relationship between MFA and adverse neonatal outcome and then to determine the extent to which health practices mediated this relationship. The level of significance was set at $\alpha = {}^1\!/_4\ 0.05$.

Neonatal outcomes were dichotomized as adverse outcome or no adverse outcome; therefore, multiple logistic regression was used to test the relationships between MFA, health practices, and neonatal outcomes. Because income and pregnancy wantedness were related to the outcome variable of an adverse neonatal outcome, they were included in subsequent regression analyses to control for their potential confounding effects. Income was dichotomized using the median of $<$\$10,000 or $>$\$10,000 total household income per year. Pregnancy wantedness was dichotomized per participant's response that the current pregnancy was wanted or participant was ambivalent about current pregnancy. Additionally, gestational diabetes and pre-eclampsia were controlled for in the regression models, given their known contribution to adverse neonatal outcomes.

## RESULTS

After initial data collection, 7.8% ($n = 13$) of study participants were diagnosed with preeclampsia, and 1.2% ($n = 2$) were diagnosed with gestational diabetes. Forty-one

TABLE 2    CLASSIFICATION OF ADVERSE NEONATAL OUTCOMES ($n = 68/166$)

| ADVERSE OUTCOMES[a] | n | % |
|---|---|---|
| SGA | 27 | 16.3 |
| LBW and SGA | 16 | 9.6 |
| Pre-term, LBW, and SGA | 6 | 3.6 |
| Pre-term and LBW | 13 | 7.8 |
| Pre-term | 6 | 3.6 |
| Total | 68 | 41.0 |

Note: SGA, small for gestational age; LBW, low birth weight.
[a]The categories of adverse outcome are mutually exclusive.

TABLE 3    CORRELATIONS AMONG THE MAIN STUDY VARIABLES ($n = 166$)

| VARIABLE | 1 | 2 | 3 | 4 |
|---|---|---|---|---|
| 1. MFA | — | | | |
| 2. Health Practices | .86* | — | | |
| 3. Adverse Neonatal Outcome[a] | −.52* | −.63* | — | |
| 4. Pregnancy Wantedness[b] | −.28* | −.34* | .19* | — |
| 5. Income[c] | .25* | .31* | −.23* | −.18* |

MFA, maternal fetal attachment
[a]Referent group was no adverse outcome.
[b]Referent group was pregnancy was wanted.
[c]Referent group was income <$10,000/year.
*p < .05.

percent ($n = 68$) of study neonates were classified as having an adverse outcome. Table 2 demonstrates the number of neonates born with adverse outcomes of LBW, pre-term birth, SGA, or a combination thereof.

The mean score on the MFAS was 84.1 ($SD = 14.2$, range: 52–116), and the median was 83.5. Analysis of the HPQ-II scores revealed a mean score of 121.2 ($SD = 19.6$, range: 78–159), and the median was 122.0.

Bivariate correlations and point biserial correlations among the main study variables are presented in Table 3. As hypothesized, there was a significant negative relationship between MFA and adverse neonatal outcomes supporting our first hypothesis. Health practices during pregnancy (mediator variable) was significantly related to MFA, the independent variable, and adverse neonatal outcomes, the dependent variable thereby supporting hypotheses 2 and 3, respectively.

The results of the logistic regression are shown in Table 4. In univariate logistic regression, MFA was regressed on adverse neonatal outcome and MFA was significantly related to adverse neonatal outcome; the odds ratio for this equation indicated that a one point increase in MFA was associated with a 9% decreased likelihood of an adverse neonatal outcome. In the second model, health practices was regressed on adverse neonatal outcome while controlling for MFA and health practices was noted to be significantly related to adverse neonatal outcome, indicating that a one point increase in the health practices scale

| TABLE 4 | SUMMARY OF LOGISTIC REGRESSION ANALYSES PREDICTING ADVERSE NEONATAL OUTCOMES* ($n = 166$) | | | | |
|---|---|---|---|---|---|
| PREDICTOR VARIABLE | ODDS RATIO | 95% CI | ADJUSTED ODDS RATIO[a] | 95% CI |
| MFA | 0.91 | 0.88–0.94 | 0.99 | 0.94–1.05 |
| Health Practices | 0.91 | 0.89–0.94 | 0.91 | 0.88–0.96 |

MFA, maternal fetal attachment.
*Referent group was no adverse outcome.
[a]Controlling for pregnancy wantedness, income, gestational diabetes, and pre-eclampsia.

score was associated with a 9% decreased likelihood of an adverse neonatal outcome. The proportion of the total effect of MFA on adverse neonatal outcomes mediated by health practices during pregnancy was 0.91. Additionally, the total indirect effect (0.56) through health practices was 10 times larger than the direct effect (0.5) between MFA and adverse neonatal outcomes. The total indirect effect through health practices remained significant with bootstrap analysis, while direct effects between MFA and adverse neonatal outcomes were nonsignificant, suggesting complete mediation through health practices. Thus, the 4th hypothesis was also supported.

# DISCUSSION

To our knowledge, this is the first study that provides strong support for the role that MFA plays both in health practices during pregnancy, and more importantly, in neonatal outcomes in a highly vulnerable population of predominantly African-American women from a low-income, urban community. Prior researchers found support for a relationship between MFA and health practices among primarily Caucasian samples (Lindgren, 2001, 2003). However, none have examined the longitudinal association between MFA and neonatal outcomes. The findings of this study highlight the significance of MFA as a predictor of neonatal health and wellbeing, and, potentially, health care costs. Neonates born SGA or at LBW tend to have longer post-partum hospitalizations and more chronic illnesses than infants born at normal weight. Thus, MFA may be an important factor contributing to the increased health care expenditures related to adverse neonatal outcomes noted in the United States.

In addition, our findings support the validity of MFA as an important health construct for African-American, low-income women. Despite considerable resources devoted to understanding and remediating the problem of perinatal health disparities, we understand relatively little about the determinants of adverse neonatal outcomes. Great effort has been focused on promoting prenatal care as a primary strategy for improving neonatal outcomes. Yet, this sample of women with a high rate of poor outcomes was receiving prenatal health care, although the content and quality of care was not assessed. The impact of MFA in this sample suggests that MFA is an important factor in our search for additional strategies beyond prenatal care.

The mediating role of health practices on the relationship between MFA and adverse neonatal outcomes was an important finding. Health practices such as assuring adequate sleep, limiting caffeine consumption, practicing safe sex, seeking advice from health care providers or social networks, and engaging in relaxing behaviors receive less attention in the literature in relation to birth outcomes than behaviors, such as tobacco use, alcohol use, and other illicit drug use. Given our knowledge that increased social support is correlated with higher MFA and overall health practices during pregnancy, an enhanced understanding of how social support may influuence the aforementioned health behaviors could be important in tailoring intervention programs (Cranley, 1984; Savage et al., 2007).

The high percentage of women whose neonates had an adverse outcome warrants special attention. In the United States, African-American women are nearly twice as likely as non-Hispanic White women (13.7% vs. 7.2%) to have a LBW baby (Mathews et al., 2011). In this sample, 21% of neonates were classified as LBW demonstrating a higher prevalence rate for LBW than previously reported though this sample was all low-income (Mathews et al., 2011). The impact of income equality on neonatal outcomes is a critical area of inquiry in the United States, due to a widening gap between rich and poor (Olson, Diekema, Elliott, & Renier, 2010). Researchers have demonstrated that income and income inequality are associated with adverse neonatal outcomes with the poorest neonates experiencing the worst outcomes (Olson et al., 2010). This is particularly concerning given recent evidence that the wealth gap between Whites and African-Americans is the largest it has been since the government began publishing such data 25 years ago (Kochar, Fry, & Taylor, 2011). Further research is necessary to better understand the contribution of income, income inequality, and financial strain to both MFA and health practices.

This study has two important limitations. First, MFA and health practices were collected via self-report measures in a cross-sectional manner making inference about their causal relationships impossible. Tobacco use and substance use, factors known to contribute to poor neonatal outcomes, may have been underreported. Second, these results are based on a convenience sample and therefore cannot be generalized beyond this group of women.

Nonetheless, this study provides compelling evidence of an important relationship among MFA, health practices, and adverse neonatal outcomes in a low-income, predominantly African-American sample. Understanding risk factors for adverse neonatal outcomes is essential to eliminate the disparities in perinatal health across racial and ethnic minorities. In this sample of mainly poor, African-American women living in an urban environment, women with higher MFA also noted better health practices and had better neonatal outcomes. Birth outcomes were explained largely by actions taken during a woman's pregnancy (e.g., substance use, maintaining prenatal appointments, risky sexual behaviors). Perhaps a more comprehensive examination of risk factors, including stress, emotional health, and financial strain, not only over the course of a pregnancy but from the pre-conception period, would reveal their influence on both MFA and birth outcomes. Future research is needed to examine additional predictors of MFA, particularly in racial and ethnic minorities at higher risk for disparate birth outcomes.

Finally, future researchers should test culturally relevant interventions aimed at improving the maternal–fetal relationship. Technological advances now allow women to detect their pregnancies earlier, and they are able to view ultrasound images of their fetus at earlier dates. Advanced technology, such as fetal imaging, prenatal diagnostics, and genetic screening, individuate the fetus from the expectant mother. Incorporating technology, with an appropriate educational component, into an intervention may serve as the impetus for adopting positive health practices at an earlier time period in pregnancy. More importantly, women at risk for poor MFA may benefit from this education thereby facilitating adequate preparation for motherhood. The limited research aimed at increasing MFA has not been supported empirically, although the samples have been quite small and lacking ethnic and/or racial diversity

(Carter-Jessop, 1981; Davis & Akridge, 1987). As research on the implications of poor MFA grows, there is a critical need for early identification and appropriate intervention.

## Conclusion

This study provides an important contribution to understanding the influence of MFA on health practices during pregnancy, and ultimately neonatal outcomes, in a sample of urban, low-income, predominantly African-American women. Women with lower MFA were less likely to engage in health promoting practices during pregnancy, and consequently, more likely to deliver neonates with adverse outcomes. Although significant strides have been made in improving maternal and infant outcomes, continued concern is needed about the widening gap in pregnancy outcomes. Continued research on the manner in which individual, environmental, and societal factors interact to contribute to poor pregnancy outcomes requires multidisciplinary research. Nurses are well positioned to lead the challenge in ensuring every woman is afforded the same opportunity for favorable maternal and neonatal outcomes.

## REFERENCES

Ahern, N. R., & Ruland, J. P. (2003). Maternal–fetal attachment in African-American and Hispanic-American women. *The Journal of Perinatal Education, 12*(4), 27–35. doi:10.1624/105812403(107044.

Alexander, G. R., Wingate, M. S., Bader, D., & Kogan, M. D. (2008). The increasing racial disparity in infant mortality rates: composition and contributors to recent US trends. *American Journal of Obstetrics and Gynecology, 198*, 51.e1–51.e59. doi:10.1016/j.ajog.2007.06.006.

Alhusen, J. L. (2008). A literature update on maternal–fetal attachment. *Journal of Obstetric, Gynecologic, and Neonatal Nursing, 37*, 315–328. doi:10.1111/j.1552-6909.2008.00241.

Andres, R. L., & Day, M. C. (2000). Perinatal complications associated with maternal tobacco use. *Seminars in Neonatology, 5*, 231–241. doi:10.1053/siny.2000.0025.

Bodnar, L. M., Ness, R. A., Markovic, N., & Roberts, J. M. (2005). The risk of preeclampsia rises with increasing prepregnancy body mass index. *Annals of Epidemiology, 15*, 475–482. doi:10.1016/ j.annepidem.2004.12.008.

Brandon, A. R., Pitts, S., Denton, W. H., Stringer, C. A., & Evans, H. M. (2009). A history of the theory of prenatal attachment. *Journal of Prenatal and Perinatal Psychology and Health, 23*, 201–222.

Carter-Jessop, L. (1981). Promoting maternal attachment through prenatal intervention. MCN. *The American Journal of Maternal Child Nursing, 6*, 107–112.

Catalano, P. M., Kirwan, J. P., Haugel-de Mouzon, S., & King, J. (2003). Gestational diabetes and insulin resistance: role in short-and long-term implications for the mother and fetus. *Journal of Nutrition, 133*, 1674S–1683S. Retrieved from http://jn. nutrition.org/content/133/5/1674S.full.pdfphtml.

Cranley, M. S. (1981). Development of a tool for the measurement of maternal attachment during pregnancy. *Nursing Research, 30*, 281–284.

Cranley, M. S. (1984). Social support as a factor in the development of parents' attachment to their unborn. *Birth Defects Original Article Series, 20*(5), 99–124.

Davis, M. S., & Akridge, K. M. (1987). The effect of promoting intrauterine attachment in primiparas on postdelivery attachment. *Journal of Obstetric, Gynecologic, and Neonatal Nursing, 16*, 430–437. doi:10.1111/j.1552-6909.1987.tb01605.x.

Feinberg, M. E., Jones, D. E., Kan, M. L., & Goslin, M. C. (2010). Effects of family foundations on parents and children: 3.5 Years after baseline. *Journal of Family Psychology, 24*(5), 532–542. doi:10.1037/a0020837.

Goldenberg, R. L., & Culhane, J. F. (2007). Low birth weight in the United States. *The American Journal of Clinical Nutrition, 85*, 584S–590S. Retrieved from http://www.ajcn.org/content/85/2/584S.long.

Halfon, N., & Lu, M. C. (2010). Gestational weight gain and birthweight. *Lancet, 376*, 937–938. doi:10.1016/S0140-6736(10)61024-0.

Hart, R., & McMahon, C. A. (2006). Mood state and psychological adjustment to pregnancy. *Archives of Women's Mental Health, 9*, 329–337. doi:10.1007/s00737-006-0141-0.

Institute of Medicine. (1988). Prenatal care: reaching mothers, reaching infants. Washington, D.C.: National Academy Press. Retrieved from http://www.nap.edu/openbook.php?record_id=731&page=R1

Kochar, R., Fry, R., & Taylor, P. (2011). Wealth gaps rise to record highs between Whites, Blacks and Hispanics. Washington, DC: Pew Research Center Publications. Retrieved from http://pewresearch.org/ pubs/2069/housing-bubble-subprime-mortgageshispanics-blacks-household-wealth-disparity

Landis, J. R., & Koch, G. G. (1977). The measurement of observer agreement for categorical data. *Biometrics, 33*, 159–174. Retrieved from http:// www.ncbi.nlm.nih.gov/pubmed/843571.

Lindgren, K. (2001). Relationships among maternal–fetal attachment, prenatal depression, and health practices in pregnancy. *Research in Nursing and Health, 24*, 203–217. doi:10.1002/nur.1023.

Lindgren, K. (2003). A comparison of pregnancy health practices of women in inner-city and small urban communities. *Journal of Obstetric, Gynecologic, and Neonatal Nursing, 32*, 313–321. doi:10.1177/0884217503253442.

Lindgren, K. (2005). Testing the health practices in Pregnancy Questionnaire-II. *Journal of Obstetric, Gynecologic, and Neonatal Nursing, 34*, 465–472. doi:10.1177/0884217505276308.

Lu, M. C., Kotelchuck, M., Hogan, V., Jones, L., Wright, K., & Halfon, N. (2010). Closing the black–white gap in birth outcomes: a life-course approach. *Ethnicity and Disease, 20*(1 Suppl 2), S2-62-76.

MacKinnon, D. P., Fairchild, A. J., & Fritz, M. S. (2007). Mediation analysis. *Annual Review of Psychology, 58*, 1–22. doi:10.1146/annurev.psych. 58.110405.085542.

Mathews, T. J., Minino, A., Osterman, M., Strobino, D., & Guyer, B. (2011). Annual summary of vital statistics: 2008. *Pediatrics, 127*, 146–157. doi:10.1542/peds.2010-3175.

Mercer, R. T. (2004). Becoming a mother versus maternal role attainment. *Journal of Nursing Scholarship, 36*, 226–232. doi:10.1111/j.15475069.2004.04042.x.

Mercer, R. T., & Walker, L. O. (2006). A review of nursing interventions to foster becoming a mother. *Journal of Obstetric, Gynecologic, and Neonatal Nursing, 35*, 568–582. doi:10.1111/j.1552-6909. 2006.00080.x.

Oken, E., Kleinman, K. P., Rich-Edwards, J., & Gillman, M. W. (2003). A nearly continuous measure of birth weight for gestational age using a United States national reference. *BMC Pediatrics, 3*, 6. doi:10.1186/1471-2431-3-6.

Olson, M. E., Diekema, D., Elliott, B. A., & Renier, C. M. (2010). Impact of income and income inequality on infant health outcomes in the United States. *Pediatrics, 126*, 1165–1173. doi:10.1542/ peds.2009-3378.

Patrick, T. E., & Bryan, Y. (2005). Research strategies for optimizing pregnancy outcomes in minority populations. *American Journal of Obstetrics and Gynecology, 192*(5 Suppl), S64–S70. doi:10.1016/j.ajog.2005.01.075.

Phares, T. M., Morrow, B., Lansky, A., Barfield, W. D., Prince, C. B., Marchi, K. S., & Kinniburgh, B. (2004). Surveillance for disparities in maternal health-related behaviors-selected states, Pregnancy Risk Assessment Monitoring System (PRAMS), 2000–2001. *MMWR Surveillance Summary, 53*(4), 1–13. Retrieved from http://www.cdc.gov/mmwr/ preview/mmwrhtml/ss5304a1.htm.

Ramsay, S. M., & Santella, R. M. (2010). The definition of life: a survey of obstetricians and neona-tologists in New York City hospitals regarding extremely premature births. *Maternal and Child Health Journal, 15*, 446–452. doi:10.1007/s10995-010-0613-8.

Rubin, R. (1967). Attainment of the maternal role: part 1: processes. *Nursing Research, 16,* 237–245.

Rubin, R. (1984). *Maternal identity and the maternal experience.* New York, NY: Springer.

Rubio, D. M., Kraemer, K. L., Farrell, M. H., & Day, N. L. (2008). Factors associated with alcohol use, depression, and their co-occurrence during pregnancy. *Alcoholism, Clinical and Experimental Research, 32,* 1543–1551. doi:10.1111/j.15300277.2008.00705.x.

Savage, C. L., Anthony, J., Lee, R., Kappesser, M. L., & Rose, B. (2007). The culture of pregnancy and infant care in African-American women: an ethnographic study. *Journal of Transcultural Nursing, 18,* 215–223. doi:10.1177/1043659607301294.

Seri, J., & Evans, J. (2008). Limits of viability: definition of the gray zone. *Journal of Perinatology, 28*(Suppl. 1), S4–S8. doi:10.1038/jp.2008.42.

Stutzman, S. S., Brown, C. A., Hains, S. M., Godwin, M., Smith, G. N., Parlow, J. L., & Kisilevsky, B. S. (2010). The effects of exercise conditioning in normal and overweight pregnant women on blood pressure and heart rate variability. *Biological Research for Nursing, 12,* 137–148. doi:10.1177/1099800410375979.

Webb, J. B., Siega-Riz, A. M., & Dole, N. (2009). Psychosocial determinants of adequacy of gestational weight gain. *Obesity, 17,* 300–309. doi:10.1038/oby.2008.490.

Widen, E., & Siega-Riz, A. M. (2010). Prenatal nutrition: a practical guide for assessment and counseling. *Journal of Midwifery and Women's Health, 55,* 540–549. doi:10.1016/j.jmwh.2010.06.017.

# C

# The Experiences of Nurse Practitioners Providing Health Care to the Homeless

*Ashley J. Seiler, MSN, FNP-C, APNP (Family Practice)[1]*
*& Vicki A. Moss, DNSc, RN (Associate Professor)[2]*

**Keywords**
Homeless; health care; nurse practitioners; qualitative analysis; descriptive phenomenology.
**Correspondence**
Ashley J. Seiler, MSN, FNP-C, APNP
Family Practice, Ministry Medical Group–Crandon
400 West Glen Street, Crandon, Wl 54520
Tel: 715-478-3318
Fax: 715-478-3325
E-mail: ashley.seiler@ministryhealth.org
Received: May 2010
Accepted: September 2010
doi:10.1111/j.1745-7599.2011. 00672.x

## ABSTRACT

**Purpose:** Homelessness is a growing public health and social concern in our society. The purpose of this qualitative descriptive study was to gain insight into the unique experiences of nurse practitioners (NPs) who provide health care to the homeless.

**Data sources:** Audio-taped, open-ended interviews were conducted with nine NPs from southeast and northeast Wisconsin.

**Conclusions:** Five themes and 13 subthemes emerged from the NPs' accounts. The main themes included: (1) why they do what they do; (2) a unique population with unique needs; (3) NP characteristics; (4) how the relationship develops; and (5) lessons learned: a relationship of reciprocity.

[1]Family Practice, Ministry Medical Group-Crandon, Crandon, Wisconsin
[2]College of Nursing, University of Wisconsin Oshkosh, Oshkosh, Wisconsin

**Implications for practice:** Study findings will assist healthcare providers to gain insight into the experience of providing health care to the homeless and learn what it takes to become successful in such an important and much needed role.

Homelessness is an increasing social and public health problem and provides unique challenges for healthcare professionals and the healthcare system (McCary & McConnell, 2005). Mullin and Ambrosia (2005) cited poverty and lack of affordable housing as the two major factors contributing to the increase in homelessness over the past 25 years; however, there are many other contributing factors such as violence in the home (Tischler, Edwards, & Vostanis, 2009), rent arrears and eviction (Bessant et al., 2002), substance abuse (Johnson & Chamberlain, 2008), and mental illness (D'Amore, Chiang, & Goldfrank, 2001). According to Metraux et al. (2001), in U.S. major cities, between 0.1% and 2.1% of the population are homeless every night, and those likely to become homeless every year include about 2.3-3.5 million persons, with 1.35 million of that number being children (Burt, Aron, & Lee, 2001). The healthcare needs of this population are complex considering the potential threats of environmental exposure, substance abuse, and violence. The health status of homeless individuals is also usually poorer than that of the general population (Zlotnick & Zerger, 2008). Many also survive on the street despite mental illness, developmental disabilities, and/or chronic physical illness (Drury, 2008).

It is because of this complexity that Drury (2008) stated that mainstream healthcare providers, unfamiliar with the socioeconomic and cultural environments in which homeless people live, may not be prepared to provide needed care. He concludes that because of the lack of understanding of homeless persons's lives and living conditions, treatment, although well intended, may not be effective. King and Wheeler (2007) stated that vulnerable medical populations are placed at a disadvantage and describe them as wounded by society. The homeless are indeed a vulnerable group. Healthcare workers may feel unprepared to care for vulnerable patients, who are more likely to be ill and have difficulty accessing care. As a result, the care that homeless patients do receive may be suboptimal.

Fortunately, a difference can be made when healthcare providers are trained to provide care for vulnerable populations (King & Wheeler, 2007).Thus, it takes a specially trained provider to be able to evaluate and address the healthcare needs of the homeless. One group of healthcare providers particularly well suited for such a responsibility is advanced practice nurses, including nurse practitioners (NPs). They bring a blend of nursing and medical care and have been shown to be cost effective (American Academy of Nurse Practitioners, 2010a; Bauer, 2010; Coddington & Sands, 2008). It has been shown that their patients use emergency rooms less, have shorter hospital stays, and spend less on medications (American Academy of Nurse Practitioners, 2010b). Satisfaction with NP care is also very high (Agosta, 2009; Coddington & Sands, 2008; Courtney & Rice, 1997; Guzik, Menzel, Fitzpatrick, & McNulty, 2009) and patient outcomes are comparable to physicians' (Agosta, 2009).

There have been several studies conducted on the role of curriculum-based exposures of students to homeless patients, service learning in the healthcare field, and the positive impact it has on their educational experience and preparation (de la Cruz, Brehm, & Harris, 2004; Hunt & Swiggum, 2007; Moskowitz, Glasco, Johnson, & Wang, 2006); and also on the experiences of registered nurses in providing health care to the homeless (Maze, 2005; Maze, 2006; Zerwekh, 2000). However, there is a lack of research on the experience of caring for the homeless from the advanced practice perspective, including that of NPs. Therefore, it was the goal of this study to address this gap in the literature in an effort to more fully understand the experiences of NPs involved in providing health care to the homeless.

## Literature Review

### Health Status of the Homeless

The health status of homeless individuals is poorer than that of the general population (Zlotnick & Zerger, 2008). The rates of both acute and chronic health problems are extremely high among the homeless; and, the majority of homeless individuals is uninsured and often lacks access to the most basic healthcare services. Zlotnick and Zerger (2008) found that homeless people are far more likely to suffer from every category of chronic health problems, with the exception of heart disease and cancer. The homeless also have higher mortality rates then the general population (Read, 2008) as well as more frequent respiratory and gastrointestinal (GI) problems, neurological conditions (Read, 2008), and infectious diseases such as tuberculosis, HIV, and pneumonia (Schanzer, Dominguez, Shrout, & Caton, 2007). Significant vision impairments have also been seen in about 40% of the homeless (Gelberg, Andersen, & Leake, 2000), with many also experiencing serious dental problems (Read, 2008). There is presently only one federally funded program, Health Care for the Homeless (HCH), that is designed specifically to provide primary health care to homeless people. Mullin and Ambrosia (2005) stated that lack of shelter and proper hygiene coupled with inadequate nutrition predisposes them to disease and illness.

A survey conducted by Zlotnick and Zerger (2008) found that in the United States 44% of homeless people using HCH clinics report their health status as *fair/poor*, as compared to 12.3% of the general population. They identified other factors responsible for poor health such as threats of violence and the potential exposure to contagious disease. Therefore, the healthcare services provided by HCH can often be a first step toward regaining housing and the ability to resume functioning within society.

Despite the services offered by the federal program HCH, many homeless individuals lack a regular source of health care and have difficulty gaining access to the services that are available. Thus, many homeless individuals use costly hospital services and emergency rooms, and as a result, receive little or fragmented health care (Zlotnick & Zerger, 2008).

### Healthcare Experiences of the Homeless

Various studies have examined the experiences of homeless patients within the healthcare system. Cocozza Martins (2008) interviewed 15 homeless adults on their experiences with the healthcare system, and found that they often waited to seek health care until a crisis occurred and faced many barriers such as feeling labeled, stigmatized, disrespected, and invisible. Cocozza Martins advocates for increasing the understanding of healthcare experiences from the homeless perspective in order to guide nursing interventions for this population.

McCormack and Gooding (1993) undertook a phenomenological study to find out what health meant to homeless individuals. They used a convenience sample of 29 homeless individuals and found that health meant having basic needs satisfied, no complaints of illness or disease, being able to function on a daily basis, and staying free from addictive substances. They also believed it was important to stay fit, exhibit good hygiene, and positive self-esteem.

Wen, Hudak, and Hwang (2007) questioned 17 homeless men and women from five Toronto shelters on their experience of "welcomeness" or "unwelcomeness" in past encounters with healthcare providers. The researchers found that most of the homeless participants perceived their experience of "unwelcomeness" within the healthcare system as acts of discrimination.The researchers recommended strategies for healthcare providers to create a welcoming experience for their homeless patients in order to make them feel empowered, listened to, and valued. This included approaching each patient with openness and humility, therefore decreasing any stereotyping related to their homeless situation.

Daiski (2007) conducted a qualitative study of 24 homeless participants and found that the homeless reported concerns about physical illness, mental health, addiction, and stress. They described feeling emotionally distressed from being socially excluded and depersonalized. They voiced wanting to find work and housing, yet felt trapped in a dehumanizing system.

Nickasch and Marnocha (2009) conducted a grounded theory study in which nine homeless individuals were interviewed on their experiences with health care. Their findings indicated that many homeless people possess an external locus of control and are unable to meet their physical need because of lack of resources, such as lack of finances to obtain transportation to medical facilities. Those interviewed also felt there was a lack of compassion for the homeless by healthcare providers.

It is evident from the results of the above studies that homeless persons encounter many obstacles in trying to obtain health care, and often when they do, they perceive the experience as negative. Cocozza Martins (2008) called for a more humanistic and empowering approach in caring for the homeless. It is imperative that changes be made to the current healthcare system in order to meet the unique needs of this population.

## The Role of the NP

Jezewski (1995) conducted a grounded theory study to explore the way nurses and others in nurse-managed shelter clinics facilitate health care for the homeless. A sample of 11 healthcare professionals including NPs, community health nurses, and a social worker were interviewed. The core category of "staying connected"was identified as the essence of facilitating care. Important aspects included the nurse's ability to stay connected by providing networks of resources and facilitating connections with appropriate medical professionals. Jezewski concluded that there are many barriers to facilitating care for the homeless population, but that nurses are well suited to overcome these barriers and can have a positive and powerful influence on the health care that these individuals receive.

Hunter, Getty, Kemsley, and Skelly (1991) undertook a descriptive study to examine healthcare and human service providers' perceptions of barriers to health care for the homeless population ($n = 122$). Their sample consisted of nursing administrators, staff nurses, human service workers, and several students. Their findings suggested that the providers were sympathetic to the homeless and believed they deserved the same social and healthcare services as others. Providers identified cost, financing, interagency referral, and lack of safe places for discharge as structural barriers. Lack of motivation for self-care and inability to follow through with treatment recommendations were characteristics perceived as client barriers by the provider participants.

Mullin and Ambrosia (2005) conducted a review of settings for delivering health care to the homeless focusing on the role of NPs. They found that recent literature supports nurse-managed, on-site care for homeless patients and that the complex psychosocial and physical needs of homeless patients can be effectively managed with the holistic model of care utilized by NPs. Mullin and Ambrosia also identified considerations to be taken when providing care to the homeless population. This included looking at the patient holistically and taking into consideration their living situation and lifestyle. Using a compassionate approach was found to be effective in providing treatment and education to not only individuals, but the homeless community in general.

Homelessness is becoming an increasing public health and social concern in our country (McCary & McConnell, 2005). Meeting the healthcare needs of the homeless requires a different approach than that of the general population, thus healthcare providers must be aware of these needs and learn how to facilitate and improve care for homeless individuals. The above review presents several studies outlining characteristics of the homeless population, their experiences within the healthcare system, and the role of NPs in providing health care to this population. However, the researcher was unable to locate any studies from the healthcare providers' perspective, including that of NPs, on the unique experience of providing health care to the homeless. The purpose of this study was to describe the experiences of NPs who provide health care to the homeless in order to gain insight into their unique experience and learn what it takes to be successful in their role.

## METHODS

### Population, Participants, and Setting

A qualitative. naturalistic approach was utilized in this study using the principles of phenomenology to guide data collection and analysis. For the purposes of this study, the target population consisted of NPs directly involved in providing health care to the homeless. The participants were obtained, using purposive and snowball sampling methodology, from NPs practicing for at least 6 months in southeast and northeast Wisconsin clinics that provided health care to the homeless.

The researcher's portal of entry for the interview process was an urban, NP-managed clinic for the homeless. The researcher had also been given the names of NPs and referred to other clinic sites directly involved in providing health care to the homeless. Nine of the 12 NPs contacted agreed to participate in the study (see Table 1).

### Data Collection Instruments

Approval from a university Institutional Review Board was obtained prior to data collection. A demographic questionnaire and an open-ended interview between the researcher and participants were used to collect data. One main question was asked at the start of the interview: "Will you please describe to me your experiences in providing health care to the homeless?" Further probe questions were also used throughout the interview. These questions included: (1) "Why do NPs who provide care to the homeless do what they do?" (2) "How is providing health care to the homeless population different from providing health care to the general population?" and (3) "What are the values/beliefs and unique characteristics of individuals devoted to serving such an underserved population?"

Each participant received an information letter that fully described the study, including the contact information of the researcher, a reminder that they could choose not to participate at any time, and that they would be able to obtain the results of the study if interested. Informed consent was obtained from each participant to complete the demographic questionnaire and to audio record the interview. All identifying data were kept

## TABLE 1 FREQUENCY AND PERCENTAGE OF DEMOGRAPHIC CHARACTERISTICS (*n* = 9)

|  | F | % |
|---|---|---|
| Gender: |  |  |
| Male | 1 | 11 |
| Female | 8 | 89 |
| Race: |  |  |
| White | 8 | 89 |
| Black | 1 | 11 |
| Marital status: |  |  |
| Single | 4 | 44.44 |
| Married | 3 | 33.33 |
| Divorced | 2 | 22.22 |
| Annual family income: |  |  |
| Less than $25,000 | 1 | 11 |
| $25,000–$49,000 | 0 | 0 |
| $50,000–$100,000 | 6 | 67 |
| Greater than $100,000 | 2 | 22 |
| Nurse practitioner position status: |  |  |
| Paid employee | 8 | 89 |
| Volunteer | 1 | 11 |

© 2012 American Academy of Nurse Practitioners, The Author(s) Seiler, A. J., & Moss, V. A. (2012). The experiences of nurse practitioners providing health care to the homeless. *Journal of the American Academy of Nurse Practitioners*, *24*(5), 303–312.

confidential in a locked file and were not including in the research report. No harm resulted from participating in the interview process. The participants benefited by sharing their first hand experiences of providing health care to the homeless and aiding the interviewer and others to gain an understanding of their role.

Field notes were collected during the interview and throughout the data collection process in order to capture characteristics of the participants and interview setting not able to be conveyed through the audiotape, as well as to record thoughts, perceptions, and ideas of the researcher. These procedures, along with the open-ended interview, provided a venue for participants to fully describe their experiences.

## Data Analysis Procedures

Data were analyzed using *descriptive phenomenology,* described by Spiegelberg as involving "direct exploration, analysis, and description of a particular phenomena, as free as possible from unexamined presuppositions, aiming at maximum intuitive presentation" (as cited in Streubert, Speziale, & Carpenter, 2007, p. 82). According to Speigelberg, "Descriptive phenomenology stimulates our perception of lived experience while emphasizing the richness, breadth, and depth of those experiences" (p. 82).

Following each interview, the audio-taped recordings were transcribed verbatim by a transcriptionist aware of the confidentiality issues and with prior experience in the management of qualitative data. The researcher then read over the transcriptions while listening to the audiotapes in order to further immerse herself in the data, correct mistakes, complete missing data, and remove any identifying information. As themes began to emerge, similar data were clustered into themes and further separated into subthemes. As the intended goal of a phenomenologically inspired study, it was the intention of this researcher to relate the emerging themes to one another and develop a meaningful report and exhaustive description of the experiences of NPs providing health care to the homeless.

## RESULTS

Five main themes and 13 subthemes emerged from data analysis of significant statements from the nine interviews (see Figure 1).

### Theme 1: Why They Do What They Do

When asked why NPs who provide health care to the homeless do what they do, the participants spoke of being able to practice the true art of nursing, making a difference, and a sense of mission fulfillment of a deeper calling.

**Subtheme 1A: Nursing at its Finest.** Providing health care to the homeless offers the NP participants the ability to practice the true art of nursing. One participant stated:

*The homeless people are extremely unique people. They are very open once you establish trust with them, and it provides an incredible nursing environment where you get to use all these extra skills, but never forget that you are a nurse.*

Another said:

*I think the homeless community offers just tremendous opportunities to help. And for the old school nursing that I'm from, that's what a nurse is about, is to help.*

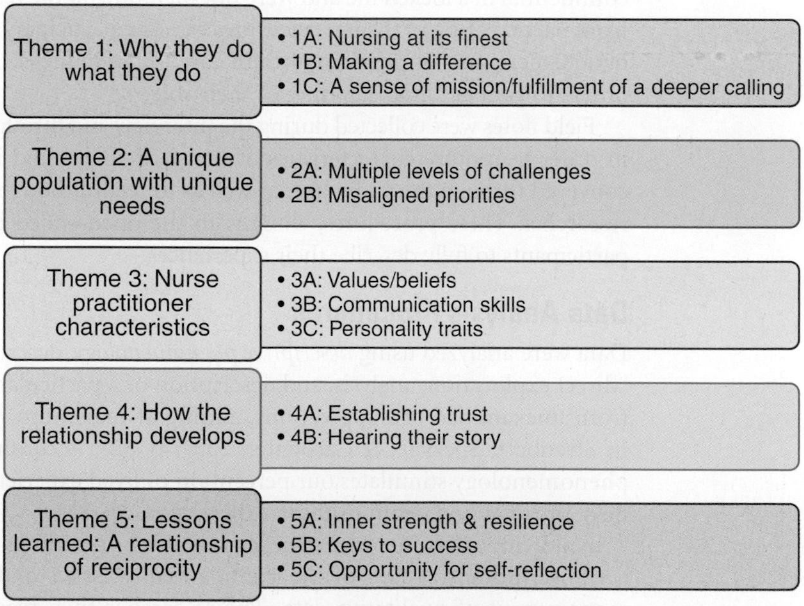

| Theme 1: Why they do what they do | • 1A: Nursing at its finest<br>• 1B: Making a difference<br>• 1C: A sense of mission/fulfillment of a deeper calling |
| --- | --- |
| Theme 2: A unique population with unique needs | • 2A: Multiple levels of challenges<br>• 2B: Misaligned priorities |
| Theme 3: Nurse practitioner characteristics | • 3A: Values/beliefs<br>• 3B: Communication skills<br>• 3C: Personality traits |
| Theme 4: How the relationship develops | • 4A: Establishing trust<br>• 4B: Hearing their story |
| Theme 5: Lessons learned: A relationship of reciprocity | • 5A: Inner strength & resilience<br>• 5B: Keys to success<br>• 5C: Opportunity for self-reflection |

**FIGURE 1** Themes and subthemes.

**Subtheme 1B: Making a Difference.** The NP participants also spoke of providing health care to the homeless as an opportunity to make a true difference in peoples' lives that truly need it. One stated:

> *There's so much need and so much difference that we can make, so I feel like my efforts reap so much reward, so it makes it the best job even though I'm exhausted at the end of the day because it is so hard.*

Another mentioned:

> *I think it's so very rewarding in the sense, for me, in the sense that you can really make a difference for somebody. And I think that's probably one of the reasons that I do it. When you can help somebody who really, really needs it, that I think is the best part about working with that population.*

**Subtheme 1C: A Sense of Mission/Fulfillment of a Deeper Calling.** Several participants felt that it was a sense of mission or the desire to fulfill a deeper calling that impelled them to provide care to such an underserved population. One NP stated:

> *I think we're very mission focused, mission driven. We have a mission, which states that we provide healthcare to underserved people who can't access traditional healthcare services. And the people who are here, including whoever provides primary care, whether it's nurse or physicians, have that philosophy. I think that's the main thing that binds us.*

Another said:

> *. . . I think they usually come from a sense of mission, so mission seems to be part of their focus as far as their work . . . It's rare that I've hired anybody where I have a sense that they just want to come and do the job and leave. It, sort of, fits with the rest of their life, which tends to be the art of caring, which is what nursing is about, practicing that art.*

Another said:

> *. . . I don't think any of them are there for the finances. I don't think any of them are there for, because it involves extra challenges, extra time. I think it is a deeper calling.*

## Theme 2: A Unique Population with Unique Needs

Interviews with the NP participants reinforced that providing health care to the homeless is different from providing health care to the general population.

**Subtheme 2A: Multiple Levels of Challenges.** The participants spoke of the complexity of providing health care to the homeless and the devastation of mental illness and substance abuse and how that leads up the severing of ties with their family and friends. One participant referred to this as *the disconnection,* another as *the downward spiral,* and another as a *lifetime of happening.* This leaves many homeless individuals with a lack of resources and disconnected from mainstream society, thus presenting a challenge to the healthcare provider on multiple levels. One participant stated:

> *The same problem is pretty universal throughout underserved people and poor people, is getting the treatment that we recommend . . . It's not just write a prescription and send someone out the door. It's helping people to find a way to get the medicines. And then,*

*since so many of . . . the homeless folks that we work with are mentally ill or chemically dependent, it's not only finding them the medicines, it's helping them to develop systems where they can take the medicines.*

Another mentioned:

*It's same thing we talked about – literacy, and how you provide education to someone who can't read, you know, or with developmental delay or mentally ill. You know, how do you get through to people like that? So, those are some of the things that I think about when I see patients.*

### Subtheme 2B: Misaligned Priorities. 
Many of the participants also spoke of some initial frustrations in trying to provide health care to the homeless and of coming to the realization and accepting that health care was not the homeless individuals' top priority. One NP stated:

*And, I really can understand how your health is not, necessarily, on your top priority list when you're thinking about housing or jobs. I mean, Maslow's hierarchy really comes into play in dealing with the homeless, and it can be a pretty frustrating experience when, you know, they come in and they've admitted to not taking their medicines, or they've lost their medicines. You know at times, you find yourself frustrated with them, and then you have to remember – that's not their priority, that's my priority.*

A second said:

*So, they come with lack of resources to get, to keep themselves healthy, probably a lack of motivation to keep themselves healthy, too, because they have other concerns. They're not interested in worrying about exercise or things like that. Their first concern in their life hasn't been their health, because they're just trying to survive.*

A third mentioned:

*. . . the main thing I take away from working with people who are homeless, a couple things. One is that their healthcare and their health, even though it's such a critical part life in their big scheme of things, when you're homeless, your health tends to take a bottom rung to finding a house, finding a place to sleep that night, finding a meal. So, it's very interesting trying to work with people who have so many other needs besides their health.*

## Theme 3: NP Characteristics
Data analysis supported the assumption that providing health care to the homeless requires healthcare providers to exhibit specific qualities, communication skills, and personality traits in order to be successful.

### Subtheme 3A: Values/Beliefs. 
The NP participants spoke of many different values and/or beliefs they themselves possessed, or that they felt were common to their profession as a whole, that allowed them to be successful in their role. One participant stated:

*I guess that is the reason I chose to work there, because I value that time spent with people is important in medical care. You need time work with them, hear their stories, try to figure out solutions to some of the issues they're going to have.*

Another said:

> I'd say as a group, I would think that NPs that care for the homeless believe in justice.
> I believe that we feel that everyone is entitled to not only healthcare, but good healthcare.
> And I think that's one of the many factors that drive us as NPs to deal with the underserved
> population.

**Subtheme 3B: Communication Skills.** The need for the healthcare provider to possess good communication skills was another resounding theme identified during analysis of the interview transcripts. One NP stated:

> . . . there's a lot more of, I hate that term, therapeutic communication, but there is. Just
> listening to people, not just rushing to make decisions for them, trying to get them involved
> in their care, what works for you?

Another said:

> . . . physicians have been really into the medical model and they're really into the disease
> process, and we have always been taught, not just as an NP, but as a nurse, to sit next to
> somebody's bedside and to be able to talk to them. I can tell you, anybody that's a long-term
> patient here, I know something about them and their family, because that's what I do,
> all that is part of their health care. To get them better, to take ownership of their health
> care, you have to really look at that person and believe in them, and I think NPs have that
> ability.

**Subtheme 3C: Personality Traits.** The participants also spoke of a variety of personality traits they felt individuals who provide health care to the homeless should have. One participant said:

> . . . when you provide care for the homeless, you have to have such a huge, broad scope
> of assessment skills and creativeness, because you can't treat their health problems like
> you would in a normal office . . . it requires that I pull into use all kinds of creativity, all
> of my assessment skills, and to really, really listen to the client to find out what options
> they have and what they really can do.

A second mentioned:

> Just a tremendous amount of patience. A tremendous desire to, I think we're all just
> excellent educators. We spend a lot of time working with people, at their level, taking into
> account – can they read, do they understand what we're saying.

A third stated:

> I would say you have to have, and people that I've known that have worked in the
> environments that I've worked in, I would say you have to have an openness to all
> kinds of patient situations, life situations, and have a desire to provide care to a
> population that's just difficult to serve, because you know that they need it.

## Theme 4: How the Relationship Develops

The fourth theme that emerged during data analysis revolved around how the relationship develops between the NP and the homeless patient.

**Subtheme 4A: Establishing Trust.** Two participants felt that establishing a relationship with the homeless patient is not unlike other relationships between healthcare providers and their patients; however, the majority of the NPs felt that it can be more challenging and take more time to establish their trust.

One NP stated:

*Here, so many of our clients have had horrifically negative experiences in the healthcare system. Plus you factor in there, mental illness, and the fact that most homeless people are homeless because they have severed all of their ties with family and friends, otherwise family and friends wouldn't let them be homeless, they would take them in. It can be very challenging, initially, to establish a relationship, so that I consider it part of the nursing skill set to be able to cull the interaction with the client, and to start out wherever they are and work with gradually moving them into a more trusting relationship.*

Another said:

*Once they understand that you're a safe place for them to talk, then they will tell you what's going on, and then you just do the best you can to help them. You have to be legitimate, you have to be sincere, because they're smart, and of course they're smart, because they've lived homeless.*

**Subtheme 4B: Hearing their Story.** A key element in developing the relationship with homeless patients identified by the participants was the importance of learning their story and acknowledging them as a person. One NP said:

*. . . there's some things I can't begin to touch, but the fact that I can hear their story, I can validate what they're saying, and acknowledge them. I think it's healing and it's the hugest thing to do . . . So, I think it's again, just time and time to just respect them as a human being and being at their level that allows you to open a lot of doors with people.*

A second stated:

*And I have found, you know, especially sometimes on our first initial visits, where we really take quality time to really listen to these individuals. And in some cases, you know, it's feeling finally they may have found a place for their home base healthcare, where they're not just another number or turned away because of their appearance or their stature or whatever.*

A third said:

*And honestly, if you asked me the most important thing I do at my job is I talk with people and allow them to share their story; and just by listening to them, that values them. I tell you, of anything I do, that's probably the most important thing that we do, is that we acknowledge them as a person.*

## Theme 5: Lessons Learned: A Relationship of Reciprocity

All NP participants have learned something about the homeless community or the homeless community has taught them something about themselves, thus their relationship with their homeless patients is one of reciprocity—both parties benefit.

**Subtheme 5A: Inner Strength and Resilience.** The NP participants were amazed by the inner strength and resilience of their homeless patients. One participant stated:

*And the other thing I take away from working with the homeless, I find it very grounding in the sense that you can see the kind of struggles that people go through, and it's a, they have amazing resilience, the people who I work with.*

Another said:

*You have so many strikes against you – no education, can't read, you have a medical problem, you have no family, you know, you have no money. You know, how do you keep going?*

A third participant spoke of getting invited into the world of the homeless community:

*One of the side benefits is that after you do this for awhile, the clients begin to invite you into their world, and it's amazing the inner strength and the survival will that our clients have, and it's amazing to get to see that again – not something you would ever, ever experience in a normal work setting.*

Others reflected upon whether they would have the strength to keep going if they were in similar situations as their patents:

*But there's always a sense that things will get better, and no matter how often they get slammed, they seem to keep bouncing back. So, I find that incredible, because I don't know if I would have that strength of will, and maybe it's just the human spirit – the will to keep going – but it's just incredible to me.*

Another said:

*I'm always amazed at how resilient they are, you know, they'll still find something to eat . . . So, these people somehow or other, they make it, they figure out some way to make it.*

**Subtheme 5B: Keys to Success.** The NP participants identified several keys to providing successful care to homeless individuals. These included recognizing one's own assumptions and biases, providing acknowledgement, being empathetic, having respect for persons, and meeting individuals at their level. For example, one participant stated:

*It's very different. I think it's very different than what people are used to. I think, it's hard to not go in judgmental when dealing with that population, and to have preconceived ideas, you know, of who they are, where they've been. So, that's something that I've been working over the years since I've been there. Just trying to see them as a person. You know how we always say – see them as a person and not a disorder – someone who has depression, not a depressed person. That kind of thing.*

Another said:

*So, in essence, I think, just like with any patient try to empathize with what their life situation is – recognizing our assumptions, our stereotypes, our judgments; recognizing that we have those things, racism or whatever that is, and not carrying that with you . . . recognizing . . . So that's deep and long, that history's long, that kind of thing.*

A third said:

*So, everyone has an interesting story. I mean, sometimes it's difficult to understand, but everyone has something, and something that motivates them, and I think just, I guess, I've always seen the homeless as people, and I have not stopped doing that.*

A fourth mentioned:

*I think it's just that when you are on the fringes of society, you become nameless, faceless, people would prefer not to really see you. And, my strong belief is that they are a human being and deserves the same kind of treatment and respect as anyone else.*

**Subtheme 5C: Opportunity for Self-Reflection.** Providing health care to the homeless, gave the NP participants the opportunity to reflect upon their own lives. One NP stated:

*I don't know if everyone feels that way, but it's like the older I became, the less enthralled with physical things and more concerned with relationships. That's why, for me, this is the best work opportunity, because again, physical possessions, making a certain amount of money, meeting productivity quotas, those aren't issues anymore, and they're not issues in the homeless population, as well.*

Another said:

*They taught me very early how superficial some of my concerns in life might be. Someone spills red wine on my new white tablecloth, and I wouldn't be happy, but you know what, I got wine and I got a tablecloth and a house to live in, and I'm getting excited when there are people sleeping out in the streets? So, they teach you so much about what really matters.*

A third mentioned:

*I always wonder, "How would I be if I had lived these people's lives?" I would probably be in the same place, so just withholding judgment, which are some of things I went in with, because you have to have that otherwise you wouldn't want to work there, you know. And again, I reiterate it's the power of the human spirit.*

A fourth said:

*I've reinforced my own listening skills, my listening ability, my patience, my own endurance, my own frailties, kind of, reaffirmed them in myself and in my own dealings with my family relations.*

# DISCUSSION

Five themes and 13 subthemes emerged from the nine NPs' accounts of their experiences providing health care to the homeless. All of the participants viewed their time providing health care to the homeless as an overall positive and rewarding experience that allowed them to practice the true art of nursing and the ability to make a true difference in peoples' lives. They also spoke of the challenges and emotional strain of their experiences which left them humbled and grounded, allowing for mutual enrichment and personal growth.

The theme "a unique population with unique needs" reinforces the challenges that healthcare providers face in providing health care to the homeless population and supports the fact that the health status of homeless individuals is poorer than that of the general population (Zlotnick & Zerger, 2008). The subtheme of "misaligned priorities" supports the findings of McCormack and Gooding's (1993) study in which "satisfying basic human needs" was identified as one of the themes essential to health; and Nickash and Marnocha's (2009) finding that most homeless individuals lack the necessary resources to meet their physical needs of shelter, air, water, and food. Indeed, it is not surprising that Maslow's hierarchy really comes into play when dealing with homeless individuals, nor that their health is not always their top priority.

The theme, "how the relationship develops" and its related subthemes, "establishing trust" and "hearing their story" identifies ways for NPs to overcome the barriers to receiving health care perceived by homeless patients as identified by Cocozza Martins (2008), and perhaps, to overcome their perceived experience of "unwelcomeness" during encounters with healthcare providers as identified by Wen, Hudak, and Hwang (2007). It also reinforces the importance of "staying connected," the core category identified by Jezewski (1995) as the essence of facilitating care for the homeless. Hopefully, these insights will help healthcare providers to provide a more welcoming experience for their homeless patients in order to make them feel empowered, listened to, and valued.

Cocozza Martins (2008) identified the theme "developing underground resourcefulness" in her study on the experiences of homeless adults in the healthcare system. This aligns with this study's theme of "inner strength and resilience" that was identified by the NP participants as one of the lessons learned during their time providing care to this population.

As Mullin and Ambrosia (2005) stated, providing care to the homeless population calls for special considerations to be taken into account. NPs must take the entire context of their patients' lives into consideration in order to find the most compassionate and effective way to treat, diagnose, and provide education for each individual.

## CONCLUSIONS

There were several limitations to the study. The first was the sample, which was quite small ($n = 9$). It became difficult to recruit more respondents in the time frame allowed. A second limitation was that all respondents were from the Midwest and the majority were women ($n = 8$). Differing results might have been obtained from other parts of the country and from a more representative male perspective. Further qualitative studies should be undertaken using a larger and more representative sample of NPs and in other urban areas of the country. Studies could also explore any similarities or differences in registered nurses and advanced practice nurses' experiences in caring for the homeless.

Homelessness is becoming an increasing public health and social concern in our country (McCary & McConnell, 2005). Meeting the healthcare needs of the homeless requires a different approach than that of the general population, thus healthcare providers must be aware of these needs and learn how to facilitate and improve care for homeless individuals. The current literature contains various studies outlining characteristics of the homeless population, their experiences within the healthcare system, and the role of NPs in providing health care to this population. However, prior to undertaking this study, the researcher was unable to locate any studies from the healthcare providers' perspective, including that of NPs, on the unique experience of providing health care to the homeless. This study helps to fill this gap in the literature and will assist healthcare providers to gain insight into the experience and learn what it takes to become successful in such an important and much needed role.

# REFERENCES

Agosta, L. (2009). Patient satisfaction with nurse-practitioner-delivered primary healthcare services. *Journal of the American Academy of Nurse Practitioners, 21*, 610–617.

American Academy of Nurse Practitioners (2010a). *Quality and cost effectiveness of NP care.* Retrieved from http://www.aanp.org

American Academy of Nurse Practitioners (2010b). *Standards of NP practice.* Retrieved from http://www.aanp.org

Bauer, J. (2010). Nurse practitioners as an underutilized resource for health reform: evidence-based demonstrations of cost-effectiveness. *Journal of the American Academy of Nurse Practitioners, 22*, 228–231.

Bessant, J., Coupland, H., Dalton, T., Maher, L., Rowe, J., & Watts, R. (2002). *Heroin users, housing and social participation: attacking social exclusion through better housing.* Australian Housing and Urban Research Institute positioning paper No. 31. RMIT Research Centre. UNSW-UWS Research Centre.

Burt, M., Aron, L. Y., & Lee, E. (2001). *Helping America's homeless: emergency shelter or affordable housing?* Washington, DC: The Urban Institute.

Cocozza Martins, D. (2008). Experiences of homeless people in the health care delivery system: a descriptive phenomenological study. *Public Health Nursing, 25*(5), 420–430.

Coddington, J. A., & Sands, L. P. (2008). Cost of health care and quality outcomes of patients in nurse-managed clinics. *Nursing Economics, 26*(2), 75–83.

Courtney, R., & Rice, C. (1997). Investigation of nurse practitioner-patient interactions: using the nurse practitioner rating form. *The Nurse Practitioner, 22*(2), 46–65.

Daiski, I. (2007). Perspectives of homeless people on their health and health needs priorities. *Journal of Advanced Nursing, 58*(3), 273–281.

D'Amore, J., Chiang, W., & Goldfrank, L. (2001). The epidemiology of the homeless population and its impact on an urban emergency department. *Academic Emergency Medicine, 8*, 1051–1055.

de la Cruz, F. A., Brehm, C., & Harris, J. (2004). Transformation in family nurse practitioner students' attitudes toward homeless individuals after participation in a homeless outreach clinic. *Journal of the American Academy of Nurse Practitioners, 16*(12), 547–553.

Drury, L. J. (2008). From homeless to housed: caring for people in transition. *Journal of Community Health Nursing, 25*, 91–105.

Gelberg, L., Andersen, R. M., & Leake, B. D. (2000). The behavioral model for vulnerable populations: application to medical care use and outcomes for homeless people. *Health Services Research, 34*(6), 1273–1302.

Guzik, A., Menzel, N., Fitzpatrick. J., & McNulty, R. (2009). Patient satisfaction with nurse practitioner and physician services in the occupational health setting. *AAOWN Journal, 57*(5), 191–197.

Hunt, R. J., & Swiggum, P. (2007). Being in another world: transcultural student experiences using service learning with families who are homeless. *Journal of Transcultural Nursing, 18*, 167–174.

Hunter, J., Getty, C., Kemsley, M., & Skelly, A. (1991). Barriers to providing health care to homeless persons: a survey of providers' perceptions. *Health Values: The Journal of Health Behavior Education, & Promotion, 15*(5), 3–11.

Jezewski, M. A. (1995). Staying connected: the core of facilitating health care for homeless persons. *Public Health Nursing, 12*(3), 203–210.

Johnson, G., & Chamberlain, C. (2008). Homelessness and substance abuse: which comes first? *Australian Social Work, 61*(4), 342–356.

King, T. E., & Wheeler, M. B. (2007). *Medical management of vulnerable and underserved patient: principles, practice, and populations.* New York, NY: McGraw-Hill Companies, Inc.

Maze, C. D. M. (2005). Registered nurses' professional rights vs. professional responsibility in caring for members of underserved and disenfranchised populations. *Journal of Clinical Nursing, 14*, 546–554.

Maze, C. D. M. (2006). Registered nurses' willingness to serve populations on the periphery of society. *Journal of Nursing Scholarship, 38*(3), 301–306.

McCary, J. M., & McConnell, J. J., (2005). Health, housing, and the heart: cardiovascular disparities in homeless people. *Circulation, 111,* 256–257.

McCormack, D., & Gooding, B. (1993). Homeless persons communicate their meaning of health. *Canadian Journal of Nursing Research, 25*(1), 33–50.

Metraux, S., Culhane, D., Raphael, S., et al. (2001). Assessing homeless population size through the use of emergency and transitional shelter services in 1998: results from the analysis of administrative data from nine U.S. jurisdictions. *Public Health Reports, 116,* 344–352.

Moskowitz, D., Glasco, J., Johnson, B., & Wang, G. (2006). Students in the community: an interprofessional student-run free clinic. *Journal of Interprofessional Care, 20*(3), 254–259.

Mullin, K. A., & Ambrosia, T. (2005). Role of the nurse practitioner in providing health care for the homeless. *American Journal for Nurse Practitioners, 9*(9), 37–44.

Nickasch, B., & Marnocha, S. K. (2009). Healthcare experiences of the homeless. *Journal of the American Academy of Nurse Practitioners, 21,* 39–46.

Read, S. (2008). Health and homelessness: whole-system perspective. *Housing, Care, and Support, 11*(1), 7–10.

Schanzer, B., Dominguez, B., Shrout, P., & Caton, C. (2007). Homelessness, health status, and health care use. *American Journal of Public Health, 97*(3), 464–468.

Streubert Speziale, H. J., & Carpenter, D. R. (2007). *Qualitative research in nursing: advancing the humanistic imperative* (4th ed.). Philadelphia, PA: Lippincott Williams & Wilkins.

Tischler, V., Edwards, V., & Vostanis, P. (2009). Working therapeutically with mothers who experience the trauma of homelessness: an opportunity for growth. *Counseling and Psychotherapy Research, 9*(1), 42–46.

Wen, C., Hudak, P., & Hwang, S. (2007). Homeless people's perceptions of welcomeness and unwelcomeness in healthcare encounters. *Journal of General Internal Medicine, 22*(7), 1011–1017.

Zerwekh, J. V. (2000). Caring on the ragged edge: nursing persons who are disenfranchised. *Advances in Nursing Science, 22*(4), 47–61.

Zlotnick, C., & Zerger, S. (2008). Survey findings on characteristics and health status of clients treated by the federally funded (US) health care for the homeless programs. *Health and Social Care in the Community, 17*(1), 18–26.

# Couple Functioning and Post-Traumatic Stress Symptoms in US Army Couples: The Role of Resilience

*Kristal C. Melvin,[1]\* Deborah Gross,[2]\*\* Matthew J. Hayat,[3]† Bonnie Mowinski Jennings,[4]‡ Jacquelyn C. Campbell[5]§*

**Abstract:** The purpose of this study was to investigate combat-related post-traumatic stress symptoms (PTSS) and couple relationships in Army couples. US Army combat veteran couples ($n = 66$ couples) completed self-report questionnaires on couple functioning, coercion, resilience, and PTSS. In 23% of the couples ($n = 15$), both members had PTSS above the clinical cut-off for suspected Post-traumatic Stress Disorder (PTSD). Higher levels of PTSS were associated with lower couple functioning and resilience. Individuals with high resilience scores reported higher couple functioning scores, regardless of PTSS

[1]Center for Nursing Science and Clinical Inquiry, Madigan Health Systems, Tacoma, WA

[2]Acute and Chronic Care, Johns Hopkins University School of Nursing, Baltimore, MD

[3]College of Nursing, Rutgers University, Newark, NJ

[4]Nell Hodgson Woodruff School of Nursing, Emory University, Atlanta, GA

[5]Community-Public Health, Johns Hopkins University School of Nursing, Baltimore, MD Accepted 16 November 2011

Published 2011. This article is a U.S. Government work and is in the public domain in the USA. Res Nurs Health 35:164–177, 2012

This research was sponsored by the TriService Nursing Research Program (TSNRP), Uniformed Services University of the Health Sciences (USUHS). However, the information, conclusions do not necessarily represent the official position or policy of, nor should any official endorsement be inferred by, the TSNRP, USUHS, the Department of Defense, or the U.S. Government.

Correspondence to Kristal C. Melvin, Center for Nursing Science and Clinical Inquiry, Madigan Health Systems, 9040 Jackson Ave, Tacoma, WA 98431.

\*Nurse Scientist Center for Nursing Science and Clinical Inquiry; Lieutenant Colonel in the United States Army Nurse Corps.

\*\*Leonard and Helen Stulman Professor in Mental Health and Psychiatric Nursing.

†Assistant Professor.

††Visiting Professor.

§Anna D. Wolf Chair and Professor.

Published online 12 December 2011 in Wiley Online Library (wileyonlinelibrary.com). DOI: 10.1002/nur.21459

($p = .004$). Future researchers should focus on the role of resilience in relation to couple functioning, and ways to amplify resilience in military couples.

**Keywords:** post-traumatic stress; resilience; couples; psychological trauma; CATS model; military

Deployments refer to military duty away from home, usually to an overseas location. There have been over 1.7 million deployments from the United States (US) to support Operation Iraqi Freedom (OIF) and Operation Enduring Freedom (OEF) in Afghanistan (Tanielian et al., 2009), with many of these representing multiple deployments for the same service member. Diagnosable Post-Traumatic Stress Disorder (PTSD), based on severity of posttraumatic stress symptoms (PTSS), is estimated to affect at least 12% of soldiers returning from OIF/OEF deployments (Milliken, Auchterlonie, & Hoge, 2007). Not only does PTSS negatively influence the military mission, but it also has profound secondary effects on the military family. For instance, in families of service members with elevated PTSS, there are increased divorce rates (Karney & Crown, 2007) as well as an increased incidence of intimate partner violence (IPV) and child abuse (Gibbs, Martin, Kupper, & Johnson, 2007; Rentz et al., 2006). In a 2008 survey of over 49,000 military spouses, 23% reported marital problems after deployment, compared with 6% reporting problems prior to deployment (Department of Defense, 2009).

Combat deployment is an expected source of stress for service members and their spouses, but recent increases in length and frequency of deployment, related to the wars in Iraq (OIF) and Afghanistan (OEF), have further strained military couples (Allen, Rhoades, Stanley, & Markman, 2010; Mansfield et al., 2010; Wheeler & Torres Stone, 2009). The OIF and OEF conflicts, presumably because of the asymmetrical and elusive nature of the enemy, have also been shown to produce higher rates of PTSS and other mental health concerns in soldiers than seen in previous wars (Fontana & Rosenheck, 2008), even in soldiers in military occupations previously regarded as safe, such as lawyers and supply clerks (Tanielian et al., 2009). In addition, PTSS in the combat veteran, with or without a diagnosis of PTSD, has been found to increase stress in military spouses (Monson, Taft, & Fredman, 2009; Sayers, 2011). Findings from a recent study in Army couples showed an inverse relationship between PTSS and couple functioning (Allen et al., 2010). This relationship has yet to be investigated while controlling for the interdependence of spouses, and potential moderators of this relationship are yet to be identified and explored. The purpose of the current study was to investigate the effect of combat-related PTSS on couple functioning in Army OIF/OEF veteran couples and the role of resilience as a moderator of this effect.

To date, few studies have been conducted to directly investigate the prevalence of stress related symptoms in spouses of OIF/OEF combat veterans; there is no agreement among reported rates of PTSS or presence of secondary traumatic stress (STS). STS is defined as clinically significant levels of PTSS without a history of direct trauma (Dekel & Solomon, 2007; Figley, 1995; Ting, Jacobson, Sanders, Bride, & Harrington, 2005). In a study of female spouses of OIF/OEF veterans conducted by Nelson-Goff, Crow, Reisbig, and Hamilton (2007, 2009), STS was found in 61% of the wives ($n = 45$). Findings from other studies, however, have shown much lower rates of STS in military spouses. For example, in a study of 295 spouses of recently returned National Guard OIF veterans, investigators found a 12.5% prevalence rate of STS (Renshaw, Rodrigues, & Jones, 2008). This lower reported rate in National Guard or Reserve families compared to active duty service member families could be due to concerns about mental health stigma upon returning to civilian jobs (Milliken et al., 2007). Alternately, there could be other confounding variables not yet explored that might affect these relationships, such as the presence of previous trauma in the wives, or of individual and/or couple resilience.

Resilience has been defined as an ability to spring back from adversity (Jacelon, 1997; Richardson, 2002; Watson Wiens & Boss, 2006), returning to the previous level of functioning or even higher (Watson Wiens & Boss, 2006). It has been conceptualized as a protective factor against adverse outcomes from traumatic events (Tusaie & Dyer, 2004). Originally conceptualized as a trait in children, resilience has more recently been defined as a dynamic process across the lifespan that can be modified and fostered through various interventions, such as cognitive behavioral therapy (Davidson et al., 2005) and training in positive coping skills (Meredith et al., 2011). Palmer (2008) proposed a theoretical pathway of risk and resilience in military families, positing that individual resilience acts as a protective factor against PTSS and other adverse mental health outcomes in military parents, which in turn protects the children from adverse outcomes. This theoretical pathway has not yet been tested.

As a preliminary step toward a better understanding of the role of resilience in levels of functioning in military families, we examined individual spouse resilience for its potential role in modifying the relationship between individual level of PTSS and couple functioning, building on the promising findings from previous studies in which individual resilience was identified as a possible protective factor in military service members (Maguen et al., 2008). This investigation is the first that we are aware of to explore the role of resilience in couple functioning in combat veteran couples from the conflicts in Iraq and Afghanistan. We chose to approach resilience as a moderator rather than a mediator because we were not sure of the causal and/or temporal nature of its relationship with PTSS. To be a mediator, a variable must occur in a specific temporal location, between the predictor and the outcome variables (Zhao, Lynch, & Chen, 2010). In our evaluation of current literature, we were unable to determine whether resilience was present in soldiers and spouses before exposure to trauma, or whether it developed as a result of adjustment to PTSS.

## CONCEPTUAL FRAMEWORK

A modified version of the Couple Adaptation to Traumatic Stress (CATS) model (Nelson-Goff & Smith, 2005) was used as the framework guiding the selection of variables for this study (see Fig. 1). We acquired verbal permission from the original author to modify the model (B. Nelson-Goff, personal communication, July 23, 2009) to be more specific to the research questions in this study. The CATS model was developed in the field of marital and family therapy and has been partially tested in female military spouses (Nelson-Goff et al., 2007, 2009). The role of resilience in couple adaptation has not been tested in previous studies, however. Nelson-Goff and Smith (2005) originally conceptualized resilience as "adaptability," 1 of 10 couple traits that comprised couple functioning. In this study, we simplified the concept of couple functioning to represent couple satisfaction, communication, conflict, and cohesion, as percieved by each partner. We assessed resilience as an individual partner dynamic process of adaptation that can be nurtured and developed, as demonstrated in at least one PTSD intervention study (Davidson et al., 2005). As a potentially alterable variable (Meredith et al., 2011), resilience may provide a target for future intervention development for military couples.

In the CATS model, predisposing factors such as age, gender, rank of the soldier, and history of previous mental or physical trauma, as well as current violence or coercion in the couple, are proposed as additional moderators of the relationship between the individual's level of functioning (PTSS) and the couple functioning. Younger age has been associated with a higher risk for developing PTSS and other mental health problems after combat exposure (LeardMann, Smith, Smith, Wells, & Ryan, 2009). Military rank has shown an inverse

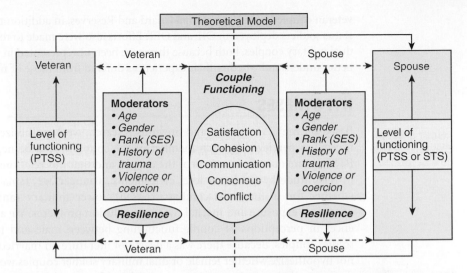

**FIGURE 1** Couple adaptation to traumatic stress (CATS) model, modified version. Note: Model modified with the permission of the original author (Nelson-Goff & Smith, personal communication, July 23, 2009) to be more specific to a military population and to answer the specific questions for this research study. Veteran = spouse who experienced combat exposure, Rank = military rank, SES = socio-economic status, Coercion = coercion or violence in the current marriage, PTSS = post-traumatic stress symptoms, STS = secondary traumatic stress. Reprinted with permission of author and publisher.

relationship with divorce rates among service members (Karney & Crown, 2007), perhaps because higher ranking service members may have postponed marriage during the early years of their military career. Because salary and education are tied to military rank, it is also an accepted proxy measure for socio-economic status (SES; MacLean & Edwards, 2010).

Differences between males and females have been shown in previous PTSD research, with females having a higher risk for developing PTSD than males, resulting from both sexual-and combat-related trauma (Tolin & Foa, 2006). This gender difference may be related to the higher lifetime risk of sexual-related trauma exposure in females than males (Campbell et al., 2003; Institute of Medicine, 2010). In addition, having a pre-combat history of trauma, such as sexual abuse, being abused as a child, or past or current IPV, has been shown to increase the risk of developing PTSD (Nemeroff et al., 2006).

The outcome variable, level of functioning, was assessed as PTSS rather than the diagnosis of PTSD for two reasons. First, symptom levels have been shown to be associated with a PTSD diagnosis (Weathers, Litz, Herman, Huska, & Keane, 1993), and second, symptom levels have been widely used in PTSD research, enabling comparison of prevalence rates across the literature.

The specific aims of the study were to: (a) investigate the relationship between individual level of PTSS and couple functioning, (b) test the moderating effects of age, gender, military rank (proxy for SES), previous trauma, violence or coercion in the marriage, and resilience, (c) explore gender differences by examining whether dual military couples (where both spouses are service members) differ on PTSS and couple functioning scores from couples where only the male spouse has been deployed, and (d) determine the prevalence of STS in civilian spouses. In this study we addressed the gaps in previous research by recruiting Army combat veteran couples from the National Guard and Reserves, in addition to active duty and retiree status soldiers deployed in OIF and OEF. Efforts also were made to recruit female soldiers and dual military couples, both because they have been unrepresented in previous research and to better understand whether their experiences differed from those of male-soldier couples.

## HYPOTHESES

Based on the CATS model and previous research, we hypothesized that (a) couple functioning as percieved by each member of the couple would be negatively associated with PTSS in one or both members of the couple, and that this relationship would be increased in magnitude by (b) lower level of resilience, younger age, female gender (regardless of whether the woman was combat exposed), lower military rank, and increased levels of trauma exposure and marital conflict resolution problems. We also examined (c) differences in perceptions of couple functioning between male and female or dual military soldier couples. Because there was a dearth of literature on married female soldiers, we did not hypothesize whether female or dual military soldier couples would exhibit more or less distress in their marriage compared to male soldier couples, but we examined and explored for differences. Based on the wide range of STS prevalence reported in the literature, we also predicted (d) the presence of STS in 12–70% of civilian spouses in our study.

## METHOD

### Participants

Inclusion criteria were (a) one or both members of the couple had been deployed to OIF or OEF while serving in the US Army, (b) both members could read and speak English, and (c) both members had been in a self-defined "committed relationship" for at least 1 year. In addition, both members of the couple had to be willing to consent to participate in the study.

Army OIF/OEF soldier couples were recruited using a variety of local and national methods, including Facebook, veteran service organization blog sites, veteran targeted publications, and fliers placed at military medical treatment facilities in the Baltimore/Washington, DC area. Interested couples made initial contact with the first author via telephone or electronic mail. Both members of the couple were screened for eligibility, with each spouse asked separately whether they were interested in participating. Surveys were mailed to both members of the couple, in separate envelopes, with instructions that questions should be answered independently and answers should not be discussed prior to returning the surveys in the pre-addressed, stamped envelope provided. Based on a power of 0.80, and an effect size of 0.70 between "distressed" and "nondistressed" couples, using couple functioning (RDAS) scores, we sought to recruit at least 45 couples.

Survey packets were mailed to 85 eligible couples. After using a maximum of four mailed reminders, 66 couples (132 respondents) returned completed surveys, for a response rate of 77.6%. Although several unmarried couples were screened, all respondent couples were married. Respondents represented all types of military status, as presented on Table 1, with over 13% identified as National Guard or Reserve soldiers. Self-identified retirees and former soldiers did not report the type of military status (e.g., active duty, reserve) during their service.

Surveys were returned by couples in which the male was the service member ($n = 39$) and in which both members of the couple were in the military ($n = 27$). Seven packets were returned by only one member of the couple and therefore were not included. To more fully

## TABLE 1    SAMPLE CHARACTERISTICS

| CATEGORY | RESPONSE | M (SD) (N = 132) |
|---|---|---|
| Age | Years | 38.91 (9.1) |
| Length of marriage | Years | 11.30 (7.7) |
| Marriages | Number of times married | 1.48 (0.77) |

| CATEGORY | RESPONSE | % (N) |
|---|---|---|
| Race | African-American/Black | 3.8 (5) |
|  | Asian/Pacific Islander | 0.7 (1) |
|  | Caucasian/White | 90.1 (119) |
|  | Other | 3.7 (5) |
|  | Unknown | 1.4 (2) |
| Ethnicity | Hispanic | 3.7 (5) |
|  | Non-Hispanic | 87.8 (116) |
|  | Unknown | 6.0 (16) |
| Education | High school diploma | 37.9 (50) |
|  | 2- or 4-year degree | 31.8 (42) |
|  | Graduate school or more | 30.3 (40) |
| Military status | Active duty | 28.8 (38) |
|  | Retired | 8.3 (11) |
|  | Left service | 18.2 (24) |
|  | National guard | 7.6 (10) |
|  | Reserves | 9.0 (8) |
|  | Civilian (spouse) | 29.5 (39) |
|  | Other service (spouse) | 1.5 (2) |
| Rank | Civilian | 31.1 (41) |
|  | Junior enlisted | 18.2 (24) |
|  | Senior enlisted | 25.0 (33) |
|  | Warrant officer | 1.5 (2) |
|  | Commissioned officer | 24.2 (32) |
| Parity | No children | 7.5 (20) |
|  | 1 | 21.2 (28) |
|  | 2 | 45.0 (54) |
|  | 3 or more | 22.7 (30) |

M, mean; SD, standard deviation; N, total sample; n, number of individual participants with this characteristic.

explore differences between types of service, we compared active duty ($n = 38$ individuals), National Guard or reserve ($n = 18$ individuals), and soldiers who had left the Army and returned to civilian life after their most recent deployment ($n = 35$ individuals).

## Measures

**Post-traumatic stress symptoms (PTSS).** For this study, PTSS was operationalized as an individual's endorsement of symptom items on the PTSD Checklist (PCL; Weathers et al., 1993) including problems with sleep, avoidance, memory, concentration, emotional connections, or mood. This measure consists of 17 items, scored on a 5-point Likert-type scale, regarding severity of various symptoms diagnostic of PTSD. The PCL has been widely used in both military and civilian populations to measure the prevalence of presumed PTSD and for group comparisons on levels of PTSS. Cronbach's α reliabilities have ranged from 0.92 in civilians to 0.97 in military populations. Validity has been supported by the statistically significant correlations between PCL scores and the Clinician-Administered PTSD Scale (CAPS; Blake et al., 1995; Elhai, Gray, Docherty, Kashdan, & Kose, 2007; Keen, Kutter, Niles, & Krinsley, 2008). The PCL scores range from 17 to 85, with higher scores indicative of greater PTSS. Recent research supports a clinical cutoff of 30 when used in military primary care settings to screen for levels of PTSS high enough to cause interpersonal problems (Bliese et al., 2008). In many studies the clinical cut-off of 50 has been used (Terhakopian, Sinaii, Engel, Schnurr, & Hoge, 2008; Wright et al., 2007). Although the higher cut-off is more specific to the diagnosis of PTSD, we chose to use the more sensitive lower number for this study, to capture more variability in levels of PTSS. The Cronbach's α was 0.96 in our sample.

**Resilience.** We conceptualized resilience as a dynamic, modifiable process. We used the Revised Connor–Davidson Resilience Scale (R-CD-RISC; Campbell-Sills, Forde, & Stein, 2009; Connor & Davidson, 2003), a 10-item scale measuring participants' perceptions of their own resilience. The R-CD-RISC is scored based on the respondent's level of agreement with items such as, "Able to adapt to change" and "Think of self as a strong person." The abbreviated scale correlated well ($r = .90$) with the original 25-item CD-RISC and showed consistently good reliability ($\alpha = .94$) in civilian populations (Campbell-Sills et al., 2009). The original version of the CD-RISC showed sensitivity to treatment effects when applied to PTSD treatment groups (Connor & Davidson, 2003). Possible scores range from 0 to 50, with a higher score indicating greater resilience. The Cronbach's α was .91 in our study sample.

**Couple functioning.** For the purposes of this study, couple functioning was defined as the degree to which the individual members of the couple were satisfied with their relationship (satisfaction), were able to successfully resolve conflict (communication, consensus, and conflict), and identified themselves as a couple (cohesion). All of these concepts were measured using the Revised Dyadic Adjustment Scale (RDAS; Heyman, Sayers, & Bellack, 1994). The RDAS is a 14-item survey that uses a 6-point Likert-type scale with options ranging from 0 to 5, providing a total range of 0–70. In addition to being much shorter than the original 32-item Dyadic Adjustment Scale (DAS; Spanier, 1976), the RDAS has shown a 0.97 correlation with the original instrument and good discrimination between distressed and non-distressed couples in civilian populations (Busby, Christensen, Crane, & Larson, 1995). Although this measure was not previously tested in military couples, it has performed well in civilian populations. The Cronbach's α was 0.84 in our study sample.

**Coercion and violence.** Disagreement and arguments are normal in couples, but some couples may have difficulty resolving these conflicts. Difficulties may be situational and temporary, or they may relate to a power imbalance and coercion in the relationship (Johnson, 2006). Relational coercion can include social isolation, rejection, or threat of physical or mental harm (Houry et al., 2008). For this study, the Women's Experience of Battery (WEB; Smith, Earp, & DeVellis, 1995) was used as a measure of coercion and violence; it reflects self-reported feelings of being controlled, manipulated or coerced, or afraid of what a partner does or will do. The WEB is a 10-item Likert-type scale. Scale scores can range from 10 to 60, with higher scores indicating more distress, and includes items such as, "I felt ashamed of the things my partner did to me" and "I hid the truth from others because I was afraid not to." The WEB has excellent sensitivity and specificity in identifying abused women (Coker, Pope, Smith,

Sanderson, & Hussey, 2001; Houry et al., 2008; Smith et al., 1995) and correlates strongly with measures of physical violence. The adapted, gender neutral version of this measure was used for this study (Houry et al., 2008). The Cronbach's α was 0.88 in our study sample.

**History of previous trauma.** Past trauma— including child abuse, natural disasters, sexual abuse, IPV, major illnesses, or injuries—has been shown to be associated with increased risk for development of PTSD. These experiences were all measured using the Traumatic Experience Questionnaire (TEQ; Vrana & Lauterbach, 1994), a self-report measure of exposure to previous trauma. Response options are counts, scoring 1 point for each exposure response, or number of years experiencing IPV or child abuse, up to a maximum of 3 points for each of the 11 items. A score of zero is possible for those with no history of trauma exposure, with a potential maximum score of 33. This survey has been used in military couples research (Hamilton, Nelson-Goff, Crow, & Reisbig, 2009; Nelson-Goff et al., 2007), but validity data are not yet available for civilian or military populations (Norris & Hamblen, 2004). All respondents completed this measure, regardless of deployment history. Cronbach's α for the TEQ was 0.46. Given the low reliability obtained for this measure, responses to the TEQ were dichotomized to reflect presence or absence of trauma rather than using the cumulative score.

## Procedures

Demographic data were collected at the initial contact with one or both spouses, and included self-reported age, gender, military status (e.g., active duty, Reserves), military rank (if applicable), race, ethnic status, current relationship status and duration, total number of marriages, number of children, and educational level. Study recruitment method also was documented (e.g., Facebook, newspaper, snowball).

The OIF/OEF soldier respondents were asked the following questions: dates of deployment, location (Iraq or Afghanistan) and job while deployed. The order of survey measures was kept constant to ensure that respondents answered questions about their lifetime history of trauma prior to answering questions about PTSS.

## Analysis

All data were entered into STATA 11 (StataCorp, 2009), with quality check of all entries by a data quality specialist. Instruments were each tested for reliability, using Cronbach's α. Respondents and non-respondents were compared on all demographic data collected during the screening process. Couples were contacted regarding missing answers, when possible. Continuous data were examined for normality.

The main outcome, couple functioning as measured by the RDAS, was evaluated in relation to hypothesis 1, using a general linear mixed model, predicted by PTSS as measured by the PCL score. Within couple correlation was accounted for by using a random effect for couple, via the xtmixed function in STATA (StataCorp, 2009). This produces a nested model, where the individual level is nested within the couple level. Moderation, as noted in hypothesis 2, was assessed using a general linear mixed model and testing for interactions.

## RESULTS

### Participants

To examine whether couple respondents differed from those who did not return surveys, sociodemographic variables were compared between responding and non-responding

## TABLE 2    COMPARISON OF STUDY VARIABLES BY GENDER OF INDIVIDUAL PARTICIPANT

| | GENDER | | | | | |
| | MALES (n = 66) | | FEMALES (n = 66) | | | |
| VARIABLE | M | SD | M | SD | STATISTIC | p |
|---|---|---|---|---|---|---|
| RDAS couple functioning score | 48.9 | 6.7 | 50.9 | 6.9 | −1.47 | .14 |
| R-CD-RISC resilience score | 30.8 | 6.7 | 30.6 | 6.4 | 0.15 | .88 |
| PCL post-traumatic symptoms | 37.6 | 16.9 | 30.3 | 15.1 | 2.68 | .008* |
| WEB violence and coercion | 13.5 | 6.5 | 15.5 | 8.3 | −0.84 | .40 |
| TEQ trauma exposure history | 9.9 | 5.9 | 6.6 | 6.0 | 3.33 | <.001* |

| | GENDER | | | | | |
| | MALES (n = 64) | | FEMALES (n = 20) | | | |
| DEPLOYED PARTICIPANTS | M | SD | M | SD | STATISTIC | p |
|---|---|---|---|---|---|---|
| Total deployments | 1.6 | 1.0 | 0.39 | 0.7 | 9.54 | <.001* |
| Total months deployed | 18.3 | 1.0 | 12.7 | 1.3 | 9.67 | <.001* |
| Months since last deployed | 34.6 | 3.1 | 51.2 | 6.4 | 1.05 | .017* |

M = mean, SD = standard deviation. Statistic = test statistic, independent sample t test used. Variables: RDAS = Revised Dyadic Adjustment Scale (Heyman et al., 1994), R-CD-RISC = Revised Connor–Davidson Resilience Scale, PCL = PTSD Checklist (Weathers et al., 1993), WEB = Women's Experience of Battery, gender neutral version (Smith et al., 1995), TEQ = Traumatic Experience Questionnaire (Vrana & Lauterbach, 1994).
*p-value <.05.

individuals. There were no statistically significant differences, although non-respondents were more likely to have missing data in regard to race ($p = .002$).

When exploring the data by the gender of the respondent, several differences became evident, as shown in Table 2. More males were combat exposed than females ($p < .01$), and they reported higher trauma scores on the trauma history measure (TEQ). In addition, when comparing only combat-exposed soldiers, males had been deployed more times and for more total months than female soldiers.

### Relationship of PTSS with Couple Functioning

To investigate the first hypothesis, that couple functioning would be negatively associated with PTSS in both members of the couple, PCL scores were regressed on couple adjustment (RDAS) scores while controlling for couple effects using a general linear mixed model. Because both spouses completed separate surveys, yet were describing the same marital relationship, this interdependence can produce significant correlations in survey scores. Therefore, our chosen analysis method accounted for interdependence of couple measures. The level of PTSS was a significant predictor of couple functioning such that higher scores on the PCL were predictive of lower scores on the RDAS ($z = 2.82$, 95% CI $[−0.17, −0.03]$, $p = .005$). This finding supports the first hypothesis.

## Moderators of the Relationship Between PTSS and Couple Functioning

The second hypothesis—that the relationship between PTSS and couple functioning would be increased in magnitude by younger age, female gender, lower rank, lower levels of resilience, increased levels of trauma exposure, and the report of coercion or violence between the spouses—was investigated using a general linear mixed model. Forward and backward stepwise selection were used, retaining only those variables with statistically significant effects. Resilience remained significant after controlling for couple effects ($z = 2.9$, $p = .004$), with resilience acting inversely on the relationship. That is, individuals with high resilience (CD-RISC) scores were less likely to have low couple functioning (RDAS) scores, regardless of PTSS (PCL) scores. Gender was also significant after controlling for couple effects ($p = .02$), such that males with high PTSS scores were likely to have lower couple functioning scores than females with the same PTSS score. Coercion and violence (WEB) remained significant ($p = .001$) and acted to increase the statistical relationship between PTSS and couple functioning, so that individuals reporting higher levels of violence and coercion reported lower couple functioning scores.

The next step in our analysis was to test for moderation by examining the statistical interaction of each proposed moderator with PTSS score and couple functioning. Interaction effects failed to reach statistical significance for any of the proposed moderators, indicating that none of these predictors acted to change the slope of the regression line of PTSS on couple functioning. The results from these analyses therefore failed to support the hypothesis for the moderating effects of resilience, age, gender, rank, trauma exposure, or reports of coercion or violence in the marriage.

## Comparisons of Male Soldier and Dual Military Couples

The data were examined in several ways to determine whether couple functioning differed between male soldier and dual military couples. First, the data were explored for gender differences by individual respondents as previously discussed (Table 2). Because this initial analysis did not address the presence or absence of clinical levels of distress, all respondents were then sorted into high or low scores for couple functioning, resilience, and PTSS, based on the clinical cut point of 30. To examine the couples as dyadic units, respondent couples were then sorted into groups based on their scores. Two couple adjustment groups were created: (a) both male and female having high couple adjustment (RDAS scores) and (b) at least one spouse reporting low couple adjustment (RDAS score <48). Similarly, couple groups were created for high and low levels of coercion, using WEB scores >20 in one or more spouses to delineate the abused versus non-abused groups and for PTSS, using PCL scores >30 (see Table 3). Chi-square analysis was used to examine group membership relationships; the results showed there were no significant differences between male and dual military couples on the likelihood of reporting lower couple functioning, higher coercion, or higher PTSS.

## Prevalence of Secondary Traumatic Stress (STS)

We investigated the presence and prevalence of STS in non-deploying spouses, with STS defined as an elevated PCL score in the absence of a history of trauma exposure. This analysis was limited to the 39 female civilian spouses, because only 2 males in this sample had not deployed to either OIF or OEF. To determine whether symptoms endorsed on the PCL were attributable to STS or could be primary PTSS, we used a two-step analysis process. First, we determined the prevalence of PTSS symptoms above the cut point of 30 on the PCL, then we controlled for the presence of trauma history in the female spouses. The prevalence of STS in the non-deployed female spouses in this study was 34%. That is, 16 of the 47 female spouses who had never deployed reported PCL scores above 30. However, when presence of previous

| TABLE 3 | STUDY MEASURE COMPARISONS BY MALE OR DUAL MILITARY COUPLE | | | | | |
|---|---|---|---|---|---|---|
| | MALE (n = 39) | | DUAL (n = 27) | | TOTALS (n = 66) | |
| COUPLE GROUPS, BY DISTRESS CUT POINTS | n | % | n | % | n | % |
| **Low couple functioning (<48 on RDAS)** | | | | | | |
| Male and female both high | 19 | 48.7 | 12 | 44.4 | 31 | 47.0 |
| At least one spouse low | 20 | 51.3 | 15 | 55.5 | 35 | 53.0 |
| $\chi^2 = 0.06, p = .81$ | | | | | | |
| **High conflict (>20 on WEB)** | | | | | | |
| Male and female both negative | 28 | 71.8 | 21 | 77.8 | 49 | 74.2 |
| At least one spouse positive | 11 | 28.2 | 6 | 22.2 | 17 | 25.8 |
| $\chi^2 = 0.22, p = .63$ | | | | | | |
| **High PTSS (>30 on PCL)** | | | | | | |
| Male and female both negative | 10 | 25.6 | 10 | 37.0 | 20 | 30.3 |
| At least one spouse positive | 29 | 74.4 | 17 | 58.7 | 46 | 69.7 |
| $\chi^2 = 0.98, p = .32$ | | | | | | |

RDAS, Revised Dyadic Adjustment Scale (Busby et al., 1995); WEB, Women's Experience of Battery scale, gender neutral version (Houry et al., 2008); PCL, Post-traumatic Stress Disorder Checklist (Weathers et al., 1993).
n = number of couples.

trauma history, as reported on the TEQ, was entered into the analysis, the prevalence of STS in the female spouses in this study was reduced to 2% ($n = 1$). All other female, non-soldier spouses with PCL scores above the cut-point reported previous traumas that could have accounted for their elevated PCL scores.

## DISCUSSION AND CONCLUSIONS

The results of this study support and expand upon recent findings that individuals with higher PTSS experience lower couple functioning (Allen et al., 2010). We also found evidence that (a) the relationship between PTSS and couple functioning remained even after controlling for the interrelated scores within couples, (b) resilience was a positive predictor of couple functioning even when individual post-traumatic stress levels were high, (c) female gender and violence or coercion in the relationship were negatively associated with couple functioning, and (d) dual military couples were at no greater risk of developing couple distress than male soldier couples. In addition, because most non-military female spouses with high PTSS scores had prior histories of trauma, our findings cast some doubt regarding the concept of STS.

Findings from this study are consistent with recent research indicating that PTSS in service members can interfere with their closest relationship, that of couplehood (Allen et al., 2010). Including both members of the couple, and controlling for the interdependence, was a strength of the current study and adds to our confidence in these findings.

The finding that couples with high resilience also had higher couple functioning despite high levels of PTSS provides a starting place for the development of preventive interventions. Investigating differences between military couples with high resilience and those with low resilience, and finding ways to increase or amplify individual and couple resilience, should be the focus of future research studies. That resilience appears to be a positive protective factor in couple functioning also sets the stage for investigating whether high levels of resilience can prevent PTSS from occurring. The findings indicate that resilience is related to PTSS and couple functioning, but they do not offer much clarity on how resilience affects these important indicators of stress and marital relationships. The eventual goal should be to develop a pre-deployment intervention or training for military couples that will help them develop or expand upon existing protective factors prior to and during deployment. However, more research is needed. Significant investments are being made in interventions designed to bolster resilience in military personnel and their families, despite the fact that we do not have a universal definition for resilience or understand much about how it is best nurtured (Meredith et al., 2011).

The investigation of moderating variables in this study adds considerably to the limited literature on the topic. The finding of increased vulnerability for PTSS and increased influence of PTSS on the couple relationship in females warrants further investigation using a larger sample of healthy female combat veterans, because previous studies of female veterans have been mostly limited to clinical populations (Feczer & Bjorklund, 2009; Nunnink, Goldwaser, Heppner, & Pittman, 2010; O'Campo et al., 2006).

Coercion and inter-personal violence, as measured by the WEB, was also a significant independent predictor of lower couple functioning in the couples in this study. Given the cross-sectional design, there is no way of knowing which variables preceded couple functioning, making mediation testing inappropriate for these data (Zhao et al., 2010). Determining the directionality of these relationships is an important goal for future research. Nonetheless, this finding suggests that we should be screening for signs of violence in clinical settings so that we can intervene as early as possible to protect both members of the couple and their children from further problems.

A finding from this study not previously reported is that PTSS demonstrated a similar effect on couple functioning in both male and dual military couples who have deployed. Approximately 11% of OIF/OEF Army soldiers are female, yet exploration of the role of PTSS in couple functioning in combat veterans of the current conflicts has been limited to a small number of studies, each with few, if any, female soldiers (Basham, 2008; Monson et al., 2009; Sayers, 2011). We sought to address this gap by over-sampling female soldiers, with 41% of our couples self-identifying as dual military (both partners in the military); 27% of the females in our sample (18 of 66) had deployed to OIF or OEF themselves. In our sample, all female soldiers were in couple relationships with male soldiers, creating a dual military partnership. Investigation of potential differences in couple functioning of female soldier and dual military couples is an important step toward developing interventions for all military couples.

The prevalence of STS in this sample was extremely low (approximately 2%). This suggests that STS may be over-estimated in studies where investigators omit measurement of primary trauma in the spouses. Measuring trauma history is important in studies of PTSS due to the possibility of retriggering symptoms as well as the risk of confounding findings.

Our findings related to low reliability of the Trauma Events Questionnaire (TEQ; Vrana & Lauterbach, 1994) in this sample warrant further investigation in larger military couple samples. We did not have a sufficient sample size to further explore the instrument through factor analysis. It is possible that our sample had higher levels and more types of trauma exposure than most military couples. A future psychometric investigation may determine whether the instrument needs to be revised for military populations.

The complex nature of how couples are affected by combat-related PTSS cannot be fully explained in this sample for several reasons. First, no male civilian spouses were recruited into this study, making it difficult to compare gender differences in secondary traumatic symptoms. A goal of future researchers in this field should be to include more civilian male spouses. Second, spouses who reported PTSS levels exceeding the clinical cut point for PTSD all reported a personal history of primary trauma, precluding our ability to determine whether their spouses' combat exposure had been the source of their symptoms. Thus, we cannot determine whether the symptoms that spouses report were (a) transmitted as STS from their combat exposed partner, (b) chronically present and linked to their own personal trauma, (c) a retriggering of previously unresolved traumatic symptoms, or (d) a combination of sources. Only a longitudinal approach to investigating military couples, with data collected at least once prior to combat exposure, could provide the information needed to determine the temporality, etiology, and transmission of PTSS.

Prevalence of PTSS in this sample (50% of civilian and 48% of combat veteran spouses met this cut in our sample) can be compared to studies using the presumptive cut off for PTSD of >30 on the PCL, as recommended for clinical settings by Bliese et al. (2008). When using the less sensitive, but more specific, cut point of 50 on the PCL, our prevalence rate was 18% for civilian and 17% for combat veteran spouses. This closely mirrors rates in a large longitudinal study of OIF/OEF veterans with positive PTSD screening rates of 16.7% for active duty and 24.5% for reserve combat veterans (Milliken et al., 2007). Our use of the more sensitive cut point of PCL >30 was consistent with our study focus on symptom level rather than PTSD diagnosis. We did not include a measure of depressive symptoms, but previous researchers have found that these symptoms often overlap or are co-morbid with PTSS, especially at low levels (Hoge, Auchertonie, & Milliken, 2006; Nemeroff et al., 2006; O'Campo et al., 2006). Therefore, the lower cut point probably captured spouses with either clinically significant depression, or a mixture of PTSS and depressive symptoms.

Cross-sectional data cannot be used to demonstrate causality, only to explore relationships between variables at a single time. The relationships described in this study should be further explored using other methods, such as longitudinal data collected before and after deployment, to better evaluate causality patterns and the presence of mediators. It is also possible that the predictor variables, such as gender, resilience, and coercion or violence, which acted as significant predictors of couple functioning in this sample, may demonstrate significant moderator effects in future studies with larger samples. For this study, sample size and power calculations were based on only the major predictor (PTSS) and outcome variable (RDAS score), and may not have been robust enough for multiple moderation testing. There also may not have been enough variability in this sample to detect differences related to resilience scores. The histograms and standard deviations showed low variability in CD-RISC scores, with a mean of 31 and standard deviation of 6.5, with scores tending toward the high end of resilience.

This sample included primarily Caucasian, non-Hispanic volunteer couples. Inferences about other racial groups should be made with caution. In addition, the recruitment methods, which required consent from both members of the couple, may have favored married couples with stronger marital relationships, as evidenced by high scores in couple satisfaction and adjustment. These couples may have been more secure in their relationship than the average military couple and more open to answering questions about their marriage. Conversely, this could be seen as a strength of the study, because couples who are doing well have the most to teach us about how to help couples who are struggling in their relationship.

Investigation of other post-combat problems, such as depression and traumatic brain injury, and their potential for affecting the couple relationship would be a logical next step in the dyadic exploration of combat veteran couples. It would be important to learn whether resilience can be protective against a range of traumas secondary to combat that are known to affect mental and physical health, couple relationships, parenting quality, and child well-being. In the meantime, nurses can best serve military couples by asking both military and civilian spouses about combat and other trauma exposures, PTSS, and violence or coercion in their relationships. Nurses and other health care professionals should also ensure accurate documentation of trauma history and referrals for treatment during interactions with military couples, as indicated.

## REFERENCES

Allen, E. S., Rhoades, G. K., Stanley, S. M., & Markman, H. J. (2010). Hitting home: relationships between recent deployment, posttraumatic stress symptoms, and marital functioning for Army couples. *Journal of Family Psychology, 24,* 280– 288. doi: 10.1037/a0019405.

Basham, K. (2008). Homecoming as safe haven or new front: attachment and detachment in military couples. *Clinical Social Work Journal, 36,* 83–96. doi: 10.1007/s10615-007-0138-9.

Blake, D. D., Weathers, F. W., Nagy, L. M., Kaloupek, D. G., Gusman, F. D., Charney, D. S., & Keane, T. M. (1995). The development of a clinician-administered PTSD scale. *Journal of Traumatic Stress, 8,* 75–90.

Bliese, P. D., Wright, K., Adler, A., Cabrera, O., Castro, C. A., & Hoge, C. (2008). Validating the Primary Care Posttraumatic Stress Disorder Screen and the Posttraumatic Stress Disorder Checklist with soldiers returning from combat. *Journal of Consulting and Clinical Psychology, 76,* 272–281. doi: 10.1037/0022-006X.76.2.272.

Busby, D. M., Christensen, C., Crane, D. R., & Larson, J. H. (1995). A revision of the Dyadic Adjustment Scale for use with distressed and non-distressed couples: construct hierarchy and multidimensional scales. *Journal of Marital and Family Therapy, 21,* 289–308.

Campbell, J. C., Garza, M. A., Gielen, A. C., O'Campo, P., Kub, J., Jones, A. S., & Jafar, E. (2003). Intimate partner violence and abuse among active duty military women. *Violence Against Women, 9,* 1072–1092. doi: 10.1177/ 1077801203255291.

Campbell-Sills, L., Forde, D. R., & Stein, M. B. (2009). Demographic and childhood environmental predictors of resilience in a community sample. *Journal of Psychiatric Research, 43,* 1007–1012. doi: 10.1016/j.jpsychires.2009.01.013.

Coker, A. L., Pope, B. O., Smith, P. H., Sanderson, M., & Hussey, J. R. (2001). Assessment of clinical partner violence screening tools. *Journal of American Medical Women's Association, 56,* 19–23.

Connor, K. M., & Davidson, J. R. T. (2003). Development of a new resilience scale: the Connor–Davidson Resilience Scale (CD-RISC). *Depression and Anxiety, 18,* 76–82. doi: 10.1002/ da.10113.

Davidson, J. R., Payne, V. M., Connor, K. M., Foa, E. B., Rothbaum, B. O., Hertzberg, M., & Weisler, R. H. (2005). Trauma, resilience and saliostasis: effects of treatment in post-traumatic stress disorder. *International Clinical Psychopharmacology, 20,* 43–48.

Dekel, R., & Solomon, Z. (2007). Secondary traumatization among wives of war veterans with PTSD. In C. Figley, & W. Nash (Eds.), *Combat stress injury: theory, research, and management* (pp. 137–157). New York, NY: Routledge, Taylor & Francis Group.

Department of Defense. (2009). *2008 Surveys of military spouses: impact of deployments on spouses and children.* Washington, DC: Department of Defense, Defense Manpower Data Center.

Elhai, J. D., Gray, M. J., Docherty, A. R., Kashdan, T. B., & Kose, S. (2007). Structural validity of the Posttraumatic Stress Disorder Checklist among college students with a trauma history. *Journal of Interpersonal Violence, 22,* 1471–1478. doi: 10.1177/0886260507305569.

Feczer, D., & Bjorklund, P. (2009). Forever changed: posttraumatic stress disorder in female military veterans, a case report. *Perspectives in Psychiatric Care, 45,* 278–291. doi: 10.1111/j.1744-6163.2009.00230.x.

Figley, C. R. (1995). Compassion fatigue as secondary traumatic stress disorder: an overview. In C. R. Figley (Ed.), *Compassion fatigue* (pp. 1–20). New York, NY: Brunner/Mazel.

Fontana, A., & Rosenheck, R. (2008). Treatment-seeking veterans of Iraq and Afghanistan: comparison with veterans of previous wars. *The Journal of Nervous and Mental Disease, 196,* 513–521. doi: 10.1097/NMD.0b013e31817cf6e6.

Gibbs, D. A., Martin, S. L., Kupper, L. L., & Johnson, R. E. (2007). Child maltreatment in enlisted soldiers' families during combat-related deployments. *The Journal of the American Medical Association, 298,* 528–535. doi: 10.1001/ jama.298.5.528.

Hamilton, S., Nelson-Goff, B. S., Crow, J. R., & Reisbig, A. M. J. (2009). Primary trauma of female partners in a military sample: individual symptoms and relationship satisfaction. *The American Journal of Family Therapy, 37,* 336–346. doi: 10.1080/ 01926180802529965.

Heyman, R. E., Sayers, S. L., & Bellack, A. S. (1994). Global marital satisfaction versus marital adjustment: an empirical comparison of three measures. *Journal of Family Psychology, 8,* 432– 446. doi: 10.1037//0893-3200.8.4.432.

Hoge, C. W., Auchertonie, J. L., & Milliken, C. S. (2006). Mental health problems, use of mental health services, and attrition from military service after returning from deployment to Iraq or Afghanistan. *The Journal of the American Medical Association, 295,* 1023–1032. doi: 10.1001/jama. 295.9.1023.

Houry, D., Rhodes, K. V., Kemball, R. S., Click, L., Cerulli, C., McNutt, L. A., & Kaslow, N. J. (2008). Differences in female and male victims and perpetrators of partner violence with respect to WEB scores. *Journal of Interpersonal Violence, 23,* 1041–1055. doi: 10.1177/0886260507313969.

Institute of Medicine. (2010). *Returning home from Iraq and Afghanistan: preliminary assessment of needs of veterans, service members, and their families.* Washington, DC: The National Academies Press. Retrieved from http://www.nap.edu

Jacelon, C. (1997). The trait and process of resilience. *Journal of Advanced Nursing, 25,* 123–129. doi: 10.1046/j.1365-2648.1997.1997025123.x.

Johnson, M. P. (2006). Conflict and control: gender symmetry and asymmetry in domestic violence. *Violence Against Women, 12,* 1003–1018. doi: 10.1177/1077801206293328.

Karney, B. R., & Crown, J. S. (2007). *Families under stress: an assessment of data, theory, and research on marriage and divorce in the military.* Santa Monica, CA: Rand Corporation. Retrieved from www.rand.org/pubs/monographs/MG599.html

Keen, S. M., Kutter, C. J., Niles, B. L., & Krinsley, K. E. (2008). Psychometric properties of PTSD Checklist in a sample of male veterans. *Journal of Rehabilitation Research & Development, 45,* 465– 474. doi: 10.1682/JRRD.2007.09.0138.

LeardMann, C. A., Smith, T. C., Smith, B., Wells, T. S., & Ryan, M. A. K. (2009). Baseline self reported functional health and vulnerability to Post-traumatic Stress Disorder after combat deployment: prospective US military cohort study. *British Medical Journal, 338,* b1273. doi:10.1136/ bmj.b1273.

MacLean, A., & Edwards, R. D. (2010). The pervasive role of rank in the health of US veterans. *Armed Forces and Society, 36,* 765–785.

Maguen, S., Turcotte, D. M., Peterson, A. L., Dremsa, T. L., Garb, H. N., McNally, R. J., & Litz, B. T. (2008). Description of risk and resilience factors among military medical personnel before deployment to Iraq. *Military Medicine, 173,* 1–9.

Mansfield, A. J., Kaufman, J. S., Marshall, S. W., Gaynes, B., Morrissey, J. P., & Engel, C. C. (2010). Deployment and the use of mental health services among US Army wives. *The New England Journal of Medicine, 362,* 101–109. doi: 10.1056/ NEJMoa0900177.

Meredith, L. S., Sherbourne, C. D., Gaillot, S., Hansell, L., Ritschard, H. V., Parker, A. M., & Wrenn, G. (2011). *Promoting psychological resilience in the U.S.* military. Santa Monica, CA: RAND Corporation.

Milliken, C. S., Auchterlonie, J. L., & Hoge, C. W. (2007). Longitudinal assessment of mental health problems among active duty and reserve component soldiers returning from the Iraq war. *The Journal of the American Medical Association, 298,* 2141–2148. doi: 10.1001/jama.298.18.2141.

Monson, C. M., Taft, C. T., & Fredman, S. J. (2009). Military-related PTSD and intimate relationships: from description to theory-driven research and intervention development. *Clinical Psychology Review, 29,* 707–714. doi: 10.1016/j.cpr.2009.09.002.

Nelson-Goff, B. S., Crow, J. R., Reisbig, A. M. J., & Hamilton, S. (2007). The impact of individual trauma symptoms of deployed soldiers on relationship satisfaction. *Journal of Family Psychology, 21,* 344–353.

Nelson-Goff, B. S., Crow, J. R., Reisbig, A. M. J., & Hamilton, S. (2009). The impact of soldiers' deployments to Iraq and Afghanistan: secondary traumatic stress in female partners. *Journal of Couple and Relationship Therapy, 8,* 291–305.

Nelson-Goff, B. S., & Smith, D. (2005). Systemic traumatic stress: the couple adaptation to traumatic stress model. *Journal of Marital and Family Therapy, 31,* 145–157. doi: 10.1111/j.1752-0606.2005.tb01552.x.

Nemeroff, C. B., Bremner, J. D., Foa, E. B., Mayberg, H. S., North, C. S., & Stein, M. B. (2006). Posttraumatic stress disorder: a state of the science review. *Journal of Psychiatric Research, 40,* 1–21. doi: 10.1016/j.jpsychires.2005.07.005.

Norris, F. H., & Hamblen, J. L. (2004). Standardized self report measures of civilian trauma and PTSD. In J. Wilson, T. M. Keane, & T. Martin (Eds.), *Assessing psychological trauma and PTSD* (pp. 63–102). New York, NY: Guilford.

Nunnink, S. E., Goldwaser, G., Heppner, P. S., & Pittman, J. O. E. (2010). Female veterans of the OEF/OIF conflict: concordance of PTSD symptoms and substance misuse. *Addictive Behaviors, 35,* 655–659. doi: 10.1016/j.addbeh. 2010.03.006.

O'Campo, P., Kub, J., Wood, A., Garza, M., Jones, S., Gielen, A. C., . . . Campbell, J. C. (2006). Depression, PTSD, and comorbidity related to intimate partner violence in civilian and military women. *Brief Treatment and Crisis Intervention, 6,* 99–110. doi: 10.1093/brief-treatment/mhj010.

Palmer, C. (2008). A theory of risk and resilience factors in military families. *Military Psychology, 20,* 205–217. doi: 10.1080/08995600802118858.

Renshaw, K. D., Rodrigues, C. S., & Jones, D. H. (2008). Psychological symptoms and marital satisfaction in spouses of Operation Iraqi Freedom veterans: relationships with spouses' perceptions of veterans' experiences and symptoms. *Journal of Family Psychology, 22,* 586–594. doi: 10.1037/ 0893-3200.22.3.586.

Rentz, E. D., Martin, S. L., Gibbs, D. A., Clinton-Sherrod, M., Hardison, J., & Marshall, S. W. (2006). Family violence in the military: a review of the literature. *Trauma Violence & Abuse, 7,* 93–108. doi: 10.1177/1524838005285916.

Richardson, G. E. (2002). The metatheory of resilience and resiliency. *Journal of Clinical Psychology, 58,* 307–321. doi: 10.1002/jclp.10020.

Sayers, S. L. (2011). Family reintegrations difficulties and couples therapy for military veterans and their spouses. *Cognitive and Behavioral Practice, 18,* 108–120. doi: 10.1016/j.cbpra.2010.03.002.

Smith, P. H., Earp, J. A., & DeVellis, R. (1995). Development and validation of the Women's Experiences with Battering (WEB) scale. *Women's Health, 1,* 273–288.

Spanier, G. B. (1976). Measuring dyadic adjustment: new scales for assessing the quality of marriage and similar dyads. *Journal of Marriage and the Family, 38*, 15–28. doi: 10.2307/350547.

StataCorp. (2009). Stata Statistical Software: release11. In *StataCorp LP*. Wiley Periodicals Inc. Published in Nursing Research and Health 2012, 35, 164–177.

Tanielian, T., Jaycox, L. H., Schell, T. L., Marshall, G. N., Burnam, M. A., Eibner, C., & Vaiana, M. E. (2009). *Invisible wounds: mental health and cognitive care needs of America's returning veterans.* Santa Monica, CA: RAND Corporation. Retrieved from http://veterans.rand.org.

Terhakopian, A., Sinaii, N., Engel, C. C., Schnurr, P. P., & Hoge, C. W. (2008). Estimating population prevalence of posttraumatic stress disorder: an example using the PTSD checklist. *Journal of Traumatic Stress, 21*, 290–300.

Ting, L., Jacobson, J. M., Sanders, S., Bride, B. E., & Harrington, D. (2005). The Secondary Traumatic Stress Scale (STSS): confirmatory factor analysis with a national sample of mental health social workers. *Journal of Human Behavior in the Social Environment, 11*, 177–194. doi: 10.1300/ J137v11n03_09.

Tolin, D. F., & Foa, E. B. (2006). Sex differences in trauma and posttraumatic stress disorder: a quantitative review of 25 years of research. *Psychological Bulletin, 132*, 959–991. doi: 10.1037/1942-9681.S.1.37.

Tusaie, K., & Dyer, J. (2004). Resilience: a historical review of the construct. *Holistic Nursing Practice, 18*, 3–8.

Vrana, S., & Lauterbach, D. (1994). Prevalence of traumatic events and posttraumatic psychological symptoms in a nonclinical sample of college students. *Journal of Traumatic Stress, 7*, 289–301. doi: 10.1007/BF02102949.

Watson Wiens, T., & Boss, P. (2006). Maintaining family resiliency before, during, and after military separation. In C. A. Castro, A. B. Adler, & T. W. Britt (Eds.), *The military family* (pp. 13–38). Westport, CT: Praeger Security International.

Weathers, F. W., Litz, B. T., Herman, D. S., Huska, J. A., & Keane, T. M. (1993, October). *The PTSD Checklist (PCL): reliability, validity and diagnostic utility.* Presented at the Annual Convention of the International Society for Traumatic Stress Studies, San Antonio, TX.

Wheeler, A. R., & Torres Stone, R. A. (2009). Exploring stress and coping strategies among National Guard spouses during times of deployment: a research note. *Armed Forces & Society, 36*, 545–557. doi: 10.1177/0095327(09344066)

Wright, K. M., Bliese, P. D., Thomas, J. L., Adler, A. B., Eckford, R. D., & Hoge, C. W. (2007). Contrasting approaches to psychological screening with U.S. combat soldiers. *Journal of Traumatic Stress, 20*, 965–975. doi: 10.1002/jts.20279.

Zhao, X., Lynch, J. G., & Chen, Q. (2010). Reconsidering Baron and Kenny: myths and truths about mediation analysis. *Journal of Consumer Research, 37*, 197–206. doi: 10.1086/651257.

# Follow-up for Improving Psychological Well Being for Women After a Miscarriage (Review)

*Fiona A Murphy[1], Allyson Lipp[2], Diane L Powles[2]*

This is a reprint of a Cochrane review, prepared and maintained by The Cochrane Collaboration and published in *The Cochrane Library* 2012, Issue 3.

## ABSTRACT

**Background.** Miscarriage is the premature expulsion of an embryo or fetus from the uterus up to 23 weeks of pregnancy and weighing up to 500 grams. International studies using diagnostic tools have identified that some women suffer from anxiety, depression and grief after miscarriage. Psychological follow-up might detect those women who are at risk of psychological complications following miscarriage. This review is necessary as the evidence is equivocal on the benefits of psychological follow-up after miscarriage.

**Objectives.** Whether follow-up affects the psychological well being of women following miscarriage.

**Search methods.** We searched the Cochrane Pregnancy and Childbirth Group's Trials Register (31 December 2011), reference lists of all retrieved papers and contacted professional and lay organisations to obtain any ongoing trials or unpublished data.

**Selection criteria.** Randomised controlled trials only.

**Data collection and analysis.** All potential trials for eligibility according to the criteria specified in the protocol by screening the titles and abstracts, retrieving full reports of

[1]College of Human & Health Science, Swansea University, Swansea, UK.
[2]Faculty of Health, Sport and Science, Department of Care Sciences, University of Glamorgan, Pontypridd, UK.
Contact address: Fiona A Murphy, College of Human & Health Science, Swansea University, Singleton Park, Swansea, West Glamorgan, SA2 8PP, UK. f.murphy@swan.ac.uk.

**Editorial group:** Cochrane Pregnancy and Childbirth Group.
**Publication status and date:** New, published in Issue 3, 2012.
**Review content assessed as up-to-date:** 31 December 2011.
**Citation:** Murphy FA, Lipp A, Powles DL. Follow-up for improving psychological well being for women after a miscarriage. *Cochrane Database of Systematic Reviews* 2012, Issue 3. Art. No.: CD008679. DOI: 10.1002/14651858.CD008679.pub2.

potentially relevant trials for assessment. All review authors extracted data and checked for accuracy. No studies were published in duplicate. When data were missing and only the abstract was available, we attempted to contact the trial authors. We resolved any disagreement through discussion.

**Main results.** Six studies involving 1001 women were included. Three trials compared one counselling session with no counselling. There was no significant difference in psychological well being including anxiety, grief, depression avoidance and self-blame. One trial compared three one-hour counselling sessions with no counselling at four and 12 months. Some subscales showed statistical significance in favour of counselling and some in favour of no counselling. The results for two trials were given in narrative form as data were unavailable for meta-analyses. One trial compared multiple interventions. The other trial compared two counselling sessions with no counselling. Neither study favoured counselling.

**Authors' conclusions.** Evidence is insufficient to demonstrate that psychological support such as counselling is effective post-miscarriage. Further trials should be good quality, adequately-powered using standardised interventions and outcome measures at specific time points. The economic implications and women's satisfaction with psychological follow-up should also be explored in any future study.

## PLAIN LANGUAGE SUMMARY

### Follow-up for Improving Psychological Well Being for Women After a Miscarriage

Miscarriage is the premature, or loss of a fetus, up to 23 weeks of pregnancy. Some women suffer from anxiety and depression after miscarriage which may be part of their grief following the loss. Psychological follow-up might detect those women who are at risk of psychological complications following miscarriage. This review of six studies, involving 1001 women, found that there is insufficient evidence from randomised controlled trials to recommend any method of psychological follow-up. Timing of the counselling interventions varied from one week following miscarriage up to 11 weeks. In all studies the interventions were delivered by different professional groups including a midwife, psychologists and nurses. Measurements of the outcomes were made from one month to 12 months after miscarriage in the different studies, which highlights the uncertainty surrounding the rate of psychological recovery following miscarriage. The two larger studies included a complex combination of interventions and outcome measures so that any potentially significant effects may have been diluted.

Further robust research is needed to determine if any recognised psychological follow-up is effective is hastening psychological recovery following miscarriage.

## BACKGROUND

### Description of the Condition

Although definitions of miscarriage vary internationally, it is defined by the World Health Organization (WHO) as the premature expulsion of an embryo or fetus from the uterus up to 23 weeks of pregnancy and weighing up to 500 grams (WHO 2001). Early pregnancy loss is defined as a confirmed empty sac or sac with fetus but with no fetal heart activity at less than 12 weeks' gestation (Farquharson 2005; RCOG 2006). It is difficult to quantify precisely how many women will have a miscarriage but in a longitudinal Swedish study, Blohm 2008 found that clinical miscarriage constituted 12% of all pregnancies, and 25%of women who had been pregnant by 39 years of age had experienced at least one miscarriage.

This review will focus on spontaneous miscarriage and will not include elective termination of pregnancy, ectopic pregnancy, stillbirth and neonatal death.

There are various categorisations of miscarriage, in that a miscarriage may be complete with all the products of conception passed or incomplete in which some of the products are retained within the uterus. There is an additional category of 'silent' miscarriage or early fetal demise in which the fetus may have been dead for some weeks but has not yet been expelled from the uterus (Trinder 2006). The characteristic symptoms of miscarriage are vaginal blood loss which may be accompanied by pain.

Physical management of women with miscarriage in the UK optimally involves rapid referral to an early pregnancy unit with ultrasound confirmation that the pregnancy is not viable. Management will depend on the category of miscarriage and the woman's clinical condition; women may be offered the option of expectant management where there is no active medical intervention with the miscarriage proceeding of its own accord. Other options are surgical management, in which the retained products of conception are evacuated usually under general anaesthetic; and medical intervention, in which medications are given to induce uterine contractions and evacuation of retained products usually without the need for surgical intervention (RCOG 2006). Systematic reviews by Nanda 2006 and Neilson 2010 suggest that all of these treatments are acceptable and women should be supported to make the choice of treatment which is most suitable for them.

Unlike physical management of women following miscarriage, the evidence on psychological management is less well developed and is the focus of this review. There has been increased awareness of the psychological consequences of miscarriage for women and their partners. International studies using diagnostic tools identified that some women suffer from anxiety and depression after miscarriage (Neugebauer 1997; Nikcevic 1999; Stirtzinger 1999). These and other feelings that women describe have been conceptualised by many as being part of a pattern of grief in response to the loss of a baby (Frost 2007; Malacrida 1998; Mander 1997). Accounts from women about their hospital experiences in one study were critical of how health professionals cared for them with little awareness of their feelings of distress and no effective interventions to support them (Stratton 2008).

## Description of the Intervention

Strategies to provide some kind of psychological follow-up after miscarriage have been proposed. However, these are characterised by their diversity both in terms of the type of follow-up and who provides it. They range from telephone counselling provided by women who have already had a miscarriage to more formal counselling programmes. The mode of intervention could be passive, such as written or electronic information, or active, via telephone, clinic appointment or one-to-one or group support.

## How the Intervention Might Work

Follow-up might detect those women who are at risk of developing or who actually have psychological complications following miscarriage such as anxiety, distress and depression. The United Kingdom RCOG guidelines (RCOG 2006) on the management of women after early pregnancy loss state that support and counselling for women after miscarriage can have significant positive effects on psychological well being. However, a Cochrane review of support after perinatal death, concluded that there is insufficient evidence that such interventions are beneficial (Flenady 2008). Similarly, Stratton 2008 in a review of hospital-based interventions, found little evidence to suggest that follow-up after miscarriage has positive outcomes. It is possible that psychological follow-up could reduce any adverse effects on women such as on their employment, relationships with their partners and other close family members.

## Why It Is Important to Do this Review

Currently once any complications are detected via follow-up, women can be referred to specific agencies which will provide interventions to manage these complications and reduce any adverse psychological outcomes following miscarriage. There is a need to systematically review the evidence on follow-up after miscarriage as it is not known which interventions are effective.

# OBJECTIVES

## Primary

To identify whether follow-up by healthcare professionals or lay organisations at any time affects the psychological well being of women following miscarriage.

## Secondary

To compare the effects of different types of interventions on the psychological well being of women following miscarriage.

# METHODS

## Criteria for Considering Studies for this Review

### Types of Studies

All published and unpublished randomised controlled trials including cluster trials that compare different methods of follow-up after miscarriage. We did not include quasi-randomised trials (e.g. trials that allocate treatment by sequential record number, sequential admitting number, by day of the week).

### Types of Participants

Females of child-bearing age experiencing miscarriage defined as premature expulsion of an embryo or fetus from the uterus up to 23 weeks of pregnancy and weighing up to 500 grams (WHO 2001).

### Types of Interventions

We considered trials if they compared interventions following miscarriage.
1. Psychological intervention versus no intervention.
2. Psychological intervention versus usual care.
3. Psychological intervention versus another psychological intervention.

### Types of Outcome Measures

*Primary Outcomes*
1. Psychological well being as defined by the trial authors.
2. Patient satisfaction as defined by the trial authors.

*Secondary Outcomes*
1. Adverse reaction to follow-up.
2. Referral to primary healthcare services.
3. Admission to hospital.
4. Costs associated with follow-up.

## Search Methods for Identification of Studies
### Electronic Searches

We contacted the Trials Search Co-ordinator to search the Cochrane Pregnancy and Child-birth Group's Trials Register (31 December 2011). The Cochrane Pregnancy and Childbirth Group's Trials Register is maintained by the Trials Search Co-ordinator and contains trials identified from:

1. quarterly searches of the Cochrane Central Register of Controlled Trials (CENTRAL);
2. weekly searches of MEDLINE;
3. weekly searches of EMBASE;
4. handsearches of 30 journals and the proceedings of major conferences;
5. weekly current awareness alerts for a further 44 journals plus monthly BioMed Central email alerts.

Details of the search strategies for CENTRAL, MEDLINE and EMBASE, the list of hand-searched journals and conference proceedings, and the list of journals reviewed via the current awareness service can be found in the 'Specialized Register' section within the editorial information about the Cochrane Pregnancy and Childbirth Group.

Trials identified through the searching activities described above are each assigned to a review topic (or topics). The Trials Search Co-ordinator searches the register for each review using the topic list rather than keywords.

### Searching Other Resources

We searched reference lists of all retrieved papers for additional studies and contacted professional and lay organisations in order to obtain any ongoing trials or unpublished data. We did not apply any language restrictions.

### Data Collection and Analysis

We assessed all potential trials for eligibility according to the criteria specified in the pro-tocol by screening the titles and abstracts. We retrieved full reports of potentially relevant trials for assessment of eligibility based on the inclusion criteria. All review authors extracted the data and checked for accuracy, and we resolved discrepancies by discussion. No studies were published in duplicate. When data were missing, or if only the abstract was available, we attempted to contact the trial authors to obtain the missing information. We resolved any disagreement through discussion or we consulted the Pregnancy and Childbirth Review Group.

*Selection of Studies.* All review authors independently assessed for inclusion all the potential studies we identified as a result of the search strategy.

*Data Extraction and Management.* We designed a form to extract data. For eligible stud-ies, all review authors extracted the data using the agreed form. We entered data into review manager software (Revman 2011) and checked for accuracy.

When information regarding any of the above was unclear, we attempted to contact authors of the original reports to provide further details.

*Assessment of risk of bias in included studies.* All review authors independently assessed risk of bias for each study using the criteria outlined in the *Cochrane Handbook for Systematic Reviews of Interventions* (Higgins 2011).

*(1) Random sequence generation (checking for possible selection bias)* We described for each included study the method used to generate the allocation sequence in sufficient detail to allow an assessment of whether it should produce comparable groups. We assessed the method as:

- low risk of bias (any truly random process, e.g. random number table; computer random number generator);
- high risk of bias (any non-random process, e.g. odd or even date of birth; hospital or clinic record number);
- unclear risk of bias.

*(2) Allocation concealment (checking for possible selection bias)* We described for each included study the method used to conceal allocation to interventions prior to assignment and assessed whether intervention allocation could have been foreseen in advance of, or during recruitment, or changed after assignment. We assessed the methods as:

- low risk of bias (e.g. telephone or central randomisation; consecutively numbered sealed opaque envelopes);
- high risk of bias (open random allocation; unsealed or nonopaque envelopes, alternation; date of birth);
- unclear risk of bias.

*(3.1) Blinding of participants and personnel (checking for possible performance bias)* We described for each included study the methods used, if any, to blind study participants and personnel from knowledge of which intervention a participant received. We consider that studies are at low risk of bias if they were blinded, or if we judge that the lack of blinding would be unlikely to affect results. We assess blinding separately for different outcomes or classes of outcomes. We assessed the methods as:

- low, high or unclear risk of bias for participants;
- low, high or unclear risk of bias for personnel.

*(3.2) Blinding of outcome assessment (checking for possible detection bias)* We described for each included study the methods used, if any, to blind outcome assessors from knowledge of which intervention a participant received. We assessed blinding separately for different outcomes or classes of outcomes. We assessed methods used to blind outcome assessment as:

- low, high or unclear risk of bias.

*(4) Incomplete outcome data (checking for possible attrition bias due to the amount, nature and handling of incomplete outcome data)* We described for each included study, and for each outcome or class of outcomes, the completeness of data including attrition and exclusions from the analysis. We stated whether attrition and exclusions were reported and the numbers included in the analysis at each stage (compared with the total randomised participants), reasons for attrition or exclusion where reported, and whether missing data were balanced across groups or were related to outcomes. Where sufficient information was reported, or could be supplied by the trial authors, we re-included missing data in the analyses which we undertook.

We assessed methods as:

- low risk of bias (e.g. no missing outcome data; missing outcome data balanced across groups);

- high risk of bias (e.g. numbers or reasons for missing data imbalanced across groups; 'as treated' analysis done with substantial departure of intervention received from that assigned at randomisation);
- unclear risk of bias.

*(5) Selective reporting (checking for reporting bias)*  We described for each included study how we investigated the possibility of selective outcome reporting bias and what we found. We assessed the methods as:

- low risk of bias (where it is clear that all of the study's prespecified outcomes and all expected outcomes of interest to the review have been reported);
- high risk of bias (where not all the study's pre-specified outcomes have been reported; one or more reported primary outcomes were not prespecified; outcomes of interest are reported incompletely and so cannot be used; study fails to include results of a key outcome that would have been expected to have been reported);
- unclear risk of bias.

*(6) Other bias (checking for bias due to problems not covered by (1) to (5) above)*  We described for each included study any important concerns we may have had about other possible sources of bias.

Was the trial stopped early due to some data-dependent process? Was there extreme baseline imbalance?

We assessed whether each study was free of other problems that could put it at risk of bias:

- low risk of other bias;
- high risk of other bias;
- unclear whether there is risk of other bias.

*(7) Overall risk of bias*  We made explicit judgements about whether studies were at high risk of bias, according to the criteria given in the *Cochrane Handbook for Systematic Reviews of Interventions* (Higgins 2011). With reference to (1) to (6) above, we assessed the likely magnitude and direction of the bias and whether we considered it was likely to impact on the findings. We explored the impact of the level of bias through undertaking sensitivity analyses - *see* Sensitivity analysis.

## Measures of Treatment Effect

*Dichotomous Data.*  For dichotomous data, we planned to present results as summary risk ratio with 95% confidence intervals.

*Continuous Data.*  For continuous data, we intended to use the mean difference if outcomes were measured in the same way between trials. We used the standardised mean difference to combine trials that measured the same outcome, but used different methods.

## Unit of Analysis Issues

*Cluster-Randomised Trials.*  If identified, we would have included cluster-randomised trials in the analyses along with individually randomised trials. We would have adjusted their sample sizes using the methods described in the *Cochrane Handbook for Systematic Reviews of Interventions* using an estimate of the intracluster correlation co-efficient (ICC) derived from the trial (if possible), or from another source. If ICCs from other sources had been used, we would have reported this and conducted sensitivity analyses to investigate the effect of variation in the ICC. If we had identified both cluster-randomised trials and individually-randomised trials, we planned to synthesise the relevant information. We considered it reasonable to combine the results from both if there was little heterogeneity between the study designs and the interaction between the effect of intervention and the choice of randomisation unit was considered to be unlikely. We also acknowledged heterogeneity in the randomisation unit and would have performed a separate sensitivity analysis to investigate the effects of the randomisation unit.

## Dealing with Missing Data

For included studies, we noted levels of attrition. We explored the impact of including studies with high levels of missing data in the overall assessment of treatment effect by using Sensitivity analysis. For all outcomes we carried out analyses, as far as possible, on an intention-to-treat basis, i.e. we attempted to include all participants randomised to each group in the analyses and all participants would have been analysed in the group to which they were allocated, regardless of whether or not they received the allocated intervention. The denominator for each outcome in each trial was the number randomised minus any participants whose outcomes were known to be missing.

## Assessment of Heterogeneity

We assessed statistical heterogeneity in each meta-analysis using the $T^2$, $I^2$ and $Chi^2$ statistics. We regarded heterogeneity as substantial if $T^2$ is greater than zero and either $I^2$ is greater than 30% or there is a low P value (less than 0.10) in the $Chi^2$ test for heterogeneity.

## Assessment of Reporting Biases

If there were 10 or more studies in the meta-analysis, we planned to investigate reporting biases (such as publication bias) using funnel plots. We would have assessed funnel plot asymmetry visually, and used formal tests for funnel plot asymmetry. For continuous outcomes, we would have used the test proposed by Egger 1997, and for dichotomous outcomes, we planned to use the test proposed by Harbord 2006. If we had detected asymmetry in any of these tests or by a visual assessment, we would have performed exploratory analyses to investigate it.

## Data Synthesis

We carried out statistical analysis using the Review Manager software (RevMan 2011). We planned to use fixed-effect meta-analysis for combining data where it was reasonable to assume that studies were estimating the same underlying treatment effect: i.e. where trials are examining the same intervention, and the trials' populations and methods were judged sufficiently similar. Where there was clinical heterogeneity sufficient to expect that the underlying treatment effects differed between trials, or if substantial statistical heterogeneity was detected, we used random-effects meta-analysis to produce an overall summary if an average treatment effect across trials was considered clinically meaningful. The random-effects summary was treated as the average range of possible treatment effects and we discussed the clinical implications of treatment effects differing between trials. If the average treatment effect was not clinically meaningful, we did not combine trials. Using random-effects analyses, the results were presented as the average treatment effect with 95% confidence intervals, and the estimates of $T^2$ and $I^2$.

## Subgroup Analysis and Investigation of Heterogeneity

If we had identified substantial heterogeneity, we would have investigated it using subgroup analyses and sensitivity analyses. We would have considered whether an overall summary was meaningful, and if it was, we would have used random-effects analysis to produce it.

We planned to carry out the following subgroup analyses.

1. Recurrent miscarriage versus sporadic miscarriage.
2. Early versus late miscarriage.
3. Pre-existing psychological condition versus no psychological condition.

We planned to use the following outcome in subgroup analysis.

- Psychological well being.

For fixed-effect meta-analyses, we planned to conduct subgroup analyses classifying whole trials by interaction tests as described by Deeks 2001. For random-effects and fixed-effect meta-analyses using methods other than inverse variance, we intended to assess differences between subgroups by inspection of the subgroups' confidence intervals; non-overlapping confidence intervals indicate a statistically significant difference in treatment effect between the subgroups.

## Sensitivity Analysis

We planned to carried out sensitivity analyses to explore the effect of trial quality separating using the 'Risk of bias' table to distinguish high-quality from low-quality trials, for example, in allocation concealment and blinding of outcome assessors.

# RESULTS

## Description of Studies

See: Characteristics of included studies; Characteristics of excluded studies.

## Results of the Search

Nineteen papers were identified in the search which covered psychological support for women who have had a miscarriage up to 23 weeks' gestation. We included six studies involving 1001 women (Adolfsson 2006; Lee 1996; Lok Hung 2006; Nikcevic 2007; Swanson 1999; Swanson 2009). We excluded the remaining 13 papers as they were either not randomised controlled trials or were not within gestation limits. Some excluded trials did not provide interventions (*see* Characteristics of excluded studies).

## Risk of Bias in Included Studies

Overall, the quality of the studies was moderate to good. Some studies were unclear regarding blinding. *See* Figure 1; 'Risk of bias' summary and Figure 2 'Risk of bias' graph and Characteristics of included studies.

*Sequence Generation.* Randomisation was adequate in all studies. We contacted one author to confirm that randomisation was by an independent person pulling one of four cards blindly from a box (Swanson 1999).

*Allocation Concealment.* This was low risk in the majority of studies and clear in only one study where allocation concealment was described in personal correspondence from the author (Swanson 1999).

*Blinding.* Following personal communication, blinding was considered adequate in one study (Adolfsson 2006) and for the remainder it was not clear that the participants, clinicians or outcome assessors were blinded. Because of the nature of the interventions, blinding was not considered crucial for the participants or clinicians.

*Incomplete Outcome Data.* Loss to follow-up, withdrawals and exclusions after randomisation were not excessive and explained in all studies. An intention-to-treat analysis was performed in one study (Lok Hung 2006).

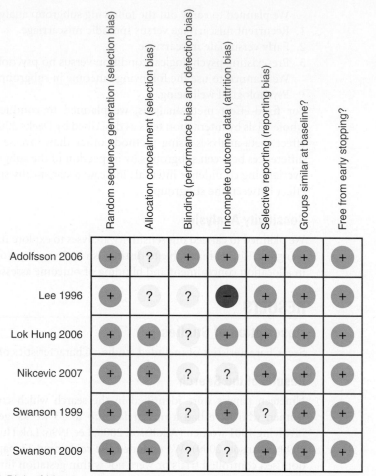

**FIGURE 1** Risk of bias summary: review authors' judgements about each risk of bias item for each included study.

***Selective Outcome Reporting.*** We were only able to access one study protocol to be assured that there was no selective outcome reporting (Lok Hung 2006). One study reported that two subscales measured were dropped from the analysis because they were confounded by alterations due to the women's pregnancy loss (Swanson 1999).

***Other Potential Sources of Bias.*** The participants in all studies were similar at baseline except for percentage of women with children (Lee 1996) and history of infertility (Lok Hung 2006) and were judged by the review authors to be at low risk of bias for this issue. As far as could be ascertained, no studies were stopped early for any reason.

## Effects of Interventions

### 1. One Counselling Session Versus No Counselling (Three Studies 236 Women) (Analysis 1.1)

#### Primary Outcomes

**Psychological well being.** This analysis included three studies with 236 women and compared one counselling session with no counselling (Adolfsson 2006; Lee 1996;

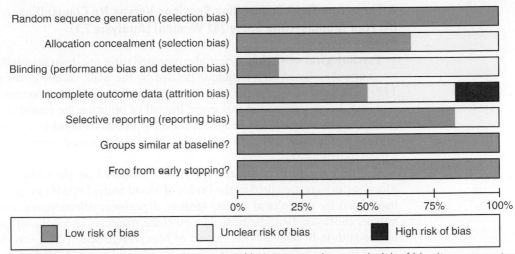

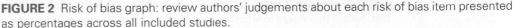

**FIGURE 2** Risk of bias graph: review authors' judgements about each risk of bias item presented as percentages across all included studies.

Nikcevic 2007). The counselling sessions were based on recognised counselling techniques and lasted 50 minutes (Nikcevic 2007) or one hour (Adolfsson 2006; Lee 1996). All three studies used a number of measures to assess psychological well being at four months after miscarriage (Analysis 1.1). For the purpose of analysis, components of the tools used to measure psychological well being are displayed separately. Two studies used the Hospital Anxiety and Depression (HADs) scale (Lee 1996; Nikcevic 2007). Both studies recognised greater than 11 as the threshold for 'caseness' with HADs. When compared with no counselling, one counselling session did not result in a statistically significant reduction in anxiety with the standardised mean difference (SMD) -0.24 (95% confidence interval (CI) -0.62 to 0.15) (Analysis 1.1.1) or depression SMD -0.25 (95% CI -0.63 to 0.14) (Analysis 1.1.2).

When combined, grief as measured on the modified Texas Grief Inventory (Nikcevic 2007) and the Perinatal Grief Scale (Swedish version) (Adolfsson 2006) showed no statistically significant reduction in grief in the counselling group (SMD -0.12; 95% CI - 0.43 to 0.20) (Analysis 1.1.3).

In addition to HADs, Lee 1996 employed the Impact of Events scale and neither of the two components measured were statistically significantly reduced in the counselling group for avoidance (SMD 0.18; 95% CI -0.45 to 0.81) (Analysis 1.1.4) and intrusion (SMD -0.42; 95% CI -1.06 to 0.22) (Analysis 1.1.5). The Perinatal grief Scale (Adolfsson 2006) measured difficulty in coping (SMD -0.08; 95% CI -0.50 to 0.34) (Analysis 1.1.6) as well as grief (see above) and despair (SMD 0.01; 95% CI -0.41 to 0.43) (Analysis 1.1.7). Neither component was statistically significantly reduced by one-hour counselling. In addition to HADs, Nikcevic 2007 used the Texas Grief Inventory which measured grief (see above), self-blame (SMD 0.03; 95% CI -0.45 to 0.51) (Analysis 1.1.8) and worry (SMD -0.42; 95% CI -0.91 to 0.06) (Analysis 1.1.9). Neither analysis showed statistically significant reduction in self-blame or worry as a result of one 50-minute counselling session.

The other primary outcome of patient satisfaction was not assessed in any of the studies.

***Secondary Outcomes.*** The other prespecified secondary outcomes were not assessed.

## 2. Three One-Hour Counselling Sessions Versus No Counselling (At Four Months) (One Study 242 Women) (Analysis 2.1)
### *Primary Outcomes*

**Psychological well being.** One study compared three one-hour counselling sessions with no counselling based on a technique devised by the main author of the study (Swanson 1999). The sessions were conducted at one, five and 11 weeks. A Solomon four group randomised design was used in this study. Instead of omitting the pretest in two of the four groups, as recommended by Solomon, the study authors delayed it. This modification was justified by the study author to reduce the risk of early focused attention on loss serving as a form of treatment.

Outcome measures comprised self-esteem measured on the 10-item Rosenberg scale. Mood states were measured by the Profile of Mood States (POMS) as 'overall mood disturbance' and six subscales of anxiety-tension, depression-dejection, anger-hostility, vigour-fatigue, confusion-bewilderment. The outcome measures of vigour-fatigue were omitted by the author. In addition, the Impact of Miscarriage Scale (IMS) was developed by the author to measure 'overall impact of miscarriage' and four subscales of 'devastating event', 'lost baby' (this refers to whether the woman views the loss as a fetus or a baby), 'personal significance' and 'feeling isolated.'

Of the scores on any of the three scales and eight subscales of all outcome measures (early and delayed measure) (22 in total), only three showed statistical significance for any intervention, either early or delayed at four months. The subscales which identified a significant result were in the measurement tool developed by Swanson 1999. These were Lost baby (early measure) which showed that those women who did not have counselling had improved psychological well being than those who had counselling (SMD 3.99; 95% CI 3.27 to 4.72) (Analysis 2.1.15) (P = 0.00001). However, those women who undertook counselling (early measure) were statistically significantly less likely to view the miscarriage as a Devastating event (SMD -2.52; 95% CI -3.08 to -1.95) (Analysis 2.1.19) (P = 0.00001). Women who undertook counselling (delayed measure) stated that they felt less isolated than women who did not (SMD -0.42; 95% CI -0.84 to -0.01) (Analysis 2.1.22) (P = 0.04). Only two of the three statistically significant results favour counselling. All three significant results were from subscales of the instrument developed by the author (IMS).

Although another study used three counselling sessions as one of the interventions measured at three and five months, data were not available for this analysis despite contact with the author (Swanson 2009).

Patient satisfaction was not assessed in this study.

***Secondary Outcomes.*** The other prespecified secondary outcomes were not assessed.

## 3. Three One-Hour Counselling Sessions Versus No Counselling (At 12 Months) (One Study 242 Women) (Analysis 3.1)

One study compared three one-hour counselling sessions with no counselling based on a technique devised by the main author of the study (Swanson 1999). The sessions were conducted at one, five and 11 weeks. To counter the potential effect of data gathering unwittingly producing a beneficial effect Solomon four group randomised design was implemented where measurements were delayed on half of the treated and half of the control group. Outcome measures comprised self-esteem measured on the 10-item Rosenberg scale. Mood states were measured by the POMS as 'over all mood disturbance' and six subscales of anxiety-tension, depression-dejection, anger-hostility, vigour-fatigue, confusion-bewilderment. The outcome measures of vigour-fatigue were omitted by the author. In addition, the IMS was developed by the author to measure 'overall impact of miscarriage' and four subscales of 'devastating event', 'lost baby', 'personal significance' and 'feeling isolated'.

Of the scores on any of the three scales and eight subscales of all outcome measures (early and delayed measure) (22 in total), only three showed statistical significance for any intervention, either early or delayed at four months. The subscales which measured a significant result were in the measurement tool (IMS) developed by Swanson 1999. At 12 months, the overall impact of miscarriage (delayed measurement) (SMD -0.43; 95% CI -0.85 to - 0.01) showed a statistically significant effect (P = 0.05) (Analysis 3.1.14) towards three one-hour counselling sessions compared with no counselling. Lost baby (delayed measurement) showed a statistically significant effect (SMD 2.15; 95% CI 1.48 to 2.82) (Analysis 3.1.16) for no counselling compared with three one-hour counselling sessions. Personal significance (delayed measurement) (SMD-0.66; 95% CI -1.09 to -0.24) (Analysis 3.1.18) and devastating event (delayed measurement) showed a statistically significant effect (SMD -0.45; 95% CI -0.87 to -0.04) (Analysis 3.1.20) towards three one-hour counselling sessions compared with no counselling. Three of the four significant results favoured counselling over no counselling. All the significant results were from a subscale of an instrument developed by the author (IMS). Significant findings at 12 months differed in that the subscale of isolation at four months was replaced by that of personal significance at 12 months.

Although another study used three counselling sessions as one of the interventions measured at 12 months, data were not available for this analysis despite contact with the author (Swanson 2009).

*Secondary Outcomes.* The other prespecified secondary outcomes were not assessed.

## 4. Two Counselling Sessions Versus No Counselling (One Study 280 Women) (Analysis 4.1)

### Primary Outcomes

**Psychological well being.** One study compared two nurse-led counselling sessions with no counselling (Lok Hung 2006). The first session was 60 minutes face-to-face counselling by a nurse counsellor before discharge. The second session was 30 minutes telephone counselling two weeks after discharge. Outcome measures were the 12-item General Health Questionnaire (GHQ-12) (caseness greater than four), the Beck Depression Inventory (BDI) (caseness greater than12) and the Dyadic Adjustment Scale (DAS) completed at six weeks, three months and six months after miscarriage.

Medians were used to express data in this study and we were unable to extract the means or obtain them despite attempts to contact the author, therefore, the results are in narrative form.

At six weeks post-miscarriage 56/132 (33.3%) women scored at least four on GHQ (median three, interquartile range (IQR) zero to six) in the counselling group compared with 60/136 (44.1%) (median three, IQR zero to seven) in the no-counselling group. Thirty-three women/132 (25%) scored at least 12 on BDI (median four, IQR two to 12) in the counselling group compared with 41/136 (30.1%) (median seven, IQR two to 13) in the no-counselling group. No significant differences were found between the counselling and control groups using an intention-to-treat analysis.

At three months post-miscarriage 32/132 (24.2%) women scored at least four on GHQ (median one, IQR 0 to three) in the counselling group compared with 42/136 (30.9%) (median one, IQR 0 to 4.75) in the no-counselling group. Twenty-four/132 (18.2%) scored at least 12 on BDI (median three, IQR 0 to seven) in the counselling group compared with

27/136 (19.9%) (median four, IQR one to 10) in the no-counselling group. No significant differences were found between the counselling and control groups using an intention-to-treat analysis.

At six months post-miscarriage, 30/132 (22.7%) women scored at least four on GHQ (median 0, IQR zero to three) in the counselling group compared with 27/136 (19.9%) (median one, IQR zero to three) in the no-counselling group. Twenty women/132 (15.2%) scored at least 12 on BDI (median two, IQR zero to seven) in the counselling group compared with 23/136 (16.9%) (median seven, IQR zero to 8.75) in the no-counselling group. No significant differences were found between the counselling and control groups using an intention-to-treat analysis.

Patient satisfaction was not assessed in this study.

*Secondary Outcomes.* The other prespecified secondary outcomes were not assessed.

## 5. Combined Caring (CC), Nurse Caring (NC), Self Caring (SC) and No Treatment (NT) (One Study 341 Women)

One study compared four interventions based on a counselling technique, videos and a workbook devised by the author (Swanson 2009). The comparisons were combined care (CC) comprising one counselling session by nurse counsellors based on the author's post-miscarriage counselling model, three 18-minute videos of the author coaching couples on ways to practice self and partner caring, plus one workbook; nurse caring (NC) comprising three one hour counselling sessions; self-care (SC) comprising three videos plus workbook; and no treatment (NT) (Swanson 2009).

Primary outcomes were measured as depression (CES-D). Women scoring 16 were associated with a higher risk of clinical depression. The secondary outcome of grief was measured by two subscales of the Miscarriage Grief Inventory; (MGI) pure grief (PG) and grief related emotions (GRE) which is adapted from the Texas Grief Inventory (TGI).

Women in all three treatment groups showed a faster rate of recovery from depression (CES-D) compared with women receiving no treatment. However, only three one-hour counselling sessions (NC) met the author's criterion for substantial evidence favouring NC over SC, CC and no treatment for accelerating resolution of depression (Bayesian Odds Ratio 7.9 median -0.7 P = 0.89).

Relative to no treatment there was, according to the author, substantial evidence that all three interventions (NC, SC, CC) hastened women's resolution of pure grief (PG) (Bayesian odds ratio 3.1 median -0.2 P = 0.76). The evidence favoured the impact of SC in hastening women's resolution of GRE (Bayesian odds ratio 3.2 median -0.2 P = 0.76).

According to Swanson 2009, there was no substantial evidence that no treatment was preferable to NC, SC or CC in accelerating women's resolution of pure grief, grief-related emotion or depression.

Patient satisfaction was not assessed in this study.

*Secondary Outcomes.* The other prespecified secondary outcomes were not assessed.

## DISCUSSION

### Summary of Main Results

There is an assumption that miscarriage is an adverse event distressing all affected women to a greater or lesser degree. Until now the extent to which psychological follow-up is necessary to reverse this state has not been examined in a Cochrane systematic review. Given the international nature of systematic reviews, the WHO definition of miscarriage was used with the limit of 23 weeks' gestation in contrast to the UK definition of 24 weeks' gestation (RCOG 2006). It is possible that a very small number of women were between 23 and 24 weeks' gestation in one study (Lok Hung 2006) although this was calculated as unlikely by the review authors, although two other studies (Neugebauer 2006; Rajan 1993) were sufficiently at risk of including women up to 28 weeks that they were excluded. Planned sensitivity analyses were not possible as no studies examined recurrent miscarriages as a specific event, differentiated between early and late miscarriages or between women with a pre-existing psychological condition and those without.

The interventions following miscarriage mainly consisted of one or a number of counselling sessions using recognised counselling techniques. Timing of the interventions varied from one week following miscarriage (Swanson 1999; Swanson 2009), up to 11 weeks (Swanson 1999; Swanson 2009). It was not possible to compare different types of psychological follow-up via a meta-analysis given the heterogeneity between studies.

In all studies the interventions were delivered by different professional groups including a midwife (Adolfsson 2006), psychologists (Lee 1996; Nikcevic 2007) and nurses (Lok Hung 2006; Swanson 1999; Swanson 2009), which may have had an impact on the way in which the intervention was delivered. No study compared professionals delivering the intervention. The time span of the studies covered more than a decade and so it is possible that psychological interventions may have changed during that period.

The major primary outcome was psychological well being. We were unable to report the majority of the studies as meta-analyses but were able to report them as forest plots with narrative. Under the primary outcome of psychological well being, a wide range of outcomes were measured from those more commonly anticipated such as grief, anxiety and depression to emotional disturbance, self-esteem and isolation. Outcome measures used included validated tools, some of which had been modified, for example, a Swedish version of the Perinatal grief Scale (Adolfsson 2006) and others which had been developed by the study authors (Impact of Miscarriage Scale Swanson 1999) (Miscarriage Grief Inventory Swanson 2009). The tools also varied in that some were generic such as the Hospital Anxiety and Depression Scale (Lee 1996; Nikcevic 2007) and others were miscarriage specific (Swanson 1999; Swanson 2009). Caseness, or the level at which women were judged to benefit from psychological follow-up using a specific tool, was not made clear in all studies. Some studies did not state whether a high score indicated psychological ill health or well being (Nikcevic 2007; Swanson 2009). All of these issues made it challenging to pool the results and compare findings.

Timing of outcome measurements differed markedly between studies from one month (Lok Hung 2006) to 12 months (Swanson 1999) highlighting the uncertainty surrounding the rate of psychological recovery following miscarriage. One study noted that anxiety, depression and grief reduced significantly in all three groups with time (Nikcevic 2007). Psychological well being was measured and improved with time which may or may not have been influenced by the intervention in four other studies (Lee 1996; Lok Hung 2006; Swanson 1999; Swanson 2009).

The possibility that the measurement of grief, depression and other associated symptoms act as part of the healing process by allowing the woman to talk about her feelings was explored in one study. The author attempted to manage this possibility by organising early or delayed measurement, but this did not make a difference to the overall results (Swanson 1999).

Generally the studies have shown that women's reactions to miscarriage vary and the extent of depression, grief and anxiety differ. Only one study showed some significant outcomes. However, they were unlikely to be of significance overall as they represented differences between delayed and early measures as well as individual subscales on a complex tool developed by the study author (Swanson 2009). No significant results were found in this study on the widely used, standardised scales.

Three studies, two of which were combined in a forest plot, measured the generic outcomes of anxiety, depression and grief. Although the results favoured counselling none were significant. The other primary outcome of patient satisfaction was not measured in any of the trials. We maintain that this is an important outcome as evidence of satisfaction alone is not a reason to provide a service. In addition, none of the secondary outcomes identified by the review authors as important were reported. They included adverse reaction to follow-up, referral to primary healthcare services, admission to hospital and costs associated with follow-up. It is possible that an adverse reaction, referral or admission to hospital following psychological follow-up is unlikely and therefore these outcomes may not be a priority outcome measure for primary studies.

## Overall Completeness and Applicability of Evidence

Our published protocol described our plan to analyse a series of major and minor outcomes. We were able to analyse one of the primary outcomes but none of the secondary outcomes were included in any studies. All eligible randomised controlled trials were included up to April 2011. The majority of studies lacked power. The two larger studies (Swanson 1999; Swanson 2009) included such a complex combination of interventions and outcome measures that any potentially significant effects may have been diluted.

## Quality of the Evidence

This review examined psychological follow-up for 1001 women after miscarriage in six randomised controlled trials. The studies were single centre, from a range of countries, over a decade and a half. Overall, the risk of bias was judged to be low, although allocation concealment and blinding was unclear as it was not stated in the majority of studies. It was recognised that given the nature of the trials, blinding of the participants and clinicians would not be possible.

## Potential Biases in the Review Process

There are a number of limitations to this review. Suprisingly, most of the studies published in the last decade did not have a published protocol and to our knowledge, had not registered their study in one of the many trial registries, indicating that a broad search strategy was still necessary. Lay organisations providing psychological follow-up were included in the search strategy, but none were found.

Strengths of this review include the methodological rigour applied, including a published protocol, data analysis and narrative, which allowed us to make the findings explicit.

## Agreements and Disagreements with other Studies or Reviews

A Cochrane review on perinatal death (Flenady 2008), has indicated that there is insufficient evidence to show that psychological follow-up improves the well being of women following perinatal death. Similarly, this review has found a lack of evidence to show that psychological follow-up is beneficial for women following miscarriage. However, some women may benefit from psychological follow-up and the review authors recommend that any service already in place should continue taking into account women's preference pending further evidence.

## AUTHORS' CONCLUSIONS

### Implications for Practice

Evidence is insufficient to demonstrate the superiority of either psychological support such as counselling or no intervention postmiscarriage. Given the equivocal evidence, women's preference should play a large role in the decision-making process.

### Implications for Research

Further evaluation of the effectiveness of psychological follow-up for women following miscarriage should be based on good quality, adequately-powered randomised trials. Future trials should use standardised interventions, standardised outcome measures at specified time points.

Women's satisfaction with psychological follow-up should be explored in future studies. Given the costs of these interventions, the economic implications for this service should also be integrated into any future study.

## ACKNOWLEDGMENTS

All authors would like to acknowledge Swansea University and the University of Glamorgan for allowing them the time to undertake the protocol and the full review. As part of the pre-publication editorial process, this review has been commented on by three peers (an editor and two referees who are external to the editorial team) and the Group's Statistical Adviser.

## REFERENCES

**References to Studies Included in this Review**

**Adolfsson 2006** (published data only)

Adolfsson, A. (2006, June). *The effect of structured second visit to midwifes in women with early miscarriages, a randomized study*. 10th International Conference of Maternity Care Researchers, Lund, Sweden.

*Adolfsson, A., Bertero, C., & Larsson, P. G. (2006). Effect of a structured follow-up visit to a midwife on women with early miscarriage: a randomized study. *Acta Obstetricia et Gynecologica Scandinavica, 85*, 330–335.

**Lee 1996** (published data only)

Lee, C., Slade, P., & Lygo, V. (1996). The influence of psychological debriefing on emotional adaptation in women following early miscarriage: a preliminary study. *British Journal of Medical Psychology, 69*(Pt 1), 47–58.

**Lok Hung 2006** (published and unpublished data)

Lok, I. H. (2006). *Psychological morbidity after miscarriage* [thesis], University of Hong Kong.

*Indicates the major publication for the study

**Nikcevic 2007** (published data only)

Nikcevic, A. V., Kuczmierczyk, A. R., & Nicolaides, K. H. (2007). The influence of medical and psychological interventions on women's distress after miscarriage. *Journal of Psychosomatic Research*, *63*(3), 283–290.

**Swanson 1999** (published data only)

Swanson, K. M. (1999). Effects of caring, measurement, and time on miscarriage impact and women's well-being. *Nursing Research*, *48*(6), 288–298.

**Swanson 2009** (published data only)

Swanson, K. M., Chen, H. T., Graham, C. J., Wojnar, D. M., & Petras, A. (2009). Resolution of depression and grief during the first year after miscarriage: a randomized controlled clinical trial of couples-focused interventions. Journal of Women's Health, 18(8), 1245–1257.

## References to Studies Excluded from this Review

**Broen 2004** (published data only)

Broen, A. N., Moum, T. R., Bødtker, A. S., & Ekeberg, O. (2004). Psychological impact on women of miscarriage versus induced abortion: a 2-year follow-up study. *Psychosomatic Medicine*, *66*(2), 265–271.

**Broen 2005** (published data only)

Broen, A. N., Moum, T. R., Bødtker, A. S., & Ekeberg, O. (2005). The course of mental health after miscarriage and induced abortion: a longitudinal, five-year follow-up study. *BMC Medicine*, *3*, 265–71.

**Cordle 1994** (published data only)

Cordle, C. J., & Prettyman, R. J. (1994). A 2-year follow-up of women who have experienced early miscarriage. *Journal of Reproductive and Infant Psychology*, *12*, 37–43.

**Jacobs 2000** (published data only)

Jacobs, J., & Harvey, J. (2009). Evaluation of an Australian miscarriage support programme. *British Journal of Nursing*, *9*(1), 2–6.

**Lefkof 2002** (published data only)

Lefkof, J., & Glazer, G. (2002). Grief after miscarriage: practical interventions can assist with far-reaching loss. *Advance for Nurse Practitioners*, *10*(10), 79–82.

**Luise 2002** (published data only)

Luise, C., Jermy, K., Collons, W. P., & Bourne, T. H. (2002). Expectant management of incomplete, spontaneous first-trimester miscarriage: outcome according to initial ultrasound criteria and value of follow-up visits. *Ultrasound in Obstetrics & Gynecology*, *19*(6), 580–582.

**Neugebauer 2006** (published data only)

Neugebauer, R., Kline, J., Markowitz, J. C., et al. (2006). Pilot randomized controlled trial of interpersonal counseling for subsyndromal depression following miscarriage. *Journal of Clinical Psychiatry*, *67*(8), 1299–1304.

**Neugebauer 2007** (published data only)

Neugebauer, R., Kline, J., Bleiberg, K., et al. (2007). Preliminary open trial of interpersonal counselling for subsyndromal depression following miscarriage. *Depression and Anxiety*, *24*(3), 219–222.

**Nikcevic 1998** (published data only)

Nikcevic, A. V., Tunkel, S. A., & Nicolaides, K. H. (1998). Psychological outcomes following missed abortions and provision of follow-up care. *Ultrasound in Obstetrics and Gynecology*, *11*(2), 123–128.

**Nikcevic 2003** (published data only)

Nikcevic, A. V. (2003). Development and evaluation of a miscarriage follow up clinic. *Journal of Reproductive & Infant Psychology*, *21*(3), 207–217.

**Rajan 1993** (published data only)

Rajan, L., & Oakley, A. (1993). No pills for heartache: the importance of social support for women who suffer pregnancy loss. *Journal of Reproductive and Infant Psychology*, *11*, 75–87.

**Sejourne 2011** (published data only)

Sejourne, N., Callahan, S., & Chabrol, H. (2011). The efficiency of a brief support intervention for anxiety, depression and stress after miscarriage [French]. Jo*urnal de Gynecologie, Obstetrique et Biologie de la Reproduction, 40*(5), 437–443.

**Thaper 1992** (published data only)

Thapar, A. K., & Thapar, A. (1992). Psychological sequelae of miscarriage: a controlled study using the General Health Questionnaire and the Hospital Anxiety and Depression scale. *British Journal of General Practice, 42*(356), 94–96.

## Additional References

**Blohm 2008**

Blohm, F., Friden, B., & Milsom, I. (2008). A prospective longitudinal population-based study of clinical miscarriage in an urban Swedish population. *BJOG: An International Journal of Obstetrics & Gynaecology, 115*(2), 176–183.

**Deeks 2001**

Deeks J. J., Altman D. G., Bradburn M. J. (2001). Statistical methods for examining heterogeneity and combining results from several studies in meta-analysis. In M. Egger, G. Davey Smith, & D. G. Altman (Eds.), *Systematic reviews in health care: meta-analysis in context.* London: BMJ Books.

**Egger 1997**

Egger M., Smith G. D., Schneider M., Minder C. (1997). Bias in meta-analysis detected by a simple, graphical test. *British Medical Journal 315*, 629–634.

**Farquharson 2005**

Farquharson, R. G., Jauniaux, E., & Exalto, N. (2005). Updated and revised nomenclature for description of early pregnancy events. *Human Reproduction, 20*, 3008–11.

**Flenady 2008**

Flenady, V., & Wilson, T. (2008). Support for mothers, fathers and families after perinatal death. *Cochrane Database of Systematic Reviews, 2008*(1). doi:10.1002/ 14651858.CD000452.pub2.

**Frost 2007**

Frost, J., Bradley, H., Levitas, R., Smith, L., & Garcia, J. (2007). The loss of possibility: scientisation of death and the special case of early miscarriage. *Sociology of Health and Illness, 29*(7), 1003–1022.

**Harbord 2006**

Harbord, R. M., Egger, M., & Sterne, J. A. (2006). A modified test for small-study effects in meta-analyses of controlled trials with binary endpoints. *Statistics in Medicine, 25*, 3443–3457.

**Higgins 2011**

Higgins, J. P. T., Green, S., (Eds.). (2011). *Cochrane Handbook for Systematic Reviews of Interventions Version 5.1.0* [updated March, 2011]. The Cochrane Collaboration. Available from www.cochrane-handbook.org.

**Malacrida 1998**

Malacrida, C. (1998). *Mourning the dreams.* Alberta Canada: Qual Institute Press.

**Mander 1997**

Mander, R. (1997). Perinatal grief: understanding the bereaved and their careers. In J. Alexander, C. Roth, & V. Levy (Eds.), *Midwifery practice* (pp. 29–50). Basingstoke, England: Macmillan.

**Nanda 2006**

Nanda, K., Peloggia, A., Grimes, D. A., Lopez, L. M., & Nanda, G. (2006). Expectant care versus surgical treatment for miscarriage. *Cochrane Database of Systematic Reviews, 2006*(2). doi:10.1002/ 14651858.CD003518.pub2.

**Neilson 2010**

Neilson, J. P., Gyte, G. M. L., Hickey, M., Vazquez, J. C., & Dou, L. Medical treatments for incomplete miscarriage (less than 24 weeks). *Cochrane Database of Systematic Reviews 2010*(1). doi:10.1002/14651858.CD007223.pub2.

**Neugebauer 1997**

Neugebauer, R., Kline, J., Shrout, P., et al. (1997). Major depressive disorder in the 6 months after miscarriage. *Journal of the American Medical Association, 277*(5), 383–388.

**Nikcevic 1999**

Nikcevic, A., Tunkel, S., & Kuczmierczyk, A. (1999). Investigation of the cause of miscarriage and its influence on women's psychological distress. *British Journal of Obstetrics and Gynaecology, 106*(8), 808–813.

**RCOG 2006**

Royal College of Obstetricians and Gynaecologists (RCOG). (2006). *Management of early pregnancy loss.* London: Royal College of Obstetricians and Gynaecologists.

**RevMan 2011**

The Nordic Cochrane Centre, & The Cochrane Collaboration. (2011). *Review manager (RevMan). 5.1.* Copenhagen: The Nordic Cochrane Centre, & The Cochrane Collaboration.

**Stirtzinger 1999**

Stirtzinger, R. M., Robinson, D. E., Stewart, D. E., & Ralevski, E. (1999). Parameters of grieving in spontaneous abortion. *International Journal of Psychiatry in Medicine, 29*, 235–249.

**Stratton 2008**

Stratton, K., & Lloyd, L. (2008). Hospital-based interventions at and following miscarriage: literature to inform a research-practice initiative. *Australian and New Zealand Journal of Obstetrics and Gynaecology, 48*, 5–11.

**Trinder 2006**

Trinder, J., Brocklehurst, P., Porter, R., Read, M., Vyas, S., & Smith, L. (2006). Management of miscarriage: expectant, medical, or surgical? results of randomised controlled trial (miscarriage treatment (MIST) trial). British Medical Journal, 332, 1235–1240.

**WHO 2001**

World Health Organization (WHO). (2001). *Definitions and indicators in family planning, maternal & child health and reproductive health: WHO regional strategy on sexual and reproductive health.* Geneva: World Health Organization.

# CHARACTERISTICS OF STUDIES

## Characteristics of Included Studies [Ordered by Study ID]

**Adolfsson 2006**

| | |
|---|---|
| Methods | Randomised controlled trial. |
| Participants | Women who had experienced complete, incomplete or missed early miscarriage before 13 weeks' gestation |
| | Inclusion criteria |
| | Visit to gynaecologic outpatient clinic to diagnose miscarriage before 13 weeks' gestation. Over 18 years of age. |
| | Swedish speaking. |
| | N = 116 commenced the study, 88 completed. |
| | Excluson criteria |
| | Pregnancy kept secret from next of kin. |
| | Extrauterine or suspicion of extrauterine pregnancy. |
| Interventions | Intervention group 1: a structured conversation with 1 midwife for 60 minutes focusing on the woman's experience of miscarriage and taking her through the process of Swanson's caring science theory. |
| | N = 43. |
| | Comparison group 2: met 1 of 5 midwives during a 30-minute visit who asked about their general health and any complications. At this visit the midwife did not ask about the woman's feelings and emotions. |
| | N = 45. |
| Outcomes | Reduction of women's grief as measured at 1 and 4 months post-miscarriage by: |
| | • Perinatal Grief Scale Swedish Short Version (PGS) at the follow-up visit to the midwife 1 month after miscarriage and at 4 months after miscarriage. The PGS has 3 subscales measuring grief, difficulty in coping and despair. |
| Notes | 1. Setting: gynaecologic clinic, south west Sweden. |
| | 2. When partners accompanied women they were reminded that the focus was on the woman. |
| | 3. Caseness threshold for PGS not stated (minimum sum 33 maximum 330). |
| | 4. No intention-to-treat analysis performed. |

### RISK OF BIAS

| BIAS | AUTHORS' JUDGEMENT | SUPPORT FOR JUDGEMENT |
|---|---|---|
| Random sequence generation (selection bias) | Low risk | Randomisation was performed in blocks of 10. |
| Allocation concealment (selection bias) | Unclear risk | Sealed envelopes, not stated as opaque. |
| Blinding (performance bias and detection bias) All outcomes | Low risk | Clinicians and outcomes assessors blinded. Participants not blinded but asked not to discuss their care during the study with other participants (personal communication with the author) |
| Incomplete outcome data (attrition bias) All outcomes | Low risk | Of the 116 included in the study, 28 did not complete either the first questionnaire or the second questionnaire |
| Selective reporting (reporting bias) | Low risk | Reports all pre-specified outcomes but we have not accessed the trial protocol |
| Groups similar at baseline? | Low risk | For age, gestational length, children, haemorrhage. |
| Free from early stopping? | Low risk | There was no statement indicating that the study was stopped early |

*Continued*

**Lee 1996**

| | |
|---|---|
| Methods | Randomised controlled trial. |
| Participants | Women who had experienced a miscarriage up to 19 weeks' gestation |
| | <u>Inclusion criteria</u> |
| | Pregnancy of 6 to 19 weeks at the time of miscarriage. |
| | No previous miscarriage. |
| | Aged 18 years or over. |
| | Able to speak and read English fluently. |
| | Had wanted pregnancy to continue. |
| | Were not under psychological or psychiatric care or taking psychoactive drugs at the time of miscarriage |
| | N = 40. |
| | <u>Exclusion criteria</u> |
| | Those who had intended to terminate the pregnancy. |
| Interventions | <u>Intervention group 1:</u> 1-hour long psychological debriefing by a female psychologist in their own home 2 weeks post-miscarriage. |
| | N = 21 |
| | <u>Comparison group 2:</u> no intervention. |
| | N = 18 |
| Outcomes | Emotional adaptation measured at 4 months post-miscarriage by: |
| | • Hospital Anxiety and Depression Scale (HADS), subscales of anxiety and depression. |
| | • Impact of Events Scale (IES), subscales of intrusion (intrusive thoughts) and avoidance. |
| | • Reaction to Miscarriage Questionnaire (RMQ) (outcomes not reported). |
| | • Perceptions of Care (POC) self-designed questionnaire (outcomes not reported). |
| | Questionnaires sent by post 2 days and 4 months post-miscarriage to all participants |
| Notes | 1. Setting Sheffield University Hospitals NHS Trust, UK. |
| | 2. Caseness threshold for HADs 11 >. |

### RISK OF BIAS

| BIAS | AUTHORS' JUDGEMENT | SUPPORT FOR JUDGEMENT |
|---|---|---|
| Random sequence generation (selection bias) | Low risk | 'Women were randomly allocated to Group 1 or Group 2.' |
| Allocation concealment (selection bias) | Unclear risk | Not stated. |
| Blinding (performance bias and detection bias) All outcomes | Unclear risk | Participants, clinicians and outcomes assessors not stated as blinded |
| Incomplete outcome data (attrition bias) All outcomes | High risk | 7 women did not return questionnaire and were excluded from the study. |
| | | 14 indicated that they did not wish to have a follow-up appointment and were excluded from the data analysis |
| Selective reporting (reporting bias) | Low risk | Reports all pre-specified outcomes but we were not able to access the trial protocol |
| Groups similar at baseline? | Low risk | 'There were no significant differences between groups on any measures taken at phase 1, except that the percentage of women with children in group 1 (38%) was significantly lower than that of women in group 2 (77.8%).' |
| Free from early stopping? | Low risk | There was no statement indicating that the study was stopped early |

**Lok Hung 2006**

| | |
|---|---|
| Methods | Randomised controlled trial. |
| Participants | Women who had experienced a miscarriage up to 24 weeks' gestation (see notes) |
| | Inclusion criteria |
| | Miscarriage before 24 weeks. |
| | N = 280 (12 withdrew after randomisation). |
| | Exclusion criteria |
| | Patients who were unwilling to participate, with actively treated psychiatric disease, non-Chinese, visitors to Hong Kong |
| Interventions | Intervention group 1 |
| | A 1-hour counselling session by a nurse following baseline questionnaire while in hospital and a second 30-minute telephone counselling session 2 weeks later. |
| | N = 132. |
| | Control group 2 |
| | 'Routine clinical practice and attended by the clinical staff as usual. No specific counseling or follow-up care was arranged.' |
| | N = 136. |
| Outcomes | Assessment of the proportion of women with psychological morbidity after miscarriage at baseline, 6 weeks, 3 and 6 months measured by: |
| | • General Health Questionnaire (GHQ-12). |
| | • Beck's Depression Inventory (BDI). |
| Notes | 1. Author reported medians and ranges only, means could not be obtained despite attempts to contact the author. |
| | 2. This study employed the UK definition of miscarriage (up to 24 weeks' gestation) whereas this review employed the WHO definition (up to 23 weeks' gestation). Demographic data reported gestational age as a mean of 9.6 weeks (SD ± 2.8). The study was therefore included on the advice of a statistician as it was thought unlikely that any women would be between 23 and 24 weeks' gestation. |
| | 3. Caseness threshold for General Health Questionnaire (GHQ-12) > 4; caseness threshold for Beck's Depression Inventory (BDI) using a threshold of > 12. |

### RISK OF BIAS

| BIAS | AUTHORS' JUDGEMENT | SUPPORT FOR JUDGEMENT |
|---|---|---|
| Random sequence generation (selection bias) | Low risk | 'Randomised using a set of sealed, opaque, sequentially numbered envelopes, each containing a computer-generated random number denoting the randomisation result.' |
| Allocation concealment (selection bias) | Low risk | 'Sealed, opaque, sequentially numbered envelopes, each containing a computer-generated random number denoting the randomisation result.' |
| Blinding (performance bias and detection bias) All outcomes | Unclear risk | Participants, clinicians and outcomes assessors not stated as blinded |
| Incomplete outcome data (attrition bias) All outcomes | Low risk | At 6 weeks there were 96 in the intervention group and 99 in the control group, at 3 months 105 and 115 and at 6 months 104 and 110 respectively. An intention-to-treat analysis was performed |
| Selective reporting (reporting bias) | Low risk | Reports all pre-specified outcomes as we were able to access the trial protocol |

*Continued*

**Lok Hung 2006—cont'd**

| | | |
|---|---|---|
| Groups similar at baseline? | Low risk | Similar for education, employment status, previous miscarriage, planned, wanted pregnancy, miscarriage symptoms, management of miscarriage. 314 women in the control group had a history of infertility compared to 187 in the counselling group |
| Free from early stopping? | Low risk | There was no statement indicating that the study was stopped early |

**Nikcevic 2007**

| | |
|---|---|
| Methods | Randomised controlled trial. |
| Participants | Women found to have a missed miscarriage at 10 to 14 weeks' gestation. |
| | <u>Inclusion criteria</u> |
| | As above. |
| | N = 80 commenced the study, 66 completed. |
| | <u>Exclusion criteria</u> |
| | Women with a history of perinatal death. |
| | Elective termination for foetal abnormality. |
| | Recurrent miscarriage. |
| | Inability to speak and read English fluently. |
| | Those under psychological or psychiatric care. |
| Interventions | <u>Intervention group 1:</u> 1 session of psychological counselling with a psychologist for 50 minutes 5 weeks after the miscarriage. |
| | N = 39. |
| | <u>Comparison group 2</u>: no psychological counselling. |
| | N = 41. |
| Outcomes | Women's distress post-miscarriage measured at 4, 7 and 16 weeks post-miscarriage by: |
| | • Hospital Anxiety and Depression Scale (HADS) subscales anxiety and depression. |
| | • Modified Texas Grief Inventory (TGI) subscales grief, self-blame and worry. |
| | • Questionnaires sent by post to all participants on diagnosis of missed miscarriage and at 4, 7 and 16 weeks. |
| Notes | 1. Setting: Harris Birthright Research Centre, UK. |
| | 2. Only women with missed miscarriage included. On diagnosis, all women were offered the option of investigations to ascertain cause. |
| | 3. An additional control group was derived non-randomly from women attending another hospital and has not been included in these results. |
| | 4. Caseness 11 > for HADs. |

**RISK OF BIAS**

| BIAS | AUTHORS' JUDGEMENT | SUPPORT FOR JUDGEMENT |
|---|---|---|
| Random sequence generation (selection bias) | Low risk | 'Randomly allocated'... 'on the basis of computer generated random number tables' |
| Allocation concealment (selection bias) | Low risk | 'At the end of the medical consultation, the doctor opened a sealed envelope and accordingly invited the women allocated to the intervention group to stay for psychological counselling.' |

**Nikcevic 2007—cont'd**

| | | |
|---|---|---|
| Blinding (performance bias and detection bias) All outcomes | Unclear risk | Participants, clinicians and outcomes assessors not stated as blinded |
| Incomplete outcome data (attrition bias) All outcomes | Unclear risk | 14 women did not complete the second and third questionnaires; 2 women from the intervention group were excluded (1 had a second miscarriage during the study and 1 had psychological counselling arranged elsewhere) |
| Selective reporting (reporting bias) | Low risk | Reports all pre-specified outcomes but we were not able to access the trial protocol |
| Groups similar at baseline? | Low risk | For age, Caucasian, married, children, miscarriage history, planned pregnancy, cause. There was a difference in those with a university education between group 1 (16) and group 2 (10) |
| Free from early stopping? | Low risk | There was no statement indicating that the study was stopped early |

**Swanson 1999**

| | |
|---|---|
| Methods | Solomon 4 group randomised experimental design with repeated measures |
| Participants | Women who had experienced a miscarriage. |
| | <u>Inclusion criteria</u> |
| | At least 18 years of age. |
| | Miscarried at 20 weeks or less. |
| | Within 5 weeks of loss. |
| | Could speak and write English. |
| | N – 242. |
| | <u>Exclusion criteria</u> |
| | Not stated. |
| Interventions | <u>Intervention group 1</u>: 1-hour long counselling sessions following Swanson's middle-range caring theory conducted by the principal investigator or a research associate at 1, 5 and 11 weeks after study entry with early measures. |
| | N = 56. |
| | <u>Intervention group 2</u>: 1-hour long counselling sessions following Swanson's middle-range caring theory conducted by the principal investigator or a research associate at 1, 5 and 11 weeks after study entry with delayed measures. |
| | N = 60. |
| | <u>Comparison group 3</u>: no counselling with early measures. |
| | N = 64. |
| | <u>Comparison group 4:</u> no counselling with delayed measures. |
| | N = 62. |

*Continued*

**Swanson 1999—cont'd**

| | |
|---|---|
| Outcomes | Women's integration of loss and emotional well-being measured at enrollment, 6 weeks, 4 months and 1 year or 4 months and 1 year post-miscarriage using the following questionnaires: |
| | • Rosenberg Self-esteem Scale, subscale self-esteem. |
| | • Profile of Mood States (POMS), subscales anxiety-tension, depression-dejection, anger-hostility, and confusion-bewilderment. |
| | • Impact of Miscarriage Scale (IMS), subscales impact of miscarriage, lost baby, personal significance, devastating event, isolated. |
| | Intervention 1 and 2 were measured 'early' immediately after enrolling, at 6 weeks, 4 months and 1 year. |
| | Comparison 3 and 4 had 'delayed' measurement at 4 months and 1 year after enrolling |
| Notes | 1. Setting: USA. |
| | 2. Solomon 4-group design comprises 2 extra control groups, which serve to reduce the influence of confounding variables and allow the researcher to test whether the pretest itself has an effect on the participants. |
| | 3. When partners accompanied women they were reminded that the purpose was to focus on the woman's experience. |
| | 4. Delayed measures implemented as empathetic data gathering may abate responses to miscarriage. |
| | 5. 1 key outcome measure (IMS) was developed and implemented by the study author. |
| | 6. Caseness not stated for any measure. |

## RISK OF BIAS

| BIAS | AUTHORS' JUDGEMENT | SUPPORT FOR JUDGEMENT |
|---|---|---|
| Random sequence generation (selection bias) | Low risk | The author was contacted and confirmed that randomisation was by an independent person pulling 1 of 4 cards blindly from a box |
| Allocation concealment (selection bias) | Low risk | Women were randomly assigned via telephone by an independent person (correspondence with author) |
| Blinding (performance bias and detection bias) All outcomes | Unclear risk | Participants, clinicians and outcomes assessors not stated as blinded |
| Incomplete outcome data (attrition bias) All outcomes | Low risk | Intervention group 1 lost 10, intervention group 2 lost 16, comparison group 3 lost 21 and comparison group 4 lost 9 to follow-up, 57 or 24% in total |
| Selective reporting (reporting bias) | Unclear risk | We were not able to access the trial protocol, but vigour and fatigue subscales were dropped 'because they were confounded by alterations in women's physical health status due to the pregnancy-related changes experienced by many women in the first year after loss' |
| Groups similar at baseline? | Low risk | There were no significant differences between groups on any recruitment criteria or demographic variables |
| Free from early stopping? | Low risk | There was no statement indicating that the study was stopped early |

**Swanson 2009**

| | |
|---|---|
| Methods | Randomised controlled clinical trial. |
| Participants | Couples of which the woman had sustained a miscarriage before 20 weeks' gestation |
| | Inclusion criteria |
| | Both agreed to participate. |
| | Reported unplanned, unexpected loss of pregnancy prior to 20 weeks' gestation. |
| | Could speak and write English. |
| | In a self-proclaimed committed relationship. |
| | Geographically accessible. |
| | Within 3 months of loss. |
| | N = 341 women (682 in total). |
| | Exclusion criteria |
| | Unmarried people aged less than 18 years. |
| Interventions | Intervention 1: nurse caring (NC) (3 1-hour counselling sessions in own home). |
| | N = 77. |
| | Intervention 2: self-caring (SC) (3 videos of Swanson coaching couples and couples speaking of their miscarriage experiences and his and hers workbooks which stimulated reflection by asking 7 daily questions, data from which were not analysed). |
| | N = 64. |
| | Intervention 3: combined caring (CC) (1-hour long counselling session plus 1 workbook given and 2 workbooks mailed). |
| | N = 63. |
| | Intervention 4: control (no treatment). |
| | N = 79 (at 13 months). |
| | All 3 interventions were based on Swanson's caring theory and comprised: |
| | week 1 - 'coming to know', week 5 - 'sharing the loss', week 11 - 'getting through it' |
| Outcomes | Depression and grief measured at baseline, 3 months, 5 months and 13 months by: |
| | • CES-D, subscale depression. |
| | • Miscarriage Grief Inventory (adapted from the Texas Grief Inventory) subscales pure grief, grief-related emotions. |
| Notes | 1. Setting: couples from the Puget Sound area of Washington, USA. |
| | 2. Both the man and woman of each couple had to participate to warrant analysis. |
| | 3. Caseness threshold CES-D '16 are associated with higher risk for clinical depression and suggest the need for further assessment'. |

## RISK OF BIAS

| BIAS | AUTHORS' JUDGEMENT | SUPPORT FOR JUDGEMENT |
|---|---|---|
| Random sequence generation (selection bias) | Low risk | Cards shuffled and box shaken vigorously. |
| Allocation concealment (selection bias) | Low risk | Upon consent random allocation via 'a strict card pulling protocol' ... 'always involved two members of staff; 1 shuffled cards, vigorously shook the box and lifted the box above the card puller's eye level and the other who reached up and blindly pulled the card out of the box' |
| Blinding (performance bias and detection bias) All outcomes | Unclear risk | Participants, clinicians and outcomes assessors not stated as blinded |

*Continued*

**Swanson 2009—cont'd**

| | | |
|---|---|---|
| Incomplete outcome data (attrition bias)<br>All outcomes | Unclear risk | 341 couples randomised, 17 couples plus 3 women and 9 men subsequently returned no data. The final analysis comprised 318 couples. 1 woman in Intervention 1 attended no NC sessions, 8 women never used their SC materials and 2 women did not participate in the CC intervention 3 |
| Selective reporting (reporting bias) | Low risk | All pre-specified outcomes appear to have been addressed, but we were not able to access the trial protocol |
| Groups similar at baseline? | Low risk | 'There were no significant differences in baseline scores attributable to randomisation'. Measured for employment, history of depression, anxiety or grief, ethnicity/race, income, age and days since loss at baseline |
| Free from early stopping? | Low risk | There was no statement indicating that the study was stopped early |

## Characteristics of Excluded Studies [Ordered by Study ID]

| STUDY | REASON FOR EXCLUSION |
|---|---|
| Broen 2004 | Not RCT, follow-up study with no intervention. |
| Broen 2005 | Not RCT, follow-up study with no intervention. |
| Cordle 1994 | Not RCT, follow-up study with no intervention. |
| Jacobs 2000 | Not RCT, qualitative evaluation of a follow-up service. |
| Lefkof 2002 | Not RCT, a review article |
| Luise 2002 | Not RCT, observational study with no intervention. |
| Neugebauer 2006 | RCT, women up to 28 weeks' gestation. |
| Neugebauer 2007 | Not RCT, a preliminary open trial. |
| Nikcevic 1998 | Not RCT, cross-sectional study. |
| Nikcevic 2003 | Not RCT, controlled intervention study. |
| Rajan 1993 | RCT, but no follow-up on pregnancy loss. |
| Sejourne 2011 | Quasi-RCT using alternation as means of randomisation. |
| Thapar 1992 | Not RCT, no intervention. |

RCT: randomised controlled trial

## DATA AND ANALYSES

### Comparison 1. One Counselling Session Versus No Counselling (At Four Months)

| OUTCOME OR SUBGROUP TITLE | NO. OF STUDIES | NO. OF PARTICIPANTS | STATISTICAL METHOD | EFFECT SIZE |
|---|---|---|---|---|
| 1 Psychological well being | 3 | | Std. Mean Difference (IV, Fixed, 95% CI) | Subtotals only |
| 1.1 Anxiety | 2 | 105 | Std. Mean Difference (IV, Fixed, 95% CI) | -0.24 [-0.62, 0.15] |
| 1.2 Depression | 2 | 105 | Std. Mean Difference (IV, Fixed, 95% CI) | -0.25 [-0.63, 0.14] |
| 1.3 Grief | 2 | 154 | Std. Mean Difference (IV, Fixed, 95% CI) | -0.12 [-0.43, 0.20] |
| 1.4 Avoidance | 1 | 39 | Std. Mean Difference (IV, Fixed, 95% CI) | 0.18 [-0.45, 0.81] |
| 1.5 Intrusion | 1 | 39 | Std. Mean Difference (IV, Fixed, 95% CI) | -0.42 [-1.06, 0.22] |
| 1.6 Difficulty in coping | 1 | 88 | Std. Mean Difference (IV, Fixed, 95% CI) | -0.08 [-0.50, 0.34] |
| 1.7 Despair | 1 | 88 | Std. Mean Difference (IV, Fixed, 95% CI) | 0.01 [-0.41, 0.43] |
| 1.8 Self blame | 1 | 66 | Std. Mean Difference (IV, Fixed, 95% CI) | 0.03 [-0.45, 0.51] |
| 1.9 Worry | 1 | 66 | Std. Mean Difference (IV, Fixed, 95% CI) | -0.42 [-0.91, 0.06] |

### Comparison 2. Three One-Hour Counselling Sessions Versus No Counselling (At Four Months)

| OUTCOME OR SUBGROUP TITLE | NO. OF STUDIES | NO. OF PARTICIPANTS | STATISTICAL METHOD | EFFECT SIZE |
|---|---|---|---|---|
| 1 Psychological well being | 1 | | Std. Mean Difference (IV, Random, 95% CI) | Subtotals only |
| 1.1 Overall emotional disturbance (early measurement) | 1 | 89 | Std. Mean Difference (IV, Random, 95% CI) | -0.14 [-0.55, 0.28] |
| 1.2 Overall emotional disturbance (delayed measurement) | 1 | 96 | Std. Mean Difference (IV, Random, 95% CI) | -0.11 [-0.51, 0.30] |
| 1.3 Anxiety (early measurement) | 1 | 89 | Std. Mean Difference (IV, Random, 95% CI) | -0.07 [-0.49, 0.34] |
| 1.4 Anxiety (delayed measurement) | 1 | 96 | Std. Mean Difference (IV, Random, 95% CI) | 0.10 [-0.30, 0.51] |
| 1.5 Depression (early measurement) | 1 | 89 | Std. Mean Difference (IV, Random, 95% CI) | -0.29 [-0.70, 0.13] |
| 1.6 Depression (delayed measurement) | 1 | 96 | Std. Mean Difference (IV, Random, 95% CI) | -0.12 [-0.53, 0.28] |
| 1.7 Anger (early measurement) | 1 | 89 | Std. Mean Difference (IV, Random, 95% CI) | -0.36 [-0.78, 0.06] |
| 1.8 Anger (delayed measurement) | 1 | 96 | Std. Mean Difference (IV, Random, 95% CI) | -0.32 [-0.72, 0.09] |
| 1.9 Confusion (early measurement) | 1 | 89 | Std. Mean Difference (IV, Random, 95% CI) | -0.02 [-0.43, 0.40] |
| 1.10 Confusion (delayed measurement) | 1 | 96 | Std. Mean Difference (IV, Random, 95% CI) | -0.04 [-0.44, 0.37] |
| 1.11 Self esteem (early measurement) | 1 | 91 | Std. Mean Difference (IV, Random, 95% CI) | 0.12 [-0.29, 0.53] |
| 1.12 Self esteem (delayed measurement) | 1 | 94 | Std. Mean Difference (IV, Random, 95% CI) | -0.07 [-0.48, 0.34] |

## Comparison 2. Three One-Hour Counselling Sessions Versus No Counselling (At Four Months)—cont'd

| OUTCOME OR SUBGROUP TITLE | NO. OF STUDIES | NO. OF PARTICIPANTS | STATISTICAL METHOD | EFFECT SIZE |
|---|---|---|---|---|
| 1.13 Overall impact of miscarriage (early measurement) | 1 | 87 | Std. Mean Difference (IV, Random, 95% CI) | 0.14 [-0.28, 0.56] |
| 1.14 Overall impact of miscarriage (delayed measurement) | 1 | 91 | Std. Mean Difference (IV, Random, 95% CI) | -0.32 [-0.74, 0.10] |
| 1.15 Lost baby (early measurement) | 1 | 90 | Std. Mean Difference (IV, Random, 95% CI) | 3.99 [3.27, 4.72] |
| 1.16 Lost baby (delayed measurement) | 1 | 93 | Std. Mean Difference (IV, Random, 95% CI) | 0.10 [-0.31, 0.51] |
| 1.17 Personal significance (early measurement) | 1 | 87 | Std. Mean Difference (IV, Random, 95% CI) | 0.35 [-0.07, 0.77] |
| 1.18 Personal significance (delayed measurement) | 1 | 92 | Std. Mean Difference (IV, Random, 95% CI) | -0.40 [-0.82, 0.02] |
| 1.19 Devastating event (early measurement) | 1 | 87 | Std. Mean Difference (IV, Random, 95% CI) | -2.52 [-3.08, -1.95] |
| 1.20 Devastating event (delayed measurement) | 1 | 92 | Std. Mean Difference (IV, Random, 95% CI) | -0.37 [-0.79, 0.05] |
| 1.21 Isolated (early measurement) | 1 | 91 | Std. Mean Difference (IV, Random, 95% CI) | -0.02 [-0.43, 0.39] |
| 1.22 Isolated (delayed measurement) | 1 | 94 | Std. Mean Difference (IV, Random, 95% CI) | -0.42 [-0.84, -0.01] |

## Comparison 3. Three One-Hour Counselling Sessions Versus No Counselling (At 12 Months)

| OUTCOME OR SUBGROUP TITLE | NO. OF STUDIES | NO. OF PARTICIPANTS | STATISTICAL METHOD | EFFECT SIZE |
|---|---|---|---|---|
| 1 Psychological well being | 1 | | Std. Mean Difference (IV, Random, 95% CI) | Subtotals only |
| 1.1 Emotional disturbance (early measurement) | 1 | 89 | Std. Mean Difference (IV, Random, 95% CI) | -0.10 [-0.51, 0.32] |
| 1.2 Emotional disturbance (delayed measurement) | 1 | 96 | Std. Mean Difference (IV, Random, 95% CI) | -0.14 [-0.54, 0.27] |
| 1.3 Anxiety (early measurement) | 1 | 89 | Std. Mean Difference (IV, Random, 95% CI) | -0.03 [-0.45, 0.39] |
| 1.4 Anxiety (delayed measurement) | 1 | 96 | Std. Mean Difference (IV, Random, 95% CI) | -0.15 [-0.56, 0.25] |
| 1.5 Depression (early measurement) | 1 | 89 | Std. Mean Difference (IV, Random, 95% CI) | -0.26 [-0.68, 0.16] |
| 1.6 Depression (delayed measurement) | 1 | 96 | Std. Mean Difference (IV, Random, 95% CI) | -0.17 [-0.57, 0.23] |
| 1.7 Anger (early measurement) | 1 | 89 | Std. Mean Difference (IV, Random, 95% CI) | -0.17 [-0.59, 0.25] |
| 1.8 Anger (delayed measurement) | 1 | 96 | Std. Mean Difference (IV, Random, 95% CI) | -0.15 [-0.56, 0.25] |

*Continued*

## Comparison 3. Three One-Hour Counselling Sessions Versus No Counselling (At 12 Months)—cont'd

| OUTCOME OR SUBGROUP TITLE | NO. OF STUDIES | NO. OF PARTICIPANTS | STATISTICAL METHOD | EFFECT SIZE |
|---|---|---|---|---|
| 1.9 Confusion (early treatment) | 1 | 89 | Std. Mean Difference (IV, Random, 95% CI) | 0.04 [-0.38, 0.46] |
| 1.10 Confusion (delayed measurement) | 1 | 96 | Std. Mean Difference (IV, Random, 95% CI) | -0.08 [-0.48, 0.32] |
| 1.11 Self esteem (early measurement) | 1 | 91 | Std. Mean Difference (IV, Random, 95% CI) | 0.13 [-0.29, 0.54] |
| 1.12 Self esteem (delayed measurement) | 1 | 94 | Std. Mean Difference (IV, Random, 95% CI) | -0.13 [-0.54, 0.28] |
| 1.13 Impact of miscarriage (early measurement) | 1 | 87 | Std. Mean Difference (IV, Random, 95% CI) | 0.12 [-0.30, 0.54] |
| 1.14 Impact of miscarriage (delayed measurement) | 1 | 91 | Std. Mean Difference (IV, Random, 95% CI) | -0.43 [-0.85, -0.01] |
| 1.15 Lost baby (early measurement) | 1 | 90 | Std. Mean Difference (IV, Random, 95% CI) | 0.0 [-0.41, 0.41] |
| 1.16 Lost baby (delayed measurement) | 1 | 68 | Std. Mean Difference (IV, Random, 95% CI) | 2.15 [1.48, 2.82] |
| 1.17 Personal significance (early measurement) | 1 | 87 | Std. Mean Difference (IV, Random, 95% CI) | 0.18 [-0.24, 0.60] |
| 1.18 Personal significance (delayed measurement) | 1 | 92 | Std. Mean Difference (IV, Random, 95% CI) | -0.66 [-1.09, -0.24] |
| 1.19 Devastating event (early measurement) | 1 | 87 | Std. Mean Difference (IV, Random, 95% CI) | 0.20 [-0.22, 0.63] |
| 1.20 Devastating event (delayed measurement) | 1 | 92 | Std. Mean Difference (IV, Random, 95% CI) | -0.45 [-0.87, -0.04] |
| 1.21 Isolated (early measurement) | 1 | 91 | Std. Mean Difference (IV, Random, 95% CI) | -0.09 [-0.50, 0.33] |
| 1.22 Isolated (delayed measurement) | 1 | 94 | Std. Mean Difference (IV, Random, 95% CI) | -0.36 [-0.77, 0.06] |

## ANALYSIS 1-1  COMPARISON 1 ONE COUNSELLING SESSION VERSUS NO COUNSELLING (AT FOUR MONTHS), OUTCOME 1 PSYCHOLOGICAL WELL BEING

Review: Follow-up for improving psychological well being for women after a miscarriage

Comparison: 1 One counselling session versus no counselling (at four months)

Outcome: 1 Psychological well being

| STUDY OR SUBGROUP | ONE COUNSELING SESSION | | NO COUNSELLING | | STD. MEAN DIFFERENCE | WEIGHT | STD. MEAN DIFFERENCE |
|---|---|---|---|---|---|---|---|
| | N | MEAN(SD) | N | MEAN(SD) | IV,FIXED,95% CI | | IV,FIXED,95% CI |
| **1 Anxiety** | | | | | | | |
| Lee 1996 | 21 | 7.4 (5.9) | 18 | 8.1 (6.2) | | 37.3 % | -0.11 [ -0.74, 0.52 ] |
| Nikcevic 2007 | 33 | 5.6 (4.5) | 33 | 7 (4.4) | | 62.7 % | -0.31 [ -0.80, 0.17 ] |
| **Subtotal (95% CI)** | **54** | | **51** | | | **100.0 %** | **-0.24 [ -0.62, 0.15 ]** |
| Heterogeneity: Chi² = 0.24, df = 1 (P = 0.63); I² =0.0% | | | | | | | |
| Test for overall effect: Z = 1.21 (P = 0.23) | | | | | | | |
| **2 Depression** | | | | | | | |
| Lee 1996 | 21 | 3.2 (4.2) | 18 | 4.8 (7) | | 36.9 % | -0.28 [ -0.91, 0.36 ] |
| Nikcevic 2007 | 33 | 2.8 (4.1) | 33 | 3.7 (3.7) | | 63.1 % | -0.23 [ -0.71, 0.26 ] |
| **Subtotal (95% CI)** | **54** | | **51** | | | **100.0 %** | **-0.25 [ -0.63, 0.14 ]** |
| Heterogencity: Chi² = 0.01, df = 1 (P = 0.90); I² =0.0% | | | | | | | |
| Test for overall effect: Z = 1.25 (P = 0.21) | | | | | | | |
| **3 Grief** | | | | | | | |
| Adolfsson 2006 | 43 | 31 (19.2) | 45 | 32.7 (20) | | 57.2 % | -0.09 [ -0.50, 0.33 ] |
| Nikcevic 2007 | 33 | 39.9 (12.4) | 33 | 42 (13.4) | | 42.8 % | -0.16 [ -0.64, 0.32 ] |
| **Subtotal (95% CI)** | **76** | | **78** | | | **100.0 %** | **-0.12 [ -0.43, 0.20 ]** |
| Heterogeneity: Chi² = 0.05, df = 1 (P = 0.82); I² =0.0% | | | | | | | |
| Test for overall effect: Z = 0.73 (P = 0.46) | | | | | | | |
| **4 Avoidance** | | | | | | | |
| Lee 1996 | 21 | 13.5 (12) | 18 | 11.4 (11.3) | | 100.0 % | 0.18 [ -0.45, 0.81 ] |
| **Subtotal (95% CI)** | **21** | | **18** | | | **100.0 %** | **0.18 [ -0.45, 0.81 ]** |
| Heterogeneity: not applicable | | | | | | | |
| Test for overall effect: Z = 0.55 (P = 0.58) | | | | | | | |
| **5 Intrusion** | | | | | | | |
| Lee 1996 | 21 | 13.2 (11.3) | 18 | 18.1 (11.5) | | 100.0 % | -0.42 [ -1.06, 0.22 ] |
| **Subtotal (95% CI)** | **21** | | **18** | | | **100.0 %** | **-0.42 [ -1.06, 0.22 ]** |
| Heterogeneity: not applicable | | | | | | | |
| Test for overall effect: Z = 1.30 (P = 0.20) | | | | | | | |
| **6 Difficulty in coping** | | | | | | | |
| Adolfsson 2006 | 43 | 21.7 (13.2) | 45 | 22.9 (15.8) | | 100.0 % | -0.08 [ -0.50, 0.34 ] |
| **Subtotal (95% CI)** | **43** | | **45** | | | **100.0 %** | **-0.08 [ -0.50, 0.34 ]** |
| Heterogeneity: not applicable | | | | | | | |
| Test for overall effect: Z = 0.38 (P = 0.70) | | | | | | | |

-2  -1  0  1  2

Favours counselling    Favours no counselling

*Continued*

## ANALYSIS 1-1 COMPARISON 1 ONE COUNSELLING SESSION VERSUS NO COUNSELLING (AT FOUR MONTHS), OUTCOME 1 PSYCHOLOGICAL WELL BEING—cont'd

| STUDY OR SUBGROUP | ONE COUNSELING SESSION | | NO COUNSELLING | | STD. MEAN DIFFERENCE | WEIGHT | STD. MEAN DIFFERENCE |
|---|---|---|---|---|---|---|---|
| | N | MEAN(SD) | N | MEAN(SD) | IV,FIXED,95% CI | | IV,FIXED,95% CI |
| 7 Despair | | | | | | | |
| Adolfsson 2006 | 43 | 20.7 (13.5) | 45 | 20.6 (13.8) | | 100.0 % | 0.01 [ -0.41, 0.43 ] |
| **Subtotal (95% CI)** | **43** | | **45** | | | **100.0 %** | **0.01 [ -0.41, 0.43 ]** |
| Heterogeneity: not applicable | | | | | | | |
| Test for overall effect: Z = 0.03 (P = 0.97) | | | | | | | |
| 8 Self blame | | | | | | | |
| Nikcevic 2007 | 33 | 5.7 (3.6) | 33 | 5.6 (3.2) | | 100.0 % | 0.03 [ -0.45, 0.51 ] |
| **Subtotal (95% CI)** | **33** | | **33** | | | **100.0 %** | **0.03 [ -0.45, 0.51 ]** |
| Heterogeneity: not applicable | | | | | | | |
| Test for overall effect: Z = 0.12 (P = 0.91) | | | | | | | |
| 9 Worry | | | | | | | |
| Nikcevic 2007 | 33 | 11.9 (3.3) | 33 | 13.5 (4.1) | | 100.0 % | -0.42 [ -0.91, 0.06 ] |
| **Subtotal (95% CI)** | **33** | | **33** | | | **100.0 %** | **-0.42 [ -0.91, 0.06 ]** |
| Heterogeneity: not applicable | | | | | | | |
| Test for overall effect: Z = 1.71 (P = 0.088) | | | | | | | |
| Test for subgroup differences: Chi$^2$ = 4.59, df = 8 (P = 0.80), I$^2$ =0.0% | | | | | | | |

-2    -1    0    1    2

Favours counselling          Favours no counselling

## ANALYSIS 2-1 COMPARISON 2 THREE ONE-HOUR COUNSELLING SESSIONS VERSUS NO COUNSELLING (AT FOUR MONTHS), OUTCOME 1 PSYCHOLOGICAL WELL BEING

Review: Follow-up for improving psychological well being for women after a miscarriage

Comparison: 2 Three one-hour counselling sessions versus no counselling (at four months)

Outcome: 1 Psychological well being

| STUDY OR SUBGROUP | COUNSELLING | | NO COUNSELLING | | STD. MEAN DIFFERENCE | WEIGHT | STD. MEAN DIFFERENCE |
|---|---|---|---|---|---|---|---|
| | N | MEAN(SD) | N | MEAN(SD) | IV,RANDOM,95% CI | | IV,RANDOM,95% CI |
| **1 Overall emotional disturbance (early measurement)** | | | | | | | |
| Swanson 1999 | 47 | 63.5 (32.1) | 42 | 68.8 (44.6) | | 100.0 % | -0.14 [ -0.55, 0.28 ] |
| **Subtotal (95% CI)** | **47** | | **42** | | | **100.0 %** | **-0.14 [ -0.55, 0.28 ]** |
| Heterogeneity: not applicable | | | | | | | |
| Test for overall effect: Z = 0.64 (P = 0.52) | | | | | | | |
| **2 Overall emotional disturbance (delayed measurement)** | | | | | | | |
| Swanson 1999 | 43 | 75.2 (36.5) | 53 | 79.2 (38) | | 100.0 % | -0.11 [ -0.51, 0.30 ] |
| **Subtotal (95% CI)** | **43** | | **53** | | | **100.0 %** | **-0.11 [ -0.51, 0.30** |
| Heterogeneity: not applicable | | | | | | | |
| Test for overall effect: Z = 0.52 (P = 0.60) | | | | | | | |
| **3 Anxiety (early measurement)** | | | | | | | |
| Swanson 1999 | 47 | 10.4 (6.7) | 42 | 10.9 (7.1) | | 100.0 % | -0.07 [ -0.49, 0.34 ] |
| **Subtotal (95% CI)** | **47** | | **42** | | | **100.0 %** | **-0.07 [ -0.49, 0.34 ]** |
| Heterogeneity: not applicable | | | | | | | |
| Test for overall effect: Z = 0.34 (P = 0.73) | | | | | | | |
| **4 Anxiety (delayed measurement)** | | | | | | | |
| Swanson 1999 | 43 | 12.3 (6.9) | 53 | 11.6 (6.6) | | 100.0 % | 0.10 [ -0.30, 0.51 ] |
| **Subtotal (95% CI)** | **43** | | **53** | | | **100.0 %** | **0.10 [ -0.30, 0.51 ]** |
| Heterogeneity: not applicable | | | | | | | |
| Test for overall effect: Z = 0.50 (P = 0.62) | | | | | | | |
| **5 Depression (early measurement)** | | | | | | | |
| Swanson 1999 | 47 | 9.2 (8.5) | 42 | 12.4 (13.4) | | 100.0 % | -0.29 [ -0.70, 0.13 ] |
| **Subtotal (95% CI)** | **47** | | **42** | | | **100.0 %** | **-0.29 [ -0.70, 0.13 ]** |
| Heterogeneity: not applicable | | | | | | | |
| Test for overall effect: Z = 1.34 (P = 0.18) | | | | | | | |
| **6 Depression (delayed measurement)** | | | | | | | |
| Swanson 1999 | 43 | 12.8 (11.7) | 53 | 14.3 (12.3) | | 100.0 % | -0.12 [ -0.53, 0.28 ] |
| **Subtotal (95% CI)** | **43** | | **53** | | | **100.0 %** | **-0.12 [ -0.53, 0.28 ]** |
| Heterogeneity: not applicable | | | | | | | |
| Test for overall effect: Z = 0.60 (P = 0.55) | | | | | | | |
| **7 Anger (early measurement)** | | | | | | | |
| Swanson 1999 | 47 | 7.7 (6.9) | 42 | 11 (11.1) | | 100.0 % | -0.36 [ -0.78, 0.06 ] |
| **Subtotal (95% CI)** | **47** | | **42** | | | **100.0 %** | **-0.36 [ -0.78, 0.06 ]** |
| Heterogeneity: not applicable | | | | | | | |
| Test for overall effect: Z = 1.67 (P = 0.094) | | | | | | | |

-4  -2  0  2  4

Favours counselling          Favours no counselling

*Continued*

## ANALYSIS 2-1　COMPARISON 2 THREE ONE-HOUR COUNSELLING SESSIONS VERSUS NO COUNSELLING (AT FOUR MONTHS), OUTCOME 1 PSYCHOLOGICAL WELL BEING—cont'd

| STUDY OR SUBGROUP | COUNSELLING | | NO COUNSELLING | | STD. MEAN DIFFERENCE | WEIGHT | STD. MEAN DIFFERENCE |
|---|---|---|---|---|---|---|---|
| | N | MEAN(SD) | N | MEAN(SD) | IV,RANDOM,95% CI | | IV,RANDOM,95% CI |
| 8 Anger (delayed measurement) | | | | | | | |
| Swanson 1999 | 43 | 10.6 (8.3) | 53 | 13.4 (9) | | 100.0 % | -0.32 [ -0.72, 0.09 ] |
| **Subtotal (95% CI)** | **43** | | **53** | | | **100.0 %** | **-0.32 [ -0.72, 0.09 ]** |
| Heterogeneity: not applicable | | | | | | | |
| Test for overall effect: Z = 1.55 (P = 0.12) | | | | | | | |
| 9 Confusion (early measurement) | | | | | | | |
| Swanson 1999 | 47 | 7.8 (4.9) | 42 | 7.9 (6.6) | | 100.0 % | -0.02 [ -0.43, 0.40 ] |
| **Subtotal (95% CI)** | **47** | | **42** | | | **100.0 %** | **-0.02 [ -0.43, 0.40 ]** |
| Heterogeneity: not applicable | | | | | | | |
| Test for overall effect: Z = 0.08 (P = 0.94) | | | | | | | |
| 10 Confusion (delayed measurement) | | | | | | | |
| Swanson 1999 | 43 | 8.6 (5.4) | 53 | 8.8 (5.5) | | 100.0 % | -0.04 [ -0.44, 0.37 ] |
| **Subtotal (95% CI)** | **43** | | **53** | | | **100.0 %** | **-0.04 [ -0.44, 0.37 ]** |
| Heterogeneity: not applicable | | | | | | | |
| Test for overall effect: Z = 0.18 (P = 0.86) | | | | | | | |
| 11 Self esteem (early measurement) | | | | | | | |
| Swanson 1999 | 48 | 33.1 (5.2) | 43 | 32.5 (4.4) | | 100.0 % | 0.12 [ -0.29, 0.53 ] |
| **Subtotal (95% CI)** | **48** | | **43** | | | **100.0 %** | **0.12 [ -0.29, 0.53 ]** |
| Heterogeneity: not applicable | | | | | | | |
| Test for overall effect: Z = 0.58 (P = 0.56) | | | | | | | |
| 12 Self esteem (delayed measurement) | | | | | | | |
| Swanson 1999 | 41 | 31.9 (5.6) | 53 | 32.3 (5.7) | | 100.0 % | -0.07 [ -0.48, 0.34 ] |
| **Subtotal (95% CI)** | **41** | | **53** | | | **100.0 %** | **-0.07 [ -0.48, 0.34 ]** |
| Heterogeneity: not applicable | | | | | | | |
| Test for overall effect: Z = 0.34 (P = 0.74) | | | | | | | |
| 13 Overall impact of miscarriage (early measurement) | | | | | | | |
| Swanson 1999 | 46 | 63.4 (14.2) | 41 | 61.2 (16.3) | | 100.0 % | 0.14 [ -0.28, 0.56 ] |
| **Subtotal (95% CI)** | **46** | | **41** | | | **100.0 %** | **0.14 [ -0.28, 0.56 ]** |
| Heterogeneity: not applicable | | | | | | | |
| Test for overall effect: Z = 0.67 (P = 0.51) | | | | | | | |
| 14 Overall impact of miscarriage (delayed measurement) | | | | | | | |
| Swanson 1999 | 39 | 57.2 (15.3) | 52 | 61.8 (13.6) | | 100.0 % | -0.32 [ -0.74, 0.10 ] |
| **Subtotal (95% CI)** | **39** | | **52** | | | **100.0 %** | **-0.32 [ -0.74, 0.10 ]** |
| Heterogeneity: not applicable | | | | | | | |
| Test for overall effect: Z = 1.49 (P = 0.14) | | | | | | | |
| 15 Lost baby (early measurement) | | | | | | | |
| Swanson 1999 | 47 | 18 (3.9) | 43 | 1.1 (4.5) | | 100.0 % | 3.99 [ 3.27, 4.72 ] |
| **Subtotal (95% CI)** | **47** | | **43** | | | **100.0 %** | **3.99 [ 3.27, 4.72 ]** |
| Heterogeneity: not applicable | | | | | | | |
| Test for overall effect: Z = 10.78 (P < 0.00001) | | | | | | | |

```
        -4    -2    0    2    4
   Favours counselling    Favours no counselling
```

## ANALYSIS 2-1    COMPARISON 2 THREE ONE-HOUR COUNSELLING SESSIONS VERSUS NO COUNSELLING (AT FOUR MONTHS), OUTCOME 1 PSYCHOLOGICAL WELL BEING—cont'd

| STUDY OR SUBGROUP | COUNSELLING | | NO COUNSELLING | | STD. MEAN DIFFERENCE | WEIGHT | STD. MEAN DIFFERENCE |
|---|---|---|---|---|---|---|---|
| | N | MEAN(SD) | N | MEAN(SD) | IV,RANDOM,95% CI | | IV,RANDOM,95% CI |
| 16 Lost baby (delayed measurement) | | | | | | | |
| Swanson 1999 | 41 | 16.8 (4.9) | 52 | 16.3 (4.7) | | 100.0 % | 0.10 [ -0.31, 0.51 ] |
| Subtotal (95% CI) | 41 | | 52 | | | 100.0 % | 0.10 [ -0.31, 0.51 ] |
| Heterogeneity: not applicable | | | | | | | |
| Test for overall effect: Z = 0.50 (P = 0.62) | | | | | | | |
| 17 Personal significance (early measurement) | | | | | | | |
| Swanson 1999 | 46 | 17.8 (4.7) | 41 | 16 (5.5) | | 100.0 % | 0.35 [ -0.07, 0.77 ] |
| Subtotal (95% CI) | 46 | | 41 | | | 100.0 % | 0.35 [ -0.07, 0.77 ] |
| Heterogeneity: not applicable | | | | | | | |
| Test for overall effect: Z = 1.62 (P = 0.11) | | | | | | | |
| 18 Personal significance (delayed measurement) | | | | | | | |
| Swanson 1999 | 40 | 15.2 (5.5) | 52 | 17.1 (4) | | 100.0 % | -0.40 [ -0.82, 0.02 ] |
| Subtotal (95% CI) | 40 | | 52 | | | 100.0 % | -0.40 [ -0.82, 0.02 ] |
| Heterogeneity: not applicable | | | | | | | |
| Test for overall effect: Z = 1.88 (P = 0.060) | | | | | | | |
| 19 Devastating event (early measurement) | | | | | | | |
| Swanson 1999 | 46 | 1.8 (4.2) | 41 | 13.2 (4.8) | | 100.0 % | -2.52 [ -3.08, -1.95 ] |
| Subtotal (95% CI) | 46 | | 41 | | | 100.0 % | -2.52 [ -3.08, -1.95 ] |
| Heterogeneity: not applicable | | | | | | | |
| Test for overall effect: Z = 8.67 (P < 0.00001) | | | | | | | |
| 20 Devastating event (delayed measurement) | | | | | | | |
| Swanson 1999 | 40 | 13 (3.9) | 52 | 14.5 (4.1) | | 100.0 % | -0.37 [ -0.79, 0.05 ] |
| Subtotal (95% CI) | 40 | | 52 | | | 100.0 % | -0.37 [ -0.79, 0.05 ] |
| Heterogeneity: not applicable | | | | | | | |
| Test for overall effect: Z = 1.75 (P = 0.081) | | | | | | | |
| 21 Isolated (early measurement) | | | | | | | |
| Swanson 1999 | 48 | 13.9 (4.2) | 43 | 14 (4.8) | | 100.0 % | -0.02 [ -0.43, 0.39 ] |
| Subtotal (95% CI) | 48 | | 43 | | | 100.0 % | -0.02 [ -0.43, 0.39 ] |
| Heterogeneity: not applicable | | | | | | | |
| Test for overall effect: Z = 0.11 (P = 0.92) | | | | | | | |
| 22 Isolated (delayed measurement) | | | | | | | |
| Swanson 1999 | 41 | 12.2 (3.8) | 53 | 13.8 (3.7) | | 100.0 % | -0.42 [ -0.84, -0.01 ] |
| Subtotal (95% CI) | 41 | | 53 | | | 100.0 % | -0.42 [ -0.84, -0.01 ] |
| Heterogeneity: not applicable | | | | | | | |
| Test for overall effect: Z = 2.01 (P = 0.044) | | | | | | | |

-4    -2    0    2    4

Favours counselling          Favours no counselling

## ANALYSIS 3-1    COMPARISON 3 THREE ONE-HOUR COUNSELLING SESSIONS VERSUS NO COUNSELLING (AT 12 MONTHS), OUTCOME 1 PSYCHOLOGICAL WELL BEING

Review: Follow-up for improving psychological well being for women after a miscarriage

Comparison: 3 Three one-hour counselling sessions versus no counselling (at 12 months)

Outcome: 1 Psychological well being

| STUDY OR SUBGROUP | COUNSELLING | | NO COUNSELLING | | STD. MEAN DIFFERENCE | WEIGHT | STD. MEAN DIFFERENCE |
|---|---|---|---|---|---|---|---|
| | N | MEAN(SD) | N | MEAN(SD) | IV,RANDOM,95% CI | | IV,RANDOM,95% CI |
| 1 Emotional disturbance (early measurement) | | | | | | | |
| Swanson 1999 | 47 | 57.3 (28.9) | 42 | 60.7 (40.9) | | 100.0 % | -0.10 [ -0.51, 0.32 ] |
| Subtotal (95% CI) | 47 | | 42 | | | 100.0 % | -0.10 [ -0.51, 0.32 ] |
| Heterogeneity: not applicable | | | | | | | |
| Test for overall effect: Z = 0.45 (P = 0.65) | | | | | | | |
| 2 Emotional disturbance (delayed measurement) | | | | | | | |
| Swanson 1999 | 43 | 61.5 (31.9) | 53 | 66.1 (34.4) | | 100.0 % | -0.14 [ -0.54, 0.27 ] |
| Subtotal (95% CI) | 43 | | 53 | | | 100.0 % | -0.14 [ -0.54, 0.27 ] |
| Heterogeneity: not applicable | | | | | | | |
| Test for overall effect: Z = 0.67 (P = 0.50) | | | | | | | |
| 3 Anxiety (early measurement) | | | | | | | |
| Swanson 1999 | 47 | 8.8 (5.6) | 42 | 9 (7.3) | | 100.0 % | -0.03 [ -0.45, 0.39 ] |
| Subtotal (95% CI) | 47 | | 42 | | | 100.0 % | -0.03 [ -0.45, 0.39 ] |
| Heterogeneity: not applicable | | | | | | | |
| Test for overall effect: Z = 0.14 (P = 0.89) | | | | | | | |
| 4 Anxiety (delayed measurement) | | | | | | | |
| Swanson 1999 | 43 | 9.9 (6.6) | 53 | 11 (7.5) | | 100.0 % | -0.15 [ -0.56, 0.25 ] |
| Subtotal (95% CI) | 43 | | 53 | | | 100.0 % | -0.15 [ -0.56, 0.25 ] |
| Heterogeneity: not applicable | | | | | | | |
| Test for overall effect: Z = 0.75 (P = 0.46) | | | | | | | |
| 5 Depression (early measurement) | | | | | | | |
| Swanson 1999 | 47 | 8 (9.1) | 42 | 11.1 (14.3) | | 100.0 % | -0.26 [ -0.68, 0.16 ] |
| Subtotal (95% CI) | 47 | | 42 | | | 100.0 % | -0.26 [ -0.68, 0.16 ] |
| Heterogeneity: not applicable | | | | | | | |
| Test for overall effect: Z = 1.22 (P = 0.22) | | | | | | | |
| 6 Depression (delayed measurement) | | | | | | | |
| Swanson 1999 | 43 | 8.7 (7.6) | 53 | 10.2 (9.6) | | 100.0 % | -0.17 [ -0.57, 0.23 ] |
| Subtotal (95% CI) | 43 | | 53 | | | 100.0 % | -0.17 [ -0.57, 0.23 ] |
| Heterogeneity: not applicable | | | | | | | |
| Test for overall effect: Z = 0.83 (P = 0.41) | | | | | | | |
| 7 Anger (early measurement) | | | | | | | |
| Swanson 1999 | 47 | 6.2 (6.3) | 42 | 7.6 (9.7) | | 100.0 % | -0.17 [ -0.59, 0.25 ] |
| Subtotal (95% CI) | 47 | | 42 | | | 100.0 % | -0.17 [ -0.59, 0.25 ] |
| Heterogeneity: not applicable | | | | | | | |
| Test for overall effect: Z = 0.81 (P = 0.42) | | | | | | | |

-2    -1    0    1    2

Favours counselling          Favours no counselling

## ANALYSIS 3-1    COMPARISON 3 THREE ONE-HOUR COUNSELLING SESSIONS VERSUS NO COUNSELLING (AT 12 MONTHS), OUTCOME 1 PSYCHOLOGICAL WELL BEING—cont'd

| STUDY OR SUBGROUP | COUNSELLING | | NO COUNSELLING | | STD. MEAN DIFFERENCE IV,RANDOM,95% CI | WEIGHT | STD. MEAN DIFFERENCE IV,RANDOM,95% CI |
|---|---|---|---|---|---|---|---|
| | N | MEAN(SD) | N | MEAN(SD) | | | |
| 8 Anger (delayed measurement) | | | | | | | |
| Swanson 1999 | 43 | 7.8 (7.5) | 53 | 9 (7.9) | | 100.0 % | -0.15 [ -0.56, 0.25 ] |
| Subtotal (95% CI) | 43 | | 53 | | | 100.0 % | -0.15 [ -0.56, 0.25 ] |
| Heterogeneity: not applicable | | | | | | | |
| Test for overall effect: Z = 0.75 (P = 0.45) | | | | | | | |
| 9 Confusion (early treatment) | | | | | | | |
| Swanson 1999 | 47 | 6.9 (4.5) | 42 | 6.7 (5.4) | | 100.0 % | 0.04 [ -0.38, 0.46 ] |
| Subtotal (95% CI) | 47 | | 42 | | | 100.0 % | 0.04 [ -0.38, 0.46 ] |
| Heterogeneity: not applicable | | | | | | | |
| Test for overall effect: Z = 0.19 (P = 0.85) | | | | | | | |
| 10 Confusion (delayed measurement) | | | | | | | |
| Swanson 1999 | 43 | 6.9 (4.8) | 53 | 7.3 (5) | | 100.0 % | -0.08 [ -0.48, 0.32 ] |
| Subtotal (95% CI) | 43 | | 53 | | | 100.0 % | -0.08 [ -0.48, 0.32 ] |
| Heterogeneity: not applicable | | | | | | | |
| Test for overall effect: Z = 0.39 (P = 0.69) | | | | | | | |
| 11 Self esteem (early measurement) | | | | | | | |
| Swanson 1999 | 48 | 33.6 (4.4) | 43 | 33 (5.1) | | 100.0 % | 0.13 [ -0.29, 0.54 ] |
| Subtotal (95% CI) | 48 | | 43 | | | 100.0 % | 0.13 [ -0.29, 0.54 ] |
| Heterogeneity: not applicable | | | | | | | |
| Test for overall effect: Z = 0.60 (P = 0.55) | | | | | | | |
| 12 Self esteem (delayed measurement) | | | | | | | |
| Swanson 1999 | 41 | 32.5 (5.3) | 53 | 33.2 (5.3) | | 100.0 % | -0.13 [ -0.54, 0.28 ] |
| Subtotal (95% CI) | 41 | | 53 | | | 100.0 % | -0.13 [ -0.54, 0.28 ] |
| Heterogeneity: not applicable | | | | | | | |
| Test for overall effect: Z = 0.63 (P = 0.53) | | | | | | | |
| 13 Impact of miscarriage (early measurement) | | | | | | | |
| Swanson 1999 | 46 | 62.8 (14.9) | 41 | 60.9 (16.3) | | 100.0 % | 0.12 [ -0.30, 0.54 ] |
| Subtotal (95% CI) | 46 | | 41 | | | 100.0 % | 0.12 [ -0.30, 0.54 ] |
| Heterogeneity: not applicable | | | | | | | |
| Test for overall effect: Z = 0.56 (P = 0.57) | | | | | | | |
| 14 Impact of miscarriage (delayed measurement) | | | | | | | |
| Swanson 1999 | 39 | 53.7 (15.1) | 52 | 60.1 (14.7) | | 100.0 % | -0.43 [ -0.85, -0.01 ] |
| Subtotal (95% CI) | 39 | | 52 | | | 100.0 % | -0.43 [ -0.85, -0.01 ] |
| Heterogeneity: not applicable | | | | | | | |
| Test for overall effect: Z = 1.99 (P = 0.046) | | | | | | | |
| 15 Lost baby (early measurement) | | | | | | | |
| Swanson 1999 | 47 | 17.9 (4.4) | 43 | 17.9 (5.1) | | 100.0 % | 0.0 [ -0.41, 0.41 ] |
| Subtotal (95% CI) | 47 | | 43 | | | 100.0 % | 0.0 [ -0.41, 0.41 ] |
| Heterogeneity: not applicable | | | | | | | |
| Test for overall effect: Z = 0.0 (P = 1.0) | | | | | | | |

-2    -1    0    1    2

Favours counselling          Favours no counselling

Continued

## ANALYSIS 3-1    COMPARISON 3 THREE ONE-HOUR COUNSELLING SESSIONS VERSUS NO COUNSELLING (AT 12 MONTHS), OUTCOME 1 PSYCHOLOGICAL WELL BEING—cont'd

| STUDY OR SUBGROUP | COUNSELLING | | NO COUNSELLING | | STD. MEAN DIFFERENCE | WEIGHT | STD. MEAN DIFFERENCE |
|---|---|---|---|---|---|---|---|
| | N | MEAN(SD) | N | MEAN(SD) | IV,RANDOM,95% CI | | IV,RANDOM,95% CI |
| **16 Lost baby (delayed measurement)** | | | | | | | |
| Swanson 1999 | 16 | 16.2 (5.1) | 52 | 5.1 (5.1) | | 100.0 % | 2.15 [ 1.48, 2.82 ] |
| **Subtotal (95% CI)** | **16** | | **52** | | | **100.0 %** | **2.15 [ 1.48, 2.82 ]** |
| Heterogeneity: not applicable | | | | | | | |
| Test for overall effect: Z = 6.27 (P < 0.00001) | | | | | | | |
| **17 Personal significance (early measurement)** | | | | | | | |
| Swanson 1999 | 46 | 16.8 (5.4) | 41 | 15.8 (5.6) | | 100.0 % | 0.18 [ -0.24, 0.60 ] |
| **Subtotal (95% CI)** | **46** | | **41** | | | **100.0 %** | **0.18 [ -0.24, 0.60 ]** |
| Heterogeneity: not applicable | | | | | | | |
| Test for overall effect: Z = 0.84 (P = 0.40) | | | | | | | |
| **18 Personal significance (delayed measurement)** | | | | | | | |
| Swanson 1999 | 40 | 13.5 (4.9) | 52 | 16.6 (4.4) | | 100.0 % | -0.66 [ -1.09, -0.24 ] |
| **Subtotal (95% CI)** | **40** | | **52** | | | **100.0 %** | **-0.66 [ -1.09, -0.24 ]** |
| Heterogeneity: not applicable | | | | | | | |
| Test for overall effect: Z = 3.08 (P = 0.0021) | | | | | | | |
| **19 Devastating event (early measurement)** | | | | | | | |
| Swanson 1999 | 46 | 14.1 (4.2) | 41 | 13.2 (4.6) | | 100.0 % | 0.20 [ -0.22, 0.63 ] |
| **Subtotal (95% CI)** | **46** | | **41** | | | **100.0 %** | **0.20 [ -0.22, 0.63 ]** |
| Heterogeneity: not applicable | | | | | | | |
| Test for overall effect: Z = 0.94 (P = 0.35) | | | | | | | |
| **20 Devastating event (delayed measurement)** | | | | | | | |
| Swanson 1999 | 40 | 12.1 (4.2) | 52 | 14.1 (4.5) | | 100.0 % | -0.45 [ -0.87, -0.04 ] |
| **Subtotal (95% CI)** | **40** | | **52** | | | **100.0 %** | **-0.45 [ -0.87, -0.04 ]** |
| Heterogeneity: not applicable | | | | | | | |
| Test for overall effect: Z = 2.13 (P = 0.033) | | | | | | | |
| **21 Isolated (early measurement)** | | | | | | | |
| Swanson 1999 | 48 | 13.6 (4.3) | 43 | 14 (4.9) | | 100.0 % | -0.09 [ -0.50, 0.33 ] |
| **Subtotal (95% CI)** | **48** | | **43** | | | **100.0 %** | **-0.09 [ -0.50, 0.33 ]** |
| Heterogeneity: not applicable | | | | | | | |
| Test for overall effect: Z = 0.41 (P = 0.68) | | | | | | | |
| **22 Isolated (delayed measurement)** | | | | | | | |
| Swanson 1999 | 41 | 12 (3.5) | 53 | 13.4 (4.2) | | 100.0 % | -0.36 [ -0.77, 0.06 ] |
| **Subtotal (95% CI)** | **41** | | **53** | | | **100.0 %** | **-0.36 [ -0.77, 0.06 ]** |
| Heterogeneity: not applicable | | | | | | | |
| Test for overall effect: Z = 1.69 (P = 0.090) | | | | | | | |

-2   -1   0   1   2

Favours counselling          Favours no counselling

**6S Hierarchy of Pre-Appraised Evidence** Model developed to assist clinicians in their search for the highest level of evidence. The main use of the 6s hierarchy is for efficiently identifying the highest level of evidence to facilitate a search on a clinical question or problem.

## A

**A Priori** From Latin: *the former;* before the study or analysis.

**Absolute Risk Reduction (ARR)** A value that gives reduction of risk in absolute terms. The ARR is considered the "real" reduction because it is the difference between the risk observed in those who did and did not experience the event.

**Abstract** A short, comprehensive synopsis or summary of a study at the beginning of an article.

**Accessible Population** A population that meets the population criteria and is available.

**Accreditation** A process in which an organization demonstrates attainment of predetermined standards set by an external nongovernmental organization responsible for setting and monitoring compliance in a particular industry sector.

**After-Only Design** An experimental design with two randomly assigned groups—a treatment group and a control group. This design differs from the true experiment in that both groups are measured only after the experimental treatment.

**After-Only Nonequivalent Control Group Design** A quasi-experimental design similar to the after-only experimental design, but subjects are not randomly assigned to the treatment or control groups.

**AGREE II Guideline** A widely used instrument to evaluate the applicability of a guideline to practice. The AGREE II was developed to assist in evaluating guideline quality, provide a methodological strategy for guideline development, and inform practitioners about what information should be reported in guidelines and how it should be reported.

**Analysis of Covariance (ANCOVA)** A statistic that measures differences among group means and uses a statistical technique to equate the groups under study in relation to an important variable.

**Analysis of Variance (ANOVA)** A statistic that tests whether group means differ from each other, rather than testing each pair of means separately. ANOVA considers the variation among all groups.

**Anecdotes** Summaries of an observation that records a behavior of interest.

**Anonymity** A research participant's protection of identity in a study so that no one, not even the researcher, can link the subject with the information given.

**Antecedent Variable** A variable that affects the dependent variable but occurs before the introduction of the independent variable.

**Assent** An aspect of informed consent that pertains to protecting the rights of children as research subjects.

**Attention Control** Operationalized as the control group receiving the same amount of "attention" as the experimental group.

**Auditability** The researcher's development of the research process in a qualitative study that allows a researcher or reader to follow the thinking or conclusions of the researcher.

## B

**Benchmarking** A systematic approach for gathering information about process or product performance and then analyzing why and how performance differs between business units.

**Beneficence** An obligation to act to benefit others and to maximize possible benefits.

**Bias** A distortion in the data-analysis results.

**Boolean Operator** Words used to define the relationships between words or groups of words in literature searches. Examples of Boolean operators are words such as "AND," "OR," "NOT," and "NEAR."

**Bracketing** A process during which the researcher identifies personal biases about the phenomenon of interest to clarify how personal experience and beliefs may color what is heard and reported.

## C

**Case Control Study** See *ex post facto study.*

**Case Study Method** The study of a selected contemporary phenomenon over time to provide an in-depth description of essential dimensions and processes of the phenomenon.

**CASP Tools** Checklists that provide an evidence-based approach for assessing the quality, quantity, and consistency of specific study designs.

**Categorical Variable** A variable that has mutually exclusive categories but has more than two values.

**Chance Error** Attributable to fluctuations in subject characteristics that occur at a specific point in time and are often beyond the awareness and control of the examiner. Also called *random error.*

**Chi-Square ($\chi^2$)** A nonparametric statistic that is used to determine whether the frequency found in each category is different from the frequency that would be expected by chance.

**Citation Management Software** Software that formats citations.

**Clinical Guidelines** Systematically developed practice statements designed to assist clinicians about health care decisions for specific conditions or situations.

**Clinical Microsystems** A QI model developed specifically for healthcare. It is considered the building block of any health care system and is the smallest replicable unit in an organization. Members of a clinical microsystem are interdependent and work together toward a common aim.

**Clinical Question** The first step in development of an evidence-based practice project.

**Close-Ended Question** Question that the respondent may answer with only one of a fixed number of choices.

**Cluster Sampling** A probability sampling strategy that involves a successive random sampling of units. The units sampled progress from large to small. Also known as *multistage sampling*.

**Cohort** The subjects of a specific group that are being studied.

**Common Cause Variation** Variation that occurs at random and is considered a characteristic of the system.

**Community-Based Participatory Research** Qualitative method that systematically accesses the voice of a community to plan context-appropriate action.

**Concealment** Refers to whether the subjects know that they are being observed.

**Concept** An image or symbolic representation of an abstract idea.

**Conceptual Definition** General meaning of a concept.

**Conceptual Framework** A structure of concepts and/or theories pulled together as a map for the study. This set of interrelated concepts symbolically represents how a group of variables relates to each other.

**Conceptual Literature** Published and unpublished non–data-based material, such as reports of theories, concepts, synthesis of research on concepts, or professional issues, some of which underlie reported research, as well as other nonresearch material.

**Concurrent Validity** The degree of correlation of two measures of the same concept that are administered at the same time.

**Conduct of Research** The analysis of data collected from a homogeneous group of subjects who meet study inclusion and exclusion criteria for the purpose of answering specific research questions or testing specified hypotheses.

**Confidence Interval** Quantifies the uncertainty of a statistic or the probable value range within which a population parameter is expected to lie.

**Confidentiality** Assurance that a research participant's identity cannot be linked to the information that was provided to the researcher.

**Consent** See *informed consent*.

**Consistency** Data are collected from each subject in the study in exactly the same way or as close to the same way as possible.

**Constancy** Methods and procedures of data collection are the same for all subjects.

**Constant Comparative Method** A process of continuously comparing data as they are acquired during research with the grounded theory method.

**Construct** An abstraction that is adapted for scientific purpose.

**Construct Validity** The extent to which an instrument is said to measure a theoretical construct or trait.

**Consumer** One who actively uses and applies research findings in nursing practice.

**Content Analysis** A technique for the objective, systematic, and quantitative description of communications and documentary evidence.

**Content Validity** The degree to which the content of the measure represents the universe of content, or the domain of a given behavior.

**Content Validity Index** A calculation that gives a researcher more confidence or evidence that the instrument truly reflects the concept or construct.

**Context** Environment where event(s) occur(s).

**Context Dependent** An observation as defined by its circumstance or context.

**Continuous Variable (Data)** A variable that can take on any value between two specified points (e.g., weight).

**Contrasted-Group Approach** A method used to assess construct validity. A researcher identifies two groups of individuals who are suspected to have an extremely high or low score on a characteristic. Scores from the groups are obtained and examined for sensitivity to the differences. Also called *known-group approach*.

**Control** Measures used to hold uniform or constant the conditions under which an investigation occurs.

**Control Chart** Used to track system performance over time. It includes information on the average performance level for the system depicted by a center line displaying the system's average performance (the mean value) and the upper and lower limits depicting one to three standard deviations from average performance level.

**Control Event Rate (CER)** Proportion of patients in a control group in which an event is observed.

**Control Group** The group in an experimental investigation that does not receive an intervention or treatment; the comparison group.

**Controlled Vocabulary** The terms that indexers have assigned to the articles in a database. When possible, it is helpful to match the words that you use in your search to those specifically used in the database.

**Convenience Sampling** A nonprobability sampling strategy that uses the most readily accessible persons or objects as subjects in a study.

**Convergent Validity** A strategy for assessing construct validity in which two or more tools that theoretically measure the same construct are administered to subjects. If the measures are positively correlated, convergent validity is said to be supported.

**Correlation** The degree of association between two variables.

**Correlational Study** A type of nonexperimental research design that examines the relationship between two or more variables.

**Credibility** Steps in qualitative research to ensure accuracy, validity, or soundness of data.

**Criterion-Related Validity** Indicates the degree of relationship between performance on the measure and actual behavior either in the present (concurrent) or in the future (predictive).

**Critical Appraisal** Appraisal by a nurse who is a knowledgeable consumer of research, and who can appraise research evidence and use existing standards to determine the merit and readiness of research for use in clinical practice.

**Critical Reading** An active interpretation and objective assessment of an article during which the reader is looking for key concepts, ideas, and justifications.

**Critique** The process of critical appraisal that objectively and critically evaluates a research report's content for scientific merit and application to practice.

**Cronbach's Alpha** Test of internal consistency that simultaneously compares each item in a scale to all others.

**Cross-Sectional Study** A nonexperimental research design that looks at data at one point in time; that is, in the immediate present.

**Culture** The system of knowledge and linguistic expressions used by social groups that allows the researcher to interpret or make sense of the world.

**Cumulative Index to Nursing and Allied Health Literature (CINAHL)** A print or computerized database; computerized CINAHL is available on CD-ROM and online.

## D

**Data** Information systematically collected in the course of a study; the plural of *datum*.

**Data-Based Literature** Reports of completed research.

**Data Saturation** A point when data collection can cease. It occurs when the information being shared with the researcher becomes repetitive. Ideas conveyed by the participant have been shared before by other participants; inclusion of additional participants does not result in new ideas.

**Database** A compilation of information about a topic organized in a systematic way.

**Debriefing** The opportunity for researchers to discuss the study with the participants; participants may refuse to have their data included in the study at this time.

**Deductive** A logical thought process in which hypotheses are derived from theory; reasoning moves from the general to the particular.

**Degrees of Freedom** The number of quantities that are unknown minus the number of independent equations linking these unknowns; a function of the number in the sample.

**Delimitations** Those characteristics that restrict the population to a homogeneous group of subjects.

**Delphi Technique** The technique of gaining expert opinion on a subject. It uses rounds or multiple stages of data collection, with each round using data from the previous round.

**Demographic Data** Data that includes information that describes important characteristics about the subjects in a study (e.g., age, gender, race, ethnicity, education, marital status).

**Dependent Variable** In experimental studies, the presumed effect of the independent or experimental variable on the outcome.

**Descriptive Statistics** Statistical methods used to describe and summarize sample data.

**Design** The plan or blueprint for conduct of a study.

**Developmental Study** A type of non-experimental research design that is concerned not only with the existing status and interrelationship of phenomena, but also with changes that take place as a function of time.

**Dichotomous Variable:** A nominal variable that has two categories (e.g., male/female).

**Directional Hypothesis** Hypothesis that specifies the expected direction of the relationship between the independent and dependent variables.

**Dissemination** The communication of research findings.

**Divergent Validity/Discriminant Validity** A strategy for assessing construct validity in which two or more tools that theoretically measure the opposite of the construct are administered to subjects. If the measures are negatively correlated, divergent validity is said to be supported.

**Domains** Symbolic categories that include the smaller categories of an ethnographic study.

## E

**Effect Size** An estimate of how large of a difference there is between intervention and control groups in summarized studies.

**Electronic Database** A database that can be accessed by computers or electronic information services.

**Electronic Index** The electronic means by which journal sources (periodicals) of data-based and conceptual articles on a variety of topics (e.g., doctoral dissertations) are found, as well as the publications of professional organizations and various governmental agencies.

**Element** The most basic unit about which information is collected.

**Eligibility Criteria** Those characteristics that restrict the population to a homogeneous group of subjects.

**Emic View** The native's or insider's view of the world.

**Empirical** The obtaining of evidence or objective data.

**Empirical Literature** A synonym for data-based literature; see *data-based literature*.

**Equivalence** Consistency or agreement among observers using the same measurement tool or agreement among alternate forms of a tool.

**Error Variance** The extent to which the variance in test scores is attributable to error rather than a true measure of the behaviors.

**Ethics** The theory or discipline dealing with principles of moral values and moral conduct.

**Ethnographic Method** A method that scientifically describes cultural groups. The goal of the ethnographer is to understand the native's view of their world.

**Ethnography/Ethnographic Method** A qualitative research approach designed to produce cultural theory.

**Etic View** An outsider's view of another's world.

**Evaluation Research** The use of scientific research methods and procedures to evaluate a program, treatment, practice, or policy outcomes; analytical means are used to document the worth of an activity.

**Evidence-Based Clinical Guidelines** A set of guidelines that allows the researcher to better understand the evidence base of certain practices.

**Evidence-Based Practice** The conscious and judicious use of the current "best" evidence in the care of patients and delivery of health care services.

**Evidence-Based Practice Guidelines** Practice guidelines developed based on research findings.

**Ex Post Facto Study** A type of nonexperimental research design that examines the relationships among the variables after the variations have occurred.

**Exclusion Criteria** Those characteristics that restrict the population to a homogeneous group of subjects.

**Existing Data** Data gathered from records (e.g., medical records, care plans, hospital records, death certificates) and databases (e.g., U.S. Census, National Cancer Data Base, Minimum Data Set for Nursing Home Resident Assessment and Care Screening).

**Experiment** A scientific investigation in which observations are made and data are collected by means of the characteristics of control, randomization, and manipulation.

**Experimental Design** A research design that has the following properties: randomization, control, and manipulation.

**Experimental Event Rate (EER)** Proportion of patients in experimental treatment groups in which an event is observed.

**Experimental Group** The group in an experimental investigation that receives an intervention or treatment.

**Expert-Based Clinical Guidelines** Guidelines developed from the combination of opinions from known experts in the field along with current research evidence.

**Exploratory Survey** A type of nonexperimental research design that collects descriptions of existing phenomena for the purpose of using the data to justify or assess current conditions or to make plans for improvement of conditions.

**External Validity** The degree to which findings of a study can be generalized to other populations or environments.

**Extraneous Variable** Variable that interferes with the operations of the phenomena being studied. Also called *mediating variable.*

## F

**Face Validity** A type of content validity that uses an expert's opinion to judge the accuracy of an instrument. (Some would say that face validity verifies that the instrument gives the subject or expert the appearance of measuring the concept.)

**Factor Analysis** A type of validity that uses a statistical procedure for determining the underlying dimensions or components of a variable.

**Field Notes** Descriptions kept by a researcher that detail the environment and nonverbal communications observed by a researcher that enrich data collected.

**Findings** Statistical results of a study.

**Fisher's Exact Probability Test** A test used to compare frequencies when samples are small and expected frequencies are less than six in each cell.

**Fittingness** Answers the following questions: Are the findings applicable outside the study situation? Are the results meaningful to the individuals not involved in the research?

**Flowchart** Depicts how a process works, detailing the sequence of steps from the beginning to the end of a process.

**Forest Plot** Also known as a blobbogram, a forest plot graphically depicts the results of analyzing a number of studies.

**Frequency Distribution** Descriptive statistical method for summarizing the occurrences of events under study.

## G

**Generalizability (Generalize)** The inferences that the data are representative of similar phenomena in a population beyond the studied sample.

**Grand Nursing Theories** Sometimes referred to as nursing conceptual models, these include the theories/models that were developed to describe the discipline of nursing as a whole.

**Grand Theory** All-inclusive conceptual structures that tend to include views on person, health, and environment to create a perspective of nursing.

**Grand Tour Question** A broad overview question.

**Grounded Theory** Theory that is constructed inductively from a base of observations of the world as it is lived by a selected group of people.

**Grounded Theory Method** An inductive approach that uses a systematic set of procedures to arrive at theory about basic social processes.

## H

**Hazard Ratio** A weighted relative risk based on the analysis of survival curves over the whole course of the study period.

**History** The internal validity threat that refers to events outside of the experimental setting that may affect the dependent variable.

**Homogeneity** Similarity of conditions. Also called *internal consistency.*

**Hypothesis** A prediction about the relationship between two or more variables.

**Hypothesis-Testing Approach** Method used when an investigator uses the theory or concept underlying the measurement instruments to validate the instrument.

**Hypothesis-Testing Validity** A strategy for assessing construct validity in which the theory or concept underlying a measurement instrument's design is used to develop hypotheses that are tested. Inferences are made based on the findings about whether the rationale underlying the instrument's construction is adequate to explain the findings.

## I

**Inclusion Criteria** See *eligibility criteria.*

**Independent Variable** The antecedent or the variable that has the presumed effect on the dependent variable.

**Inductive Reasoning** A logical thought process in which generalizations are developed from specific observations; reasoning moves from the particular to the general.

**Inferential Statistics** Procedures that combine mathematical processes and logic to test hypotheses about a population with the help of sample data.

**Information Literacy** The skills needed to consult the literature and answer a clinical question.

**Informed Consent** An ethical principle that requires a researcher to obtain the voluntary participation of subjects after informing them of potential benefits and risks.

**Institutional Review Boards (IRBs)** Boards established in agencies to review biomedical and behavioral research involving human subjects within the agency or in programs sponsored by the agency.

**Instrumental Case Study** Research that is done when the researcher pursues insight into an issue or wants to challenge a generalization.

**Instrumentation** Changes in the measurement of the variables that may account for changes in the obtained measurement.

**Integrative Review** Synthesis review of the literature on a specific concept or topic.

**Internal Consistency** The extent to which items within a scale reflect or measure the same concept.

**Internal Validity** The degree to which it can be inferred that the experimental treatment, rather than an uncontrolled condition, resulted in the observed effects.

**Interpretive Phenomenology** An approach to research that "seeks to reveal and convey deep insight and understanding of the concealed meanings of everyday life experiences" (deWitt & Ploeg, 2006, pp. 216-217).

**Interrater Reliability** The consistency of observations between two or more observers; often expressed as a percentage of agreement between raters or observers or a coefficient of agreement that takes into account the element of chance. This usually is used with the direct observation method.

**Interval Measurement** Level used to show rankings of events or objects on a scale with equal intervals between numbers but with an arbitrary zero (e.g., centigrade temperature).

**Intervening Variable** A variable that occurs during an experimental or quasi-experimental study that affects the dependent variable.

**Intervention** Deals with whether or not the observer provokes actions from those who are being observed.

**Intervention Fidelity** The process of enhancing the study's internal validity by ensuring that the intervention is delivered systematically to all subjects.

**Interview Guide** A list of questions and probes used by interviews that use open-ended questions.

**Interviews** A method of data collection in which a data collector questions a subject verbally. Interviews may be in person or performed over the telephone, and they may consist of open-ended or close-ended questions.

**Intrinsic Case Study** Research that is undertaken to gain a better understanding of the essential nature of the case.

**Item to Total Correlation** The relationship between each of the items on a scale and the total scale.

## J

**Justice** The principle that human subjects should be treated fairly.

## K

**Kappa** Expresses the level of agreement observed beyond the level that would be expected by chance alone. Kappa (K) ranges from +1 (total agreement) to 0 (no agreement). K greater than .80 generally indicates good reliability. K between .68 and .80 is considered acceptable/substantial agreement. Levels lower than .68 may allow tentative conclusions to be drawn when lower levels are accepted.

**Key Informants** Individuals who have special knowledge, status, or communication skills, and who are willing to teach the ethnographer about the phenomenon.

**Knowledge-Focused Triggers** Ideas that are generated when staff read research, listen to scientific papers at research conferences, or encounter evidence-based practice guidelines published by government agencies or specialty organizations.

**Kuder-Richardson (KR-20) Coefficient** The estimate of homogeneity used for instruments that use a dichotomous response pattern.

## L

**Lean** A QI model that focuses on eliminating waste from the production system by designing the most efficient and effective system. It is sometimes referred to as the Toyota Quality Model.

**Level of Significance (Alpha Level)** The risk of making a type I error, set by the researcher before the study begins.

**Levels of Evidence** A rating system for judging the strength of a study's design.

**Levels of Measurement** Categorization of the precision with which an event can be measured (nominal, ordinal, interval, and ratio).

**Likelihood Ratios** Provide the nurse with information about the accuracy of a diagnostic test and can also help the nurse to be a more efficient decision maker by allowing the clinician to quantify the probability of disease for any individual patient.

**Likert-Type Scales** Lists of statements for which respondents indicate whether they "strongly agree," "agree," "disagree," or "strongly disagree."

**Limitation** Weakness of a study.

**Literature Review** A systematic and critical appraisal of the most important literature on a topic.

**Lived Experience** In phenomenological research, a term used to refer to the focus on living through events and circumstances (prelingual) rather than thinking about these events and circumstances (conceptualized experience).

**Longitudinal Study** A nonexperimental research design in which a researcher collects data from the same group at different points in time.

## M

**Manipulation** The provision of some experimental treatment, in one or varying degrees, to some of the subjects in the study.

**Matching** A special sampling strategy used to construct an equivalent comparison sample group by filling it with subjects who are similar to each subject in another sample group in relation to preestablished variables, such as age and gender.

**Maturation** Developmental, biological, or psychological processes that operate within an individual as a function of time and are external to the events of the investigation.

**Mean** A measure of central tendency; the arithmetic average of all scores.

**Measurement** The standardized method of collecting data.

**Measurement Effects** Administration of a pretest in a study that affects the generalizability of the findings to other populations.

**Measurement Error** The difference between what really exists and what is measured in a given study.

**Measures of Central Tendency** Descriptive statistical procedure that describes the average member of a sample (mean, median, and mode).

**Measures of Variability** Descriptive statistical procedure that describes how much dispersion there is in sample data.

**Median** A measure of central tendency; the middle score.

**Mediating Variable** A variable that intervenes between the independent and dependent variable.

**Meta-Analysis** A research method that takes the results of multiple studies in a specific area and synthesizes the findings to make conclusions regarding the area of focus.

**Meta-Summary** Integrations that are approximately equal to the sum of parts, or the sum of findings across reports in a target domain of research.

**Meta-Synthesis** Integrates qualitative research findings on a topic and is based on comparative analysis and interpretative synthesis.

**Methodological Research** The controlled investigation and measurement of the means of gathering and analyzing data.

**Microrange Theory** The linking of concrete concepts into a statement that can be examined in practice and research.

**Middle Range Nursing Theories** Theories that contain a limited number of concepts and are focused on a limited aspect of reality.

**Modality** The number of peaks in a frequency distribution.

**Mode** A measure of central tendency; the most frequent score or result.

**Model** A symbolic representation of a set of concepts that is created to depict relationships.

**Mortality** The loss of subjects from time 1 data collection to time 2 data collection.

**Multiple Analysis of Variance (MANOVA)** A test used to determine differences in group means; used when there is more than one dependent variable.

**Multiple Regression** Measure of the relationship between one interval level dependent variable and several independent variables. Canonical correlation is used when there is more than one dependent variable.

**Multistage Sampling (Cluster Sampling)** Involves a successive random sampling of units (clusters) that programs from large to small and meets sample eligibility criteria.

**Multitrait-Multimethod Approach** A type of validity that uses more than one method to assess the accuracy of an instrument (e.g., observation and interview of anxiety).

**Multivariate Statistics** A statistical procedure that involves two or more variables.

**Naturalistic Setting** An environment of familiar "day to day" surroundings.

**Negative Likelihood Ratio (LR)** The LR of a negative test indicates the accuracy of a negative test result by comparing its performance when the disease is absent to that when the disease is present. The better test to use to rule out disease is the one with the smaller likelihood ratio of a negative test.

**Negative Predictive Value** Expresses the proportion of those with negative test results who truly do not have the disease.

**Network Sampling (Snowball Effect Sample)** A strategy used for locating samples that are difficult to locate. It uses social networks and the fact that friends tend to have characteristics in common; subjects who meet the eligibility criteria are asked for assistance in getting in touch with others who meet the same criteria.

**Nominal** The level of measurement that simply assigns data into categories that are mutually exclusive.

**Nominal Measurement** Level used to classify objects or events into categories without any relative ranking (e.g., gender, hair color).

**Nondirectional Hypothesis** Indicates the existence of a relationship between the variables but does not specify the anticipated direction of the relationship.

**Nonequivalent Control Group Design** A quasi-experimental design that is similar to the true experiment, but subjects are not randomly assigned to the treatment or control groups.

**Nonexperimental Research Design** Research design in which an investigator observes a phenomenon without manipulating the independent variable(s).

**Nonparametric Statistics** Statistics that are usually used when variables are measured at the nominal or ordinal level because they do not estimate population parameters and involve less restrictive assumptions about the underlying distribution.

**Nonprobability Sampling** A procedure in which elements are chosen by nonrandom methods.

**Normal Curve** A curve that is symmetrical about the mean and is unimodal.

**Null Hypothesis** A statement that there is no relationship between the variables and that any relationship observed is a function of chance or fluctuations in sampling.

**Null Value** In an experiment, when a value is obtained that indicates that there is no difference between the treatment and control groups.

**Number Needed to Treat** The number of people who need to receive a treatment (or intervention) in order for one patient to receive any benefit.

**Objective** Data that are not influenced by anyone who collects the information.

**Objectivity** The use of facts without distortion by personal feelings or bias.

**Observation** A method for measuring psychological and physiological behaviors for the purpose of evaluating change and facilitating recovery.

**Observed Score** The actual score obtained in a measurement.

**Observed Test Score** Derived from a set of items actually consists of the true score plus error.

**Odds Ratio (OR)** An estimate of relative risk used in logistic regression as a measure of association; describes the probability of an event.

**One-Group (Pretest-Posttest) Design** Design used by researchers when only one group is available for study. Data are collected before and after an experimental treatment on one group of subjects. In this type of design, there is no control group and no randomization.

**Open-Ended Question** Question that the respondent may answer in his or her own words.

**Operational Definition** The measurements used to observe or measure a variable; delineates the procedures or operations required to measure a concept.

**Opinion Leaders** From the local peer group, viewed as a respected source of influence, considered by associates as technically competent, and trusted to judge the fit between the innovation and the local situation.

**Ordinal** The level of measurement that systematically categorizes data in an ordered or ranked manner. Ordinal measures do not permit a high level of differentiation among subjects.

**Ordinal Measurement** Level used to show rankings of events or objects; numbers are not equidistant, and zero is arbitrary (e.g., class ranking).

**Paradigm** From Greek: *pattern*; it has been applied to science to describe the way people in society think about the world.

**Parallel Form Reliability** See *alternate form reliability*.

**Parameter** A characteristic of a population.

**Parametric Statistics** Inferential statistics that involve the estimation of at least one parameter, require measurement at the interval level or above, and involve assumptions about the variables being studied. These assumptions usually include the fact that the variable is normally distributed.

**Participant Observation** When the observer keeps field notes (a short summary of observations) to record the activities, as well as the observer's interpretations of these activities.

**Pearson Correlation Coefficient (Pearson *r*)** A statistic that is calculated to reflect the degree of relationship between two interval level variables. Also called *Pearson Product Moment Correlation Coefficient.*

**Percentile** Represents the percentage of cases a given score exceeds.

**Performance Measurement** A tool that tracks an organization's performance using standardized measures to document and manage quality.

**Phenomena** Those things that are perceived by our senses (e.g., pain, losing a loved one).

**Phenomenological Method** A process of learning and constructing the meaning of human experience through intensive dialogue with persons who are living the experience.

**Phenomenological Research** Phenomenological research is based on phenomenological philosophy and is research aimed at obtaining a description of an experience as it is lived in order to understand the meaning of that experience for those who have it.

**Phenomenology** A qualitative research approach that aims to describe experience as it is lived through, before it is conceptualized.

**Philosophical Beliefs** The system of motivating values, concepts, principles, and the nature of human knowledge of an individual, group, or culture.

**Philosophical Research** Based on the investigation of the truths and principles of existence, knowledge, and conduct.

**Pilot Study** A small, simple study conducted as a prelude to a larger-scale study that is often called the "parent study."

**Plan-Do-Study-Act (PDSA) Improvement Cycle** The last step of the Improvement Model.

**Population** A well-defined set that has certain specified properties.

**Positive Likelihood Ratio (LR)** The LR of a positive test indicates the accuracy of a positive test result by comparing its performance when the disease is present to that when the disease is absent. The best test to use for ruling in a disease is the one with the largest likelihood ratio of a positive test.

**Positive Predictive Value** Expresses the proportion of those with positive test results who truly have disease.

**Power Analysis** The mathematical procedure to determine the number for each arm (group) of a study.

**Predictive Validity** The degree of correlation between the measure of the concept and some future measure of the same concept.

**Prefiltered Evidence** Evidence for which an editorial team has already read and summarized articles on a topic and appraised its relevance to clinical care.

**Primary Source** Scholarly literature that is written by the person(s) who developed the theory or conducted the research. Primary sources include eyewitness accounts of historic events, provided by original documents, films, letters, diaries, records, artifacts, periodicals, or audio/video recordings.

**Probability** The probability of an event is the event's long-run relative frequency in repeated trials under similar conditions.

**Probability Sampling** A procedure that uses some form of random selection when the sample units are chosen.

**Problem-Focused Triggers** Those that are identified by staff through quality improvement, risk surveillance, benchmarking data, financial data, or recurrent clinical problems.

**Program** A list of instructions in a machine-readable language written so that a computer's hardware can carry out an operation; software.

**Prospective Study** Nonexperimental study that begins with an exploration of assumed causes and then moves forward in time to the presumed effect.

**Psychometrics** The theory and development of measurement instruments.

**Public Reporting** Provides objective information to promote consumer choice, guide QI efforts, and promote accountability for performance among providers and delivery organizations. It also allows organizations to compare their performance across standard measures against their peer organizations locally and nationally.

**Purpose** That which encompasses the aims or objectives the investigator hopes to achieve with the research, not the question to be answered.

**Purposive Sampling** A nonprobability sampling strategy in which the researcher selects subjects who are considered to be typical of the population.

## Q

**Qualitative Measurement** The items or observed behaviors are assigned to mutually exclusive categories that are representative of the kinds of behavior exhibited by the subjects.

**Qualitative Research** The study of research questions about human experiences. It is often conducted in natural settings, and uses data that are words or text, rather than numerical, in order to describe the experiences that are being studied.

**Quality Health Care** Care that is safe, effective, patient-centered, timely, efficient, and equitable.

**Quality Improvement (QI)** The systematic use of data to monitor the outcomes of care processes as well as the use of improvement methods to design and test changes in practice for the purpose of continuously improving the quality and safety of health care systems.

**Quantitative Measurement** The assignment of items or behaviors to categories that represent the amount of a possessed characteristic.

**Quantitative Research** The process of testing relationships, differences, and cause and effect interactions among and between variables. These processes are tested with either hypotheses and/or research questions.

**Quasi-Experiment** Research designs in which the researcher initiates an experimental treatment, but some characteristic of a true experiment is lacking.

**Quasi-Experimental Design** A study design in which random assignment is not used, but the independent variable is manipulated and certain mechanisms of control are used.

**Questionnaires** Paper-and-pencil instruments designed to gather data from individuals about knowledge, attitudes, beliefs, and feelings.

**Quota Sampling** A nonprobability sampling strategy that identifies the strata of the population and proportionately represents the strata in the sample.

## R

**Random Error** Error that occurs when scores vary in a random way. Random error occurs when data collectors do not use standard procedures to collect data consistently among all subjects in a study.

**Random Selection** A selection process in which each element of the population has an equal and independent chance of being included in the sample.

**Randomization** A sampling selection procedure in which each person or element in a population has an equal chance of being selected to either the experimental group or the control group.

**Randomized Controlled Trial (RCT)** A research study using a true experimental design.

**Range** A measure of variability; difference between the highest and lowest scores in a set of sample data.

**Ratio** The highest level of measurement that possesses the characteristics of categorizing, ordering, and ranking, and also has an absolute or natural zero that has empirical meaning.

**Ratio Measurement** Level that ranks the order of events or objects, and that has equal intervals and an absolute zero (e.g., height, weight).

**Reactivity** The distortion created when those who are being observed change their behavior because they know that they are being observed.

**Recommendation** Application of a study to practice, theory, and future research.

**Refereed Journal or Peer-Reviewed Journal** A scholarly journal that has a panel of external and internal reviewers or editors; the panel reviews submitted manuscripts for possible publication. The review panels use the same set of scholarly criteria to judge if the manuscripts are worthy of publication.

**Relationship/Difference Studies** Studies that trace the relationships or differences between variables that can provide a deeper insight into a phenomenon.

**Relative Risk (RR)** Risk of event after experimental treatment as a percentage of original risk.

**Relative Risk Reduction (RRR)** A helpful tool to indicate how much of the baseline risk (the control group event rate) is removed as a result of having the intervention.

**Reliability** The consistency or constancy of a measuring instrument.

**Reliability Coefficient** A number between 0 and 1 that expresses the relationship between the error variance, the true variance, and the observed score. A zero correlation indicates no relationship. The closer to 1 the coefficient is, the more reliable the tool.

**Repeated Measures Studies** See *longitudinal study*.

**Representative Sample** A sample whose key characteristics closely approximate those of the population.

**Research** The systematic, logical, and empirical inquiry into the possible relationships among particular phenomena to produce verifiable knowledge.

**Research Hypothesis** A statement about the expected relationship between the variables; also known as a *scientific hypothesis*.

**Research Literature** A synonym for data-based literature.

**Research Problem** Presents the question that is to be asked in a research study.

**Research Question** A key preliminary step wherein the foundation for a study is developed from the research problem and results in the research hypothesis.

**Research Utilization** A systematic method of implementing sound research-based innovations in clinical practice, evaluating the outcome, and sharing the knowledge through the process of research dissemination.

**Research-Based Protocols** Practice standards that are formulated from findings of several studies.

**Respect for Persons** The principle that people have the right to self-determination and to treatment as autonomous agents; that is, they have the freedom to participate or not participate in research.

**Respondent Burden** Occurs when the length of the questionnaire or interview is too long or the questions too difficult for respondents to answer in a reasonable amount of time considering their age, health condition, or mental status.

**Retrospective Data** Data that have been manifested, such as scores on a standard examination.

**Retrospective Study** A nonexperimental research design that begins with the phenomenon of interest (dependent variable) in the present and examines its relationship to another variable (independent variable) in the past.

**Review of the Literature** An extensive, systematic, and critical review of the most important published scholarly literature on a particular topic. In most cases it is not considered exhaustive.

**Risk** Potential negative outcome(s) of participation in research study.

**Risk/Benefit Ratio** The extent to which the benefits of the study are maximized and the risks are minimized such that the subjects are protected from harm during the study.

**Root Cause Analysis (RCA)** A structured method used to understand sources of system variation that lead to errors or mistakes, including sentinel events, with the goal of learning from mistakes and mitigating hazards that arise as a characteristic of the system design.

**Run Chart** A graphical data display that shows trends in a measure of interest; trends reveal what is occurring over time.

## S

**Sample** A subset of sampling units from a population.

**Sampling** A process in which representative units of a population are selected for study in a research investigation.

**Sampling Error** The tendency for statistics to fluctuate from one sample to another.

**Sampling Frame** A list of all units of the population.

**Sampling Interval** The standard distance between the elements chosen for the sample.

**Sampling Unit** The element or set of elements used for selecting the sample.

**Saturation** See *data saturation*.

**Scale** A self-report inventory that provides a set of response symbols for each item. A rating or score is assigned to each response.

**Scientific Approach** A logical, orderly, and objective means of generating and testing ideas.

**Scientific Hypothesis** The researcher's expectation about the outcome of a study; also known as the *research hypothesis*.

**Scientific Literature** A synonym for data-based literature; see *data-based literature*.

**Scientific Observation** Collecting data about the environment and subjects. Data collection has specific objectives to guide it, is systematically planned and recorded, is checked and controlled, and is related to scientific concepts and theories.

**Secondary Analysis** A form of research in which the researcher takes previously collected and analyzed data from one study and reanalyzes the data for a secondary purpose.

**Secondary Source** Scholarly material written by a person(s) other than the individual who developed the theory or conducted the research. Most are usually published. Often a secondary source represents a response to or a summary and critique of a theorist's or researcher's work. Examples are documents, films, letters, diaries, records, artifacts, periodicals, or tapes that provide a view of the phenomenon from another's perspective.

**Selection** The generalizability of the results to other populations.

**Selection Bias** The internal validity threat that arises when pretreatment differences between the experimental group and the control group are present.

**Self-Report** Data collection methods that require subjects to respond directly to either interviews or structured questionnaires about their experiences, behaviors, feelings, or attitudes. These are commonly used in nursing research and are most useful for collecting data on variables that cannot be directly observed or measured by physiological instruments.

**Semiquartile Range** A measure of variability; range of the middle 50% of the scores. Also known as *Semi-interquartile Range*.

**Sensitivity** The proportion of those with disease who test positive.

**Simple Random Sampling** A probability sampling strategy in which the population is defined, a sampling frame is listed, and a subset from which the sample will be chosen is selected; members are randomly selected.

**Situation-Specific Theories** More specific theories than middle range theories, they are composed of a limited number of concepts. They are narrow in scope, explain a small aspect of phenomena and processes of interest to nurses, and are usually limited to specific populations or field of practice.

**Snowball Effect Sampling (Network Sampling)** A strategy used for locating samples difficult to locate. It uses the social network and the fact that friends tend to have characteristics in common; subjects who meet the eligibility criteria are asked for assistance in getting in touch with others who meet the same criteria.

**Solomon Four-Group Design** An experimental design with four randomly assigned groups—the pretest-posttest intervention group, the pretest-posttest control group, a treatment or intervention group with only posttest measurement, and a control group with only posttest measurement.

**Specificity** The proportion of those without disease who test negative. It measures how well the test rules out disease when it is really absent; a specific test has few false positive results.

**Split-Half Reliability** An index of the comparison between the scores on one half of a test with those on the other half to determine the consistency in response to items that reflect specific content.

**Stability** An instrument's ability to produce the same results with repeated testing.

**Standard Deviation (SD)** A measure of variability; measure of average deviation of scores from the mean.

**Statistic** A descriptive index for a sample such as a sample mean or a standard deviation.

**Statistical Hypothesis** States that there is no relationship between the independent and dependent variables. The statistical hypothesis also is known as the null hypothesis.

**Stratified Random Sampling** A probability sampling strategy in which the population is divided into strata or subgroups. An appropriate number of elements from each subgroup are randomly selected based on their proportion in the population.

**Survey Studies** Descriptive, exploratory, or comparative studies that collect detailed descriptions of existing variables and use the data to justify and assess current conditions and practices, or to make more plans for improving health care practices.

**Survival Curve** A graph that shows the probability that a patient "survives" in a given state for at least a specified time (or longer).

**Systematic** Data collection carried out in the same manner with all subjects.

**Systematic Error** Attributable to lasting characteristics of the subject that do not tend to fluctuate from one time to another. Also called *constant error*.

**Systematic Review** Process where investigators find all relevant studies, published and unpublished, on the topic or question, at least two members of the review team independently assess the quality of each study, include or exclude studies based on preestablished criteria, statistically combine the results of individual studies, and present a balanced and impartial evidence summary of the findings that represents a "state of the science" conclusion about the evidence supporting benefits and risks of a given health care practice.

**Systematic Sampling** A probability sampling strategy that involves the selection of subjects randomly drawn from a population list at fixed intervals.

## T

**t Statistic** Commonly used in nursing research; it tests whether two group means are more different than would be expected by chance. Groups may be related or independent.

**Target Population**  A population or group of individuals that meet the sampling criteria.

**Test**  A self-report inventory that provides for one response to each item that the examiner assigns a rating or score. Inferences are made from the total score about the degree to which a subject possesses whatever trait, emotion, attitude, or behavior the test is supposed to measure.

**Test-Retest Reliability**  Administration of the same instrument twice to the same subjects under the same conditions within a prescribed time interval, with a comparison of the paired scores to determine the stability of the measure.

**Testability**  Variables of proposed study that lend themselves to observation, measurement, and analysis.

**Testing**  The effects of taking a pretest on the scores of a posttest.

**Text**  Data in a contextual form; that is, narrative or words that are written and transcribed.

**Theme**  A label that represents a way of describing large quantities of data in a condensed format.

**Theoretical Framework**  Theoretical rationale for the development of hypotheses.

**Theoretical Literature**  A synonym for conceptual literature; see *conceptual literature*.

**Theory**  Set of interrelated concepts, definitions, and propositions that present a systematic view of phenomena for the purpose of explaining and making predictions about those phenomena.

**Time Series Design**  A quasi-experimental design used to determine trends before and after an experimental treatment. Measurements are taken several times before the introduction of the experimental treatment, the treatment is introduced, and measurements are taken again at specified times afterward.

**Transferability**  See *fittingness*.

**Treatment Effect**  The impact of the independent variable/intervention on the dependent variable.

**Triangulation**  The expansion of research methods in a single study or multiple studies to enhance diversity, enrich understanding, and accomplish specific goals.

**True (Classic) Experiment**  Also known as the *pretest-posttest control group design*. In this design, subjects are randomly assigned to an experimental or control group, pretest measurements are performed, an intervention or treatment occurs in the experimental group, and posttest measurements are performed.

**Trustworthiness**  The rigor of the research in a qualitative research study.

**Type I Error**  The rejection of a null hypothesis that is actually true.

**Type II Error**  The acceptance of a null hypothesis that is actually false.

## V

**Validity**  Determination of whether a measurement instrument actually measures what it is purported to measure.

**Variable**  A defined concept.

## W

**Web Browser**  Software program used to connect or "read" the World Wide Web (www).

Note: Page numbers followed by f, t, and b indicate figures, tables, and boxes.